Communications in Computer and Information Science **1024**

Commenced Publication in 2007
Founding and Former Series Editors:
Phoebe Chen, Alfredo Cuzzocrea, Xiaoyong Du, Orhun Kara, Ting Liu,
Krishna M. Sivalingam, Dominik Ślęzak, Takashi Washio, and Xiaokang Yang

Editorial Board Members

More information about this series at http://www.springer.com/series/7899

Alberto Cliquet Jr. · Sheldon Wiebe ·
Paul Anderson · Giovanni Saggio ·
Reyer Zwiggelaar · Hugo Gamboa ·
Ana Fred · Sergi Bermúdez i Badia (Eds.)

Biomedical Engineering Systems and Technologies

11th International Joint Conference, BIOSTEC 2018
Funchal, Madeira, Portugal, January 19–21, 2018
Revised Selected Papers

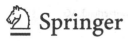 Springer

Editors
Alberto Cliquet Jr.
University of Sao Paulo
São Paulo, Brazil

Sheldon Wiebe
University of Saskatchewan
Saskatoon, Canada

Paul Anderson
College of Charleston
Charleston, SC, USA

Giovanni Saggio
University of Rome Tor Vergata
Rome, Italy

Reyer Zwiggelaar
Aberystwyth University
Aberystwyth, UK

Hugo Gamboa
LIBPhys
New University of Lisbon
Lisbon, Portugal

Ana Fred
Instituto de Telecomunicações
and Instituto Superior Técnico
Lisbon, Portugal

Sergi Bermúdez i Badia
Madeira Interactive Technologies Institute
Universidade da Madeira
Funchal, Portugal

ISSN 1865-0929   ISSN 1865-0937 (electronic)
Communications in Computer and Information Science
ISBN 978-3-030-29195-2   ISBN 978-3-030-29196-9 (eBook)
https://doi.org/10.1007/978-3-030-29196-9

Preface

The present book includes extended and revised versions of a set of selected papers from the 11th International Joint Conference on Biomedical Engineering Systems and Technologies (BIOSTEC 2018), held in Funchal, Madeira, Portugal, during January 19–21, 2018. BIOSTEC is composed of five co-located conferences, each specialized in a different knowledge area, namely, BIODE-VICES, BIOIMAGING, BIOINFORMATICS, BIOSIGNALS, and HEALTH-INF.

BIOSTEC 2018 received 344 paper submissions from 50 countries, of which only 7% are included in this book. This reflects our care in selecting those contributions. These papers were selected by the conference chairs and their selection is based on a number of criteria that include the classifications and comments provided by the Program Committee members, the session chairs' assessment, and the program chairs' meta review of the papers that were included in the technical program. The authors of selected papers were invited to submit a revised, extended, and improved version of their conference paper, including at least 30% new material.

The purpose of the BIOSTEC joint conferences is to bring together researchers and practitioners, including engineers, biologists, health professionals, and informatics/ computer scientists. Research presented at BIOSTEC included both theoretical advances and applications of information systems, artificial intelligence, signal processing, electronics, and other engineering tools in areas related to advancing biomedical research and improving healthcare.

These advances and improvements are to answer modern requests relevant in the medical field that have not been evolving as rapidly as in other fields. Different examples can be made: aviation evolved from the first flight of the Wright brothers in 1903 to the current tests for commercial space flights; the automotive evolved from the first model-T by Ford in 1908 to the current electric motor Model 3 by Tesla; radio-communications evolved from the bulky radio stations by Marconi company in 1897 to the current foldable smartphone models Mate X and Galaxy X by Huawei and Samsung, respectively. Conversely, the hospital model is pretty similar today as it was in the seventeenth century: rooms with beds where patients are lying down and medical doctors come to visit. Fortunately, new technologies are continuously evolving, allowing medical doctors to count on new and more objective measures of biomarkers for different pathologies (objectively-based rather than subjectively-based diagnostics), medical treatments that are considerable more focused on the individual rather than the pathology (personalized medicine), and new wearable technology for non-invasive measures to allow for telemedicine, without forcing the patient to go every-time to the hospital (home-care treatment).

Within Medical Imaging, there is a continued rapid development in using large datasets and high computational processes in data analysis and evaluation. Artificial Intelligence interests have increased significantly to the point where large multinational companies are significantly investing in developing products that could potentially automate some of the work done at clinical level. I think in the future there will be two major disruptive scientific developments within the world of Medical Imaging. One, mentioned above, is the use of artificial intelligence in medical imaging systems. The other is the integration of targeted contrast or therapeutic agents that will provide some functional imaging or therapeutic component to anatomical imaging and may be very disease specific.

Within this framework, this book includes different, meaningful contributions, from new technologies for objective measurements, to new algorithms to manage medical records, to predictive algorithms, and so forth.

We would like to thank all the authors for their contributions and also to the reviewers who have helped to ensure the quality of this publication.

January 2018

Alberto Cliquet Jr.
Sheldon Wiebe
Paul Anderson
Giovanni Saggio
Reyer Zwiggelaar
Hugo Gamboa
Ana Fred
Sergi Bermúdez i Badia

Organization

Conference Co-chairs

Hugo Gamboa — LIBPHYS-UNL/FCT, New University of Lisbon, Portugal

Ana Fred — Instituto de Telecomunicações/IST, Lisbon University, Portugal

Sergi Bermúdez i Badia — Madeira Interactive Technologies Institute, Universidade da Madeira, Portugal

Program Co-chairs

BIODEVICES

Alberto Cliquet Jr. — University of São Paulo and University of Campinas, Brazil

BIOIMAGING

Sheldon Wiebe — University of Saskatchewan, Canada

BIOINFORMATICS

Paul Anderson — College of Charleston, USA

BIOSIGNALS

Giovanni Saggio — University of Rome Tor Vergata, Italy

HEALTHINF

Reyer Zwiggelaar — Aberystwyth University, UK

BIODEVICES Program Committee

Nizametin Aydin	Yildiz Technical University, Turkey
Steve Beeby	University of Southampton, UK
Dinesh Bhatia	North Eastern Hill University, India
Luciano Boquete	Alcala University, Spain
Jan Cabri	Norwegian School of Sport Sciences, Norway
Carlo Capelli	Norwegian School of Sport Sciences, Norway
Youngjae Chun	University of Pittsburgh, USA
Alberto Cliquet Jr.	University of São Paulo and University of Campinas, Brazil
Albert Cook	Faculty of Rehabilitation Medicine, University of Alberta, Canada

Dong Ik Shin	Asan Medical Center, South Korea
Filomena Soares	Algoritmi Research Centre, UM, Portugal
Akihiro Takeuchi	Kitasato University School of Medicine, Japan
Marco Tatullo	Tecnologica Research Institute, Italy
John Tudor	University of Southampton, UK
Egon L. van den Broek	Utrecht University, The Netherlands
Renato Varoto	University of Campinas, Brazil
Pedro Vieira	Faculdade de Ciências e Tecnologia, Universidade Nova de Lisboa, Portugal
Bruno Wacogne	FEMTO-ST, UMR CNRS 6174, France
Hakan Yavuz	Çukurova Üniversity, Turkey
Alberto Yufera	Instituto de MIcroelectronica de Sevilla, Universidad de Sevilla, Spain
Xian-En Zhang	Institute of Biophysics, Chinese Academy of Sciences, China

BIOIMAGING Program Committee

Anna Chiara De Luca	IBP-CNR, Italy
Sameer Antani	National Library of Medicine, National Institutes of Health, USA
Peter Balazs	University of Szeged, Hungary
Grégory Barbillon	EPF Ecole d'Ingénieurs, France
Richard Bayford	Middlesex University, UK
Alpan Bek	Middle East Technical University, Turkey
Obara Boguslaw	University of Durham, UK
Alexander Bykov	University of Oulu, Optoelectronics and Measurement Techniques Laboratory, Finland
Enrico Caiani	Politecnico di Milano, Italy
Begoña Calvo	University of Zaragoza, Spain
Alessia Cedola	CNR, Institute of Nanotechnology, Italy
Heang-Ping Chan	University of Michigan, USA
Chung-Ming Chen	National Taiwan University, Taiwan
Guanying Chen	Harbin Institute of Technology and SUNY Buffalo, China
Miguel Coimbra	IT, University of Porto, Portugal
Giacomo Cuttone	INFN, Laboratori Nazionali del Sud Catania, Italy
Alexandre Douplik	Ryerson University, Canada
Wolfgang Drexler	Medical University Vienna, Austria
Karen Drukker	The University of Chicago, USA
Edite Figueiras	Champalimaud Foundation, Portugal
Costel Flueraru	National Research Council of Canada, Canada
Dimitrios Fotiadis	University of Ioannina, Greece
Carlos Geraldes	Universidade de Coimbra, Portugal
P. Gopinath	Indian Institute of Technology Roorkee, India
Dimitris Gorpas	Technical University of Munich, Germany

Jan Schier	The Institute of Information Theory and Automation of the Czech Academy of Sciences, Czech Republic
Gregory Sharp	Massachusetts General Hospital, USA
Leonid Shvartsman	Hebrew University, Israel
Arcot Sowmya	UNSW, Australia
Chi-Kuang Sun	National Taiwan University, Taiwan
Piotr Szczepaniak	Institute of Information Technology, Lodz University of Technology, Poland
Pablo Taboada	University of Santiago de Compostela, Spain
Jie Tian	Chinese Academy of Sciences, China
Arkadiusz Tomczyk	Institute of Information Technology, Lodz University of Technology, Poland
Ibtisam Tothill	Cranfield University, UK
Muhammed Toy	Istanbul Medipol University, Turkey
Carlos M. Travieso	University of Las Palmas de Gran Canaria, Spain
Benjamin Tsui	Johns Hopkins University, USA
Vladimír Ulman	Faculty of Informatics, Masaryk University, Czech Republic
Sandra Ventura	School of Health - Escola Superior de Saüde do Politécnico do Porto, Portugal
Vijay Vijay	Massachusetts Institute of Technology, USA
Irina Voiculescu	University of Oxford, UK
Yuanyuan Wang	Fudan University, China
Quan Wen	University of Electronic Science and Technology of China, China
Sheldon Wiebe	University of Saskatchewan, Canada
Lei Xi	University of Electronic Science and Technology of China, China
Hongki Yoo	Hanyang University, South Korea
Zeyun Yu	University of Wisconsin at Milwaukee, USA
Jiangbo Zhao	University of Adelaide, Australia

BIOIMAGING Additional Reviewers

| Xiaoli Qi | Johns Hopkins University, USA |

BIOINFORMATICS Program Committee

Allen Adum	Nnamdi Azikiwe University, Nigeria
Afiahayati Afiahayati	Universitas Gadjah Mada, Indonesia
Tatsuya Akutsu	Kyoto University, Japan
Jens Allmer	Hochschule Ruhr West, University of Applied Sciences, Germany
Paul Anderson	College of Charleston, USA
Francois Andry	Philips, France
Sameer Antani	National Library of Medicine, National Institutes of Health, USA

Yannis Kalaidzidis	Max Planck Institute Molecular Cell Biology and Genetic, Germany
Michael Kaufmann	Witten/Herdecke University, Germany
Natalia Khuri	Wake Forest University, USA
Inyoung Kim	Virginia Tech, USA
Jirí Kléma	Czech Technical University in Prague, Faculty of Electrical Engineering, Czech Republic
Malgorzata Kotulska	Wroclaw University of Technology, Poland
Ivan Kulakovskiy	Russia
Carlile Lavor	University of Campinas, Brazil
Antonios Lontos	Frederick University, Cyprus
Pawel Mackiewicz	Faculty of Biotechnology, Wroclaw University, Poland
Paolo Magni	Università degli Studi di Pavia, Italy
Thérése Malliavin	CNRS/Institut Pasteur, France
Elena Marchiori	Radboud University, The Netherlands
Andrea Marin	University of Venice, Italy
Majid Masso	George Mason University, USA
Petr Matula	Faculty of Informatics, Masaryk University, Czech Republic
Giancarlo Mauri	Università di Milano Bicocca, Italy
Nikolaos Michailidis	Aristoteles University of Thessaloniki, Greece
Paolo Milazzo	Università di Pisa, Italy
Pedro Monteiro	INESC-ID/IST, Universidade de Lisboa, Portugal
Monica Mordonini	Universitá Degli Studi Di Parma, Italy
Vincent Moulton	University of East Anglia, UK
Helder Nakaya	University of Säo Paulo, Brazil
David Naranjo-Hernández	University of Seville, Spain
Jean-Christophe Nebel	Kingston University, UK
José Oliveira	University of Aveiro, DETI/IEETA, Portugal
Hakan Orer	Koc University, Turkey
Giulia Paciello	Politecnico di Torino, Italy
Taesung Park	Seoul National University, South Korea
Oscar Pastor	Universidad Politécnica de Valencia, Spain
Marco Pellegrini	Consiglio Nazionale delle Ricerche, Italy
Matteo Pellegrini	University of California, Los Angeles, USA
Horacio Pérez-Sánchez	Catholic University of Murcia, Spain
Nadia Pisanti	Università di Pisa, Italy
Olivier Poch	ICube, UMR 7357 CNRS, Université de Strasbourg, France
Alberto Policriti	Università degli Studi di Udine, Italy
Gianfranco Politano	Politecnico di Torino, Italy
Giuseppe Profiti	University of Bologna, Italy
Maria Psiha	Ionian University, Greece
Junfeng Qu	Clayton State University, USA
Javier Reina-Tosina	University of Seville, Spain
Laura Roa	University of Seville, Spain

Simona Rombo	Dipartimento di Matematica e Informatica, Università degli Studi di Palermo, Italy
Eric Rouchka	University of Louisville, USA
Claudia Rubiano Castellanos	Universidad Nacional de Colombia, Colombia
Carolina Ruiz	WPI, USA
J. Salgado	University of Chile, Chile
Alessandro Savino	Politecnico di Torino, Italy
Noor Akhmad Setiawan	Universitas Gadjah Mada, Indonesia
João Setubal	Universidade de São Paulo, Brazil
Christine Sinoquet	University of Nantes, France
Neil Smalheiser	University of Illinois Chicago, USA
Pavel Smrz	Brno University of Technology, Czech Republic
Gordon Smyth	Walter and Eliza Hall Institute of Medical Research, Australia
Yinglei Song	Jiansu University of Science and Technology, China
David Svoboda	Masaryk University, Czech Republic
Peter Sykacek	University of Natural Resources and Life Sciences, Austria
Gerhard Thallinger	Graz University of Technology, Austria
Takashi Tomita	Japan Advanced Institute of Science and Technology, Japan
Alexander Tsouknidas	Aristotle University of Thessaloniki, Greece
Gabriel Valiente	Technical University of Catalonia, Spain
Juris Viksna	Institute of Mathematics and Computer Science, University of Latvia, Latvia
Arndt von Haeseler	Center for Integrative Bioinformatics Vienna, Austria
Sebastian Will	Universität Leipzig, Germany
Yanbin Yin	University of Nebraska, USA
Malik Yousef	Zefat Academic College, Israel
Erliang Zeng	University of Iowa, USA
Wen Zhang	Icahn School of Medicine at Mount Sinai, USA
Leming Zhou	University of Pittsburgh, USA
Jiali Zhuang	Molecular Stethoscope Inc., USA

BIOINFORMATICS Additional Reviewers

Artem Kasianov	VIGG, Russia
Michalis Michaelides	The University of Edinburgh, UK
Cátia Vaz	INESC-ID, Portugal

BIOSIGNALS Program Committee

Bruce Denby	Université Pierre et Marie Curie, France
Robert Allen	University of Southampton, UK
Alexandre Andrade	Faculdade de Ciências da Universidade de Lisboa, Portugal

Mochammad Ariyanto	Diponegoro University, Indonesia
Sridhar Arjunan	RMIT University, Australia
Joonbum Bae	UNIST, South Korea
Richard Bayford	Middlesex University, UK
Eberhard Beck	Brandenburg University of Applied Sciences, Germany
Philipp Beckerle	TU Darmstadt, Germany
Peter Bentley	UCL, UK
Santosh Bothe	NMIMS Deemed to be University, India
Bethany Bracken	Charles River Analytics Inc., USA
Maurizio Caon	University of Applied Sciences and Arts Western Switzerland, Switzerland
Guy Carrault	University of Rennes 1, France
Maria Claudia Castro	Centro Universitário FEI, Brazil
Marcus Cheetham	University of Zurich, Switzerland
Gaurav Chitranshi	HCL Technologies Ltd., Technical Excellence Group, Uttar Pradesh, India
Bruno Cornelis	Vrije Universiteit Brussel (VUB), Belgium
Jan Cornelis	VUB, Belgium
Adam Czajka	University of Notre Dame, USA
Christakis Damianou	Cyprus University of Technology, Cyprus
Justin Dauwels	Nanyang Technological University, Singapore
Gert-Jan de Vries	Philips Research - Healthcare, The Netherlands
Petr Dolezel	University of Pardubice, Czech Republic
Pier Emiliani	Italian National Research Council (CNR), Italy
Pedro Encarnação	Universidade Católica Portuguesa, Portugal
Poree Fabienne	Université de Rennes 1, France
Luca Faes	Università degli Studi di Trento, Italy
Dimitrios Fotiadis	University of Ioannina, Greece
Takuya Funatomi	Nara Institute of Science and Technology, Japan
Javier Garcia-Casado	Universitat Politècnica de València, Spain
Arfan Ghani	Coventry University, UK
James Gilbert	University of Hull, UK
Didem Gokcay	Middle East Technical University, Turkey
Pedro Gómez Vilda	Universidad Politécnica de Madrid, Spain
Inan Güler	Gazi University, Turkey
Thomas Hinze	Friedrich Schiller University Jena, Germany
Roberto Hornero	University of Valladolid, Spain
Donna Hudson	University of California San Francisco, USA
Bart Jansen	Vrije Universiteit Brussel, Belgium
Gordana Jovanovic Dolecek	Institute INAOE, Mexico
Tzyy-Ping Jung	University of California San Diego, USA
Natalya Kizilova	Warsaw University of Technology, Poland
Dagmar Krefting	HTW Berlin - University of Applied Sciences, Germany
Vaclav Kremen	Czech Technical University in Prague, Czech Republic
Lenka Lhotska	Czech Technical University in Prague, Czech Republic

Ana Tomé	University of Aveiro, Portugal
Carlos M. Travieso	University of Las Palmas de Gran Canaria, Spain
Ahsan Ursani	Mehran University of Engineering and Technology, Pakistan
Pedro Vaz	University of Coimbra, Portugal
Giovanni Vecchiato	National Research Council, Italy
Jacques Verly	University of Liege, Belgium
Yuanyuan Wang	Fudan University, China
Quan Wen	University of Electronic Science and Technology of China, China
Didier Wolf	Research Centre for Automatic Control, CRAN CNRS UMR 7039, France
Chia-Hung Yeh	National Sun Yat-sen University, Taiwan
Rafal Zdunek	Wroclaw University of Technology, Poland
Wei Zhang	Swiss Federal Institute of Technology Lausanne, Switzerland
Aneeq Zia	Georgia Institute of Technology, USA

BIOSIGNALS Additional Reviewers

Francesco Carrino	University of Applied Sciences and Arts Western Switzerland, Switzerland
Luca Gerardo Giorda	BCAM Basque Center for Applied Mathematics, Spain

HEALTHINF Program Committee

Anurag Agrawal	CSIR Institute of Genomics and Integrative Biology, Center for Translational Research in Asthma & Lung, India
Francois Andry	Philips, France
Wassim Ayadi	LERIA, University of Angers, France and LaTICE, University of Tunis, Tunisia
Payam Behzadi	Shahr-e-Qods Branch, Islamic Azad University, Iran
Bert-Jan van Beijnum	University of Twente, The Netherlands
Sorana Bolboaca	Iuliu Hatieganu University of Medicine and Pharmacy, Romania
Alessio Bottrighi	Universitá del Piemonte Orientale, Italy
Andrew Boyd	University of Illinois at Chicago, USA
Klaus Brinker	Hamm-Lippstadt University of Applied Sciences, Germany
Edward Brown	Memorial University, Canada
Eric Campo	LAAS CNRS, France
Guilherme Campos	IEETA, Portugal
Marc Cavazza	University of Greenwich, UK
Rui César das Neves	Directorate-General of Health, Portugal
James Cimino	School of Medicine at the University of Alabama at Birmingham, USA

José Oliveira	University of Aveiro, DETI/IEETA, Portugal
Agnieszka Onisko	Faculty of Computer Science, Bialystok University of Technology, Poland
Thomas Ostermann	Witten/Herdecke University, Germany
Nelson Pacheco da Rocha	University of Aveiro, Portugal
Rui Pedro Paiva	University of Coimbra, Portugal
Sotiris Pavlopoulos	ICCS, Greece
Alejandro Pazos Sierra	University of A Coruña, Spain
José Pazos-Arias	University of Vigo, Spain
Fabrizio Pecoraro	National Research Council, Italy
Liam Peyton	University of Ottawa, Canada
Enrico Piras	Fondazione Bruno Kessler, Italy
Arkalgud Ramaprasad	University of Illinois at Chicago, USA
Grzegorz Redlarski	Gdansk University of Technology, Poland
Ita Richardson	University of Limerick, Ireland
Marcos Rodrigues	Sheffield Hallam University, UK
Alejandro Rodríguez González	Centro de Tecnología Biomédica, Spain
Elisabetta Ronchieri	INFN, Italy
Carolina Ruiz	WPI, USA
Renato Sabbatini	The Edumed Institute, Brazil
George Sakellaropoulos	University of Patras, Greece
Ovidio Salvetti	National Research Council of Italy (CNR), Italy
Akio Sashima	AIST, Japan
Bettina Schnor	Potsdam University, Germany
Yuval Shahar	Ben Gurion University, Israel
Aziz Sheikh	Centre of Medical Informatics, University of Edinburgh, UK
Berglind Smaradottir	University of Agder, Norway
Äsa Smedberg	Stockholm University, Sweden
Jiangwen Sun	Old Dominion University, USA
Lauri Tuovinen	Dublin City University, Ireland
Mohy Uddin	King Abdullah International Medical Research Center (KAIMRC), Saudi Arabia
Gary Ushaw	Newcastle University, UK
Aristides Vagelatos	CTI, Greece
Egon L. van den Broek	Utrecht University, The Netherlands
Sitalakshmi Venkatraman	Melbourne Polytechnic, Australia
Francisco Veredas	Universidad de Málaga, Spain
Dagmar Waltemath	University of Rostock, Germany
Szymon Wilk	Institute of Computing Science, Poznan University of Technology, Poland
Janusz Wojtusiak	George Mason University, USA
Jitao Yang	China

Lixia Yao   Mayo Clinic, USA
Xuezhong Zhou   Beijing Jiaotong University, China
André Züquete   IEETA, IT, Universidade de Aveiro, Portugal

HEALTHINF Additional Reviewers

Luca Piovesan   Università del Piemonte Orientale, Italy

Invited Speakers

Anatole Lécuyer   Inria Rennes/IRISA, Hybrid Research Team, France
Corina Sas   Lancaster University, UK
Dinesh Kumar   RMIT University, Australia
Maximiliano Romero   Università Iuav di Venezia, Italy

Contents

Bioinformatics Models, Methods and Algorithms

Health Informatics

Biomedical Electronics and Devices

Fiber Bragg Based Sensors for Foot Plantar Pressure Analysis

Arnaldo G. Leal-Junior[1], M. Fátima Domingues[2], Rui Min[3],
Débora Vilarinho[4], Antreas Theodosiou[5], Cátia Tavares[4],
Nélia Alberto[2], Cátia Leitão[4], Kyriacos Kalli[5],
Anselmo Frizera-Neto[1], Paulo André[6], Paulo Antunes[2,4],
and Carlos Marques[2,4(✉)]

[1] Telecommunications Laboratory, Electrical Engineering Department,
Federal University of Espírito Santo, Fernando Ferrari Avenue, Vitoria,
ES 29075-910, Brazil
[2] Instituto de Telecomunicações, Campus Universitário de Santiago,
3810-193 Aveiro, Portugal
carlos.marques@ua.pt
[3] ITEAM Research Institute, Universitat Politècnica de València,
Valencia, Spain
[4] Department of Physics and I3N, University of Aveiro,
Campus Universitário de Santiago, 3810-193 Aveiro, Portugal
[5] Photonics and Optical Sensors Research Laboratory (PhOSLab),
Cyprus University of Technology, 3036 Limassol, Cyprus
[6] Instituto de Telecomunicações and Department of Electrical and Computer
Engineering, Instituto Superior Técnico, University of Lisbon,
1049-001 Lisbon, Portugal

Abstract. Gait analysis is of major importance in physical rehabilitation scenarios, lower limbs diseases diagnosis and prevention. Foot plantar pressure is a key parameter in the gait analysis and its dynamic monitoring is crucial for an accurate assessment of gait related pathologies and/or rehabilitation status evolution. It is therefore critical to invest effort in research for foot plantar analysis technologies. From that perspective, optical fiber sensors appear to be an excellent solution, given their sensing advantages for medical applications, when compared with their electronic counterparts. This chapter explores the use of optical fiber Bragg grating (FBG) sensors, both in plastic and silica optical fiber, to dynamically monitor the foot plantar pressure. An array of FBGs was integrated in a specially designed cork insole, with the optical sensors placed at key pressure points for analysis. Both insoles, containing plastic and silica optical fiber sensors, were tested for dynamic gait monitoring and body center of mass displacement, showing the reliability of this sensing technology for foot plantar pressure monitoring during gait motion.

Keywords: Fiber Bragg Gratings · Foot plantar pressure · Polymer optical · Fiber · Silica optical fiber · Gait analysis

© Springer Nature Switzerland AG 2019
A. Cliquet jr. et al. (Eds.): BIOSTEC 2018, CCIS 1024, pp. 3–25, 2019.
https://doi.org/10.1007/978-3-030-29196-9_1

1 Introduction

Improvements to the quality of life and advances in medicine have resulted in the continuous increase of population lifetimes with enhancements to aging, and this requires the rigorous health monitoring of elderly citizens [1]. Thus, there is a demand for continuous and dynamic health monitoring systems for the assessment and control of the person's physical incapacities [2].

Motion is among the different, key monitoring parameters for human health assessment, and in particular gait analysis is an important indicator of the health condition of a person. As part of the gait analysis method, foot plantar pressure can provide a foot pressure distribution map, where the development or evolution of foot ulcerations, of particular importance for diabetes patients, can be assessed [3]. The foot plantar pressure is an indicator of the gait pattern, which can provide information for the clinicians regarding a gait related pathology [4]. In addition, gait pattern analysis is needed for the application of robotic control devices used for gait assistance [5].

Generally, plantar pressure monitoring is performed with force plates or platforms. Although they can provide accurate measurements of the 3-D dynamics of the foot, they lack portability [6], which is undesirable for dynamic applications, such as in wearable robotics, and they cannot be employed as wearable sensors for remote monitoring. In addition, when a platform is fixed on the ground, the patient may alter their natural gait pattern in order to place the foot within the platform boundaries, which leads to incorrect evaluation of the patient [7]. Although the platform can be hidden in the ground to reduce this effect, several tests need to be performed to obtain a natural gait pattern with the foot within the platform boundaries, which results in a time-consuming process [8].

To mitigate the platform's limitations, instrumented insoles were developed, to be used inside a shoe, thereby resulting in a portable device that could assess the human gait outside the laboratory environment [6]. The advantageous features of instrumented insoles allow the plantar pressure assessment to occur in daily activities, which may lead to a better approximation of the natural gait pattern of the patients or users. However, insoles are generally based on electronic sensors, which, in some cases, lack in stability and resistance to impact loads and so can present measurement errors and inconsistencies [6].

In comparison with electronic sensors, optical fiber sensors (OFSs) present intrinsic advantages related to their compactness, lightweight, multiplexing capabilities, electrical isolation, electromagnetic field immunity and biocompatibility [9]. By exploiting these advantages, OFSs have been applied for the measurement of temperature [10], strain [11], humidity [12], refractive index [13], angle [14], liquid level [15] and pressure [16].

There are two major types of optical fibers: silica optical fibers (SOFs) and polymer optical fibers (POFs). Although SOFs offer lower optical attenuation, POFs have advantages regarding their material features [17]. These features include higher strain limits, higher fracture toughness, flexibility in bending and impact resistance [17]. However, the glass transition temperature of the POFs is only about 100 °C, which leads to a variation of their properties and can limit their applications at temperatures exceed the glass transition temperature [18].

There are many different approaches and mechanisms for optical fiber sensing that may include the measurement of intensity-variation [19], the use of interferometers for phase measurements [20], nonlinear effects [21] and wavelength modulation or change [22]. The latter option uses fiber Bragg gratings (FBGs), which are periodic perturbations of the refractive index of the fiber core along the longitudinal axis of the optical fiber, where a specific wavelength (the Bragg wavelength) is reflected [23]; this is essentially a wavelength selective mirror. Such a grating structure can be obtained by using lasers to modify the optical fiber, and this can take several forms, such as ultraviolet (UV) laser irradiation through a phase mask [23] or direct-write of the grating pattern in the fiber core using a femtosecond (fs) laser [24]. In FBG-based sensors, the shift of the reflected wavelength as a function of the monitored parameter is evaluated. The FBG is intrinsically sensitive to temperature and strain, following Eq. (1) [25]:

$$\Delta\lambda = [(\alpha + \xi)\Delta T + (1 - P_e)\Delta\varepsilon]\lambda_B \tag{1}$$

where $\Delta\lambda$ is the Bragg wavelength shift, λ_B is the Bragg wavelength, P_e is the photoelastic constant, α is the thermal expansion coefficient of the fiber, ξ is the thermo-optic coefficient, ΔT is the temperature variation and $\Delta\varepsilon$ is the strain variation. Furthermore, the FBG may be embedded in different structures to measure parameters such as force or pressure. For instance, if the FBG is embedded in a diaphragm, the pressure applied to the diaphragm can result in fiber strain following Hooke's law [26].

This chapter discusses the use of a FBG-based sensor network for plantar pressure monitoring, by taking advantage of the special properties provided by OFSs, and in particular FBG-based sensors. The focus of our application considers the increasing demand for monitoring physical parameters for elderly citizens and populations in general. The sensor network is compact and portable and this was achieved by embedding the sensors in a cork insole. In order to address the advantages offered by both SOFs and POFs and to compare their performance, the instrumented insole was developed first with FBGs inscribed in SOFs, followed by a similar system developed with POFs.

After this initial introduction, Sect. 2 presents an overview of foot biomechanics including its structure, movements and plantar pressure distribution during the gait motion. This section also comprises/contains the system requirements, the insole production and tests protocols. In Sect. 3, the insole development with SOFs is discussed, whereas in Sect. 4, the FBG-based insole with POFs is proposed. Finally, the main conclusions are presented in Sect. 5.

2 System Requirements and Insole Production

2.1 Foot Plantar Pressure Overview

The human foot provides the support and balance when a person is in a standing position and acts to ensure body stabilization during the gait motion [27]. In order to provide such crucial role in daily activities and locomotion, the foot is a multi-articular structure comprising soft tissues, bones and joints. In total, the human foot has 26 bones, which are divided as 7 tarsals, 5 metatarsals and 14 phalanges. Regarding the joints, there are the ankle, subtalar, midtarsal, tarsometatarsal, metatarsophalangeal and interphalangeal [27]. Such a complex structure is divided in to four main segments: hindfoot, midfoot, forefoot and phalanges, which are presented in Fig. 1.

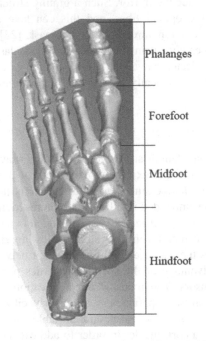

Phalanges

Forefoot

Midfoot

Hindfoot

Fig. 1. Top view of the left foot structure divided in to the four main segments.

Extrinsic and intrinsic muscles are responsible for the control of the joints presented in Fig. 1, which provide support for the foot and its motion [6]. The human motion generally occurs in 3 planes of motion, which are defined as sagittal, frontal and transverse planes [28]. The foot movements that occur in the sagittal plane are the plantarflexion and dorsiflexion (Fig. 2(a)), whereas in the transversal plane, there is the foot abduction and adduction (Fig. 2(b)). In addition, the movements in the frontal plane are the foot inversion and eversion (Fig. 2(c)). There is also a combination of these movements (pronation and supination). The foot is pronated when there is simultaneous abduction, eversion and dorsiflexion. On the other hand, the foot is supinated when the opposite occurs, i.e., it is simultaneously adducted, inverted and plantar flexed [27].

Conventionally, the gait cycle is delimited from the initial contact with one foot until the same foot touches the ground again, and this is divided in stance and swing phases [28]. The percentage of each phase varies with the gait velocity, but generally the stance phase represents 62% of the cycle [29]. Both stance and swing phases have

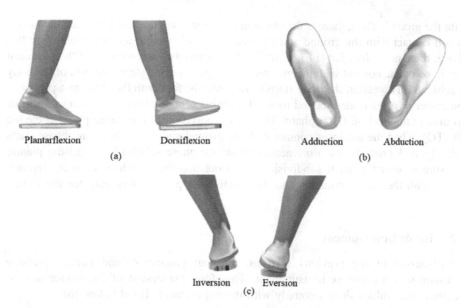

Plantarflexion Dorsiflexion Adduction Abduction

(a) (b)

Inversion Eversion

(c)

Fig. 2. Representation of different movements for the foot: (a) plantarflexion and dorsiflexion, (b) adduction and abduction and (c) inversion and eversion.

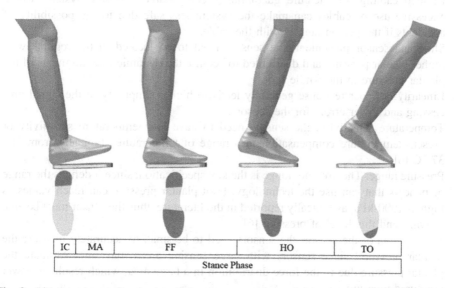

| IC | MA | FF | HO | TO |

Stance Phase

Fig. 3. Plantar pressure distribution during the stance phase of the gait cycle. The length of each subdivision is presented for illustration proposes only and the actual length of each phase varies with the person's gait.

subdivisions [6], nevertheless we will only present those of the stance phase, since this is the one detected by the proposed insole. Regarding the adopted stance phase subdivisions, it begins with the initial contact (IC), which is the first contact of the foot with the ground. Then, there is the maximum weight acceptance (MA) when the heel is in full contact with the ground and the entire person's weight applied. Following this phase, there is the foot flat (FF), which is characterized by the rotation of the foot until it is in complete contact with the ground. In this gait event, a stable support of the body is achieved. Thereafter, the body starts to roll over the foot with the ankle as a pivot and the center of mass is also moved forward. In this event, the heel loses contact with the ground, at the heel off (HO) phase. The final subdivision of the stance phase is the toe off (TO), when the toe loses contact with the ground and, then, the swing phase starts [6]. Figure 3 presents the aforementioned stance phase subdivisions and the plantar pressure involved at each subdivision. We note that the length of each subdivision varies with the gait parameters and the subdivision presented is only for illustration proposes.

2.2 Insole Development

As discussed in the previous sections, the gait parameters and plantar pressure assessment is a complex measurement. Therefore, the design of the device able to monitor such values should comply with the requirements listed below [6]:

- Lightweight: the insole weight is important for the user mobility and should not change his/her natural gait pattern.
- Limited cabling: this feature guaranties a comfortable and safe system, where excessive use of cables can make the system less safe due to the possibility of accidents if the person tangles with the cables.
- Shoe and sensor placement: the sensors need to be located in the regions with higher plantar pressure and distributed to acquire the dynamic measurements of the plantar pressure in the whole foot.
- Linearity: a linear response generally leads to higher simplicity in the signal processing and lower errors for the sensors.
- Temperature sensitivity: the sensors need to have low temperature sensitivity or present temperature compensation in a range of temperatures typically from 26–37 °C [6].
- Pressure range: The pressure range is the key specification, since it defines the range of patients that can use the technology. Foot plantar pressure can reach values as high as 1900 kPa, as typically reported in the literature, thus the sensor must be able to withstand this level of pressure [6].
- Sensing area of the sensor: the sensors need to be small to accurately measure the plantar pressure, since sensors with large sensing areas may underestimate the plantar pressure due to the force distribution in a large area, which results in lower measured pressure.
- Operating frequency: since the gait is a dynamic event, a precise plantar pressure assessment involves sampling frequencies as high as 200 Hz [6].

In order to achieve the requirement regarding the sensor positioning, 5 sensing points were chosen, following the regions known to have higher plantar pressure, as defined in [30]. The 5 sensing regions were chosen to coincide with the key regions in a distributed manner, as shown in Fig. 4.

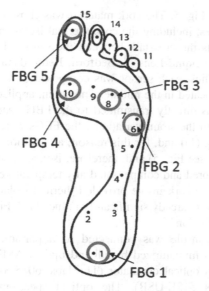

Fig. 4. Plantar pressure region and the chosen measurement points.

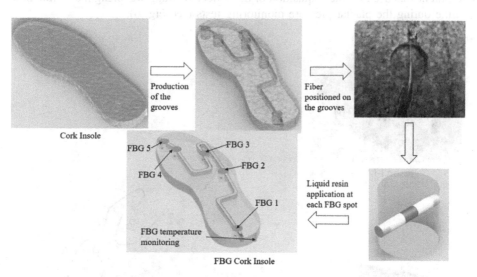

Fig. 5. Instrumented cork insole production steps.

The 5 FBGs sensors, distributed according to Fig. 4, were embedded in a cork insole with 10-mm thickness. The fabrication methodology for both SOF and POF-based FBG-embedded insoles was similar, with the type of fiber used representing the main difference between the insoles [1, 31]. The first step for the instrumented insole fabrication was to machine a cork plate to give it an insole shape. Then, a groove with 2.5-mm depth and 2.0-mm width was carved in to the cork sole, paving the way to place the optical fiber. In the key points of analysis, a cylinder of 10-mm diameter was also carved, as shown in Fig. 5. The cork material was chosen to produce the insoles due to desirable properties, including the cork thermal isolation, malleability and low Poison ratio that prevents the crosstalk between the sensors [1, 32]. In each carved cylinder, an epoxy resin (Liquid Lens™, Bedford, Bedfordshire, UK) was applied to encapsulate the FBGs. Thus, each sensor was composed of a cylindrical epoxy resin structure with the FBG located in the middle. The strain, applied in the resin when the cylinder was pressed, was directly transmitted to the FBG, leading to a Bragg wavelength shift. In addition to the strain variations, the FBGs were also sensitive to temperature changes (see Eq. (1)) and, for this reason, an additional FBG was positioned on the side of the insole (see Fig. 5) and, therefore, isolated from the plantar pressure. This isolated FBG monitored and compensated any temperature effects in the sensors' response. Nevertheless, the cork insole provided thermal isolation to the sensors and the temperature effects were already significantly reduced [1]. Figure 5 summarizes the instrumented insole production.

The FBG-embedded insole was connected to a portable interrogation system composed of a battery, a miniaturized broadband optical ASE module (B&A Technology Co., As4500), an optical circulator (Thorlabs, 6015-3), and an optical spectrometer (Ibsen, I-MON 512E-USB). The optical spectrometer operated with a maximum acquisition rate of 960 Hz and a wavelength resolution of 5 pm. This equipment was used for the acquisition of the reflected Bragg wavelength as a function of time during the plantar pressure monitoring tests (see Fig. 6).

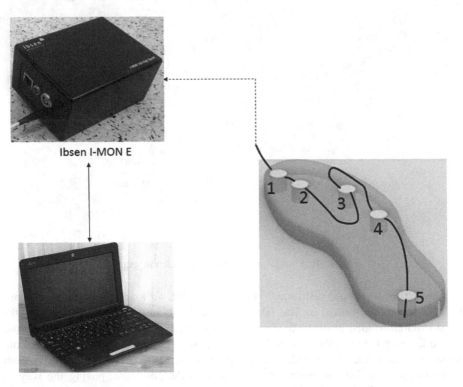

Ibsen I-MON E

Fig. 6. Schematic representation of the instrumented insole monitoring system.

2.3   Experimental Protocols

In the first test, the FBG array with sensing elements were calibrated in a universal mechanical testing machine (Shimadzu® AGS-5Knd, Columbia, SC, USA) from 0 to 1500 kPa, as shown in Fig. 7. The loads were applied independently at each sensing point, FBG 1 to FBG 5, using a probe with a diameter of 10 mm (the same diameter as the epoxy resin cylinder). The response of each sensor with respect to predefined pressures was acquired, it was possible to evaluate each sensors' sensitivity and linearity. In addition, the characterization tests were made at a constant temperature of 22 °C to reduce the effect of this parameter in the sensors' response.

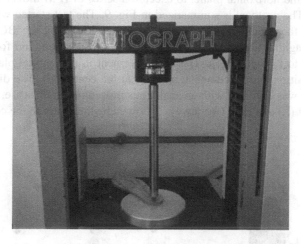

Fig. 7. Experimental setup for the FBG-based instrumented insole pressure characterization.

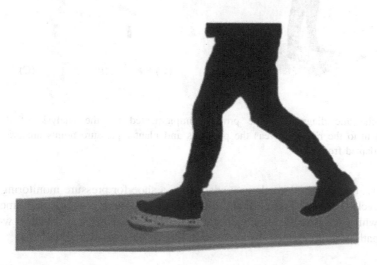

Fig. 8. Experimental setup for the proof-of-concept test with the instrumented insole acting as a fixed platform (adapted from [1]).

The second proposed test was the evaluation of plantar pressure during a normal gait, but with the insole fixed to the ground (as a force platform). This test was made as a proof-of-concept for the proposed FBG-embedded sensor system. The response of each sensing point, as well as the sum of all sensors were analyzed, and the tests were repeated 5 times. Figure 8 shows a schematic representation of this test protocol.

In the third test, the body center of mass (BCM) displacements for different movement planes was evaluated. The movements are in the frontal plane, following the movement of the subject's torso to left and right and on the sagittal plane, where the volunteer was requested to move the body forward and backward. The subject was asked to stand on the sensing platform, with one foot on the sensing area and the other leveled in the same horizontal plane, to execute a series of B M movements (of ~3-s duration each). The protocol is summarized in Fig. 9. The test started with the subject standing still at the center position (C). This was followed by the BCM movement forward in the sagittal plane to achieve the anterior (A) position, and followed by the movement back to the center (C). The last movement in the sagittal plane was to the posterior (P) position and, once again, arriving at the center (C). The displacement in the frontal plane was executed with an analogous procedure. In this case, the BCM was moved to the left (L) and right (R), always followed by the return to the center position.

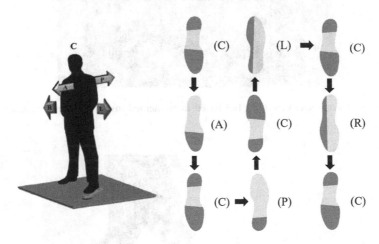

Fig. 9. Schematic diagram of the protocol implemented for the analysis of the BCM displacement to the right, whereas the positions and plantar pressure points are presented to the left (adapted from [1]).

Finally, the proposed insole was adapted to a shoe for pressure monitoring during the gait cycle (Fig. 10), as a portable solution for the plantar pressure assessment. The subject, whilst wearing the shoe with the instrumented insole, was asked to walk in a straight path with predefined distance, while the gait cycles were analyzed.

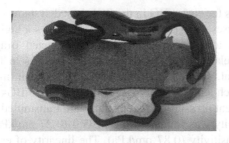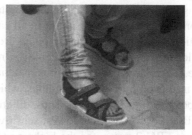

Fig. 10. FBG-embedded insole positioned inside a shoe for plantar pressure monitoring during the gait motion.

3 SOF-FBG-Based Instrumented Insole

The first approach analyzed was the FBG-embedded insole with the Bragg gratings inscribed in SOF, in this case GF1-photosensitive optical fiber (Thorlabs), using the "phase mask technique". The laser employed was an UV pulsed KrF excimer laser (Bragg Star Industrial-LN), operating at 248 nm, applying pulses with energy of 5 mJ and repetition rate of 500 Hz. The gratings had a physical length of 1.5 mm. The phase masks that were used were customized for 248-nm UV lasers in order to produce FBGs in the 1550-nm spectral region (Ibsen Photonics). Figure 11 shows the reflection spectrum of an FBG array with the 5 sensing elements, inscribed in the SOF with the aforementioned setup.

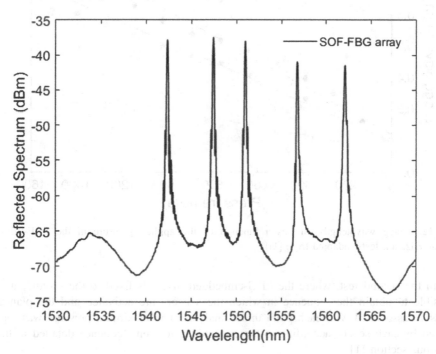

Fig. 11. Reflection spectrum of the FBG array inscribed in the SOF.

Figure 12 shows the calibration results for each FBG in the SOF-based system. The sensors display a linear response in all cases. However, the sensitivity shows a higher variation between each sensor point. Besides the differences in the reflected Bragg wavelength, this discrepancy could be related with the incorporation process in the insole. Since the cork is a porous material, different amounts of the epoxy resin may have infiltrated into its surroundings, which leads to different positions of the FBGs in the epoxy resin cylinders [1]. Thus, different pressure-induced strains are transmitted to the FBG. In this case, the lowest sensitivity was found for the FBG 4 (0.27 pm/kPa), whereas FBG 2 presented the highest sensitivity (0.87 pm/kPa). The linearity of each sensor was also analyzed considering its determination coefficient (R^2), shown in Fig. 12. In this case, all the sensors showed a linearity greater than 0.990, except the FBG 4. The low linearity (0.956) could be related with the incorporation process of the grating in to the cork insole, as discussed above.

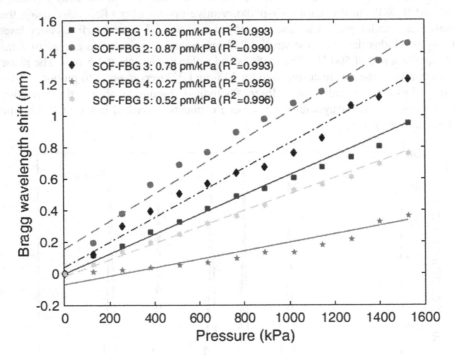

Fig. 12. Bragg wavelength shift as a function of the applied pressure in the SOF-FBGs characterization tests (adapted from [1]).

In the second test, where the FBG-embedded insole is fixed to the ground, it is possible to obtain the sequence in which the sensors are activated and the plantar pressure associated with each point under analysis. The maximum pressure was registered by each sensor according to the expected gait event sequence detailed in the previous section [1].

The stance period is initiated when the heel touches the ground, IC; after the contact of the heel with the ground, there is the first peak in the sensors responses (MA phase); in these events, FBG 1 presents the highest pressure. The foot is then moved toward a stable support position for the body in which the hip joint becomes aligned with the ankle joint (FF phase), where all five FBGs are under pressure. Thereafter, the heel loses contact with the ground in the HO phase, which results in a drop in the pressure measured by FBG 1, the pressure in the FBG 2 is also reduced, whereas the FBGs 3, 4 and 5 show an increase in the measured pressure. Finally, there is the TO phase, where all FBGs presents null pressure, which indicates that the foot is not in contact with the ground and the swing phase is about to start. Figure 13 shows the response of each FBG during a complete phase stance. In addition, the gait events detected are shown with respect to the stance phase percentage.

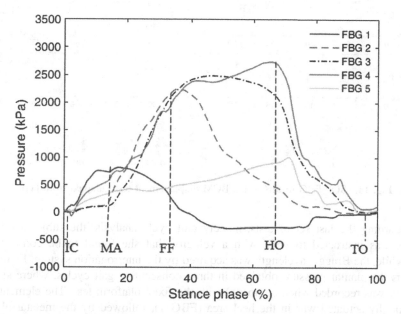

Fig. 13. Plantar pressure during the stance phase in the force platform application (adapted from [1]).

Regarding the BCM displacement tests, the Bragg wavelength shift of each sensor is presented as a function of time in Fig. 14. In the first pose (C), corresponding to the subject without BCM displacement, all the sensors are activated. Then, in the anterior movement (A), there is an increase of the pressure in the sensors positioned in the metatarsal and toe areas (FBGs 4 and 5), while the sensor placed in the heel section indicates a decrease of the plantar pressure when compared with the position (C). Similarly, during the BCM posterior displacement (P), the opposite occurs, with increase of the pressure in FBG 1 and 2. Regarding the frontal plane displacements, when the BCM is dislocated to the right, there is an increase of the pressure in FBG 2, whereas FBG 4 experiences an increase in the pressure when the BCM is moved to the right.

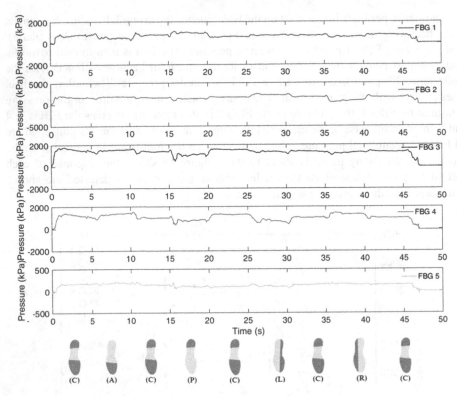

Fig. 14. SOF-FBG results in the BCM displacement test (adapted from [1]).

Regarding the last set of tests, namely gait cycle analysis, the subject, a 45-kg female, was instructed to walk with a velocity that she found to be comfortable. Meanwhile, the Bragg wavelength was acquired by the interrogation system. Figure 15 presents the plantar pressure obtained in three consecutive gait cycles, where similar behavior was recorded when compared with the fixed platform test. The element that was initially actuated was in the heel area (FBG 1), followed by the metatarsal area (FBG 2, 3 and 4) and, finally, the element in the toe (FBG 5), at the conclusion of the stance phase. Moreover, the different phases in the gait cycle can be identified, namely the stance phase (this characterizes $\sim 68\%$ of the cycle) and the swing phase. The duration of the stance phase can be related to the subject gait velocity and spatial parameters [29]. The swing phase is characterized by the absence of measured pressure by the instrumented insole.

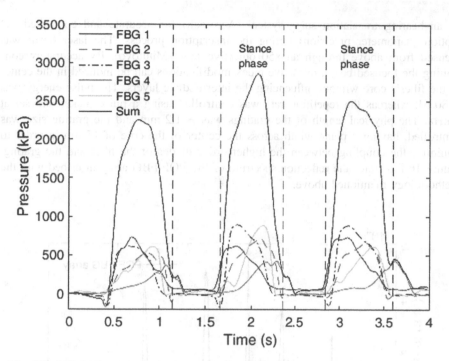

Fig. 15. SOF-FBG results in the in-shoe gait monitoring application (adapted from [1]).

4 POF-FBG-Based Instrumented Insole

After the initial development of a FBG-embedded insole using SOFs, the next version of the instrumented insole was based on POFs. The advantages of using POFs in the plantar pressure assessment are related to the material having a lower Young's modulus that leads to a higher sensitivity compared with the similar SOF sensors. In addition, POFs can withstand strain of approximately 10%, whereas SOF typically have strain limits of ~1% [17]. Thus, in a rough estimation, the insole based on POFs can support a pressure 10 times greater than the SOF-based device, assuming that both sensors are incorporated into the insole under the same conditions. These latter advantages mean that the POF-based insole can be used with patients having greater body mass.

The FBG sensors employed in the experiments were inscribed in a gradient index multimode CYTOP fiber (Chromis Fiberoptics Inc., Warren, NJ, USA) with core diameter of 120 μm, a 20 μm cladding layer, and an additional polyester and poly-carbonate over-cladding structure to protect the fiber, resulting in a total diameter of 490 μm [33]. For the POF-FBG inscription, the plane-by-plane femtosecond laser inscription method was used [24]. Regarding the setup for the gratings inscription, a fs laser system (HighQ laser femtoREGEN) operating at 517 nm with 220 fs pulses duration was used to modify the material [24]. All the inscriptions were performed without removing the outer protection jacket, and the fiber samples were immersed in matching oil between two thin glass slides. In addition, the samples were mounted on an air-bearing translation stage system (Aerotech) for accurate and controlled 2D motion (nanometer precision) during the inscription process. The laser beam was focused from above through an x50 objective lens (Mitutoyo). By accurately controlling the focused beam, refractive index modifications can be induced in the center of the fiber's core without influencing the intermediate layers. The pulse energy was ~80 nJ, whereas the repetition rate was controlled using a pulse picker and set at 5 kHz. The physical length of the gratings was ~1.2 mm and the grating size was controlled, having a plane width across the center of the core of 15 μm in order to minimize the coupling between the higher order modes of the fiber and the grating. Figure 16 illustrates the reflection spectrum of the POF-FBG array inscribed with the methodology mentioned above.

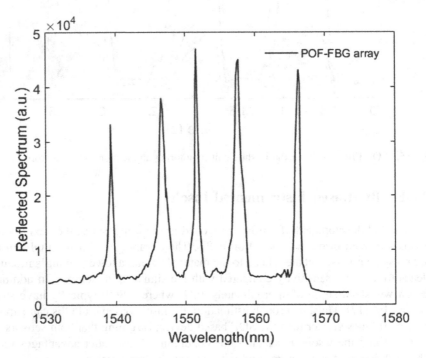

Fig. 16. Reflection spectrum of the FBG array inscribed in the POF.

Following the grating inscription, the FBGs were incorporated in the cork insole as presented in Sect. 2, and the tests were made with the protocols already discussed in the same section and also applied to the SOF-based insole. Therefore, the first test was the calibration of each POF-FBG in the universal mechanical testing machine. The calibration for all sensing elements are depicted in Fig. 17, where a linear dependence of the Bragg wavelength shift with the applied pressure is obtained (mean R^2 higher than 0.990).

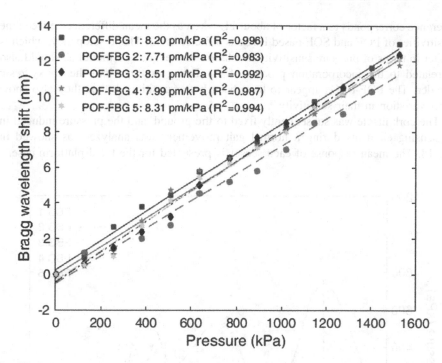

Fig. 17. Bragg wavelength shift as a function of the applied pressure in the POF-FBGs characterization tests.

In order to have a broader comparison with the SOF-based sensor system, Table 1 summarizes the sensitivity coefficients for all POF and SOF sensors. By comparing the values obtained for the SOF-based insole, the POF-FBG insole shows higher sensitivity for all the 5 FBGs, as anticipated based on the material advantages. The lowest sensitivity obtained for the POF-FBGs is 7.71 pm/kPa, whereas, for the silica FBGs is 0.27 pm/kPa. Regarding the mean value of pressure sensitivity, the values obtained are 8.14 pm/kPa and 0.61 pm/kPa, for the POF-FBGs and SOF-FBGs, respectively. The Young's modulus of the CYTOP is ~ 4 GPa and the silica is ~ 70 GPa [34]. Thus, this

Table 1. Pressure sensitivities obtained at the sensor characterization.

FBG	Pressure sensitivity (pm/kPa)	
	POF	SOF
1	8.31	0.62
2	7.99	0.87
3	8.51	0.78
4	7.71	0.27
5	8.20	0.52

difference corresponds to a factor of about 11, whereas the mean difference between the sensitivities of POF and SOF-based FBGs is a factor of 13. This discrepancy, which is greater in terms of pressure sensitivity in relation to the Young's modulus, should also be related to the incorporation process of the Bragg gratings into the epoxy resin cylinder. The POF-FBGs appear to have been better positioned, thus they also show lower variation in their sensitivity.

The cork insole was subsequently fixed to the ground, and the pressure induced in the sensing elements during a normal gait movement was analyzed, as showed in Fig. 18. The mean response of each sensor is presented for the fixed platform case.

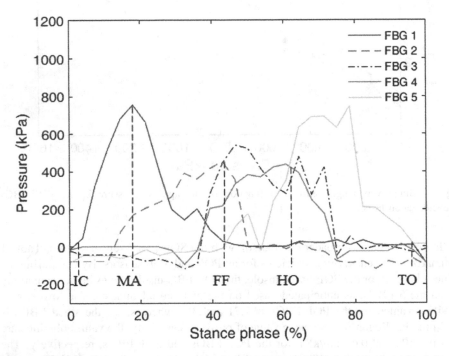

Fig. 18. POF-FBGs response of the tests using the FBG-embedded insole as a fixed force platform.

In Fig. 18, it is possible to observe the activation time for each sensor and its relation to the stance phase of the gait cycle. The FBG 1, located at the heel region, shows a pressure increasing at the beginning of the cycle (IC phase). In addition, FBG 1 exhibits a peak in the MA phase, where there is also an increase of the pressure exerted in the FBG 2, while the other sensors (FBG 3, 4 and 5) do not show a significant variation in the pressure. As the stance phase continues, the responses of FBGs 2, 3 and 4 show a pressure increase, whereas the FBGs 1 and 5 localized in heel and toe regions, respectively, show lower pressure responses than the sensors in the midfoot and forefoot regions. Such behavior is related to the FF phase and, as the cycle continues, there is a decrease in the pressure of the FBGs 1 and 2 until it reaches a null value in the HO phase. Finally, there is a peak in the FBG 5 (localized in the toe region) and, when its pressure response starts to drop, there is the TO phase, which also indicates the beginning of the swing phase, where all FBGs present negligible pressure values.

The third static test is the assessment of the BCM displacements both in the body sagittal plane, by moving it forward and backwards, and in the frontal plane, with the subject moving the torso from the left to the right and vice-verse. The results for this protocol are presented in Fig. 19.

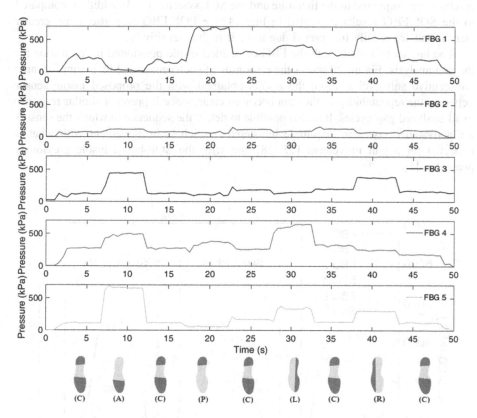

Fig. 19. POF-FBG responses for the BCM displacement tests.

In the center position (C), there is a pressure increase in all POF-FBGs. Regarding the tests on the sagittal plane, the sensors positioned in the metatarsal and toe areas show higher pressure in the anterior movement (A), when compared to the sensors in the heel and midfoot sections. On the other hand, during the posterior displacement of the BCM (P), the pressure increases on FBG 1, positioned at the heel area, whereas the pressure values at the toe and metatarsal areas decrease. However, due to the high sensor sensitivity and fiber positioning in the insole, it is not possible to activate only the heel and toe regions. Thus, the sensors on the metatarsal and midfoot regions are also activated. This is more evident on the anterior movement, since the subject presents more difficulty to maintain her balance during the test. In the displacements within the frontal plane (left and right displacements), the sensor placed in position 2 records the increase of pressure, when the BCM is displaced to the left (L). Analogously, FBGs 3 and 4 show a pressure increase when the BCM is moved to the right (R). Since the BCM displacement is a combined movement, where the whole foot is involved, there is also the activation of FBGs 1 and 5, positioned on the heel and toe, respectively. In summary, the results obtained on both sagittal and frontal planes show that the proposed sensor system is able to track the BCM displacement with similar results when compared to the literature and the SOF system [35]. In addition, compared to the SOF-FBG results presented in Fig. 14, the POF-FBG response show greater clarity, and are readily interpreted due to their higher sensitivity.

The last set of tests is with the FBG-embedded insole positioned inside a shoe for the gait analysis. Figure 20 shows the responses of each sensor and their sum for three consecutive gait cycles. From the results obtained with the proposed insole sensor network, the repeatability of the data becomes clear, since it presents similar response in all analyzed gait cycles. It is also possible to detect the sequence in which the sensors are activated (maximum amplitude registered), which is in agreement with what is expected for a gait movement [27, 28] and with the SOF-based insole previously presented [1].

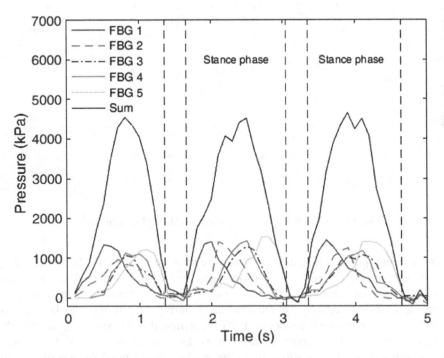

Fig. 20. POF-based instrumented insole response for the plantar pressure assessment during the gait.

At the beginning of the stance phase of the gait cycle, the heel starts its contact with the floor and FBG 1 is activated. The other FBGs respond in sequence with the evolution of the cycle, i.e., first the FBG 1 shows a pressure increase and, as the cycle continues, FBGs 2, 3, 4 and 5 are activated. When all the sensors record negligible pressure, we know that this coincides with the start of the swing phase of the gait cycle. The sum of all sensors is also presented, where we observe the combined effect of the plantar pressure response. In addition, it is possible to infer that the sensors present high repeatability, which is actually limited by the human's ability to repeat the motion, since different gait cycles may not be identical, even for the same person [28]. The dynamic measurements show the capability of the proposed system to detect the subdivisions of the stance phase, discussed in Sect. 2. Such features of the proposed sensor system not only can aid in the detection of gait related pathologies, but also can be applied on the controllers of wearable robots for gait assistance and in eHealth architectures [5, 36].

In general, the results obtained in the POF-based instrumented sole show that in addition to the advantages related to the material features, the employed POF is easier to handle and to incorporate in the cork insole when compared with the SOF system.

To conclude, it is worth to mention that we adopted a 5 FBGs sensors solution embedded in a cork insole with 10-mm thickness and such a thickness can slightly influence and change the walking efforts/capabilities of the walkers. However, from the results of this work, it maintains the same pattern of reaction force found in other systems, for example. Also, 10-mm thickness of the insole is only slightly larger than the conventional insoles. So, if there is influence, we can assume that it is relatively negligible in the context of the work presented here and, the results support this, since we find the same pattern in the ground reaction force curves.

5 Conclusions

The fast technological evolution we have been witnessing in the past decades offers several benefits to healthcare systems and diagnosis methodologies. The presented sensing platforms are reliable and accurate technologies for gait disorder diagnoses and physical rehabilitation evolution analysis. The discussed solutions show a level of performance that meets the electronics devices currently available in the market, with the additional OFS inherent advantages.

Furthermore, the OFS insoles can act as eHealth enablers, in an architecture comprising of a small interrogator system (adapted to a belt), a wireless transceiver and a cloud-based monitoring application [36]. Such architectures can be used to register, in real time, the plantar pressure of users, thereby emitting alerts in case of abnormal values, or even automatically requesting for emergency services in the extreme events, such as the case of a fall. This technology is a very promising eHealth tool.

Acknowledgments. CAPES (88887.095626/2015-01); FAPES (72982608); CNPq (304192/2016-3 and 310310/2015-6); FCT (SFRH/BPD/101372/2014 and SFRH/ BPD/109458/2015); Fundação para Ciência e a Tecnologia/Ministério da Educação e Ciência (UID/EEA/50008/2013); European Regional Development Fund (PT2020 Partnership Agreement); FCT, IT-LA

(PREDICT scientific action); Fundamental Research Funds for the Heilongjiang Provincial Universities (KJCXZD201703).

References

1. Domingues, M.F., et al.: Insole optical fiber Bragg grating sensors network for dynamic vertical force monitoring. J. Biomed. Opt. **22**(9), 91507 (2017)
2. Korhonen, I., Pärkkä, J., Van Gils, M.: Health monitoring in the home of the future. IEEE Eng. Med. Biol. Mag. **22**(3), 66–73 (2003)
3. Morag, E., Cavanagh, P.R.: Structural and functional predictors of regional peak pressures under the foot during walking. J. Biomech. **32**, 359–370 (1999)
4. Leal-Junior, A.G., Frizera, A., Avellar, L.M., Marques, C., Pontes, M.J.: Polymer optical fiber for in-shoe monitoring of ground reaction forces during the gait. IEEE Sens. J. **18**(6), 2362–2368 (2018)
5. Villa-Parra, A., Delisle-Rodriguez, D., Souza Lima, J., Frizera-Neto, A., Bastos, T.: Knee impedance modulation to control an active orthosis using insole sensors. Sensors **17**(12), 2751 (2017)
6. Hadi, A., Razak, A., Zayegh, A., Begg, R.K., Wahab, Y.: Foot plantar pressure measurement system: a review. Sensors **12**, 9884–9912 (2012)
7. Sanderson, D.J., Franks, I.M., Elliott, D.: The effects of targeting on the ground reaction forces during level walking. Hum. Mov. Sci. **12**(3), 327–337 (1993)
8. Ballaz, L., Raison, M., Detrembleur, C.: Decomposition of the vertical ground reaction forces during gait on a single force plate. J. Musculoskelet. Neuronal Interact. **13**(2), 236–243 (2013)
9. Webb, D.J.: Fibre Bragg grating sensors in polymer optical fibres. Meas. Sci. Technol. **26**(9), 92004 (2015)
10. Zhu, T., Ke, T., Rao, Y., Chiang, K.S.: Fabry-Perot optical fiber tip sensor for high temperature measurement. Opt. Commun. **283**(19), 3683–3685 (2010)
11. Minakawa, K., Mizuno, Y., Nakamura, K.: Cross effect of strain and temperature on Brillouin frequency shift in polymer optical fibers. J. Light. Technol. **35**(12), 2481–2486 (2017)
12. Rajan, G., Noor, Y.M., Liu, B., Ambikairaja, E., Webb, D.J., Peng, G.D.: A fast response intrinsic humidity sensor based on an etched singlemode polymer fiber Bragg grating. Sens. Actuators A Phys. **203**, 107–111 (2013)
13. Zhong, N., Liao, Q., Zhu, X., Zhao, M., Huang, Y., Chen, R.: Temperature-independent polymer optical fiber evanescent wave sensor. Sci. Rep. **5**, 1–10 (2015)
14. Leal-Junior, A., Frizera, A., Marques, C., José Pontes, M.: Polymer-optical-fiber-based sensor system for simultaneous measurement of angle and temperature. Appl. Opt. **57**(7), 1717 (2018)
15. Diaz, C.A.R., et al.: Liquid level measurement based on FBG-embedded diaphragms with temperature compensation. IEEE Sens. J. **18**(1), 193–200 (2018)
16. Ishikawa, R., et al.: Pressure dependence of fiber Bragg grating inscribed in perfluorinated polymer fiber. IEEE Photonics Technol. Lett. **29**(24), 2167–2170 (2017)
17. Peters, K.: Polymer optical fiber sensors—a review. Smart Mater. Struct. **20**(1), 13002 (2010)
18. Leal-Junior, A.G., Marques, C., Frizera, A., Pontes, M.J.: Dynamic mechanical analysis on a polymethyl methacrylate (PMMA) polymer optical fiber. IEEE Sens. J. **18**(6), 2353–2361 (2018)

19. Leal-Junior, A., Frizera-Neto, A., Marques, C., Pontes, M.: Measurement of temperature and relative humidity with polymer optical fiber sensors based on the induced stress-optic effect. Sensors 18(3), 916 (2018)
20. Liu, Y., Peng, W., Liang, Y., Zhang, X., Zhou, X., Pan, L.: Fiber-optic Mach-Zehnder interferometric sensor for high-sensitivity high temperature measurement. Opt. Commun. 300, 194–198 (2013)
21. Mizuno, Y., Hayashi, N., Fukuda, H., Song, K.Y., Nakamura, K.: Ultrahigh-speed distributed Brillouin reflectometry. Light Sci. Appl. 5(12), e16184 (2016)
22. Perrotton, C., Javahiraly, N., Slaman, M., Dam, B., Meyrueis, P.: Fiber optic surface plasmon resonance sensor based on wavelength modulation for hydrogen sensing. Opt. Express 19(S6), A1175 (2011)
23. Luo, Y., Yan, B., Zhang, Q., Peng, G.-D., Wen, J., Zhang, J.: Fabrication of polymer optical fibre (POF) gratings. Sensors 17(3), 511 (2017)
24. Theodosiou, A., Lacraz, A., Stassis, A., Koutsides, C., Komodromos, M., Kalli, K.: Plane-by-plane femtosecond laser inscription method for single-peak bragg gratings in multimode CYTOP polymer optical fiber. J. Light. Technol. 35(24), 5404–5410 (2017)
25. Cusano, A., Cutolo, A., Albert, J.: Fiber Bragg Grating Sensors: Market Overview and New Perspectives. Bentham Science Publishers, Potomac (2009)
26. Ashby, M.F.: Materials Selection in Mechanical Design. Elsevier, Cambridge (2005)
27. Abboud, R.J.: (i) relevant foot biomechanics. Orthopaedics 16, 165–179 (2002)
28. Kirtley, C.: Clinical Gait Analysis: Theory and Practice. Elsevier, Philadelphia (2006)
29. Liu, Y., Lu, K., Yan, S., Sun, M., Lester, D.K., Zhang, K.: Gait phase varies over velocities. Gait Posture 39(2), 756–760 (2014)
30. Shu, L., Hua, T., Wang, Y., Li, Q., Feng, D.D., Tao, X.: In-shoe plantar pressure measurement and analysis system based on fabric pressure sensing array. IEEE Trans. Inf. Technol. Biomed. 14(3), 767–775 (2010)
31. Vilarinho, D., et al.: POFBG-embedded cork insole for plantar pressure monitoring. Sensors 17(12), 2924 (2017)
32. Vilarinho, D., et al.: Foot plantar pressure monitoring with CYTOP Bragg Gratings sensing system. In: Proceedings of the 11th International Joint Conference on Biomedical Engineering Systems and Technologies, vol. 1, no. Biostec, pp. 25–29 (2018)
33. Thorlabs, Graded-Index Polymer Optical Fiber (GI-POF). https://www.thorlabs.com/catalogPages/1100.pdf. Accessed 17 May 2018
34. Antunes, P., Domingues, F., Granada, M., André, P.: Mechanical properties of optical fibers, pp. 1–15. INTECH Open Access Publisher (2012)
35. Suresh, R., Bhalla, S., Hao, J., Singh, C.: Development of a high resolution plantar pressure monitoring pad based on fiber Bragg grating (FBG) sensors. Technol. Health Care 23, 785–794 (2015)
36. Domingues, M.F., et al.: Insole optical fiber sensor architecture for remote gait analysis - an eHealth solution. IEEE Internet Things J. 6, 207–214 (2017)

A New Compact Optical System Proposal and Image Quality Comparison Against Other Affordable Non-mydriatic Fundus Cameras

David Melo[1,2]([envelope]), Filipe Soares[2], Simão Felgueiras[2], João Gonçalves[2], and Pedro Vieira[1]

[1] Department of Physics, Faculdade de Ciências e Tecnologia, Universidade Nova de Lisboa, Quinta da Torre, 2829-516 Caparica, Portugal
ds.melo@campus.fct.unl.pt
[2] Fraunhofer Portugal AICOS, Rua Alfredo Allen, 455/461, 4200-135 Porto, Portugal

Abstract. Imaging the eye retina is critical to diagnose various pathologies, particularly Diabetic Retinopathy, which is the leading cause of avoidable blindness in the world. The image acquisition through table-top fundus cameras is the preferred method for retinopathy screening. However, these devices require expertise for operation, limiting its broad application. In this paper, two handheld fundus camera prototypes developed by Fraunhofer AICOS (EyeFundusScope Compact and EyeFundusScope Standard) have their optical capabilities compared, not only between each other but also with another commercially available camera. Field-of-view measurements are performed, as well as a subjective analysis on eye model images acquired with each of prototypes. Besides the comparison between handheld devices in the same experimental setup, conceptual specification on the prototype and optical system for the Compact version are described in order to demonstrate the most relevant issues to be considered when developing a valuable instrument for diabetic retinopathy screening and diagnosis.

Keywords: Diabetic retinopathy · Fundus camera design · Handheld devices

1 Introduction

1.1 Diabetic Retinopathy

The eye retina is the only structure in the body where vessels can be directly seen, without intrusive procedures. Imaging this structure is extremely important in the diagnosis of various pathologies, particularly Diabetic Retinopathy. This is a microvascular disease caused by the diabetes mellitus condition, affecting 76% of the diabetic patients for longer than 20 years [6] and being the leading cause of blindness in adults with working age [5]. It is characterized by the loss of perycites

© Springer Nature Switzerland AG 2019
A. Cliquet jr. et al. (Eds.): BIOSTEC 2018, CCIS 1024, pp. 26–48, 2019.
https://doi.org/10.1007/978-3-030-29196-9_2

and by a progressive capillary occlusion that occurs mostly without symptoms. The capillary occlusion can lead to retinal ischemia and to the breakdown of the blood-retinal-barrier [28].

The disease can be divided in two different stages: Non-proliferative and Proliferative [15]. The first is characterized by abnormalities in the blood vessels materialized in the leakage of substances from the lumen of the vessels to the retinal epithelium. The leakages may be the blood itself leading to microaneurysms and intraretinal hemorrhages, and lipids leading to hard and soft Exudates [8,10,15]. The Proliferative stage is characterized by the creation of new blood vessels surrounding occluded regions (neovascularization). The new blood vessels, being more fragile than the previous ones, increase the risk of bleeding and do not solve retinal ischemia [10]. In the Proliferative stage there is also the formation of fibrous tissue that while contracting can provoke retinal detachment [23].

Several types of instruments can perform ophthalmological examination, but for the diagnosis of Diabetic Retinopathy the use of Fundus Camera is preferred [25].

The asymptomatic profile of the initial progression of diabetic retinopathy is problematic for diagnostic purposes. On the other hand, the success of early treatment provides a large incentive to implement population-based screening programs for diabetic patients. In these programs, images of the patient retinas are acquired and assessed by qualified technicians and ophthalmologists, which lead to high costs due to the required use of expensive and bulky equipment, and the laborious task of manual analysis by scarcely available medical personnel. The prototypes EyeFundusScope, currently under investigation by Fraunhofer Portugal AICOS, aims to address these issues by researching on a self-contained solution comprising automated retinopathy detection with a low cost optical attachment to a smartphone for retinal image acquisition. The major goal is to improve patient access to early treatment and decrease the burden of screening actions on healthcare systems, mainly in medically underserved areas. The prototype described in this paper being compact, easy to transport, easy to mount and revealing good image quality can be a good tool for the accomplishment of these objectives.

1.2 Fundus Camera

A Fundus Camera is a device that allows the observation of the structures and the blood vessels in the ocular fundus, being employed in the diagnosis of several pathologies (like Diabetic Retinopathy, described in Sect. 1.1) [21].

When compared with other eye examination devices, a Fundus Camera enables patient documentation and easy follow, as well as allowing analysis of a great extent of the patient retina, due to the wide field-of-view empowered by the usage of indirect ophthalmoscopy principles, hardly achievable with direct ophthalmoscopy methods [2,22].

The importance of the fundus examination can be seen in many medicine fields and not only in ophthalmology. Since the retina is the human body structure where the vessels can more easily be seen with no use of ionizing radiation [21], fields like Neurology and Cardiology can also use the capabilities of a Fundus Camera [19]. A handheld portable Fundus Camera can also be a crucial tool in the development of telemedicine [21].

In this work, to diminish the production costs, only the fundamental components of a Fundus Camera were used. When compared with the version presented in Melo et al. on the paper "Optical Design of a Compact Image Acquisition Device for Mobile Diabetic Retinopathy Screening", [17] the final optical system used in the compact version of the prototype has some improvements. To prevent the existence of brighter spots in the final image obtained, circular polarizers were added to the optical path avoiding that light reflected from the cornea or from the back of the objective lens could reach Smartphone CMOS and an iris (or aperture stop) to limit the smartphone angle of view only to the required for a 40°. The usefulness of polarizers in ophthalmology, specifically in fundus imaging will be discussed in the Sect. 2.4. The software used for the Optical Simulation was BEAM IV, an Optical Ray Tracer developed by Stellar Software. Figure 1 shows a diagram with the refractive components that are fundamentally present in a Fundus Camera.

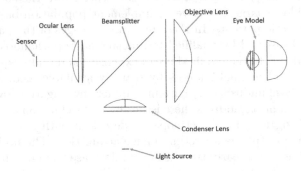

Fig. 1. Demonstration of the fundamental components in the Fundus Camera prototype [17].

The usage of smartphone cameras as sensors is justified by its continuous evolution. An evolution on the sensor can lead to a better image quality, and consequently to an improved performance on the image analysis algorithms, associated with the smartphone applications.

1.3 Optical Principles

To reach an optimal optical system several lenses types were tested. To simulate them according to the characteristics supplied by the manufacturers, the thin lens approximation was used. This approximation neglects the thickness of the lens and considers that the unit planes pass through the axial point of the infinitely thin lens [13]. Considering that the media on both sides of the lens is the same, the following equation can be used to describe it [3].

Lens-Maker's Formula

$$P_{lens} = \frac{n_{lens} - n_0}{n_0}\left(\frac{1}{R_1} - \frac{1}{R_2}\right) \tag{1}$$

Where n_0 is the refractive index of the surrounding medium, the air in this case, equal to 1, n_{lens} is the refractive index of the lens, R_1 is the radius of curvature of the first surface and R_2 is the radius of curvature of the second surface. The P_{lens} is the refractive power in diopters.

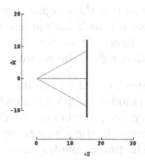

Fig. 2. Demonstration of the 4-extremes model along the x-axis [17].

To simulate a Fundus Camera optical system, the optical path taken by the rays is separated in two different ones by the usage of a beamsplitter [30]. The path that describes how the rays illuminate the retina is called *illumination path* and the path describing how the rays go from the retina to the smartphone camera is called *imaging path*. To simulate them two different approaches were tested, the *4-extreme model* for the illumination, and the *parallel rays model* for the imaging path (see Fig. 2). The 4-extreme model assumes that the light source emits from a single point with a certain aperture previously declared by the manufacturer. The angles for which the relative luminous intensity is bellow half the maximum intensity can be neglected.

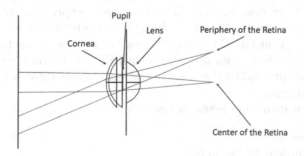

Fig. 3. Demonstration of the parallel rays model. In this figure rays are focused on the retina, leaving the pupil collimated and parallel [17].

The parallel rays model assumes that when two rays focused at some point reach a lens they are collimated and leave the lens with the same direction and parallel with each other. In Fig. 3 one of the applications of this model is demonstrated, showing rays focused at some point, leaving the pupil parallel.

1.4 Related Work

Recently, the features of handheld Fundus Camera prototypes have increased significantly when compared with the traditional tabletop fundus cameras [30], proving as an helpful instrument in the diagnosis of many pathologies related with the retina and facilitating telemedicine applications [14, 24]. This improvement of the capabilities of handheld devices led to a variety of different approaches. Some examples that reflect the recent scientific development are:

- Nonmydriatic Fundus Camera Based on the Raspberry Pi® Computer: Uses the Raspberry Pi® camera module coupled with a Condenser Lens to perform fundus imaging with a very low production cost [26].
- Eye-Selfie: By using internal fixation points as targets, it allows a self-performed acquisition of the fundus photography, completely by the patient [27].

There are already, some fundus imaging devices available in the market but most, present one of the following issues:

- Low Field Of View, as for the D-EYE ophthalmoscope [9].
- Require pupil dilation, as for the Volk inView [32].
- High price, as for the Volk Pictor Plus [33].

This year, Optomed commercialized a new device for fundus imaging named Optomed Aurora [18]. It presents better features than any other fundus camera available, showing a Field-of-View of $50 \times 40°$. To ensure that the examiner capability for identification of eye smallest structures isn't diminished by increasing the Field-of-view, a screen correspondingly large is used. Besides fundus imaging, the fundus camera also allows the observation of the surface of the eye and surrounding areas. This way it is versatile enough to be an exceptional tool for the screening of eye diseases. The User Interface comprises a rotary encoder, capacitive touch buttons and battery charging indicator LEDs.

The selection of the OICO Fundus Camera for the comparison tests described in the Sect. 3 is justified by its similarities with EFS prototypes, namely its low-cost, high availability and by the usage of the smartphone camera for acquisition of the fundus images.

OICO fundus camera presents as main features:

- Field-of-View: 35°
- Sensor Resolution: 12 Megapixel
- Minimum Pupil Size: 3.4 mm
- Capture Mode: Infrared for guidance and Color for acquisition

The system we propose differs from the previous approaches by using a smartphone for non-mydriatic, high field-of-view retinal image acquisition. The use of a smartphone instead of custom electronic devices for image capture and processing allows a substantial decrease in costs while allowing for a very high image quality and resolution, thus guaranteeing the cost-effectiveness of the overall solution.

2 Compact System Design

2.1 Eye Model

To guarantee a satisfactory field-of-view, an accurate model of the eye is needed. The eye has two refractive lenses, the cornea and the crystalline lens. Based on literature [1] and following a similar approach to [29], a model of the eye was created in BEAM IV considering the radius of curvature, diameter and asphericity coefficients of all structures relevant for human eye modeling. The pupil has been designed with a 4 mm diameter to simulate a non-mydriatic acquisition with no visible light and is coincident with the lens anterior surface. The chromatic aberrations from the eye were neglected as the change in diopters at different wavelengths were not considered significant in the scope of this work [1].

The refractive indexes for each medium are:

- Cornea: 1.376
- Aqueous Humour: 1.366
- Lens: 1.406
- Vitreous Humour: 1.336

The defined refractive surfaces of the eye, as represented in Fig. 4, are:

- Corneal Anterior surface: Diameter = 11.50 mm
  Radius of Curvature = 7.75 mm
  Asphericity coefficient = −0.2

- Corneal Posterior surface:
  Diameter = 11.50 mm
  Radius of Curvature = 6.8 mm
  Asphericity coefficient = 0

- Pupil/Lens Anterior surface:
  Diameter = 4 mm
  Radius of Curvature = 10 mm
  Asphericity coefficient = −0.94

- Lens Posterior Surface:
  Diameter = 9 mm
  Radius of Curvature = −6 mm
  Asphericity coefficient = 0.96

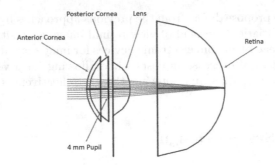

Fig. 4. BEAM IV simulation of the eye model used with collimated rays being focused on the retina [17].

– Retina:
  Diameter $= 24\,mm$
  Radius of Curvature $= 12\,mm$
  Asphericity coefficient $= 0$

2.2 Illumination Path

For the illumination path the main goal is a 40° field-of-view with a uniform illumination of the retina. The diagram of the illumination path is represented in Fig. 5. The image is obtained using a White LED but, to allow a non-mydriatic acquisition, a Near Infrared (NIR) LED is used, helping the examiner to perform alignment of the device with the eye and to find the area of the retina to be imaged. As in most fundus cameras, there is a lens above the light source to collimate the rays and another lens to focus the rays [30].

To obtain a field-of-view of 40° there is a constraint that the relationship $\frac{WD}{2f}$ should be equal to or larger than sin(20), where WD stands for Working Diameter and f means the effective focal length of the lens. This condition, coupled with the demand of minimization of spherical aberrations makes Aspheric lenses the only suitable option for the focusing of the rays when reaching the retina.

The lenses for the illumination path of the optical system described in this paper were the ones used in Melo et al. [17], a Thorlabs aspheric lens with 50.00 mm diameter, 40.00 mm focal length and SLAH-64 glass type as an objective and for collimation of the light rays an Edmund Optics Plano-Convex Lens with 25.4 mm diameter, 38.1 mm focal length and N-BK7 glass type. Even though the lenses are the same when compared with the optical system, the usage of the polarizer lead to a different placement of both lenses. The condenser lens was brought down so the polarizers could fit the system while the objective lens was placed to the right of its initial position. So, despite using the same set of lenses the optical system shown in Fig. 5, has several different features.

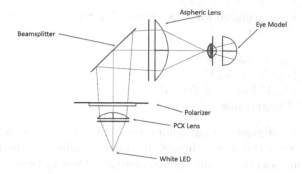

Fig. 5. Visible Light illumination path and components used. (Color figure online)

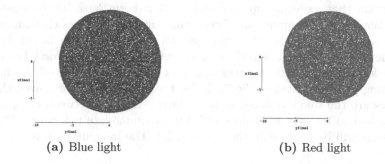

(a) Blue light   (b) Red light

Fig. 6. The retinal area illuminated, also called retinal illumination profile, is described, for the configuration represented in Fig. 5 at both ends of the visible electromagnetic spectrum. (Color figure online)

As the white light emitted by the LED has a continuous emission spectrum, measurements at both ends of the visible spectrum are needed. The mean percentage of rays for both wavelengths (blue - 486.13 nm, red - 656.27) reaching the retina for the white visible LED, is about 90% of the ones emitted. The illumination profile is uniform, as can be observed in Fig. 6 for blue and red light. The mean value was also calculated between the illumination half-angle of both wavelengths and was 20.58° leading to a total field-of-view of 41.16°.

2.3   Imaging Path

For the imaging path the key features desired are the almost complete fulfillment of the Smartphone Camera sensor angle-of-view, the minimization of aberrations and an accurate focusing of the rays in the retina. In order to perform ray tracing analysis of the imaging path, two pairs of parallel rays going from the smartphone camera to the back of the eye were considered, one pair parallel with the optical axis and the other with an angle close to the value of the vertical angle of view of the smartphone.

The system was optimized for a LG Nexus 5X camera whose relevant specifications are:

- Horizontal Angle of View: 68.2°
- Vertical Angle of View: 53.1°
- Sensor Size: 1/2.3″ (6.17 × 4.55 mm)
- Resolution: 12 Megapixels

The final optical system must guarantee that the Vertical Angle of View is mostly filled with the retinal image, in order to allow the highest possible retinal resolution, essential for the clinical analysis of fine features. The objective lens had already been defined by the simulations of the illumination path so it was necessary to test which lens could best fulfill our needs as an ocular. The solution that we came up was with a Best-Form lens. These lenses are manufactured with a conjunction of curvatures in both surfaces that minimizes monochromatic aberrations. They were proven to operate better in this type of applications than regular Plano-Convex Lenses [17]. So a Best-Form Lens with 40.0 mm focal length, 25.0 Diopters and 25.4 diameter was tested, leading to the imaging path presented in Fig. 7. As for the illumination path, even though the lenses are the same, changes in the relative distance between components were required so the system could physically accommodate polarizers. The use of polarizers will be justified in the Subsect. 2.4. The imaging path is presented in Fig. 7.

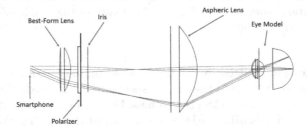

Fig. 7. Parallel rays model. In this model the progression of two pairs of parallel rays is studied, one parallel with the optical axis and the other with an angle of 22°. The goal is to ensure that both pairs have their focal point as close to the retina as possible. In this configuration 83% of the smartphone vertical angle of view is approximately used.

Only 83% of the smartphone vertical angle of view is used because the Best-Form Lenses required for the reduction of spherical aberrations are only available with relatively small diameters, making it difficult to use much wider angles. Besides that 83% of the smartphone camera 12 Megapixels resolution can be considered sufficient for fundus imaging. The iris (or aperture stop) in Fig. 7 has 25 mm of inner diameter and a thickness of 1 mm. Its purpose is to stop the rays at a wider angle than the necessary for a field-of-view of 40°, preventing reflections and the imaging of not illuminated areas of the retina.

2.4   Polarizers

Polarizers are, by definition, optical filters where the transmission of light is dependent on its polarization. Being really helpful to block light with a specific polarization having many application in fields like microscopy and photography. Light reflected from dielectric surfaces, like water, glass or the human cornea has its electrical vector parallel with that surface so get linearly polarized [7].

Polarizers are usually named after the polarization of light transmitted by it. The two most applied types of polarizers are linear and circular. Circular polarizers are composed of one linear polarizer followed by a retarder (or quarter wave-plate). When the angle between the axis of the retarder and the axis of the linear polarizer is 90°, the light becomes circularly polarized being right-handed or left-handed polarized, depending on the relative orientation between components [20].

Taking advantage of the polarization state changes light suffers along the optical path, polarizers can be a great tool in the prevention of undesired reflections from reducing the quality of the final image obtained, ensuring that only light coming from the fundus reach the Smartphone CMOS. Linearly polarized light when reflected from a dielectric surface keeps its polarization state. This property can be explored using one polarizer right above the condenser lens to make light linearly polarized and the other on the imaging path right before the ocular lens. According to several papers light reaching the fundus is scattered on the retina and by other the human eye structures, thus becoming depolarized [4,31]. So polarizers must be perpendicularly oriented so light coming from the illumination path polarizer without any depolarization is blocked. This way, light that is reflected from the cornea and the back of the objective lens, is blocked by the polarizer. Using polarizers this way is often named crossed polarizers technique [30].

2.5   Imaging Path for Eyes with Refractive Errors

Eyes with refractive errors present different optical characteristics and so the distance between lenses in the optical system must be adjustable to compensate this.

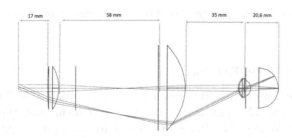

Fig. 8. The distances between each components to image an eye without refractive errors.

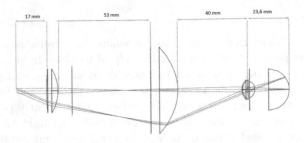

Fig. 9. The distances between each components to image an eye with refractive errors (Myopia).

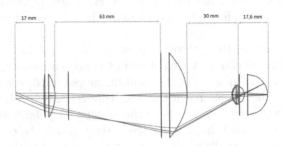

Fig. 10. The distances between each components to image an eye with refractive errors (Hyperopia).

As the smartphone camera is able to change its focus target distance, the refractive errors were only simulated in the range −5D to +5D. Since one of the possible cause of refractive errors is the size of the eyeball, for the simulation of Myopia the retina was moved 3 mm away from the refractive center of the eye. Concerning the simulation of Hyperopia the eyeball was shortened 3 mm.

In Fig. 8, the system configuration for an eye without any refractive error is shown. In Figs. 9 and 10, diagrams showing the adjustments done to compensate these refractive errors are shown.

For the Myopic eye the error is corrected by moving the Objective Lens 5 mm away from the eye.

Concerning the Hyperopic eye, the Objective lens is approximated 5 mm to the eye.

2.6   Mechanical Prototyping

The optical system previously described was implemented in a 3D printed prototype (Figs. 11 and 12). The design of the mechanical prototype was developed using Solid Works. The important goals for this prototype are to allow the arrangement of the desired lens, a support for the smartphone that ensures that the camera is centered with the optical path, and the adjustment of the objective lens. Due to the need of physical space for the placement of polarizers

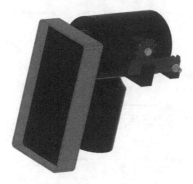

Fig. 11. Mechanical prototype showing both the smartphone support and the rack and pinion mate.

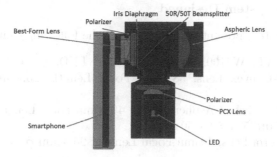

Fig. 12. Section view of the prototype.

and consequent changes on the optical system, when compared with Melo et al. [17] version, several alterations are observable on the 3D printed mechanical prototype. Although some features, like the Rack and Pinion system to allow the examiner to precisely search for the working distance, were preserved.

Other solution to allow the movement of the lens would be by the use of threaded surfaces in both sides, so the rotation of the objective ensures a change in the working distance. This approach was rejected because it is expected the future implementation of a piece leaning against the patient forehead, to guarantee the centering with the Optical Path. The rotation of this piece, in contact with the patient, would not be comfortable or, possibly, safe.

Some other changes were performed in the mechanical prototype design like the implementation of a new case for smartphone support printed in flexible material (FilaFlex) to ensure that smartphone edges weren't damaged. A Solid-Works fastening tool named lip and groove was used in the connection between parts with the goal of preventing external light from entering the mechanical case and create unnatural reflections.

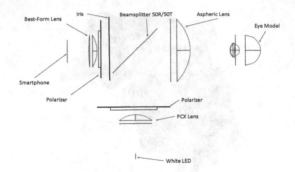

Fig. 13. Complete Optical System.

2.7 Complete System Designed

The Complete System presented in Fig. 13 has the following elements:

- Visible LED - VLHW4100, Ultrabright White LED.
- N-BK7 Plano-Convex Lens, 38.1 mm Focal Length, 25.4 mm ϕ, VIS-NIR Coated.
- S-LAH64 CNC-Polished Aspheric Lens, 40.0 mm Focal Length, 50 mm ϕ.
- Beamsplitter 50R/50T 50 × 50 mm.
- N-BK7 Best-Form Lens, 40 mm Focal Length, 25.4 mm ϕ.
- Polarizers.

In this setup the distance between the prototype and the human eye is intended to be 31.5 mm.

The main features of the developed system are:

- About 40° field-of-view.
- Non-Mydriatic Acquisition, for a 4 mm pupil size, achievable by using the NIR LED for guidance.
- No significant aberrations (Spherical and Chromatic).
- Uniform Illumination of the Retina.
- Simple and affordable lens system.

3 Handheld Devices Comparison

In this Sect. 3 different handheld devices are compared. To allow an accurate measurement of the Field-of-View, photographs of graph paper are obtained with each of the 3 prototypes. Besides that, images of an eye model (Model Eye Ophthalmoscope Trainer by HEINE) are analyzed and sharpness of the photographs on specific regions is evaluated. Some post-processing is also applied to the images in order to address the quality of the illumination each prototype supplies. The Optomed Aurora Fundus Camera [18], considered the one with better specifications commercially available wasn't considered in this comparison due to its high cost and low availability.

The three prototypes to be compared are:

- EFS Compact Version;
- EFS Standard Version;
- OICO Fundus Camera.

The prototypes were tested under the same conditions at Fraunhofer Portugal Association facilities in Porto, more specifically in the OpenLab.

3.1 Field-of-View

The Retinal area whose observation is possible is one of the most important features of a Fundus Camera.

The setup for calculation of the FOV comprises a 38.1 mm focal length lens and graph paper. The lens was placed in front of the prototype on the plane where the illumination circle of confusion was minimum and the graph paper was placed in front of the lens at its focal distance (as close to 38.1 mm as possible). The setup for the FOV image acquisition is presented on Fig. 14.

The Total Field of view values obtained for each fundus camera were:

- EFS Compact Version - 45 × 45°;
- EFS Standard Version - 45 × 45°;
- OICO Fundus Camera - 37 × 30°;

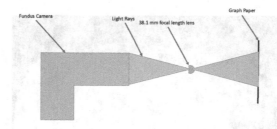

Fig. 14. Diagram of the optical setup for Field of View measurement.

3.2   Eye Model Photos

Images of an eye model were obtained with each one of the 3 different devices. The sharpness of the pictures was qualitatively evaluated and consequently also the suitability of each of the systems for Diabetic Retinopathy Screening. The pictures are shown in Figs. 15 and 16.

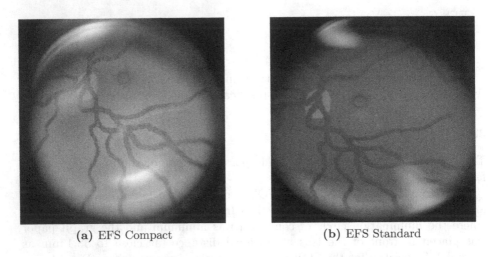

(a) EFS Compact   (b) EFS Standard

Fig. 15. Model Eye photograph acquired for each EFS prototype.

The differences in the acquirable Field of View as described in the Sect. 3.1 are easily noticeable. The purple spots on the image of the Fig. 15a are caused by back reflections of the objective lens and by reflections from the refractive lens of the eye model, analogous to the cornea in the human eye.

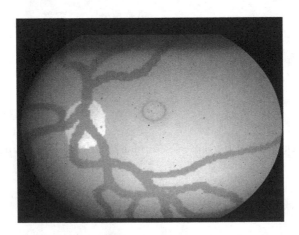

Fig. 16. Model Eye photographs obtained with OICO Fundus Camera.

Even though these reflections can diminish the final quality of the images obtained the sharpness of the image is noticeable when specific regions are zoomed in. Figure 17 allow a comparison between the sharpness of the vessels near the optic disk.

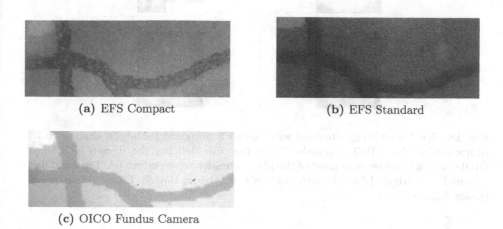

(a) EFS Compact   (b) EFS Standard

(c) OICO Fundus Camera

Fig. 17. Photos acquired with each of the prototypes with zoom in after the acquisition.

The chromatic changes observable on Fig. 17a also show that polarizers are not working properly, as they don't block light coming from the back of the objective lens.

As for the EFS Standard (Fig. 17b), even though, the reflections are not as representative, the illumination intensity seems lower than for the others. Considering the low reflection ratio of the retina, this could be a problem when imaging real human eyes [16].

3.3   Retinal Illumination

To properly illuminate the retina is one of the fundamental challenges when designing a fundus camera, so, a Java open-source software named ImageJ was used to calculate the mean pixel intensity for the images presented in Sect. 3.2. The images were also split in the 3 RGB channels in order to find out any possible saturation and to check the differences between each prototype. As an example, the images obtained for the EFS Standard Eye Model photograph are presented in Fig. 18.

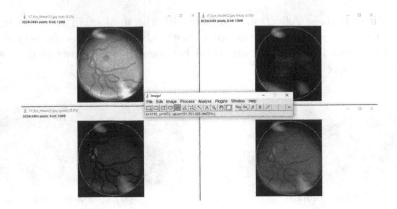

Fig. 18. Eye Model image obtained with the EFS Standard prototype along with its projection on the 3 RGB channels. The yellow line delimits the Region of Interest (ROI) in which the measurement of the pixel intensity were performed. Top Left: Red Channel; Top Right: Blue Channel; Bottom Left: Green; Bottom Right: All channels. (Color figure online)

The red channel of the image obtained with the OICO Fundus Camera presented an artifact at the center of the image, most likely derived from red channel saturation. This problem may be solved by the appliance of a "bluish" White-Balance. White-Balance is a tool normally used to balance the colors, approximating the colors shown in the photographs to the colors of the actual objects. For of Retinal Photography, the normally used White-Balance increases lower wavelengths prevalence over higher wavelengths so, the previously referred red channel saturation effect (Fig. 19) can be minimized [11].

The results obtained for mean pixel intensity on each one of the 3 channels are presented in the following table (Table 1):

Table 1. Comparison on Mean Pixel Intensity for each of the RGB channels using the 3 prototypes.

Prototype	Channel			
	All	Red	Green	Blue
EFS Compact	129	142	100	144
EFS Standard	70	158	30	21
OICO Fundus Camera	180	218	144	177

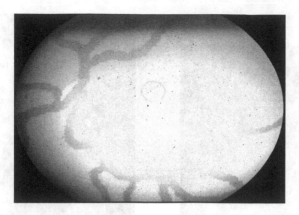

Fig. 19. Red Channel image obtained with the OICO Fundus Camera showing saturation on the middle of photograph.

Besides the calculation of the mean pixel intensity the image was transformed to YUV (in which Y is the variable Luminance, U and V are chromaticity coordinates) so the relative luminance of the 3 images could be directly obtained. As the relative luminance along the object to be imaged (fundus) is not constant (vessels are less bright than retinal epithelium), and the regions of the eye model obtained with each prototype are different, the luminance values presented in Table 2 aren't directly proportional to the illumination intensity. Although, the margin by which they differ, ascertains what was previously predicted on the Sect. 3.2.

Table 2. Comparison on Luminance value for each of the RGB channels using the 3 prototypes.

Prototype	Mean luminance
EFS Compact	0,469
EFS Standard	0,26
OICO Fundus Camera	0,669

The values suggest that OICO Fundus Camera allows an higher illumination intensity than EFS prototypes, and that between EFS prototypes, the EFS Compact has higher illumination intensity than the EFS Compact. The images obtained are presented in Fig. 20.

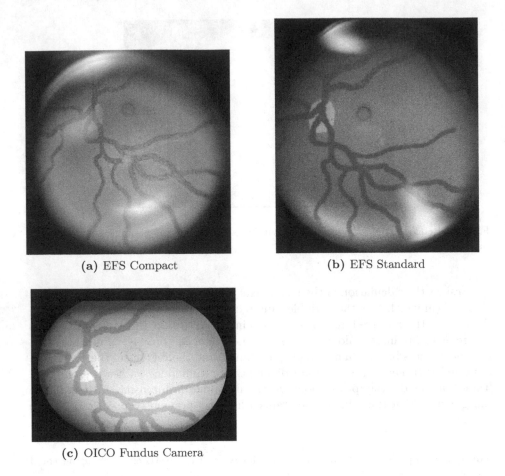

(a) EFS Compact

(b) EFS Standard

(c) OICO Fundus Camera

Fig. 20. Luminance images for on the photographs of the Fig. 15.

4   Conclusions

Some of the tasks described as future work in Melo et al. [17], were performed and are described in this paper. The Compact prototype has been printed (Fig. 21) and eye model photographs were obtained with the prototype containing the Optical system described in this paper.

The fact that the prototype is 3D-printed (rapid prototyping) supports one of the most important features of the work here presented, the use of the smartphone, for both imaging and processing.

Considering the continuous evolution of smartphone cameras, in the future, this approach may provide a great enhancement on the quality of the images obtained which will, undoubtedly allow an easier detection of fundus structures that regular healthcare personnel, and not only ophthalmologist experts are

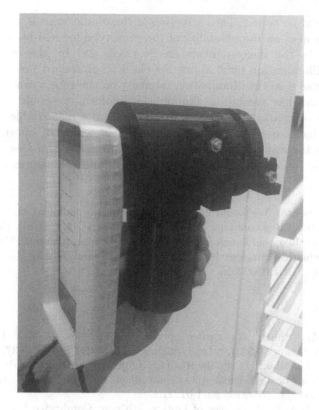

Fig. 21. EFS Compact prototype.

aware of. This way, this smartphone-based prototype can become a valuable tool for non-experts.

The fact that the prototype is 3D-printed, besides enforcing rapid prototyping, allows an easier dissemination which could make it a really helpful tool on the prevention of ophthalmic pathologies as: Diabetic Retinopathy (DR), Glaucoma, Age-Related Macular Degeneration, Cardiovascular diseases, Cerebrovascular diseases on medically underserved areas.

It can be concluded that the optical system designed showed satisfactory capabilities in experimental tests, when compared with two other affordable optical systems. The images obtained suggest that the required resolution for the detection of some of the smallest features with interest for Diabetic Retinopathy was achieved.

As future work, to diminish the reflections, an anti-reflective coating should be applied to the lenses, specially on the objective lens, the most likely cause of the purplish blurs on the final image obtained with the Compact Version Fig. 15a. To understand which set of polarizers would help the most on the minimization of back and corneal reflections, an appropriate experimental test set for polarizers comparison should be established and executed. Not only circular, but also linear polarizers should be tested. The correction of these reflections is considered one major improvement on the reliability of the prototype for real-life use cases.

According to the measurements on Sect. 3.3, and by the observation of Fig. 15b, the illumination light source for the EFS Standard prototype should also be reevaluated so the illumination intensity on the retina can be increased.

Also, features like resolution, illumination uniformity should be addressed with a proper comparison test set in order to acquire measurable information on these handheld systems capabilities for the screening of ophthalmological diseases. Later the results obtained should be compared to the ones regarded for fundus cameras, according to the ISO norm for Fundus Cameras - ISO 10940 [12].

Acknowledgements. We would like to acknowledge the financial support obtained from North Portugal Regional Operational Programme (NORTE 2020), Portugal 2020 and the European Regional Development Fund (ERDF) from European Union through the project Symbiotic technology for societal efficiency gains: Deus ex Machina (DEM), NORTE-01-0145-FEDER-000026.

References

1. Atchison, D., Smith, G.: Optics of the Human Eye, p. 259. Butterworth-Heinemann, Oxford (2000). https://doi.org/10.1016/B978-0-7506-3775-6.50001-8
2. Benbassat, J., Polak, B.C.P., Javitt, J.C.: Objectives of teaching direct ophthalmoscopy to medical students. Acta Ophthalmol. **90**(6), 503–507 (2012). https://doi.org/10.1111/j.1755-3768.2011.02221.x
3. Born, M., Wolf, E.: Principles of Optics, 7th edn. Cambridge University Press, Cambridge (1999)
4. Bueno, J.M.: Depolarization effects in the human eye. Vis. Res. **41**(21), 2687–2696 (2001). https://doi.org/10.1016/S0042-6989(01)00167-5. http://www.sciencedirect.com/science/article/pii/S0042698901001675
5. Bunce, C., Wormald, R.: Leading causes of certification for blindness and partial sight in England & Wales. BMC Public Health **6**, 58 (2006). https://doi.org/10.1186/1471-2458-6-58
6. Cheung, N., Mitchell, P., Wong, T.Y.: Diabetic retinopathy. Lancet **376**(9735), 124–136 (2010). https://doi.org/10.1016/S0140-6736(09)62124-3
7. Cronin, T.W., Shashar, N.: The linearly polarized light field in clear, tropical marine waters: spatial and temporal variation of light intensity, degree of polarization and e-vector angle. J. Exp. Biol. **204**(14), 2461–2467 (2001). http://jeb.biologists.org/content/204/14/2461
8. Cunha-Vaz, J.: Characterization and relevance of different diabetic retinopathy phenotypes. Dev. Ophthalmol. **39**, 13–30 (2007). https://doi.org/10.1159/000098497
9. D-EYE S.r.l.: D-EYE Ophthalmoscope. https://www.d-eyecare.com/#vision
10. Giancardo, L.: Automated fundus images analysis techniques to screen retinal diseases in diabetic patients. Docteur de l ' université Automated Fundus Images Analysis Techniques to Screen Retinal Diseases in Diabetic Patients (2012)
11. Hubbard, L.D., et al.: Brightness, contrast, and color balance of digital versus film retinal images in the age-related eye disease study 2. Invest. Ophthalmol. Vis. Sci. **49**(8), 3269 (2008). https://doi.org/10.1167/iovs.07-1267

12. Ophthalmic instruments - Fundus cameras. Standard, International Organization for Standardization, Geneva, CH (2009)
13. Jenkins, F., White, H.: Fundamentals of Optics. McGraw-Hill, New York (1957). https://books.google.pt/books?id=SAwJAQAAIAAJ
14. Jin, K., Lu, H., Su, Z., Cheng, C., Ye, J., Qian, D.: Telemedicine screening of retinal diseases with a handheld portable non-mydriatic fundus camera. BMC Ophthalmol. **17**(1), 89 (2017). https://doi.org/10.1186/s12886-017-0484-5
15. Kauppi, T.: Eye Fundus Image Analysis for Automatic Detection of Diabetic Retinopathy (2010)
16. van de Kraats, J., Berendschot, T.T., van Norren, D.: The pathways of light measured in fundus reflectometry. Vis. Res. **36**(15), 2229–2247 (1996). https://doi.org/10.1016/0042-6989(96)00001-6
17. Melo, D., Costa, J., Soares, F., Vieira, P.: Optical design of a compact image acquisition device for mobile diabetic retinopathy screening. In: Proceedings of the 11th International Joint Conference on Biomedical Engineering Systems and Technologies, BIODEVICES, vol. 1, pp. 63–70. INSTICC, SciTePress (2018). https://doi.org/10.5220/0006592200630070
18. Optomed Oy Ltd.: Optomed Aurora. https://www.optomed.com/optomedaurora
19. Patton, N., Aslam, T., MacGillivray, T., Pattie, A., Deary, I.J., Dhillon, B.: Retinal vascular image analysis as a potential screening tool for cerebrovascular disease: a rationale based on homology between cerebral and retinal microvasculatures. J. Anat. **206**(4), 319–348 (2005). https://doi.org/10.1111/j.1469-7580.2005.00395.x. http://www.ncbi.nlm.nih.gov/pmc/articles/PMC1571489/, 15817102[pmid]
20. Peli, E.: Ophthalmic applications of circular polarizers. J. Am. Optom. Assoc. **57**, 298–302 (1986)
21. Pérez, M.A., Bruce, B.B., Newman, N.J., Biousse, V.: The use of retinal photography in non-ophthalmic settings and its potential for neurology. Neurologist **18**(6), 350–355 (2012). https://doi.org/10.1097/NRL.0b013e318272f7d7. http://www.ncbi.nlm.nih.gov/pmc/articles/PMC3521530/, 23114666[pmid]
22. Phillips, C.I.: Dilate the pupil and see the fundus. Br. Med. J. (Clin. Res. Ed.) **288**(6433), 1779–1780 (1984). http://www.ncbi.nlm.nih.gov/pmc/articles/PMC1441835/, 6428541[pmid]
23. do Prado, R.S., Figueiredo, E.L., Magalhaes, T.V.B.: Retinal detachment in preeclampsia. Arquivos brasileiros de cardiologia **79**(2), 183–186 (2002). https://doi.org/10.1590/S0066-782X2002001100011. http://ovidsp.ovid.com/ovidweb.cgi?T=JS&PAGE=reference&D=med4&NEWS=N&AN=12219193
24. Quellec, G., Bazin, L., Cazuguel, G., Delafoy, I., Cochener, B., Lamard, M.: Suitability of a low-cost, handheld, nonmydriatic retinograph for diabetic retinopathy diagnosis. Transl. Vis. Sci. Technol. **5**(2), 16 (2016). https://doi.org/10.1167/tvst.5.2.16
25. Salz, D.A., Witkin, A.J.: Imaging in diabetic retinopathy. Middle East Afr. J. Ophthalmol. **22**(2), 145 (2015)
26. Shen, B.Y., Mukai, S.: A portable, inexpensive, nonmydriatic fundus camera based on the raspberry pi® computer. J. Ophthalmol. **2017**(3), 5 (2017). https://doi.org/10.1155/2017/4526243. http://www.sciencedirect.com/science/article/pii/S0022231399005992
27. Swedish, T., Roesch, K., Lee, I., Rastogi, K., Bernstein, S., Raskar, R.: EyeSelfie: self directed eye alignment using reciprocal eye box imaging. ACM Trans. Graph. **34**(4), 58 (2015)

28. Tarr, J.M., Kaul, K., Chopra, M., Kohner, E.M., Chibber, R.: Pathophysiology of diabetic retinopathy. ISRN Ophthalmol. **2013**, 1–13 (2013). https://doi.org/10.1155/2013/343560
29. Tocci, M.: How to model the human eye in zemax (2007). http://www.zemax.com/kb/articles/186/1/How-to-Model-the-Human-Eye-in-ZEMAX/Page1.html
30. Tran, K., Mendel, T.A., Holbrook, K.L., Yates, P.A.: Construction of an inexpensive, hand-held fundus camera through modification of a consumer "point-and-shoot" camera. Invest. Ophthalmol. Vis. Sci. **53**(12), 7600–7607 (2012)
31. Tuchin, V.V.: Polarized light interaction with tissues. J. Biomed. Opt. **21**, 1–37 (2016). https://doi.org/10.1117/1.JBO.21.7.071114
32. Volk Optical Inc.: Volk InView. https://volk.com/index.php/volk-products/ophthalmic-cameras/volk-inview.html
33. Volk Optical Inc.: Volk Pictor Plus. https://volk.com/index.php/volk-products/ophthalmic-cameras/volk-pictor-plus-digital-ophthalmic-imager.html

Design and Optimization of an Open Configuration Microfluidic Device for Clinical Diagnostics

A. S. Moita(✉) ⓘ, F. Jacinto, F. Mata, and A. L. N. Moreira

IN+ - Center for Innovation, Technology and Policy Research,
Instituto Superior Técnico, Universidade de Lisboa, Av. Rovisco Pais,
1049-001 Lisbon, Portugal
anamoita@tecnico.ulisboa.pt

Abstract. This paper addresses the design and optimization of an electrowetting chip to transport biosamples in microdroplets, for future integration in a microfluidic device for cancer diagnostics. Materials and chip configuration are optimized to obtain a sustainable system, requiring low voltage to transport the microdroplets. Within this scope, droplet dynamic behavior is accurately described and considered in the design of the chip. Hence, in a first approach, a basic chip configuration is designed, and experiments are performed to determine the basic size and positioning of the electrodes, as a function of droplets diameter and displacement velocity. Then these basic dimensions are used in a numerical model, to optimize the chip configuration (e.g. distance between electrodes, thickness of the dielectric). The model includes effects of droplet evaporation by mass diffusion, which are experimentally validated. Overall the results confirm the potential of this model as a design tool for effective chips.

Keywords: Lab-on-a-chip · Droplet based microfluidics ·
Clinical diagnostics · Chip design and test ·
Experimental and numerical approaches

1 Introduction

Biomicrofluidics, towards the development of lab-on-chip devices, have opened a wide range of possibilities for sample manipulation and biochemical analysis, offering portability, flexibility, reduced use of samples and of reagents and the possibility to perform several programmed operations, which conventionally required expensive equipment and highly skilled personnel [1]. More recently, several studies in the literature report the development of lab-on-chips for future clinical diagnostics. Such lab-on-chips under development can perform blood samples separation, isolation of specific cells for further analysis, diagnostics based, for instance, on DNA analysis and cell sorting [2], but are not yet fully functional or validated for clinical use. Furthermore, most of these devices are based on microchannel flows. This configuration is known to have some problems related to clogging and maintenance difficulties [3]. In this context, droplet based digital microfluidics offers an appealing alternative solution. Particularly, open configuration electrowetting systems, in which the electrodes and

A. Cliquet jr. et al. (Eds.): BIOSTEC 2018, CCIS 1024, pp. 49–64, 2019.
https://doi.org/10.1007/978-3-030-29196-9_3

counter electrodes are gathered in a single plate over which the droplet is transported, can fully take advantage of the aforementioned positive characteristics of digital microfluidics, but have still several technical difficulties to overcome. The most adequate electrodes configuration depends on the wetting properties of the dielectric material covering the electrodes and on the particular wetting and physico-chemical properties of the samples [3–5]. Furthermore, previous studies report the affinity of the dielectrics with the biosamples, e.g. proteins, which may locally alter the wettability at the droplet-dielectric surface interface, thus affecting the effectiveness of droplet transport [4, 6].

Finally, although the physics governing EWOD – Electrowetting on Dielectric apis already quite well described, as recently reviewed for instance in [7], details on the fabrication of the devices are still scarcely reported. Relating the fundamentals with device fabrication, however is not always easy and erroneous relations may ultimately preclude the development of an efficient device, as explained for instance by Li *et al.* [8].

In this context, the present paper addresses the design and test of a simple lab-on-chip configuration, aiming at the future development of a microfluidic device applied for cancer diagnostics, using cell and rheological properties from pleural fluids. The diagnostics explores the basic principles earlier reported, for instance by e Gosset *et al.* [9]. Hence succeeding previous work [5], which introduced the microfluidic device, and focused on the effects of the properties of the dielectrics and of the biosamples, this work focuses now on the configuration of the transport section of the microfluidic device, namely on the dimensions and positioning of the electrodes. Firstly, an experimental approach is followed to infer on the basic dimensions, allowing the best performance, evaluated based on droplet dynamics. Then, a numerical model is devised and used to optimize the basic configuration taken from the experimental approach. The model includes evaporative effects by mass diffusion, which, as revised in previous work [4, 5, 10] can be significant and affect the working conditions of the device, under harsh environmental conditions of temperature and relative humidity. The results of the model, which are validated based on experimental results are relevant for point-of-care applications (e.g. providing diagnostic possibilities in developing countries).

The fabrication of the chip is usually performed on a trial-and-error basis, not considering droplet dynamics. Consequently, chips are custom made for particular applications, without specific care on the selection of the materials or on the energy required to effectively manipulate the droplet in an efficient and sustainable way. In this work, given that droplet dynamics, related to the fluids rheology is useful for the diagnostics itself, using the parameters describing droplet dynamics (spreading diameter, spreading velocity and contact angles) to optimize the size and position of the electrodes is a relevant approach, as the chip is configured, from the start, as a function of the parameters useful for the diagnostics.

2 Materials and Methods

2.1 Experimental Procedure

Simple test chips are composed by arrays of interdigited coplanar electrodes printed on a 0.6 μm aluminium film by lithography and wet etch on a glass substrate with 102×45 mm^2 and 700 μm of width. A thin film of a dielectric material (e.g. PDMS – Polydimethylsiloxane, SU8, Teflon) was deposited on the chip assembly. Following some basic dimensioning, as reported by [11], different basic configurations were firstly assayed, where the width of the electrodes w, was varied between 120 μm and 1400 μm, for a fixed distance between them of 2a = 60 μm.

A Sorensen DCR600-.75B power supply was used to actuate the chips with DC current. The applied voltage was varied from 0 to 245 V. The switching frequency, which was programmed using a square wave, as in [12], was varied between 0 and 400 Hz.

Biofluid droplets of 1.5–5 μL volume were deposited on the top of the chips which were then actuated under different working conditions.

The test chips were enclosed in a Perspex chamber, previously saturated with the biofluid and under continuous monitoring of temperature and relative humidity of the surrounding air, using a DHT 22 Humidity & Temperature Sensor. Under these conditions, temperature was measured at a sample rate of 0.5 Hz, with an accuracy of ±0.5 °C. The relative humidity was measured also at a sample rate of 0.5 Hz, within 2–5% accuracy. The temperature was observed to be constant within T = 20 ± 3 °C and relative humidity was kept constant varied, under controlled conditions, between 70% and 99%.

The performance of the chips was evaluated based on the dynamic behaviour of the actuated droplets. Hence, quantities such as the spreading diameter (diameter of the droplet as it spreads on the surface), the contact angles under actuation and the displacement velocity of the droplet were evaluated based on the post processing of high-speed images, taken at 2200 fps using a Phantom v4.2 from Vision Research Inc., with 512×512 pixels@2100fps resolution. For the present optical configuration, the spatial resolution is 25 μm/pixel and the temporal resolution is 0.45 ms. The post-processing was performed using an in-house routine developed in Matlab. Temporal evolution of the contact (spreading and receding) diameters was presented as the average curve of at least 6 events (6 droplets), obtained under similar experimental conditions. Afterwards, maximum/averaged values were taken to obtain the discrete values for the velocity and for D/D$_0$.

Contact angle measurements were averaged from twelve events. Static and quasi-static angles were measured using an optical tensiometer (THETA, from Attention). For detailed characterization of the liquid-solid contact region and contact angle measurements with high spatial accuracy, an additional technique was used: the 3D Laser Scanning Fluorescence Confocal Microscopy 3D LSFCM, as described in detail in [13]. The measurements were performed with a laser with 552 nm wavelength, set for the power of 10.50 mW (3.00% of its maximum power) and gain of the photomultiplier (PMT) of 550 V. These values were set after a sensitivity analysis on the contrast of the image (before the post-processing) and on the Signal to Noise Ratio (SNR). The images were recorded in the format 1024 × 1024 and the scanning frequency was set to 400 Hz. The z-step was fixed in 1 μm for all the measurements. The pixel size achieved in this technique was, for the worse resolution 5.42 μm, but can be as small as 500 nm. A fluorescent dye - Rhodamine B (Sigma Aldrich) was used, which was chosen taken into account its excitation and emission wavelengths, to be compatible with the wavelengths available in the Laser Scanning Confocal Microscope (Leica SP8), but also due to particular characteristics of the experimental conditions, in the present study. For the concentrations used here (0.0007936 mg/ml < Concentration < 0.496 mg/ml) the physico-chemical properties of the working fluid are not altered by the presence of the dye. The images taken with the confocal microscope were also post-processed to evaluate the evaporative mass rate, as described in [chap4biodevices].

Surface and droplet temperatures were complementary monitored using an infrared IR-high speed camera (ONCA-MWIR-InSb from Xenics - ONCA 4696 series), which was placed above the device. Configuration and calibration procedures are described in [14]. The biofluids used here were a solution of GFP – Green Fluorescent Protein, (produced and purified in house) with 1.71×10^{-3} mM concentration and GFP expressing *E. Coli* suspensions, with concentrations of 1×10^9 cells/mL and 2×10^9 cells/mL. The solutions were characterized in terms of density, surface tension and viscosity, as summarized in Table 1 and following the procedures described in [4] and in [10]. All the solutions depicted a Newtonian behaviour, from the rheological point of view, with a dynamic viscosity very close to that of water ($\mu = 1 \times 10^{-3}$ Nsm^{-2}).

Table 1. Physico-chemical properties of the GFP solution used in the present work [15].

Solution	Density ρ [kgm^{-3}]	Surface tension σ_{lv} [mNm^{-1}]
GFP (1.71×10^{-3} mM)	998	72.2 ± 0.7
E. Coli (1×10^9 cells/mL)	991	71.8 ± 0.3
E. Coli (2×10^9 cells/mL)	982	61.3 ± 0.2

2.2 Numerical Methods

The simulations were performed using COMSOL Multiphysics 4.3b. The numerical domain considered was a 0.655 mm radius sphere (droplet domain) within an air domain of $3.21 \times 1.6 \times 3$ mm^3. The electrostatic boundary conditions are an electrical potential imposed to the electrode on the right (positive x-axis) and a ground (0 V) imposed the electrode on the left [12]. The mesh is composed of 67025 tetrahedral elements, being refined at the liquid-solid and liquid-vapor interfaces.

The Maxwell stress tensor is used to determine the electrostatic force actuating on the droplet, integrated on its surface. Thus, the electrostatic force was calculated by integrating [15]:

$$n_1 T_2 = -\frac{1}{2} n_1 (E \cdot D) + (n_1 \cdot E) D^T \tag{1}$$

on the surface of the droplet, where E is the electric field, D the electric displacement, and n_1 the outward normal from the object. Using the Maxwell stress tensor for a 2D configuration, the volume force was calculated as the first derivative of this tensor.

Phase Field User Interface was used to track the liquid-air interface, for a laminar flow, using the incompressible formulation of the Navier-Stokes Eqs. (2) and (3) [15]:

$$\rho\frac{\partial u}{\partial t} + \rho(u \cdot \nabla) = \nabla \cdot \left[-pI + \mu\left(\nabla u + \nabla u^T\right)\right] + F_g + F_g + F_{ext} + F \tag{2}$$

$$\nabla \cdot u = 0 \tag{3}$$

The phase field method adds the following equations also defined in [15]:

$$\frac{\partial \Phi}{\partial t} + u \cdot \nabla \Phi = \nabla \cdot \frac{\gamma\lambda}{\varepsilon^2}\nabla\psi \tag{4}$$

$$\psi = -\nabla \cdot \varepsilon^2\nabla\Phi + \left(\Phi^2 - 1\right)\Phi + \left(\frac{\varepsilon^2}{\lambda}\right)\frac{\partial f_{ext}}{\partial \Phi} \tag{5}$$

where the quantity λ (SI unit: N) is the mixing energy density and ε (SI unit: m) is a capillary width that scales with the thickness of the interface. These two parameters are related to the surface tension coefficient, σ (SI unit: N/m), through equation [15]:

$$\sigma = \frac{2\sqrt{2}}{3}\frac{\lambda}{\sigma} \tag{6}$$

The volume fraction of air (fluid 2) is computed as [15]:

$$V_f = \min(\max([1+f]/2], 0, 1) \tag{7}$$

where the min and max operators are used so that the volume fraction has a lower limit of 0 and an upper limit of 1. The density is then computed, as in [15] by:

$$\rho = \rho_1 + (\rho_2 - \rho_1)V_f \tag{8}$$

and the dynamic viscosity according to [15]:

$$\mu = \mu_1 + (\mu_2 - \mu_1)V_f \tag{9}$$

where ρ_1 and ρ_2 are the densities and μ_1 and μ_2 are the dynamic viscosities of fluid 1 (biofluids) and fluid 2 (air), respectively.

As aforementioned, mass effusion was included in the numerical model developed here, being evaluated using the diffusion-convection equation [15]:

$$\frac{\partial c_i}{\partial t} + \nabla \cdot (-D_i\nabla c_i) + u \cdot \nabla c_i = 0 \tag{10}$$

which includes the transport mechanisms of diffusion and convection. Here c_i is the concentration of the species, D_i denotes the diffusion coefficient and u is the velocity vector. The diffusion coefficient is 2.6×10^{-5} m²/s, the initial water concentration in the surrounding air is 0.27688 mol/m³ (relative humidity of 0.29) and the droplet surface concentration is HR.psat/(Rconst.T), where HR.psat is the relative humidity at the saturation pressure (for the temperature T), Rconst is the ideal gases constant and T the temperature of the droplet surface. The boundary conditions consider no liquid flux for all the surfaces, except for the droplet/air interfaces.

Detailed description of the numerical methods is described in [15].

3 Results and Discussion

As detailed in [10], the microfluidic device under development has three main sections: the transport section, the diagnostics section and the sorting/collecting section. This paper will focus on the configuration of the first, given the paramount role of an effective transport and manipulation of the samples in the entire device. Within this scope, the results section is organized in the following items: Subsect. 3.1 summarizes the paramount role of the wetting properties of the dielectric material to be used in the chip, following our previous results reported in [4, 5, 10]. This sub-section also emphasizes the relevance of precluding surface contamination, not only to avoid its obvious influence in the analysis to be performed in the diagnostic section, but also to avoid its negative effect in the device efficacy to manipulate the sample droplet.

The selected materials are then used to make a first batch of test chips, which will be tested in Subsect. 3.2. These chips are assayed to describe the dynamic behavior of the biofluid droplets and to use this characterization (spreading diameters, contact angles, droplets' velocity) to obtain a rough first estimative of the positioning and size of the electrodes. These results are then introduced as input values, in the numerical model, which is used in Subsect. 3.3 to optimize the chip configuration.

3.1 Selection of the Working Materials for the Transport Section: The Role of Wettability and Surface Contamination

As referred in the Introduction, this paper mainly focuses on the development of an efficient transport section in the microfluidic device, which is capable of transporting the samples from the region where they are collected to the diagnostics/sensing area. Selecting the materials to use is a paramount and challenging step. The material should be biocompatible, but adsorption should be avoided, as it may alter the diagnostics. Furthermore, in the present device, the microdroplets have to transport cells, so they are quite large (of the order of hundreds of diameters). Thus, any resistance that the surface my offer to the droplet motion will require an additional external actuation, increasing the applied voltage.

Vieira *et al.* [5] and Mata *et al.* [16] performed an extensive literature review on the most usual dielectric materials used in electrowetting chips and selected the most suitable materials, based on the dynamic response of the actuated biofluid droplets. Hence, the chosen materials should be repellent to the biofluid droplets (hydrophobic or superhydrophobic, i.e. depicting contact angles higher than 120° or 150°, respectively), to promote their spreading (allowing the droplets to easily touch consecutive electrodes) and should depict very low contact angle hysteresis (preferably lower than 11°), since the energy dissipated at the droplet-surface contact line is proportional to the hysteresis. Furthermore, some authors (e.g. [6]) report the frequent adsorption of the biocomponents (mainly of the proteins) by most of the usual dielectric materials, which decreased locally the contact angle, promoting surface energy dissipation and restricting the motion of the droplet. In this context, our previous studies [4, 5, 10] evidence that the dielectric material (typically best results were obtained with PDMS – Polydimethylsiloxane and with Teflon) may adsorb the biocomponents, mainly the proteins, which locally decrease the contact angle of the microdroplets, leading to an irreversible spreading of the droplet, which does not recoil afterwards. The presence of the proteins was confirmed by Laser Scanning Fluorescence Confocal Microscopy, in a custom-made method devised in [4], which allows to visualize the footprint of the droplets and correlate the quantity of the adsorbed substances with the intensity signal received. It is worth mentioning that in this previous work, the biofluids were similar to those used in the current study.

[4, 5, 10] further confirm that coating the dielectric with a thin layer of Glaco©, a perfluoroalkyltrichlorosilane combined with perfluoropolyether carboxylic acid and a fluorinated solvent [17], turns the dielectric substrates superhydrophobic and reduces the protein adsorption. These effects combined, consequently reduce the contact angle hysteresis and, consequently, energy dissipation at the contact line, thus promoting droplet motion.

3.2 Basic Dimensioning of the Size and Position of the Electrodes

Once the dielectric materials were selected and the aforementioned issues were solved, the configuration of the chip was designed, defining the size and positioning of the electrodes. A first approach was made experimentally to provide a basic dimensioning that could be used as an input in the model described in Subsect. 2.2.

The motion of the droplet requires it to be in contact with at least two electrodes, which are actuated according to an imposed switching frequency. The imposed duty cycle, which acts as the switching frequency between electrodes, was programmed to vary between 0 Hz and 400 Hz, so one can infer on the effect of this frequency on the dynamic response of the droplet. Following the recommendations of [11] to evaluate the chip capacitance, the distance between electrodes a should be much smaller than their width w. So, after some preliminary calculations, four basic configurations were tested, namely, $w = 120$ μm, 800 μm, 1200 μm and 1400 μm, with a fixed distance between electrodes, $2a = 60$ μm.

The chips performance was evaluated based on the dynamic response of the droplets under actuation, namely quantifying the spreading diameter, made non-dimensional with the initial diameter of the deposited droplet, the contact angles measured under actuation and the droplet displacement velocity. For these assays the droplets used were formed from a solution of GFP (1.71×10^{-3} mM). The main objective is to set the width and distance between the electrodes which maximizes droplet spreading diameter and velocity for various conditions of imposed frequency and imposed voltage. The latter should be as low as possible, for the reasons afore-mentioned in the Introduction.

Figure 1 shows the temporal evolution of the droplet spreading diameter, under actuation at different applied voltages, made non-dimensional with its initial diameter at t = 0 ms (before actuation). Here, the dielectric substrate, PDMS is still not coated. Hence, the results emphasize the irreversibility on droplet motion due to the high adhesion force of the PDMS substrate: after the spreading of the droplet, up to its maximum diameter, this strong adhesion due to the high contact angle hysteresis (larger than 20°, as reported in previous work – [10]) promotes energy dissipation at the contact line, thus restraining the spreading motion of the droplet. The energy dissipation during this motion precludes the recoiling, thus turning the motion of the droplet irreversible. Consequently, it is difficult for the droplet to be transported to the subsequent electrodes and the voltages applied are very high.

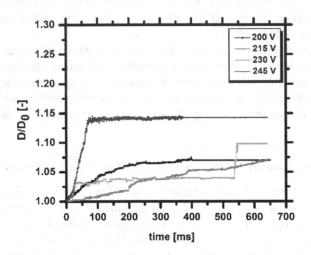

Fig. 1. Temporal evolution of the spreading diameter for 350 Hz of a GFP droplet, for the configuration 2a = 60 μm and w = 1400 μm. The dielectric substrate is PDMS. The volume of the liquid droplet is 1.8 μL [15].

These results are consistent with those reported in Fig. 2, which depicts the temporal evolution of the spreading diameter for different imposed frequencies.

The current configuration requires very high imposed voltages (above 200 V), being limited to 245 V, as above this value, the dielectric breakdown occurs leading to electrolysis inside the droplet, which in turn generates a violent droplet disintegration, in agreement with the observations reported, for instance by Mugele and Baret [18] and by Cooney et al. [19]. The results overall suggest that droplet motion is not much affected by the imposed frequency.

The dynamic behaviour of the droplet is illustrated here for 230 V, but consistently similar results were observed for other applied voltages, in steps of 15 V between 200 and 245 V.

In fact, Fig. 3 shows in a more intuitive representation the effect of the applied voltage and imposed frequency for various chip configurations, i.e. for different electrode widths. In agreement with Figs. 1 and 2, the results reported in Fig. 3 support that droplet dynamics is nearly independent from the imposed frequency. However, one may notice a weaker response of the droplet to low frequencies (50 Hz) and a swifter response for frequencies between 100–300 Hz (Fig. 3b), although it is not possible to identify a monotonic trend between the frequency and the spreading diameter or the velocity. On the other hand, maximum spreading diameters are observed for the highest imposed frequency (400 Hz), but the droplet depicts a lower response in time (Fig. 3a). This trend is attributed to the imposed electric force that must overcome the resistance to droplet motion associated to the energy dissipation on the surface. The velocities obtained here are lower than those reported in other studies in the literature [12, 19, 20], as the chips configuration is not optimized yet. Also, most of the fluids used in the aforementioned studies are salt solutions and not biofluids.

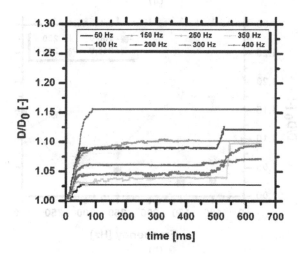

Fig. 2. Temporal evolution of the spreading diameter of a GFP droplet on a PDMS substrate, actuated at 230 V for different imposed frequencies, for the configuration $2a = 60$ μm and $w = 1400$ μm. The volume of the liquid droplet is 1.8 μL [15].

To infer on the influence of the electrodes width on the dynamic response of the droplets, four alternative electrode configurations were tested. Comparative results between the different configurations are presented in Fig. 4, which depicts the contact line velocity and the maximum spreading diameter, as a function of the imposed frequency. The results highlight that the configuration with $w = 120$ μm provides the worst droplet response to the electrostatic actuation, expressed by the low values of the spreading velocity and of the non-dimensional spreading diameter D/D_0. The response of the droplet under actuation on all the other configurations is very similar, being however, overall more regular for the chip with $w = 1200$ μm, mainly regarding the values achieved for the maximum diameter.

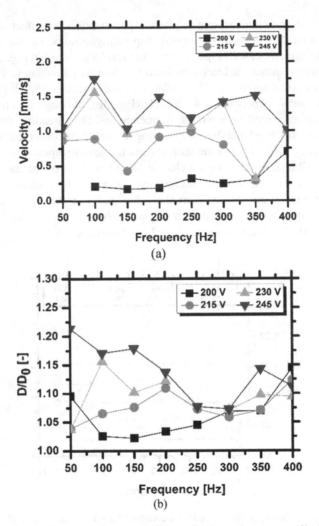

Fig. 3. (a) Spreading velocity of the contact line and (b) maximum spreading dimensionless diameter of a GFP droplet on PDMS, moving between coplanar electrodes for the configuration $2a = 60$ μm and $w = 1400$ μm, for different applied voltages and an imposed frequency. The volume of the liquid droplet is 1.8 μL [15].

Consistently with the analysis performed so far, the set of plots shown here does not identify a monotonic trend between the spreading velocity and diameter and the imposed frequency; it mainly indicates a slower response for very low frequencies (50 Hz) and faster response (with larger spreading diameters) for higher imposed frequencies. These plots suggest that, regardless of the imposed frequencies, the configurations with $w = 1200$ μm and $w = 1400$ μm provide a slightly better dynamic response, which enables droplet motion. However, overall, and for the range of dimensions tested here, the width of the electrodes seems to play a secondary role in the transport of the microdroplets.

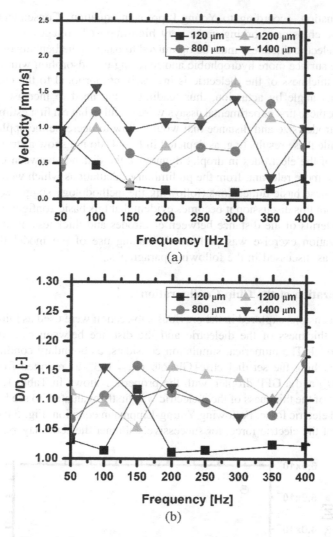

Fig. 4. (a) Spreading velocity and (b) maximum spreading dimensionless diameter of a GFP droplet on PDMS, moving between coplanar electrodes for the different configurations, for an imposed frequency of 350 Hz and an imposed electric potential of 230 V. The volume of the liquid droplet is 1.8 μL [15].

For all the configurations tested and discussed in the previous paragraphs, the dielectric material used was PDMS, with a thickness of 30 μm. This thickness was set following the values reported in the literature and due to some limitations of the microfabrication method, which did not allow a deposition of a thinner dielectric layer. As aforementioned, our previous results showed improvements in the transport efficiency of the droplet by coating the dielectric with the chemical compound called Glaco®.

However, in the current case, the Glaco® coating increases substantially the thickness of the dielectric layer, turning difficult for the droplet to respond to the electrical actuation, according to Young-Lippmann equation. Consequently, despite functional, the chips are working under very high imposed voltages and frequencies. Hence, the dielectric thickness must be optimized to balance the benefits of the coating in turning the surface more hydrophobic and reducing the adsorption with the fact that an increased thickness of the dielectric is inversely proportional to the change in the droplet contact angle by actuation, thus leading to the need to increase the applied voltage. Also, these first experimental assays were useful to have a first estimative of the range of electrodes size and distance that would allow to decrease the applied voltage. However, while these results (e.g. as depicted in Fig. 4) do not show a strong influence of the width of the electrodes in droplet dynamics, the distance between electrodes is expected to be more relevant, from the preliminary calculations which were performed to determine these basic dimensions (following the methodology suggested by [11]).

Hence, from this discussion it becomes evident that this basic configuration must be optimized in terms of the distance between electrodes and thickness of the dielectric. Such optimization exercise was performed, making use of the model described in Subsect. 2.2, as discussed in the following paragraphs.

3.3   Optimization of the Chip Configuration

The basic dimensions explored in the previous sub-section were used as initial guests to optimize the thickness of the dielectric and the distance between electrodes, in the numerical model. The numerical simulation considers, as boundary conditions a contact angle matching the set dielectric+Glaco® ($\theta_e = 153°$, as reported from previous studies [5, 10]) and a GFP droplet, with the properties shown in Table 1.

The effect of the thickness of the dielectric was firstly evaluated, to see how it affects the generated electric force. Following Young-Lippmann equation, Fig. 5 clearly shows the increase of the electric force, for successively thinner dielectric layers.

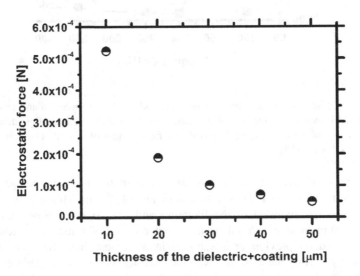

Fig. 5. Electric force generated, as a function of the thickness of the dielectric (dielectric +Glaco®).

With this new thickness of the dielectric, the distance between electrodes was also optimized, computing the generated electric force, as a function of the distance between electrodes. The results depicted in Fig. 6 show that the distance 2*a* considered in the experimental approach was over dimensioned and that the optimum distance which maximizes the electric force generated is around 10 μm. The values obtained for the electric force are in qualitative agreement with those reported by Di Virgilio [21], with a similar geometry.

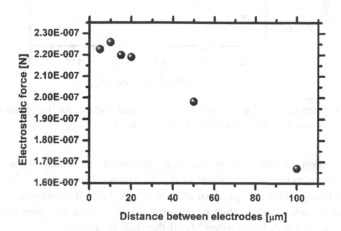

Fig. 6. Electric force generated by the electrodes configuration, as a function of the distance between electrodes for the fixed optimized dielectric thickness (10 μm) [15].

With this optimized geometry, much lower values of the applied voltage (nearly 70 V) can already generate a force with a magnitude high enough to move the droplet. This is evident from Fig. 7, which depicts the electric force generated as a function of the applied voltage (for the fixed optimum dielectric thickness depicted in Fig. 5) and the resulting initial velocity of the droplet. The variation in the values of the generated force are probably due to the fact that the imposed voltage is always considered as the minimum possible. However, a complete study on this issue will be presented in a future work.

After this optimization process, it is worth mentioning that the imposed frequency could even be lowered than the 50 Hz, without affecting droplet motion, probably because the optimum conditions of wettability (superhydrophobicity) and reduced adsorption/contamination of the dielectric substrates, allow the regular motion of the droplet with reduced adhesion and energy dissipation. Hence, for the lowest applied voltage of 70 V, the imposed frequency could be lowered down to 9 Hz, matching the very low values achieved by Fan et al. [12]. Overall, the dynamic behaviour of the droplet is in qualitative agreement with that reported in the simulations of [21].

Despite preliminary, these results are quite promising, considering that the dielectric thickness can still be further reduced, although with care, to avoid the occurrence of dielectric breakdown [17].

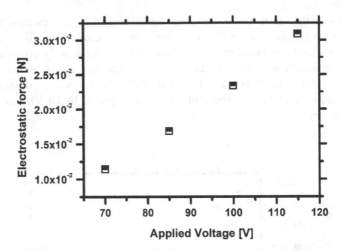

Fig. 7. Electric force generated as a function of the applied voltage, for the optimum dielectric thickness (10 μm) and distance between electrodes (10 μm).

The new patch of chips being currently produced are following a fabrication method allowing a more precise control of the thickness of the dielectric layer, to meet the numerical results. This new patch of chips will now be tested following a procedure similar to that reported here to then be integrated in the more complex design of the entire microdevice, towards the assembly of the final prototype.

To conclude, one must also refer that regarding the effect of mass diffusion, the model predicts a non-negligible mass evaporation by diffusion, for ambient temperatures above 20 °C and relative humidity below 80%, which agrees well with the experimental analysis previously reported in [10].

4 Conclusions

The intensive research in the development of microfluidics for biomedical applications have mostly focused on the end user, leaving the fabrication procedures in a secondary plane. However, a careful design and the development of systematic fabrication procedures are vital to obtain sustainable and efficient devices, with significant cost reductions, which is able to manipulate the samples with minimum external actuation. Within this scope, the present paper concerns the design and optimization of a microfluidic device based on an open configuration system, where the samples are transported in microdroplets by electrostatic actuation. The paper focuses on the section that transports and manipulates the samples, which will be integrated in the entire device in the near future. The final microfluidic device will be used for the early diagnostics of cancer from pleural fluids. As droplet dynamics will be used as part of the diagnostic procedure, this study proposes a design method based on the dynamic behavior of the microdroplets under actuation, to design the size and position of the electrodes. Hence, post-processing of the images taken by combining high-speed visualization with infrared high-speed thermography and with 3D Laser Scanning Fluorescence Confocal Microscopy are used to evaluate quantitatively the spreading and receding diameter and droplet displacement velocity under electrostatic actuation. These quantities were then used, in a first approach, to determine basic dimensions (electrodes width and distance between them). Afterwards, a numerical model was devised and use to optimize these basic dimensions.

The results confirm the efficacy of the coating determined in our previous studies, in turning the surfaces of the dielectric substrates superhydrophobic and in minimizing their contamination with the biocomponents. Consequently, droplet manipulation became much easier. However, the increased thickness of the dielectric caused by the application of this additional coating was requiring the application of high voltages to manipulate the microdroplets. The numerical model allowed to optimize all the design parameters of the chip, including the thickness of the dielectric substrate, allowing droplet manipulation at 70 V and 9 Hz of external actuation, against the more than 200 V and 400 Hz which were required before the optimization. It is worth mentioning that the devised model includes effects of droplet evaporation by mass diffusion, which are experimentally validated.

Overall these positive results confirm the high potential of this model as a design tool for the development of effective chips.

Acknowledgements. The authors are grateful to Fundação para a Ciência e Tecnologia (FCT) for financing A. S. Moita's contract and exploratory research project through the recruitment programme FCT Investigator (IF 00810-2015). The authors further acknowledge the contribution of Prof. Susana Freitas and her team from INESC-MN for the microfabrication of the test chips.

References

1. Yager, P., et al.: Microfluidic diagnostic technologies for global public health. Nature **442**(7101), 412–418 (2006)
2. Dance, A.: The making of a medical microchip. Nature **545**, 512–514 (2017)
3. Geng, H., Feng, J., Stabryl, L.M., Cho, S.K.: Dielectrowetting manipulation for digital microfluidics: creating, transporting, splitting, and merging droplets. Lab Chip **17**, 1060–1068 (2017)
4. Moita, A.S., Laurência, C., Ramos, J.A., Prazeres, D.M.F., Moreira, A.L.N.: Dynamics of droplets of biological fluids on smooth superhydrophobic surfaces under electrostatic actuation. J. Bionic Eng. **13**, 220–234 (2016)
5. Vieira, D., Mata, F., Moita, A.S., Moreira, A.L.N.: Microfluidic prototype of a lab-on-chip device for lung cancer diagnostics. In: Proceedings of the 10th International Joint Conference on Biomedical Engineering Systems and Technologies, BIODEVICES, Porto, Portugal, 21–23 February 2017, vol. 1, pp. 63–68 (2017). https://doi.org/10.5220/0006252700630068. ISBN 978-989-758-216-5
6. Yoon, J.Y., Garrel, R.L.: Preventing biomolecular adsorption in electrowetting-based biofluidic chips. Anal. Chem. **75**, 5097–5102 (2003)
7. Nelson, W.C., Kim, C.-J.: Droplet actuation by electrowetting-on-dielectric (EWOD): a review. J. Adhesion Sci. Tech. **26**, 1747–1771 (2012)

8. Li, Y., Fu, Y.Q., Brodie, S.D., Alghane, M., Walton, A.J.: Integrated microfluidics system using surface acoustic wave and electrowetting on dielectrics technology. Biomicrofluidics 6, 012812 (2012)
9. Gosset, G.R., et al.: Hydrodynamic stretching of single cells for large population mechanical phenotyping. PNAS 109(20), 7630–7635 (2009)
10. Moita, A.S., Vieira, D., Mata, F., Pereira, J., Moreira, A.L.N.: Microfluidic devices integrating clinical alternative diagnostic techniques based on cell mechanical properties. In: Peixoto, N., Silveira, M., Ali, Hesham H., Maciel, C., van den Broek, Egon L. (eds.) BIOSTEC 2017. CCIS, vol. 881, pp. 74–93. Springer, Cham (2018). https://doi.org/10.1007/978-3-319-94806-5_4
11. Chen, J.Z., Darhuber, A.A., Troian, S.M., Wagner, S.: Capacitive sensing of droplets for microfluidic devices based on thermocapillary actuation. Lab Chip 4(5), 473–480 (2004)
12. Fan, S.-K., Yang, H., Wang, T.-T., Hsu, W.: Asymmetric electrowetting-moving droplets by a square wave. Lab Chip 7(10), 1330–1335 (2007)
13. Vieira, D., Moita, A.S., Moreira, A.L.N.: Non-intrusive wettability characterization on complex surfaces using 3D Laser Scanning Confocal Fluorescence Microscopy. In: Proceedings of 18th International the Symposium on Applications of Laser and Imaging Techniques to Fluid Mechanics, Lisbon, Portugal, 4–7 July (2016)
14. Teodori, E., Pontes, P., Moita, A.S., Moreira, A.L.N.: Thermographic analysis of interfacial heat transfer mechanisms on droplet/wall interactions with high temporal and spatial resolution. Exp. Thermal Fluid Sci. 96, 284–294 (2018)
15. Jacinto, F., Moita, A.S., Moreira, A.L.N.: Design, test and fabrication of a droplet based microfluidic device for clinical diagnostics. In: Proceedings of the 11th International Conference on Biomedical Electronics and Devices, BIODEVICES 2018, Funchal, Madeira, 19–21 January, vol. 1, pp. 88–95 (2018). ISBN 978-989-758-277-6
16. Mata, F., Moita, A.S., Kumar, R., Cardoso, S., Prazeres, D.M.F, Moreira, A.L.N.: Effect of surface wettability on the spreading and displacement of biofluid drops in electrowetting. In: Proceedings of ILASS – Europe 2016, 27th Annual Conference on Liquid Atomization and Spray Systems, Brighton, UK, 4–7 September 2016 (2016). ISBN 978-1-910172-09-4
17. Kato, M., Tanaka, A., Sasagawa, M., Adachi, H.: Durable automotive windshield coating and the use thereof. US Patent, 8043421 B2 (2008)
18. Mugele, F., Baret, J.C.: Electrowetting: from basics to applications. J. Phys.: Condens. Matter 17, R705–R774 (2005)
19. Cooney, C.G., Chen, C.Y., Emerling, M.R., Nadim, A., Sterling, J.D.: Electrowetting droplet microfluidics on a single planar surface. Microfluid. Nanofluid. 2(5), 435–446 (2006)
20. Sen, P., Kim, C.-J.C.: Capillary spreading dynamics of electrowetted sessile droplets in air. Langmuir 25(8), 4302–4305 (2009)
21. Di Virgilio, V.: Contactless electrowetting. Ph.D. thesis, Universitat Politècnica de Catalunya, Catalunya, Spain (2015)

Bioimaging

Transferability of Deep Learning Algorithms for Malignancy Detection in Confocal Laser Endomicroscopy Images from Different Anatomical Locations of the Upper Gastrointestinal Tract

Marc Aubreville[1]([envelope]), Miguel Goncalves[2], Christian Knipfer[3,4],
Nicolai Oetter[4,5], Tobias Würfl[1], Helmut Neumann[6], Florian Stelzle[4,5],
Christopher Bohr[7], and Andreas Maier[1,4]

[1] Pattern Recognition Lab, Computer Science,
Friedrich-Alexander-Universität Erlangen-Nürnberg, Erlangen, Germany
marc.aubreville@fau.de
[2] Department of Otorhinolaryngology, Head and Neck Surgery, University Hospital
Erlangen, Friedrich-Alexander-Universität Erlangen-Nürnberg, Erlangen, Germany
[3] Department of Oral and Maxillofacial Surgery,
University Medical Center Hamburg-Eppendorf, Hamburg, Germany
[4] Erlangen Graduate School in Advanced Optical Technologies (SAOT),
Friedrich-Alexander-Universität Erlangen-Nürnberg, Erlangen, Germany
[5] Department of Oral and Maxillofacial Surgery, University Hospital Erlangen,
Friedrich-Alexander-Universität Erlangen-Nürnberg, Erlangen, Germany
[6] First Department of Internal Medicine, University Medical Center Mainz,
Johannes Gutenberg-Universität Mainz, Erlangen, Germany
[7] Department of Otorhinolaryngology, Head and Neck Surgery,
Universität Regensburg, University Hospital, Regensburg, Germany

Abstract. Squamous Cell Carcinoma (SCC) is the most common cancer type of the epithelium and is often detected at a late stage. Besides invasive diagnosis of SCC by means of biopsy and histo-pathologic assessment, Confocal Laser Endomicroscopy (CLE) has emerged as noninvasive method that was successfully used to diagnose SCC in vivo. For interpretation of CLE images, however, extensive training is required, which limits its applicability and use in clinical practice of the method. To aid diagnosis of SCC in a broader scope, automatic detection methods have been proposed. This work compares two methods with regard to their applicability in a transfer learning sense, i.e. training on one tissue type (from one clinical team) and applying the learnt classification system to another entity (different anatomy, different clinical team). Besides a previously proposed, patch-based method based on convolutional neural networks, a novel classification method on image level (based on a pre-trained Inception V.3 network with dedicated preprocessing and interpretation of class activation maps) is proposed and evaluated.

The newly presented approach improves recognition performance, yielding accuracies of 91.63% on the first data set (oral cavity) and

© Springer Nature Switzerland AG 2019
A. Cliquet jr. et al. (Eds.): BIOSTEC 2018, CCIS 1024, pp. 67–85, 2019.
https://doi.org/10.1007/978-3-030-29196-9_4

92.63% on a joint data set. The generalization from oral cavity to the second data set (vocal folds) lead to similar area-under-the-ROC curve values than a direct training on the vocal folds data set, indicating good generalization.

Keywords: Confocal Laser Endomicroscopy · Transfer learning · Head and neck squamous cell carcinoma

1   Introduction

Squamous cell carcinoma (SCC) is the most common kind of cancer of the epithelium, which accounts for over 90% of all cancer types in the oral cavity and pharynx [7], as well as for almost the totality of malignancies in the larynx [24]. For SCC, the incidence rates are higher for men in their 6th and 7th decade, and long-term tabacco and alcohol consumption are regarded as the most important risk factors [15,30]. Only one third of the patients with head and neck cancer is diagnosed in an early tumor stadium (T1), and thus treatment options are reduced and the need for more radical surgical treatment is often increased [17].

The gold standard of diagnosis is the invasive biopsy of the epithelial tissue with subsequent histopathological assessment. The biopsies and (part) resections of mutated tissue provide information about surgical margins, i.e. healthy tissue is biopsied to demonstrate the disease has not spread beyond the resection area. However, due to the invasiveness a limitation in the sample size and quantity can hinder the finding of accurate resection margins and limit monitoring of these lesions. The resection volume is correlated with the severity of functional disorders (e.g. concerning swallowing, speech, voice). Thus, for surgical removal of SCC, the resection volume should be as low as reasonably possible while completely removing the tumor. A non- or minimally invasive in-vivo characterization of microstructures would be a significant asset for the early diagnosis of SCC while at the same time reducing the aforementioned risks. Further, it could significantly help to improve tumor follow-up monitoring of possible local recurrence, reducing the risk accompanying unnecessary biopsies.

One non-invasive method that has successfully been used to differentiate micro-cellular structures is Confocal Laser Endomicroscopy (CLE) [8,18,21]. For this fluorescence imaging method, laser light in the cyan color spectrum is emitted by a laser diode and directed towards the tissue under investigation by means of a fiber bundle, which is typically inserted into cavities of the body using the accessory channel of an endoscope [4]. The resolution of CLE is high, providing magnifications of up to 1000x [21] and enabling sub-cellular imaging in real-time. A contrast agent (typically fluorescein) is applied intravenously prior to the examination in order to stain the intercellular space and hence outline the cell borders.

CLE is being successfully used in diagnostics of the intestine in clinical practice [18]. It was reported, that probe-based CLE (pCLE) can also successfully be used for assessment of malignancy of SCC of the vocal folds [8,9] as well as in epithelium of the oral cavity [21]. However, it is also known that interpretation of CLE images requires significant training [20]. An automatic interpretation and classification of CLE images could thus help to spread this non-invasive method in screening more widely, and also improve identifying the exact location of tumor (margins) in pre- or intra-operative use.

The main research question for this work (and the preliminary work in [1]) is, how well a classification system learnt from one CLE data set (acquired in the oral cavity) can be applied to another data set (acquired from the vocal folds), and vice versa. Since, in both cases, epithelial tissue is investigated, a robust algorithm should be able to apply knowledge acquired in one domain in the other domain. This would provide a strong hint of generalization towards other locations of the upper aero-digestive tract with similar but not identical epithelia.

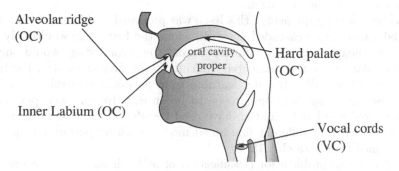

Fig. 1. Anatomical locations/examined measurement points from the oral cavity and the upper aero-digestive and respiratory tract (adapted from [1]).

2 Related Work

Deep learning methods, such as convolutional neural networks (CNN) have recently been used in a variety of image recognition tasks. For the application of cancer recognition, it was shown that, given sufficient training material, they can be used to differentiate various subtypes of skin cancer from photography images [6]. In the field of bright light microscopy, CNN-based methods are predicted to become the leading pattern recognition tool [31].

For the processing and analysis of CLE images, a number of algorithmic approaches have been proposed to date. Our work group was among the first to automatically detect malignancies using manually designed features for classification with support vector machine (SVM) or random forest [12]. They used a patch extraction from the round pCLE field of view to classify OSCC images from clinically normal epithelium [12]. Using the same tool chain, Vo et al. showed that this detection methodology is also applicable to the detection of SCC of the vocal folds [29]. On a larger (and thus more realistic) data set of OSCC, the performance of these algorithms decreased, however [2]. We were able to show, that the usage of a CNN for classification of extracted patches greatly improves performance [2].

One major issue with most medical images is the quantity of data of a specific class for training. For deep networks, the number of parameters increases significantly with every layer, and so does the network's capacity to memorize single instances. An increased quantity of parameters often has a negative effect on generalization, and can lead to over-fitting the training data, in cases where the training data set is limited, which is also true for our (and other authors') CLE data sets. One method to cope with this issue is the reduction of input size of the network, in conjunction with patch extraction from the image and subsequent fusion of separate classification outcomes. This has the additional advantage, that a large portion of the area of the round CLE field of view can be investigated. The amount of patches per image further increases the total batch size for training of the algorithm.

Another way of approaching this issue was proposed by Murthy *et al.*: They proposed a two-staged cascaded network, where the first stage would only perform a classification with low confidence, and the second stage would only be trained on data that was considered difficult by the first stage [16]. For many image recognition tasks, transfer learning from networks pre-trained on large data bases (e.g. ImageNet) has proven to be an effective and well performing approach. Izadyyazdanabadi *et al.* have used transfer learning on CLE images, and have shown that different fine-tuned models each outperformed the same model trained from scratch [11].

As stated, one problem for classification of pCLE images is the round field of view (see e.g. Fig. 2). Because of this, besides patch-based methods [12,29] that extract rectangular patches from the round image area, all image-scale classification approaches known today use squared center crop of the overall image, which reduces the available data for classification [2,16,27].

Since the magnification of pCLE is very high and matching with histology images is almost impossible, image segmentation data of malignancy is hard to derive for the expert, so data sets typically have only image labels. Differentiation of diagnostic vs. non-diagnostic (e.g. artifact-tainted) image parts, however, can be performed by a CLE expert. This sub-image classification can be done supervised (as proposed by Stoeve *et al.* for motion artifacts [27]), or also *weakly* supervised (as proposed by Izadyyazdanabadi *et al.*) [10]. Even for the case of malignancy classification, however, a sub-image classification would be interesting for the observer, as it helps interpretation of the image and the classification result.

3   Material

For this work we used CLE sequences from four anatomical locations (see Fig. 1): Our original data set consists of images from three clinically normal sites within the oral cavity and, additionally, data from a verified SCC lesion site. Our secondary data set was recorded on epithelium of the vocal cords.

All images were acquired using a pCLE system (Cellvizio, Mauna Kea Technologies, Paris, France). Written informed consent was obtained from all patients prior to the study. Also prior to the study, approval was granted by the respective institutional review board. Research was carried out in accordance with the Code of Ethics of the World Medical Association (Declaration of Helsinki) and the ethical guidelines of the Friedrich-Alexander-Universität Erlangen-Nürnberg.

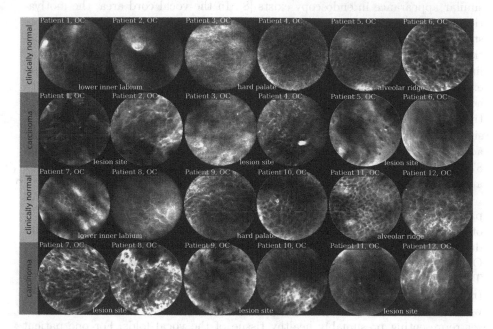

Fig. 2. Selected CLE Images acquired from the oral cavity (OC). First and third row show images from clinically normal regions, second and fourth row show images from lesion sites later diagnosed as OSCC.

3.1 Oral Cavity (OC)

For this study, we included 116 image sequences from 12 subjects with histo-pathologically verified HNSCC in the oral cavity that were recorded at the Department of Oral and Maxillofacial Surgery (University Hospital Erlangen). The study was approved by the IRB of the University of Erlangen-Nürnberg (reference number: 243_12 B).

The investigation was conducted chair-side on conscious patients prior to histo-pathological assessment and surgical procedure for removal of the tissue. Imaging was performed on three non-affected sites, i.e. the alveolar ridge, the lower inner labium and the hard palate (see Fig. 1). Oetter *et al.* conducted a CLE expert recognition assessment based on a subset of the data set used in this work (95 CLE sequences) and found an accuracy of 92.3% [21].

3.2   Vocal Cords (VC)

The promising results in other anatomical areas motivated the acquisition of CLE images for diagnosis of SCC of the vocal folds, which is the most prevalent form of cancer of the laryngeal tract [23]. When first symptoms occur, the primary investigation method is white light endoscopy, which is however known to be insufficient for diagnosis, since a great number of non-malign alterations with similar appearance in endoscopy exists [8]. In the vocal cord area, the motivation for non-invasive micro-structural analysis, as provided by CLE, is even more striking, since extensive sampling of tissue by means of biopsy can cause functional problems such as voice modifications or chronic hoarseness [5]. Besides its limitations, it was successfully shown that – given sufficient training – human experts are able to classify SCC from CLE image sequences successfully, with accuracies between 91.38% and 96.55% [9]. Goncalves et al. found a significant training effect (as described by Neumann [20]) when judging CLE images on a single still image base. On a similar, different data set with 7 patients, they found accuracies by Ear, Nose and Throat (ENT) specialists to be between 58.1% and 87.1%, where the non-CLE experienced doctors had a mean accuracy of 67.7% and those with profound CLE experience one of 82.2% [8].

For this work, 73 image sequences from five patients were recorded. All patients underwent biopsy subsequent to CLE and were diagnosed with SCC of the vocal folds using the gold-standard of histo-pathology. The images of this data set have been acquired during micro-laryngoscopy at the Department of Otorhinolaryngology, Head and Neck Surgery (University Hospital Erlangen). The study was approved by the IRB of the University of Erlangen-Nürnberg (reference number: 60_14 B). For each patient, the contra-lateral vocal cord that was in each case macroscopically unaffected was also recorded, building a data set representing presumably healthy tissue of the vocal folds. For one patient (patient 5, see Fig. 3), no sequences with histo-pathology-confirmed SCC were available when this data set was created.

All images were pre-selected by a clinical expert in CLE imaging. This was done to remove diagnostically useless images, e.g. when the probe was not in contact with the tissue. After this cleaning step, the total number of images of this data set is 4,425. Vo et al. have done previous investigations on this data set, and found accuracies in grading of between 86.4% and 89.8% [29] using a patch-based method where they found best results for a support vector machine classifier with a feature set based on gray-level co-occurrence matrices [12].

3.3   Image Quality and Artifact Occurrence

As described by Neumann et al. and also Izadyyazdanabadi et al., CLE images are tainted by a range of deteriorations that impede image quality [11,19]. A significant part of images within the CLE sequences show low signal to noise ratios, which renders them unusable for either human or algorithmic evaluation. The reasons behind are manifold: the concentration of contrast agent might be insufficient in the tissue under the probe, the contact to the tissue might be lost,

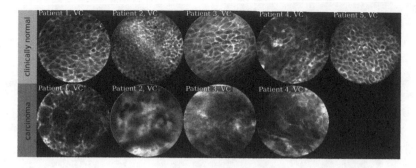

Fig. 3. Selected CLE Images acquired from the vocal fold area. In the top row, presumably healthy images are depicted that were taken from the clinically normal contralateral vocal cord of patients with epithelial cancer one of the both vocal cords (shown in the bottom row). Note that for patient 5, only images showing clinically normal tissue were available.

or the tissue perfusion with blood containing contrast agent might be too low. All of these factors can rarely be determined in retrospect. We found that low signal to noise ratio seems to be correlated with SCC image sequences. However, for the sake of robustness we assume that this is a non-causal relationship. Thus, very noisy images that were judged to be of no diagnostic use were removed from the data sets after manual inspection.

Comparing the images in Figs. 2 and 3, for clinically normal (and presumably healthy) tissue we find a large difference in contrast for some regions. While for images acquired from the alveolar ridge (rows 1 and 3, columns 5–6 in Fig. 2) and the vocal folds (top row in Fig. 3), contrast is generally good and cell outlines can be clearly spotted for most images, we find a much broader spread in image quality for images acquired at the hard palate and the lower inner labium (rows 1 and 3, columns 1–4 in Fig. 2).

In CLE images, the raw pixel value represents the optical (fluorescent) response to the laser light excitation. The optical receiver and analog to digital converter of the CLE scanner in use have a broad dynamic response. Thus, all images presented in this work and also in the CellVizio software are automatically compressed in their value range to fit the 8 bit gray level range of today's screens and to increase contrast for the viewer. The median raw pixel value, however, is indicative of the amount of fluorescent light that was picked up by the scanner, and as such also related to the signal-to-noise-ratio of the image. We use median, as it is more robust to the (typically sparsely distributed) very bright areas representing micro-vessels filled with contrast agent, as e.g. in row 2, column 4 of Fig. 2. We evaluated the median raw pixel value on images for all anatomical regions separately (see Fig. 4). For images acquired from the hard palate and the lower inner labium, we find a significantly different distribution than for both other anatomical locations, in that the prevalence of images with low median value (and thus likely low SNR) is much higher for these regions. In contrast, the vocal fold and alveolar ridge area both have a rather low amount

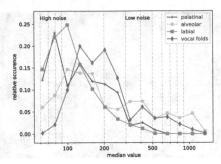

Fig. 4. Normalized histogram of the median value for the different classes of clinically normal tissue from both data sets. Due to the wide range of pixel values, the histogram is given at log scale (from: [1]).

of noisy images. This underlines our visual observation derived from the representative images in Fig. 2.

This difference can likely be attributed to the different anatomical properties of the tissue at the respective locations: Epithelium exposed to higher mechanical stress (in our case: usually due to chewing), is known to have a higher degree of cornification [26]. The vocal cords, due to not being exposed to mechanical stress, consist of multiple layers of uncornified squamous epithelium [25]. The alveolar ridge, located in the vestibule and outside of the *oral cavity proper* (where food is grinded and predigested), is normally not subject to high levels of mechanical stress. The hard palate, in contrast, is part of the chewing process and known to have a high degree of cornification [14]. The inner lip (labium), also located in the vestibule, is generally not considered a cornified epithelium. The images in our oral cavity data set, however, were taken at the intersection of mucous epithelial tissue in the vestibule and the skin-covered outer lip, which has an epidermal layer which is associated with a high level of cornification [25].

4   Methods

In this paper, we want to compare two methods of detection that differ significantly in their structure. Firstly, we assess a patch-based method using a CNN for individual classification of the patches (see Fig. 5 and [2] for further details). The patch classification is projected on the originating image coordinates, thereby deriving a probability map PM_{ppf}. Subsequently, the maps are fused to a single scalar for each class, denoted as image probability P_{ppf}. We denote this approach *patch probability fusion* (ppf). The approach is subject to the supposition that image labels can always be assumed to be also correct for individual patch labels, which, in our experience, holds true for a vast majority of images in our data set, since rarely the actual margin of a tumor is shown within an image with normal tissue structure in one part and malignant structural changes in the other.

Secondly, we perform a classification on image level, where a preprocessed complete image is fed through a deep network based on the stem of an Inception V.3 network [28] which will be described in detail in Sect. 4.3.

4.1 Experimental Setup

We performed five data experiments for this study:

Algorithmic Generalization. One major question is, how well the algorithms work on both data sets, when trained and evaluated on the same data set (using leave-1-patient-out (LOPO) cross-validation). This experiment aims to give us hints about algorithmic robustness.

1 (OC) Training on 11 patients of the OC data set, test on 1 patient (LOPO cross-validation).
2 (VC) Training on 4 patients of the VC data set, test on 1 patient (LOPO cross-validation).

The results given for these experiments represent an evaluation on the concatenated result vector of all cross-validation steps.

Medical Data Generalization. Since in both data sets, epithelium was scanned using the same technology, we assumed that classification knowledge acquired from one domain could generalize to the other domain.

3 (OC/VC) Training on all patients of the OC data set, test on all patients of the VC data set.
4 (VC/OC) Training on all patients of the VC data set, test on all patients of the OC data set.

Finally, we concatenated both data sets and performed yet another LOPO cross-validation on the joint data set.

5 (OC+VC) Training on 16 patients of the concatenated data set, test on 1 remaining patient (LOPO cross-validation).

4.2 Training of the Patch Classifier

We trained the patch classification network for a fixed number of 60 epochs, using an 3-fold augmented data set with random rotations of multiples of $\pi/2$ on patch level. All network weights have been initialized randomly. We used cross-entropy loss with the ADAM optimizer (learning rate: 10^{-2}).

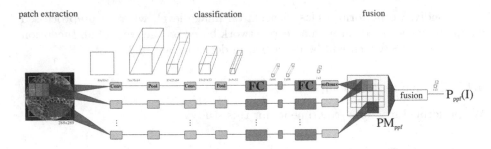

Fig. 5. Overview of the patch probability fusion (ppf) method [2]. Patches are extracted from the image, classified by a DNN using two layers of convolutional, pooling and finally two fully connected (FC) layers and subsequently probabilities are fused to a per-image probability.

4.3   Whole Image Classification with Activation Maps

Especially in the medical domain, two important requirement towards examination methodology are predictability and transparency. This contrasts with deep networks, essentially representing a complex function with unknown content and trained numerically. Therefore, insight into the method is difficult to attain. Especially since for domains where image quantity is low, overfitting plays an important role, medical experts and authorities may demand insights into intermediate classification results. As such, the aforementioned patch probability fusion (ppf) approach gives insights into classification results of different areas of the image, but its receptive field is also limited to the patches it classifies. The human expert, however, will always assess the whole image, and consequently also the labels are (for our data set) given only on image level.

One hint towards understanding image-level classification was given by Oquab *et al.* [22], a method that is commonly denoted as *weakly-supervised* learning. Their idea was to use a convolutional neural network that consists only of convolutional layers and pooling/striding operations. This leaves intact the localization of the image. Next, a global pooling operation is employed, resulting in an $1 \times 1 \times C$ image, where C is the number of channels/filters of the previous layer. Then, a final fully connected layer creates the mapping towards the output classes (see classification branch in Fig. 6). This approach has some nice properties: Since all operators are agnostic of the position on the actual image and all image regions are included into the final classification with equal weight, it is ensured that similar structures are recognized equally and a certain translational robustness can thus be expected. During inference, a second branch is added to the network prior to the average pooling layer, which maps the activations of said layer to class activity maps for each class, that can be easily visualized and gives insights into possible interpretations of the recognition.

Weakly supervised classification is especially useful, if only image-labels are available, but information about the subparts of the image would be informative. In our database of CLE images, we have these image-level class labels, as no further annotation was made available or is feasible to perform, since structures acquired during CLE image acquisition are hard to be identified exactly in the H&E-stained histology images that were taken as diagnostic samples from the same area.

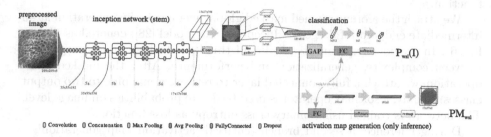

Fig. 6. Overview of the proposed whole image classification approach. Preprocessed images are fed through the stem of a pre-trained Inception V.3 network, then a convolutional (Conv) layer, a global average pooling (GAP) operation and finally a fully connected (FC) layer are attached. During inference, a class activation map is derived.

For the case of CLE the round circle of view is a challenge for image-level algorithms, due to steep edges on the corner. To circumvent this, we employ a preprocessing scheme described in Sect. 4.4 which ensures similar statistical probabilities across the whole image.

Still, since the newly created border area does not contain useful information, we aim to limit the networks attention to the area inside of the circle. For this, we suggest to use masking operations within the network, preceding the global average pooling (GAP) layer. The masking operation cuts position-dependent fragments out of the original image, that are due to the nature of being located just before the GAP layer, however, no longer dependent on the actual position.

We denote the respective previous layer of a network to be $\mathbf{U}$ with its elements $u_{i,j,c}$. The average pooling operation $F_{\mathrm{GAP}} : \mathbf{U} \to \mathbf{V}$, with $\mathbf{U} \in \mathbb{R}^{W \times H \times C}$, $\mathbf{V} \in \mathbb{R}^{1 \times 1 \times C}$ and $W \times H$ being the spatial resolution of the network and v_C being the elements of $\mathbf{V}$ is defined as:

$$v_c = \frac{1}{W \cdot H} \sum_{j}^{W} \sum_{i}^{H} u_c(i,j) \tag{1}$$

In order to restrict the attention of the algorithm to areas that have a valid image, we apply a masked average pooling operation $F_{\mathrm{MAP}} : \mathbf{U} \to \mathbf{V}'$ with $\mathbf{V}' \in \mathbb{R}^{1 \times 1 \times C}$ the elements of the resulting vector v'_c as:

$$v_c^* = \frac{1}{\sum_{i}^{W} \sum_{j}^{H} \delta(i,j)} \sum_{j}^{W} \sum_{i}^{H} \delta(i,j) \cdot u_c(i,j) \tag{2}$$

with:

$$\delta(i,j) = \sigma \left(r^2 - \left(j - \frac{H}{2} \right)^2 - \left(i - \frac{W}{2} \right)^2 \right) \tag{3}$$

where r is a constraining radius of the field of view, and $\sigma(x)$ is the step function.

We attach the aforementioned masked global average pooling operation at an intermediate endpoint of Szegedy's Inception V.3 model [28], denoted as *6b* (see Fig. 6). In previous experiments, we found this layer to be a good compromise between complexity, generalization and performance. After the masked GAP operation, we attach a fully connected layer to retrieve a mapping to two output classes. Finally, a softmax operator is used to derive probabilities on image level. The network is trained using binary cross-entropy as loss function.

During inference, a second branch (entitled 'activation map generation' in Fig. 6) is added just before the GAP operation, starting with a fully connected layer with shared weights to the fully connected layer in the classification branch. After the softmax, a class activation map of size 17×17 can be retrieved.

4.4   Preprocessing of the Image Classifier

To avoid problems in optimization due to the steep edges of the round field of view of pCLE images, we performed a circular extrapolation, as described in the following steps:

- Transformation of the image using a linear to polar transformation.
- Concatenation of the image in polar representation with its flipped version (along the distance axis).
- Transformation into the linear domain.
- Cropping of the square representing the original image coordinates.

This creates a mirroring around the circle that is defined using the radius in the linear to polar transformation. An example preprocessed image can be seen in Fig. 6.

4.5   Training of the Whole Image Classifier

Using Inception V.3 [28] as its base topology, the network capacity of the image classifier is significantly higher than that of the patch classifier. To leverage transfer learning, we initialize this network stem with pre-trained values acquired on the ImageNet database. With this, we try to benefit from the knowledge about shapes that can be derived from the real-world images used for pre-training this stem. We assume that this knowledge generalizes better than any conclusions that the model would derive from CLE data, so we train the stem with a reduced learning rate (10^{-4} vs. 10^{-6}).

In order to avoid overfitting, we make use of an early stopping mechanism. For this, two patients of the training data set (for the VC data set: 1 patient, due to its smaller size) are used as validation set. The training is initially run for 2 epochs. After the third and every following epoch, the classifier is evaluated for performance on the validation data set. In case of performance decrease, coefficients from the last epoch are restored and training is stopped. We allow for a maximum of 10 epochs, which was in practice never reached in our experiments. We assume that a validation on a different patient should allow to draw conclusions about overfitting within the same data collective. Further, we arbitrary rotation (before the preprocessing) as augmentation during training.

5   Results

Overall Results

Both algorithmic approaches seem to be applicable to both data sets with overall comparable results. The image-based classification yields better results for the oral cavity data set (AUC of 0.9687 vs. 0.9550, see Table 1), while the overall results are similar for the vocal cords data set (AUCs of 0.9484 vs. 0.9550).

For the medical data generalization task, which was the main research question in this work, we find a good performance for both algorithms when trained on the OC data set and applied on the VC data set. In contrast, the generalization from vocal folds to oral cavity performs significantly worse, and even more so for the whole image classification method.

Not surprisingly, we find that the overall performance of both approaches benefits from the larger (joint) data set in the OC+VC experiment.

Table 1. Results of all image and patch based (ppf) tests. For the cross validation cases OC, VC and OC+VC, the results were calculated on the concatenated result vector of all cross validation steps.

Condition	Accuracy (%)		Precision (%)		Recall (%)		ROC AUC (%)	
	ppf	image	ppf	image	ppf	image	ppf	image
OC	88.34% [2]	91.63 %	85.40%	91.06%	91.10%	91.43%	0.9550	**0.9687**
VC	91.39 %	89.97%	93.64%	93.66%	92.03%	89.50%	0.9484	**0.9550**
OC/VC	89.45 %	86.33%	87.47%	82.33%	96.37%	98.58%	0.9548	**0.9644**
VC/OC	68.53%	61.68%	60.81%	55.60%	95.63%	97.43%	**0.8484**	0.7694
OC+VC	90.81%	92.63%	90.12%	92.89%	92.59%	93.04%	0.9697	**0.9762**

Single Patient Results

Investigating single patient results, we find significant differences between individual patients. Where overall accuracies of some patients were approaching perfect recognition, others showed mediocre performance – this is most striking in the VC data set (see Fig. 7).

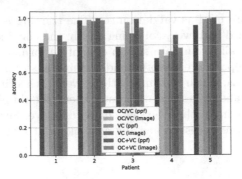

Fig. 7. Accuracy for all patients with both classes of the vocal fold data set.

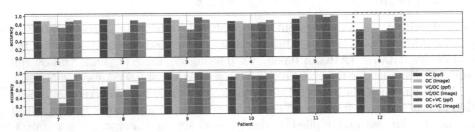

Fig. 8. Accuracy for all patients of the oral cavity data set. While for most patients, image level recognition and ppf method have similar results, patient 6 shows significantly improved results for the proposed approach.

We further find that classification results on one particular patient in cross validation (patient 6, see Fig. 8) benefit significantly from the whole image approach in both, the OC and the OC+VC experiment. This seems to be of strong influence on the overall increased performance for this condition. In the image probabilities produced by both approaches for this patient, we find that the ppf approach produces a significant amount of false positives (Fig. 9, $P_{ppf} > 0.5$ in clinically normal images), resulting in a low accuracy of 65.93%. While this might seem like a training anomaly at first, it is present in both, the concatenated OC+VC data set as well as the OC data set alone. In contrast, for the whole image recognition method, the accuracy for this patient is 91.91%.

6   Discussion

The results indicate that the recognition worked overall well for both methods. Both methods were applicable on both data sets, with slight advantages for the image level recognition proposed in this work. The prediction from VC data set to the OC data set, however, did not lead to satisfactory results. While differences in data set size might account for some loss of generalization, it is presumably not the only reason that the classifier trained on the VC data set shows significantly decreased performance on the OC data set. The much lower

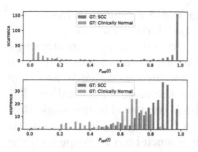 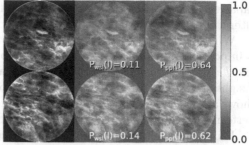

(a) Histogram of probabilities. Top: Proposed image classification method, bottom: patch-based method

(b) Example original images (left) with class map of the proposed image classification method (middle) and the ppf method (right).

Fig. 9. Comparison of results for both algorithmic approaches for patient 6 of the OC data set. As the histogram indicates, a high number of false positives is produced by the patch-based approach, leading to a decreased accuracy (65.93% vs. 91.91%). (Color figure online)

precision (see Table 1) in this experiment suggests the interpretation, that the underlying image material also differs significantly, which is backed up by our visual and statistical analysis from Sect. 3.3. Further, the anatomical differences (especially w.r.t cornification of tissue) influence these images in an explicable manner. With this, we would expect that a classification system trained on uncornified epithelial tissue would likely not be applicable directly to cornified epithelial tissue. Since the OC data set contains both tissue manifestations, the observed generalization (cf. Table 1) to the VC data set that contains only uncornified epithelium appears likely.

While images acquired from patient 6 (as depicted in Fig. 9) are certainly not showing perfectly ordered epithelial tissue, they represent a physiological variation. In this case, the whole image approach with its much wider algorithmic receptive field can make use of the overall image information and classify most images correctly. The distribution also shows a difference between a final softmax (as in the image level classification) and an averaging over different softmax outputs: the amount of samples with low confidence scores is extremely limited in the upper plot, while the averaging by the ppf method in the lower plot generates a more widespread distribution. The color-coded class map in Fig. 9(b) also indicates that, while certain low-contrast parts of the image are assigned higher class probabilities for carcinoma in the whole image approach, they do not influence the overall probability (color coded in the background of the image).

Furthermore, as both algorithmic approaches profit from an enhanced data set, it is obvious that the limited size of our current data set cannot provide a final answer to the question of algorithmic generalization. The whole image approach introduced in this paper, however, has the much higher algorithmic capacity and should thus be able to adjust to a wider range of physiological alterations, as could be expected when the data set further increases.

While our approach is related to weakly supervised image segmentation, it is important to state that we did not aim to segment the image between *cancer* and *healthy* regions. The reason to use this architecture was rather to give more insights into image cues, used by the method for the image classification. This shows also the close relation between both methods compared in this work: Both perform averaging of some kind of class maps on the complete image, while the GAP-based global feature averaging can encode a much broader scope on image level, as the final mapping to the output classes is only performed with the final fully connected layer. It is worth pointing out that without this layer, both approaches are similar (if we ignore the different filter layers). While patch based approaches usually have a higher flexibility in handling (such as, e.g. for class distribution equalization during training), the image-based approaches with an average pooling layer have a higher computational performance.

A major limitation of our study is that we do not have histo-pathological proof for any of our clinically normal CLE images, since extraction of tissue from clinically normal regions would be ethically questionable, and histo-pathology confirmed squamous cell carcinoma for all patients in our data set. However, we are confident that a larger data set that our research group is preparing to record will also include verified healthy tissue.

It must be stated, however, that it is questionable if a negative diagnosis for SCC can be retrieved using CLE alone. CLE has a limited penetration depth, and thus tumors that spread within the submucosa could be invisible for CLE. A combination with other methods, such as Raman spectroscopy [13] or Optical Coherence Tomography [3] could yield improved results.

The results of this study imply that our method could generalize well for all kinds of epithelial cancer diagnosis where CLE is applicable. This would, however, obviously be a too broad statement given the limited amount of patient data available for this work. Our future work will thus focus on the acquisition of a larger and more diverse data set. The fact that the concatenated data set improved performance for both domains indicates that an enlarged data set will improve performance as well as robustness.

7 Summary

In this work we evaluated two approaches for automatic classification of confocal laser endomicroscopy images for the detection of head and neck squamous cell carcinoma, with a focus on the ability to generalize knowledge learnt from one anatomical location (oral cavity) to another (vocal folds).

The patch-based classification approach and the newly introduced whole image classification system both show good performance when evaluated on the same entity. The image-based classification system showed better performance (accuracy of 91.63% vs. 88.34%) on one of the data sets, whereas results on the other data set were similar.

The generalization tasks, where a classification system learnt from CLE images of the oral cavity was applied on vocal fold CLE images, showed promising results. Concatenation of both data sets led to an overall improved accuracy of 92.63% with the image classification system. We expect that a further increase of data amount will significantly improve performance on this recognition task.

References

1. Aubreville, M., et al.: Patch-based carcinoma detection on confocal laser endomicroscopy images - a cross-site robustness assessment. In: Proceedings of the 11th International Joint Conference on Biomedical Engineering Systems and Technologies, BIOIMAGING, vol. 2, pp. 27–34. INSTICC, SciTePress (2018). https://doi.org/10.5220/0006534700270034
2. Aubreville, M., et al.: Automatic classification of cancerous tissue in laser endomicroscopy images of the oral cavity using deep learning. Sci. Rep. **7**(1), s41598–017 (2017). https://doi.org/10.1038/s41598-017-12320-8
3. Betz, C.S., et al.: Optical diagnostic methods for early tumour diagnosis in the upper aerodigestive tract. HNO **64**(1), 41–48 (2016). https://doi.org/10.1007/s00106-015-0104-8
4. Chauhan, S.S., et al.: Confocal laser endomicroscopy. Gastrointest. Endosc. **80**(6), 928–938 (2014). https://doi.org/10.1016/j.gie.2014.06.021
5. Cikojević, D., Glunčić, I., Pešutić-Pisac, V.: Comparison of contact endoscopy and frozen section histopathology in the intra-operative diagnosis of laryngeal pathology. J. Laryngol. Otol. **122**(8), 836–839 (2008). https://doi.org/10.1017/S0022215107000539
6. Esteva, A., et al.: Dermatologist-level classification of skin cancer with deep neural networks. Nature **542**(7639), 115–118 (2017). https://doi.org/10.1038/nature21056
7. Forastiere, A., Koch, W., Trotti, A., Sidransky, D.: Head and neck cancer. N. Engl. J. Med. **345**(26), 1890–1900 (2001). https://doi.org/10.1056/NEJMra001375
8. Goncalves, M., Iro, H., Dittberner, A., Agaimy, A., Bohr, C.: Value of confocal laser endomicroscopy in the diagnosis of vocal cord lesions. Eur. Rev. Med. Pharmacol. Sci. **21**, 3990–3997 (2017)
9. Goncalves, M., et al.: Probe-based confocal laser endomicroscopy in detecting malignant lesions of the vocal folds. Acta Otorhinolaryngol. Ital. (2019). https://doi.org/10.14639/0392-100X-2121
10. Izadyyazdanabadi, M., et al.: Weakly-supervised learning-based feature localization for confocal laser endomicroscopy glioma images. In: Frangi, A.F., Schnabel, J.A., Davatzikos, C., Alberola-López, C., Fichtinger, G. (eds.) MICCAI 2018. LNCS, vol. 11071, pp. 300–308. Springer, Cham (2018). https://doi.org/10.1007/978-3-030-00934-2_34
11. Izadyyazdanabadi, M., et al.: Improving utility of brain tumor confocal laser endomicroscopy: objective value assessment and diagnostic frame detection with convolutional neural networks. In: Proceedings of the SPIE, vol. 10134, p. 101342J (2017). https://doi.org/10.1117/12.2254902
12. Jaremenko, C., et al.: Classification of confocal laser endomicroscopic images of the oral cavity to distinguish pathological from healthy tissue. In: Handels, H., Deserno, T.M., Meinzer, H.-P., Tolxdorff, T. (eds.) Bildverarbeitung für die Medizin 2015. INFORMAT, pp. 479–485. Springer, Heidelberg (2015). https://doi.org/10.1007/978-3-662-46224-9_82

13. Knipfer, C., et al.: Raman difference spectroscopy: a non-invasive method for identification of oral squamous cell carcinoma. Biomed. Opt. Express **5**(9), 3252–3265 (2014). https://doi.org/10.1364/BOE.5.003252

14. Lüllmann-Rauch, R., Paulsen, F.: Taschenlehrbuch Histologie, 4th edn. Thieme, Stuttgart (2012)

15. Maier, H., Dietz, A., Gewelke, U., Heller, W., Weidauer, H.: Tobacco andalcohol and the risk of head and neck cancer. Clin. Investig. **70**(3–4), 320–327 (1992). https://doi.org/10.1007/BF00184668

16. Murthy, V.N., Singh, V., Sun, S., Bhattacharya, S., Chen, T., Comaniciu, D.: Cascaded deep decision networks for classification of endoscopic images. In: Proceedings of the SPIE, vol. 10133 (2017). https://doi.org/10.1117/12.2254333

17. Muto, M.: Squamous cell carcinoma in situ at oropharyngeal and hypopharyngeal mucosal sites. Cancer **101**(6), 1375–1381 (2004). https://doi.org/10.1002/cncr.20482

18. Neumann, H., Kiesslich, R., Wallace, M.B., Neurath, M.F.: Confocal laser endomicroscopy: technical advances and clinical applications. Gastroenterology **139**(2), 388–392.e2 (2010). https://doi.org/10.1053/j.gastro.2010.06.029

19. Neumann, H., Langner, C., Neurath, M.F., Vieth, M.: Confocal laser endomicroscopy for diagnosis of barrett's esophagus. Front. Oncol. **2** (2012). https://doi.org/10.3389/fonc.2012.00042

20. Neumann, H., Vieth, M., Atreya, R., Neurath, M.F., Mudter, J.: Prospective evaluation of the learning curve of confocal laser endomicroscopy in patients with IBD. Histol. Histopathol. **26**(7), 867–872 (2011). https://doi.org/10.14670/HH-26.867

21. Oetter, N., et al.: Development and validation of a classification and scoring system for the diagnosis of oral squamous cell carcinomas through confocal laser endomicroscopy. J. Transl. Med. **14**(1), 1–11 (2016). https://doi.org/10.1186/s12967-016-0919-4

22. Oquab, M., Bottou, L., Laptev, I., Sivic, J.: Is object localization for free? - weakly-supervised learning with convolutional neural networks. In: Proceedings of IEEE Conference on Computer Vision and Pattern Recognition, pp. 685–694. IEEE (2015). https://doi.org/10.1109/CVPR.2015.7298668

23. Parkin, D.M., Bray, F., Ferlay, J., Pisani, P.: Global cancer statistics, 2002. CA: Cancer J. Clin. **55**(2), 74–108 (2005). https://doi.org/10.3322/canjclin.55.2.74

24. Robert Koch Institut: Zentrum für Krebsregisterdaten: Krebs in Deutschland für 2013/2014, 11th edn. Robert Koch Institut, Berlin (2017)

25. Rohen, J.W.: Histologische Differentialdiagnose, 5th edn. Schattauer, Stuttgart (1994)

26. Rohen, J.W., Lütjen-Drecoll, E.: Funktionelle Histologie, 4th edn. Schattauer, Stuttgart (2000)

27. Stoeve, M., et al.: Motion artifact detection in confocal laser endomicroscopy images. Bildverarbeitung für die Medizin 2018. INFORMAT, pp. 328–333. Springer, Heidelberg (2018). https://doi.org/10.1007/978-3-662-56537-7_85

28. Szegedy, C., et al.: Going deeper with convolutions. In: 2015 IEEE Conference on Computer Vision and Pattern Recognition (CVPR), September 2015. https://doi.org/10.1109/CVPR.2015.7298594

29. Vo, K., Jaremenko, C., Bohr, C., Neumann, H., Maier, A.: Automatic classification and pathological staging of confocal laser endomicroscopic images of the vocal cords. Bildverarbeitung für die Medizin 2017. INFORMAT, pp. 312–317. Springer, Heidelberg (2017). https://doi.org/10.1007/978-3-662-54345-0_70

30. Westra, W.H.: The pathology of HPV-related head and neck cancer: implications for the diagnostic pathologist. Semin. Diagn. Pathol. **32**(1), 42–53 (2015). https://doi.org/10.1053/j.semdp.2015.02.023
31. Xing, F., Xie, Y., Su, H., Liu, F., Yang, L.: Deep learning in microscopy image analysis: a survey. IEEE Trans. Neural Netw. Learn. Syst. **PP**(99), 1–19 (2017). https://doi.org/10.1109/TNNLS.2017.2766168

Min-Cut Segmentation of Retinal OCT Images

Bashir Isa Dodo$^{(\boxtimes)}$, Yongmin Li, Khalid Eltayef, and Xiaohui Liu

Brunel University London, UB8 3PH London, UK
{Bashir.Dodo,Yongmin.Li,Khalid.Eltayef,XiaoHui.Liu}@brunel.ac.uk

Abstract. Optical Coherence Tomography (OCT) is one of the most vital tools for diagnosing and tracking progress of medication of various retinal disorders. Many methods have been proposed to aid with the analysis of retinal images due to the intricacy of retinal structures, the tediousness of manual segmentation and variation from different specialists. However image artifacts, in addition to inhomogeneity in pathological structures, remain a challenge, with negative influence on the performance of segmentation algorithms. In this paper we present an automatic retinal layer segmentation method, which comprises of fuzzy histogram hyperbolization and graph cut methods. We impose hard constraints to limit search region to sequentially segment 8 boundaries and 7 layers of the retina on 150 OCT B-Sans images, 50 each from the temporal, nasal and center of foveal regions. Our method shows positive results, with additional tolerance and adaptability to contour variance and pathological inconsistence of the retinal structures in all regions.

Keywords: Retinal layer segmentation ·
Optical Coherence Tomography · Graph-cut · Image analysis

1 Introduction

Segmentation using graph cut methods depends on the assignment of appropriate weight during graph construction. The paths obtained by the shortest path algorithms have no optimal way of handling inconsistencies (such as the irregularity in OCT images), as thus it sometimes obtains the wrong paths, which we call the "wrong short-cuts". To avoid the wrong short-cuts, we reassign the weights to promote the homogeneity between adjacent edges using fuzzy histogram hyperbolization. In other words, the edges with high value get higher weights, while those with low values become lower. The idea behind this weight reassignment is that, the transition between layers of OCT images which are from dark to light or vice versa are improved. This means we can better identify the layers by searching for the changes or transitions between layer boundaries. Additionally, we take into account the transition between the layers is in most cases very smooth, making it quite difficult to segment the layers. Now if we re-emphasize on this changes, such that they become clearer, this aids the algorithm in successful segmentation and avoiding wrong short-cuts.

© Springer Nature Switzerland AG 2019
A. Cliquet jr. et al. (Eds.): BIOSTEC 2018, CCIS 1024, pp. 86–99, 2019.
https://doi.org/10.1007/978-3-030-29196-9_5

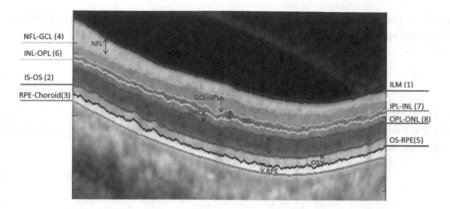

Fig. 1. Illustration of the 8 boundaries and 7 retinal layers segmented in the study. The numbers in brackets are the sequential order of the segmentation [8].

In this paper we take into account the effect of promoting continuity and discontinuity, in addition to adding hard constraints based on the structure of retina to segment 7 retinal layers including the Nerve Fibre Layer (NFL), the Ganglion Cell to Layer-Inner Plexiform Layer (GCL+IPL), the Inner Nuclear Layer (INL), the Outer Plexiform Layer (OPL), the Outer Nuclear Layer to Inner Segment (ONL+IS), the Outer Segment (OS) and the Retinal Pigment Epithelium (RPE) by detecting eight (8) layer boundaries. The locations of these layers and boundaries in an OCT image are illustrated in Fig. 1.

This paper is organized as follows. In Sect. 2, we review background information on the Graph-Cut segmentation method and the previous work in retinal layer segmentation. Section 3 describes the proposed segmentation method. Section 4 presents experimental results on 150 OCT images and finally conclusions are drawn in Sect. 5.

2   Background

2.1   The Graph-Cut Method

Graph-Cut is an optimization method that provides solution to many computational problems including image processing and computer vision as first reported by [23]. In the context of image processing, a graph G is a pair (ν, ε) consisting of a node (referred to as Vertex in 3D nested grid) set ν and an edge set $\varepsilon \subset \nu \times \nu$. The source s and the sink t are the two main terminal nodes. The edge set comprises of two type of edges: the spatial edges $en = (r, q)$, where $r, q \in \nu \backslash \{s \backslash t\}$, stick to the given grid and link two neighbor grid nodes r and q except s and t; the terminal edges or data edges, i.e. $e_s = (s, r)$ or $e_t = (r, t)$, where $r \in \nu \backslash \{s \backslash t\}$, link the specified terminal s or t to each grid node p respectively. Each edge is assigned a cost $C(e)$, assuming all are non-negative i.e. $C(e) \geq 0$. A cut, also known as the s-t cut, splits the image into two disjoint sets of s and t. It partitions the spatial grid nodes of Ω into disjoint groups, whereby one belongs to source and the other belongs to the sink, such that

$$\nu = \nu_s \bigcup \nu_t, \nu_s \bigcap \nu_t = \emptyset \tag{1}$$

We then introduce the concept of max-flow/min-cut [10]. The max-flow calculates the maximum amount of flow allowed to pass from the source s to the sink t based on edges capacity, and is formulated by:

$$\max_{p_s} \sum_{v \in \nu \setminus \{s,t\}} p_s(v) \tag{2}$$

For each cut, the energy is defined as the sum of the costs C(e) of each edge e $\in \varepsilon_{st} \subset \varepsilon$, where its two end points belong to two different partitions. Hence the problem of min-cut is to find two partitions of nodes such that the corresponding cut-energy is minimal,

$$\min_{\varepsilon_{st} \subset \varepsilon} \sum_{e \in \varepsilon_{st}} C(e) \tag{3}$$

Additional insightful literature detailing the concept of graph-cut for image segmentation can be found in [4,15,29].

2.2   Segmentation of Retinal Layers

The segmentation of retinal layers has drawn a large number of researches, since the introduction of Optical Coherence Tomography (OCT) [13]. Manual segmentation of retinal OCT images is intricate and requires automated methods of analysis [1]. Various methods have been proposed to help with OCT image segmentation. In particular, the main discussions are on the number of layers, computational complexity, graph formulation and mostly now optimization and machine learning approaches. In this regard a multi-step approach was developed by [2]. However the results obtained were highly dependent on the quality of images and the alterations induced by retinal pathologies. A 1-D edge detection algorithm using the Markov Boundary Model [16], which was later extended by [3] to obtain the optic nerve head and RNFL. Seven layers were obtained by [5] using a peak search interactive boundary detection algorithm based on local coherence information of the retinal structure. The Level Set method was used by [19,26–28] which were computationally expensive compared to other optimization methods. Graph based methods in [11,12,20–22] have reported successful segmentation results, with varying success rates. Recently, [9] proposed a method using the Fuzzy Histogram Hyperbolization (FHH) to improve the image quality, then embedded the image into the continuous max-flow to simultaneously segment 4 retinal layers.

   In recent years, researchers have been inquisitive on the use of gradient information derived from the retinal structures. This information has been utilised with the Graph-Cut method, where the retinal architecture and dynamic programming were deployed to limit the search space and reduce computational time respectively [6]. This method was recently extended to the 3D volumetric analysis by [24] in OCTRIMA 3D with edge map and convolution kernel in addition to hard constraints in calculating weights. The OCTRIMA 3D approach also exploited spatial dependency between adjacent frames to reduce processing time. Combination of methods including Edge detection and polynomial fitting [18] and machine learning with random forest classifier [17] were yet other approaches proposed to obtain the retinal layers from gradient information. The use of OCT gradient information is primarily due to the transition that occurs in the vertical direction at each layer boundary, thereby attracting segmentation algorithms to exploit this advantage. Our method takes into account the retinal structure and gradient information, but more importantly, the re-assignment of weights in the adjacency matrix is paramount to the success of our graph-cut approach.

3   The Proposed Method

In this section we explain the components of our approach to segmenting 8 retinal layer boundaries from OCT B-Scan images. A schematic representation of these components is illustrated in Fig. 2.

3.1   Pre-processing

Like most medical images, OCT suffer from a granular pattern called speckle noise. This noise is very common in OCT images, which has negative effects on further processing, for example, the retinal OCT images have low Signal to Noise Ratio (SNR) due to the strong amplitude of speckle noise. Various methods have been used to handle the presence of noise. In this work, we pre-process the images with a Gaussian filter to suppress the speckle noise and enhance the retinal layer boundaries, which is important for the weight calculation in the next stage. This also reduces false positive in the segmentation stage. An example of a pre-processed image compared to its original is shown in Fig. 3.

3.2   Graph Formulation

In this stage we obtain the vertical gradient of the image, normalize the gradient image to values in the range of 0 to 1, and then obtain the inverse of the normalized image gradient. Example of the gradient images are shown in Fig. 4. The two normalized gradient images are then used to obtain two separate undirected adjacency matrices, where Fig. 4(left) contains information of light-dark transitions while Fig. 4(right) contains information for transition from dark-light. The adjacency matrices are formulated with the following equation adapted from [6]:

$$w_{ab} = 2 - g_a - g_b + w_{min} \qquad (4)$$

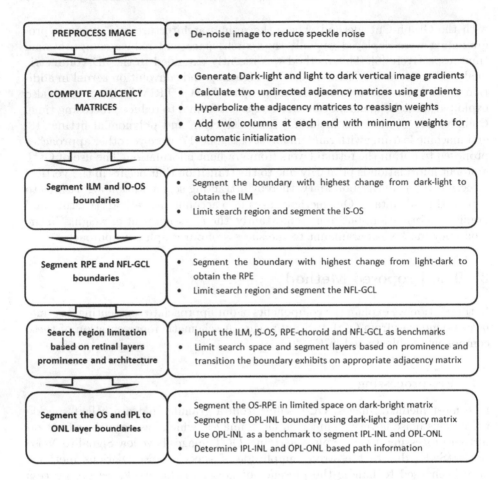

Fig. 2. Main steps of segmentation algorithm schematic representation [8].

where w_{ab}, g_a, g_b and w_{min} are the weights assigned to the edge connecting any two adjacent nodes a and b, the vertical gradient of the image at node a, the vertical gradient of the image at node b, and the minimum weight added for system stabilization. To improve the continuity and homogeneity in the adjacency matrices they are hyperbolized, firstly by calculating the membership function with the fuzzy sets Eq. (5) [25] and then transformed with Eq. (6).

$$w'_{ab} = \frac{w_{ab} - w_{mn}}{w_{mx} - w_{mn}}. \tag{5}$$

where w_{mn} and w_{mx} represents the maximum and minimum values of the adjacency matrix respectively. The adjacency matrices are then transformed with the following equation:

$$w''_{ab} = (w'_{ab})^{\beta} \tag{6}$$

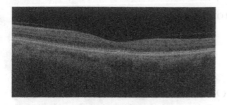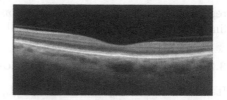

Fig. 3. Image pre-processing: original image corrupted with speckle noise (left) compared to filtered image by Gaussian (right) [8].

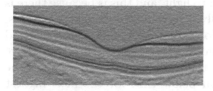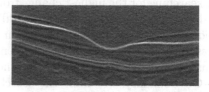

Fig. 4. Image gradients used in generating dark-bright adjacency matrix (left) and bright-dark adjacency matrix (right) [8].

where w'_{ab} is the membership value from (5), and β, the fuzzifier is a constant. Considering the number of edges in an adjacency matrix, we use a constant β instead of calculating the fuzziness. The main reason is to reduce computational time and memory usage. The resulting adjacency matrices are such that we reassign the weights, and the edges with high weights get higher values while those with low values get lower edge weights. Our motive here is that if we re-emphasize continuity or discontinuity, the algorithm would perform better, wherein our method we improve both by transforming the matrices. The region of the layers get similar values, while that of the background gets lower along the way. This is more realistic and applicable in this context (as the shortest path is greedy search approach), because at the boundary of each layer there is a transition from bright to dark or dark to bright, and therefore improving it aids the algorithm in finding correct optimal solutions that are very close to the actual features of interest.

The weight calculation is followed by several sequential steps of segmentation that we discuss in the next few subsections. We adopt layer initialization from [6], where two columns are added to either side of the image with minimum weights (w_{min}), to enable the cut move freely in those columns. We base this initialization from the understanding that each layer spans horizontally across the image, and that the graph-cut method prefers paths with minimum weights. We utilize the Djikstra's algorithm [7] in finding the minimum weighted path in the graph, which corresponds to layer boundaries. To segment multiple regions, we use an iterative search in limited space because graph-Cut methods are optimal at finding one boundary at a time. Limiting the region of search is a complex task, it requires prior knowledge and is dependent on the structure of the features or regions of interest. More information on automatic layer initialization and region limitation can be obtained from [6,14].

3.3   ILM and IS-OS Segmentation

It is commonly accepted that the NFL, IS-OS and RPE exhibit high reflectivity in an OCT image [6,18,24]. Taking this reflectivity and the dark-bright adjacency matrix into account, we identify the ILM and IS-OS boundaries using Dijkstra's algorithm [7]. More specifically, the ILM (vitreous-NFL) boundary is segmented by searching for the highest change from dark to light, and this is because there is a sharp change in the transition. Additionally, it is amidst extraneous features, above it is the background region in addition to no interruption of the blood vessels, as can be seen in the gradient image in Fig. 4(right). All of the above reasons make it easier to segment the ILM than other layers. To segment the IS-OS boundary, We limit the search region below ILM for the next highest change from dark-bright. We then use the mean value of the vertical axis of the paths obtained, as a precaution to confirm which layer was segmented, because the ILM is above the IS-OS take (similar to [6]).

3.4   RPE and NFL-GCL Segmentation

As mentioned in the previous subsection, RPE is one of the most reflective layers. The RPE-Choroid boundary exhibits the highest bright-dark layer transition as can be seen in Fig. 4(left). Besides, it is better to search for the transition from bright-dark for the RPE based on experimental results, interference of blood vessels and the disruption of hyper-reflective pixels in the choroid region. Therefore searching for the highest bright-dark transition is ideal for the RPE most especially to adapt to noisy images. Now to segment the NFL-GCL boundary we limit the search space between ILM to IS-OS and utilize the bright-dark adjacency matrix to find the minimum weighted path. The resulting path is the NFL-GCL boundary, as it is one of the most hyper-reflective layers. Furthermore, the NFL-GCL and IS-OS boundaries exhibit the second highest bright-dark and dark-bright transition respectively in an OCT image. If we limit our search space to regions below the ILM and above the RPE, the resulting bright-dark and dark-bright minimum paths are the NFL-GCL and IS-OS respectively. It is also significant to note we use the paths obtained from one adjacency matrix to limit the region on either of the matrices. This is feasible because the paths are (x, y) coordinates and the matrices are of the same size. For example, in finding the NFL-GCL boundary on the bright-dark adjacency matrix, we use paths of the ILM and IS-OS obtained from the dark-bright matrix to limit the search region.

3.5   OS and IPL to ONL Segmentation

Now that we have segmented the most prominent boundaries, we use them as benchmarks to limit the search space in order to segment the OS-RPE, IPL-INL,

INL-OPL, and OPL-ONL. We obtain the OS-RPE boundary by searching for the dark-bright shortest path between IS-OS and the RPE-Choroid. As for the remaining boundaries, we first segment the INL-OPL by searching for the shortest path between NFL-GCL and IS-OS on the dark-bright adjacency matrix, primarily because it exhibits a different transition from the IPL-INL and OPL-ONL boundaries. Consequently, the IPL-INL and OPL-ONL boundaries are obtained by limiting the region of path search between INL-OPL and NFL-GCL, and INL-OPL and IS-OS regions respectively, on the bright-dark adjacency matrix.

3.6 Avoiding the Cortical Vitreous

The vitreous cortex depicts a layer-like structure, just above the ILM, which lures the algorithm into finding unintended boundaries as illustrated in Fig. 5. To handle this issue, we impose a hard constraint to restrict all paths between the ILM to RPE boundaries inclusive. This is because the ILM exhibits the highest transition from dark-bright, while the RPE exhibits the highest transition from bright-dark. This helps the algorithm in avoiding features that imitate the retinal structures.

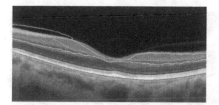 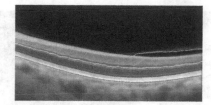

Fig. 5. Error in segmentation caused by vitreous cortex at temporal region (left) and Nasal region (right).

4   Experimental Results

The performance evaluation of our proposed method was tested on a dataset of 150 B-scan OCT images centred on the macular region. The data was collected in Tongren Hospital with a standard imaging protocol for retinal diseases such as glaucoma. Each B-scan image has a resolution of 512 pixels in depth and 992 pixels across section with 16 bits per pixel. Prior to segmenting the images, we cropped 15% percent of the image height from the top to remove regions with low signal and no features of interest. The ground truth images used in our experiments were manually labeled under the supervision of clinical experts. We segment seven retinal layers automatically using MATLAB 2016a software. Using a computer with Intel i5-4590 CPU, clock of 3.3 GHz, and 8 GB RAM memory, the average computational time was 4.25 s per image. The method obtains the boundaries in the order from ILM(Vitreous-NFL), IS-OS, RPE-Choroid, NFL-GCL, OS-RPE, INL-OPL, IPL-INL to OPL-ONL respectively. The locations of

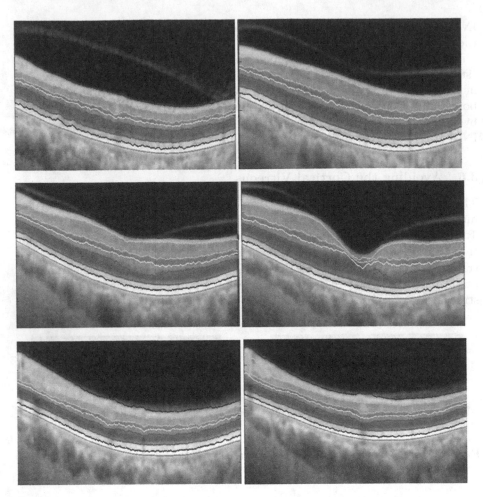

Fig. 6. Segmentation results of 8 boundaries and 7 layers. Boundaries from top to bottom, the segmented boundaries are ILM, NFL-GCL, IPL-INL, INL-OPL, OPL-ONL, IS-OS, OS-RPE and RPE-Choroid [8].

these boundaries and the sequential segmentation order of the 8 retinal layer boundaries and underlying 7 layers were shown earlier in Fig. 1, and we show output sample of results achieved in Fig. 6.

To evaluate the proposed method we calculate the Root Mean Squared Error (RMSE), and Mean Absolute Deviation (MAD) by (7). Table 1 shows output of the mean and standard deviation of both MAD and RMSE, for the seven layers targeted in this study.

$$MAD(GT, SEG) =$$

$$0.5 * \left(\frac{1}{n} \sum_{i=1}^{n} d(pt_i, SEG) + \frac{1}{m} \sum_{i=1}^{m} d(ps_i, GT) \right)$$

$$RMSE = \sqrt{\frac{1}{n} \sum_{i=1}^{n} (SEG_i - GT_i)^2}$$

$$Dice \qquad = \frac{2 \mid GT_i \cap SEG_i \mid}{\mid GT_i \mid + \mid SEG_i \mid}$$

(7)

where SEG_i is the pixel labelled as retinal Layer (foreground) by the proposed segmentation method and GT_i is the true retinal layers pixel in the manually annotated image (ground truth) image. In computing the MAD pt_i and ps_i represent the coordinates of the images, while $d(pt_i, SEG)$ is the distance of pt_i to the closest pixel on SEG with the same segmentation label, and $d(ps_i, GT)$ is the distance of ps_i to the closest pixel on GT with the same segmentation label. n and m are the number of points on SEG and GT respectively. For all layers our method has performed well. Especially considering the low value of NFL for both MAD and RMSE. The high value in ONL+IS is due to the presence of high noise and lower reflectivity of the boundaries within the region, however, this is still considerably low.

Table 1. Performance evaluation: Mean and Standard Deviation (STD) of RMSE and MAD for 7 retinal layers on 150 SD-OCT B-Scan images (Units in pixels) [8].

RetinalLayer	MeanMAD	MeanRMSE	STDMAD	STDRMSE
NFL	0.2689	0.0168	0.0189	0.0121
GCL+IPL	0.5938	0.0432	0.0592	0.0382
INL	0.6519	0.0387	0.0792	0.0612
OPL	0.5101	0.0446	0.0410	0.0335
ONL+IS	0.6896	0.0597	0.0865	0.0329
OS	0.4617	0.0341	0.0360	0.0150
RPE	0.4617	0.0341	0.0360	0.0150

Furthermore, The retinal nerve fibre layer thickness (RNFLT), the area between ILM and NFL-GCL, is critical in diagnosing ocular diseases, including glaucoma. For this reason, we evaluated the RNFLT with four additional criteria, namely, accuracy, sensitivity (true positive rate (TPR)), error rate (FPR) and the Dice index (coefficient). These measurements are computed with the

Table 2. Mean for accuracy, sensitivity, error rate and Dice coefficient of the Retinal Nerve Fibre Layer Thickness (RNFLT) and their respective standard deviation (STD). [8].

Criteria	Mean	STD
Accuracy	0.9816	0.0375
Sensitivity	0.9687	0.0473
Error Rate	0.0669	0.0768
Dice	0.9746	0.0559

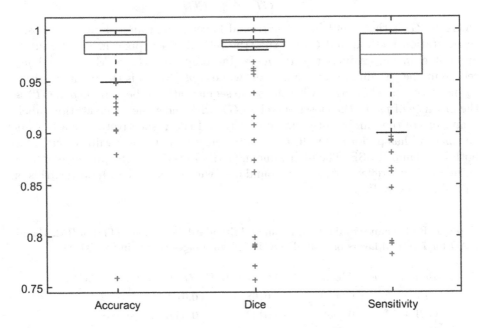

Fig. 7. Box plot for values distribution of Accuracy, Dice coefficient and Sensitivity of RNFLT from Table 2.

following equations while the Dice is computed from (7):

$$Accuracy = \frac{TP + TN}{(TP + FP + FN + TN)}$$

$$Sensitivity(TPR) = \frac{TP}{(TP + FN)} \qquad (8)$$

$$ErrorRate(FPR) = \frac{FP}{(FP + TN)}$$

where TP, TN, FP and FN refers to true positive, true negative, false positive and false negative respectively. Distinctively, TP represents the number of pixels which are part of the region that are labeled correctly by both the method and the ground truth. TN represents the number of pixels which are part of the background region and labeled correctly by both the method and the ground truth. FP represents the number of pixels labeled as a part of the region by the method but labeled as a part of the background by the ground truth. Finally, FN represents the number of pixels labeled as a part of the background by the system but labeled as a part of the region in ground truth. The Mean and standard Deviation of applying the above criteria on the achieved results for the RNFLT are shown in Table 2, and the distribution of these values in Fig. 7.

Some of the facts we draw from the results in Table 2 and their distribution Fig. 7 are as follows:

1. The method achieves more than 95% accuracy in most images
2. The method obtain paths very close to the actual retinal boundaries by achieving mean sensitivity of ≈97% over 150 images, which portrays adaptability to contours of the retinal layers.
3. The distribution of the dice score in Fig. 7 further attests to the statements in 2 above, i.e there is high overlap between the manual annotation and results obtained by our method.

5 Conclusions

We have presented a comprehensive approach towards retinal OCT image analysis. Our fully automatic method is capable of segmenting 7 retinal layers across 8 layer boundaries. The core of the method is the integration of the adjacency matrices from vertical gradients with improved weight calculation into a sequential process of the Graph-Cut framework using Dijkstra's algorithm [7]. Categorically, the sequential segmentation process is based on the unique characteristics of reflectivity of different retinal layers and their transitions at the boundaries. We have applied the proposed method to a dataset of 150 OCT B-scan images, with successful segmentation results. Additionally, quantitative evaluation indicates that the segmentation measurement is very close to the ground-truth. Furthermore, it is evident prior knowledge plays an essential role in segmentation. Therefore studies on how to automatically derive this information from images and electronic health records will be necessary because this information can be useful in optimizing image analysis algorithms, particularly methods of statistical based modelling.

References

1. Baglietto, S., Kepiro, I.E., Hilgen, G., Sernagor, E., Murino, V., Sona, D.: Segmentation of retinal ganglion cells from fluorescent microscopy imaging. In: Proceedings of the 10th International Joint Conference on Biomedical Engineering Systems and Technologies (BIOSTEC 2017), pp. 17–23 (2017). https://doi.org/10.5220/0006110300170023

2. Baroni, M., Fortunato, P., La Torre, A.: Towards quantitative analysis of retinal features in optical coherence tomography. Med. Eng. Phys. **29**(4), 432–441 (2007). https://doi.org/10.1016/j.medengphy.2006.06.003
3. Boyer, K.L., Herzog, A., Roberts, C.: Automatic recovery of the optic nervehead geometry in optical coherence tomography. IEEE Trans. Med. Imaging **25**(5), 553–570 (2006). https://doi.org/10.1109/TMI.2006.871417
4. Boykov, Y., Jolly, M.P.: Interactive graph cuts for optimal boundary & region segmentation of objects in N-D images. In: Proceedings Eighth IEEE International Conference on Computer Vision, ICCV 2001, vol. 1(July), pp. 105–112 (2001). https://doi.org/10.1109/ICCV.2001.937505
5. Cabrera Fernández, D., Salinas, H.M., Puliafito, C.A.: Automated detection of retinal layer structures on optical coherence tomography images. Opt. Express **13**(25), 10200 (2005). https://doi.org/10.1364/OPEX.13.010200
6. Chiu, S.J., Li, X.T., Nicholas, P., Toth, C.A., Izatt, J.A., Farsiu, S.: Automatic segmentation of seven retinal layers in SDOCT images congruent with expert manual segmentation. Opt. Express **18**(18), 19413–19428 (2010). https://doi.org/10.1364/OE.18.019413
7. Dijkstra, E.W.: A note on two problems in connexion with graphs. Numer. Math. **1**(1), 269–271 (1959)
8. Dodo, B.I., Li, Y., Eltayef, K., Liu, X.: Graph-cut segmentation of retinal layers from OCT images. In: Proceedings of the 11th International Joint Conference on Biomedical Engineering Systems and Technologies. BIOIMAGING, vol. 2, pp. 35–42. INSTICC, SciTePress (2018). https://doi.org/10.5220/0006580600350042
9. Dodo, B.I., Li, Y., Liu, X.: Retinal OCT image segmentation using fuzzy histogram hyperbolization and continuous max-flow. In: 2017 IEEE 30th International Symposium on Computer-Based Medical Systems (CBMS), pp. 745–750. IEEE (2017)
10. Ford, L.R., Fulkerson, D.R.: Maximal flow through a network. J. Can. de mathématiques **8**, 399–404 (1956). https://doi.org/10.4153/CJM-1956-045-5
11. Garvin, M.K., Abràmoff, M.D., Wu, X., Russell, S.R., Burns, T.L., Sonka, M.: Automated 3-D intraretinal layer segmentation of macular spectral-domain optical coherence tomography images. IEEE Trans. Med. Imaging **28**(9), 1436–1447 (2009). https://doi.org/10.1109/TMI.2009.2016958
12. Haeker, M., Wu, X., Abràmoff, M., Kardon, R., Sonka, M.: Incorporation of regional information in optimal 3-D graph search with application for intraretinal layer segmentation of optical coherence tomography images. In: Karssemeijer, N., Lelieveldt, B. (eds.) IPMI 2007. LNCS, vol. 4584, pp. 607–618. Springer, Heidelberg (2007). https://doi.org/10.1007/978-3-540-73273-0_50
13. Huang, D., et al.: Optical coherence tomography. Sci. (New York, N.Y.) **254**(5035), 1178–1181 (1991). https://doi.org/10.1126/science.1957169
14. Kaba, D., et al.: Retina layer segmentation using kernel graph cuts and continuous max-flow. Opt. Express **23**(6), 7366–7384 (2015). https://doi.org/10.1364/OE.23.007366
15. Kolmogorov, V., Zabih, R.: What energy functions can be minimized via graph cuts? IEEE Trans. Pattern Anal. Mach. Intell. **26**(2), 147–159 (2004). https://doi.org/10.1109/TPAMI.2004.1262177
16. Koozekanani, D., Boyer, K., Roberts, C.: Retinal thickness measurements from optical coherence tomography using a Markov boundary model. IEEE Trans. Med. Imaging **20**(9), 900–916 (2001). https://doi.org/10.1109/42.952728
17. Lang, A., et al.: Retinal layer segmentation of macular OCT images using boundary classification. Biomed. Opt. Express **4**(7), 1133–1152 (2013). https://doi.org/10.1364/BOE.4.001133

18. Lu, S., Yim-liu, C., Lim, J.H., Leung, C.K.S., Wong, T.Y.: Automated layer segmentation of optical coherence tomography images. In: Proceedings - 2011 4th International Conference on Biomedical Engineering and Informatics, BMEI 2011, vol. 1, no. 10, pp. 142–146 (2011). https://doi.org/10.1109/BMEI.2011.6098329
19. Novosel, J., Vermeer, K.A., Thepass, G., Lemij, H.G., Vliet, L.J.V.: Loosely coupled level sets for retinal layer segmentation in optical coherence tomography. In: IEEE 10th International Symposium on Biomedical Imaging, pp. 998–1001 (2013)
20. Salazar-Gonzalez, A., Kaba, D., Li, Y., Liu, X.: Segmentation of the blood vessels and optic disk in retinal images. IEEE J. Biomed. Health Inform. 18(6), 1874–1886 (2014)
21. Salazar-Gonzalez, A., Li, Y., Liu, X.: Automatic graph cut based segmentation of retinal optic disc by incorporating blood vessel compensation. J. Artif. Intell. Soft Comput. Res. 2(3), 235–245 (2012)
22. Salazar-Gonzalez, A.G., Li, Y., Liu, X.: Retinal blood vessel segmentation via graph cut. In: International Conference on Control Automation Robotics and Vision, pp. 225–230 (2010)
23. Seheult, A., Greig, D., Porteous, B.: Exact maximum a posteriori estimation for binary images. J. R. Stat. Soc. 51(2), 271–279 (1989)
24. Tian, J., Varga, B., Somfai, G.M., Lee, W.H., Smiddy, W.E., DeBuc, D.C.: Real-time automatic segmentation of optical coherence tomography volume data of the macular region. PLoS ONE 10(8), 1–20 (2015). https://doi.org/10.1371/journal.pone.0133908
25. Tizhoosh, H.R., Krell, G., Michaelis, B.: Locally adaptive fuzzy image enhancement. In: Reusch, B. (ed.) Fuzzy Days 1997. LNCS, vol. 1226, pp. 272–276. Springer, Heidelberg (1997). https://doi.org/10.1007/3-540-62868-1_118
26. Wang, C., Kaba, D., Li, Y.: Level set segmentation of optic discs from retinal images. J. Med. Syst. 4(3), 213–220 (2015)
27. Zhang, Y.-J. (ed.): ICIG 2015. LNCS, vol. 9217. Springer, Cham (2015). https://doi.org/10.1007/978-3-319-21978-3
28. Wang, C., Wang, Y., Li, Y.: Automatic choroidal layer segmentation using Markov random field and level set method. IEEE J. Biomed. Health Inform. 21, 1694–1702 (2017)
29. Yuan, J., Bae, E., Tai, X.C., Boykov, Y.: A study on continuous max- flow and min-cut approaches. In: 2010 IEEE Conference, vo. 7, pp. 2217–2224 (2010)

An Optimized Method for 3D Body Scanning Applications Based on KinectFusion

Faraj Alhwarin[✉], Stefan Schiffer, Alexander Ferrein, and Ingrid Scholl

Mobile Autonomous Systems and Cognitive Robotics Institute (MASCOR),
FH Aachen University of Applied Sciences, Aachen, Germany
{alhwarin,s.schiffer,ferrein,scholl}@fh-aachen.de
http://www.mascor.fh-aachen.de

Abstract. KinectFusion is a powerful method for 3D reconstruction of indoor scenes. It uses a Kinect camera and tracks camera motion in real-time by applying ICP method on successive captured depth frames. Then it merges depth frames according their positions into a 3D model. Unfortunately the model accuracy is not sufficient for body scanner applications because the sensor depth noise affects the camera motion tracking and deforms the reconstructed model. In this paper we introduce a modification of the KinectFusion method for specific 3D body scanning applications. Our idea is based on the fact that, most body scanners are designed so that the camera trajectory is a fixed circle in the 3D space. Therefore each camera position can be determined as a rotation angle around a fixed axis (rotation axis) passing through a fixed point (rotation center). Because the rotation axis and the rotation center are always fixed, they can be estimated offline while filtering out depth noise through averaging many depth frames. The rotation angle can be also precisely measured by equipping the scanner motor with an angle sensor.

Keywords: Specified KinectFusion · Body scanner · 3D reconstruction

1 Introduction

3D reconstruction is one of the fundamental challenging problems in computer vision and computer graphics, which is faced in many fields including robotics, 3D scanning and virtual reality. The 3D reconstruction is usually achieved by registering 2D projections of the scene captured from different points of view by a moving camera or a set of static cameras. In general, 3D reconstruction involves two problems to be solved: depth recovery from 2D images and camera motion tracking. If the 2D images overlap and the relative camera positions are known, the scene depth can be recovered using multi view stereo (MVS) techniques [1,2]. For camera motion tracking, the camera has to move slightly or it must have a sufficient frame rate to guarantee overlapping of successive captured images. The relative motion from frame to frame can then be estimated

© Springer Nature Switzerland AG 2019
A. Cliquet jr. et al. (Eds.): BIOSTEC 2018, CCIS 1024, pp. 100–113, 2019.
https://doi.org/10.1007/978-3-030-29196-9_6

by using structure from motion (SfM) techniques [3,4]. Bundle adjustment or pose graph optimization are usually used to refine camera motion tracking [5,6].

Generally, 3D reconstruction can be realized by combining SfM and MVS. Once the relative camera poses are determined, recovered depth frames are transformed according to their poses and merged together into a common 3D volume to generate a 3D model of the scene.

Based on the density of image features used for camera motion estimation and depth recovering, 3D reconstruction methods can be typically classified into two main classes: *sparse* and *dense* reconstruction.

In the case of sparse reconstruction, camera motion and/or depth recovery are estimated by comparing many of the local features extracted from the images. Therefore, the quality of the reconstructed model depends on the quality and distinctiveness of used features and in turn depends on the texture content of the scene. Furthermore, the model is incomplete and of poor quality.

Even though sparse methods such as Monocular SLAM [7,8] are successfully used in robotic applications, e.g. for self-localisation, mapping and collision avoidance, they are completely unsuitable for 3D scanning applications.

Dense reconstruction methods usually start with matching sparse features to compute relative camera positions. Then the depth of all image points computed by dense stereo vision [9,10] or provided by a 3D imaging sensor like Kinect camera [11,12] are used to refine camera motion tracking using bundle adjustment.

Although it is possible to reconstruct the scene completely using dense approaches, but they are impractical for 3D scanning applications because, firstly the quality of the model is unacceptable due to the accumulation of errors while camera motion tracking, and secondly the processing time is extremely excessive.

Using the KinectFusion method [13,14], it is possible to determine camera motion from depth images such as those from a Kinect sensor by Microsoft in real time and simultaneously create a 3D model of the scene by integrating depth information into a truncated signed distance function (TSDF) volume. Using the Iterative Closest Point (ICP) method, correspondences in 3D point clouds are found and used for camera motion tracking. In contrast to other 3D reconstruction methods that track camera movement from frame to frame, KinectFusion tracks camera motion from frame to model increasing the reliability of tracking, since depth noise is reduced while reconstructing model by averaging of all previous depth frames. In KinectFusion, finding correspondences, estimating camera motion and generating 3D model can be parallelized efficiently on GPU hardware, which makes it real-time adaptable.

Generally, KinectFusion suffers from two main weaknesses. The first point is that the camera motion tracking requires the scene to be rich in asymmetrical geometric shapes. Otherwise the registration procedure can not converge to a unique solution. For example, the motion of a camera can not be tracked if it moves in parallel to a plane or rotates around a spherical or cylindrical surface. The other weakness is because of the depth noise of the Kinect camera, which ranges in ± 5 mm. The depth noise affects the camera motion tracking and in turn degrades the quality of reconstructed 3D model.

Recently, many methods have been proposed to extend KinectFusion. [15] extended the KinectFusion algorithm to work with multiple sensors simultaneously. [16] extended the KinectFusion method by visual odometry to avoid camera motion tracking failure at regions of low geometric features. In [17] KinectFusion is modified to enhance 3D reconstruction of non-rigid objects. In [18], KinectFusion was improved by running scanning process twice. In the first run, the circular trajectory of the camera is estimated. In the second run, the model is constructed while correcting depth data using the estimated camera trajectory. [19] improved KinectFusion by using graph based-optimization to refine sensor pose estimation. In [20], the authors proposed a method to optimize KinectFusion for a 3D body scanner by simplifying camera motion tracking assuming that camera moves on a circle around the object to be scanned. The camera motion tracking was split in two steps: firstly, the scanner was calibrated offline by estimating the circle center and circle axis while averaging depth errors, and secondly, the ICP method was modified to determine camera location on the circle by estimating a rotation angle. As a result, the quality of reconstructed model by this method was enhanced when compared to the original KinectFusion method, because depth noise impact was limited on rotation angle.

In this paper we introduce an approach to further improve on the method proposed in [20]. Our contribution is twofold: We first propose a novel procedure for accurate calibration of the body scanner using a precise 3D model of a display dummy. Second, we eliminate the influence of depth noise on rotation angle by equipment of the body scanner with a rotary encoder to directly measure rotation angle (dispensing with the ICP based rotation angle estimation).

The rest of paper is organized as follows. In the next Sect. 2 the KinectFusion method is presented briefly. In Sect. 3, we present our method in detail. In Sect. 4, we evaluate our method by comparing it to the KinectFusion method. Finally, we conclude the paper in Sect. 5.

2   KinectFusion Algorithm

KinectFusion algorithm, introduced in [13, 14] is considered as a quantum leap in the field of 3D reconstruction. It is the first algorithm that allows the 3D reconstruction of an indoor scene and generates a 3D model with fairly good quality in real time. As its name implies, KinectFusion uses a Kinect camera and fuses depth frames into a 3D volumetric data structure after estimating their relative positions.

The main novelty of KinectFusion is the way how to track camera motion. Unlike all the other 3D reconstruction methods that track camera motion frame-by-frame, KinectFusion tracks camera motion from frame to model; it compares the last frame with a 3D model that includes all previous frames. This technique for camera motion tracking greatly improves the quality of the model because it eliminates the accumulation of errors completely.

As presented in [13], KinectFusion consists of four main steps: (1) Surface measurement, (2)surface reconstruction update, (3) surface prediction and (4) sensor pose estimation. In first step, a 3D surface is computed from the raw depth data and the intrinsic parameter of the camera, and represented as vertex and normal maps. Before computing 3D surface, a bilateral filter is applied on the raw depth image to reduce depth noise while keeping depth edges fairly sharp. In the second step, the computed surface is used to update reconstructed 3D model. The computed 3D surface is transformed to a global reference coordinate system and integrated into 3D volumetric data structure called truncated signed distance function (TSDF) by averaging it with all previous surfaces. In the third step, a 3D surface is predicted by rendering TSDF volume into a virtual camera, and represented by predicted vertex and normal maps. The predicted vertex and normal maps are used in the last step to estimate sensor pose by registering them to current computed surface. While sensor pose estimation, it is assumed that camera slightly moves, which allows the use of fast projective data association method [21] and point-plane metric [22].

3   Optimized Body Scanner

As mentioned above, most of 3D scanners are designed so that the sensor trajectory is a fixed circle surrounding the object to be scanned. In general, the sensor pose relative to a reference coordinate system, is given by a 6 DoF transformation. This transformation consists of 6 parameters (3 parameters for rotation and 3 for displacement) that have to be determined to estimate the sensor pose. In original KinectFusion algorithm, ICP method is used to estimate these parameters using depth data of successive images. Because the depth data of Kinect sensor is highly noisy, all the transformation parameters will be affected.

Considering that the sensor moves on a fixed circle while scanning, the sensor pose can be split into three parameters: (1) a 3D vector to describe the circle axis, (2) a 3D vector to describe the circle center and (3) an angle determining the sensor position on the circle. Therefore, the sensor pose estimation process can be done in two steps: First calibrate the body scanner by determining the axis and center vectors, and second estimate the rotation angle. Since the axis and the center of rotation are fixed as long as the scanner setup is not changed, they can be estimated offline by averaging many depth frames, which leads to reduce depth noise effects on them significantly.

Once the axis and center vectors are precisely determined, the sensor pose is reduced to one parameter (rotation angle) that can be measured directly by a rotary encoder.

Body Scanner Calibration. In this context we mean with scanner calibration, the determination of the axis and the center of rotation that define the scanner set-up. In order to calibrate the scanner, we use a display dummy and its 3D model (see Fig. 1(a)), which is precisely reconstructed by a laser scanner with a precision of 0.1 mm. To start the calibration process, the dummy is placed in

front of the camera and then we capture a depth image that can be converted
to a point cloud as shown in Fig. 1(b). After that we align the point cloud to the
3D model of the dummy using ICP method to get an initial transformation that
determine the initial camera position relative to the dummy position. Figure 1
shows the 3D model and the point cloud captured by Kinect camera and the
alignment of 3D model and the point cloud.

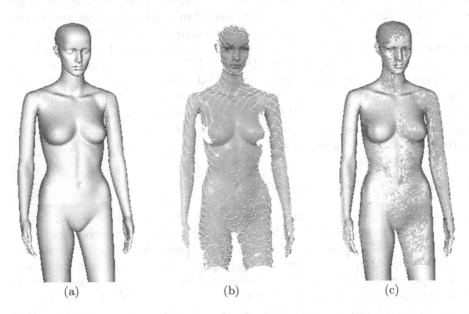

(a)   (b)   (c)

Fig. 1. Body scanner calibration using 3D model of display dummy: (a) 3D model of
used dummy (b) Point cloud captured using Kinect camera (c) registering point cloud
to 3D model to determine the camera position.

After that we start rotating the camera around the dummy. At each captured
depth frame, we register the point cloud to the 3D model of the dummy using
ICP method and we get a transformation that describe the pose of the camera
in current frame. Assuming that the initial position of the camera in the first
frame (reference frame) is in the origin, so we can calculate the positions of the
camera in other frames by transforming the origin point with the corresponding
transformation. As a result, we get a series of 3D points that determine the
locations of the camera during the rotation around the dummy. These points
form together a circular point cloud. Using RANSAC method, a circle can be
estimated by fitting a circle through the circular point cloud. Figure 2(b) shows
the camera trajectory computed during scanner calibration.

The parameters of this circle determine the center and axis of the scanner
and they do not change as long as the set-up of the scanner is not changed. Once
the scanner is precisely calibrated, the camera pose is defined by only a rotation
angle, instead of a 6DoF transformation as it is in general case.

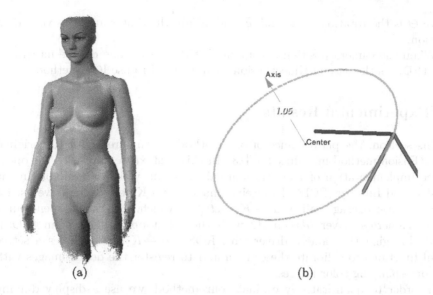

(a)   (b)

Fig. 2. Body scanner calibration using 3D model of display dummy: (a) some point clouds of Kinect camera registered to dummy model and merged to gather, (b) camera trajectory computed while scanner calibration.

Determination of Rotation Angle. To determine the rotation angle, the scanner motor is equipped with an angle sensor (incremental rotary encoder), which can provide the angular position of the motor with a precision of $360 \cdot 10^{-6}$. The rotary encoder is driven by an Arduino board and a pulse counter. The pulse counter is used to count the pulses generated by the sensor and the number of pulses is passed to Arduino board by Serial Peripheral Interface (SPI) bus. To communicate with the Arduino, we use the ROS-Serial package. ROS-Serial manages the communication with Arduino via USB port and allows receiving and sending data messages by ROS publish/subscribe mechanism. Using ROS-Serial, the angular position of the motor can be published onto a ROS topic. To obtain the camera rotation angle we need to synchronize the image capturing with the output of the angle sensor.

ROS provides a message filters package which collects commonly used message filtering algorithms including the time synchronizer filter. Time synchronizer filter takes in messages of different types from multiple sources, and outputs them only if they are received with the same time stamp.

In this paper, we used the time synchronizer filter to synchronize motor angle messages and Kinect depth image messages to determine the rotation angle for each captured depth frame.

Once the motor angle at a depth frame is measured, we can compute the camera position at that frame directly:

$$P = T(\overrightarrow{c}) * R(\Theta, \overrightarrow{a}) * T^{-1}(\overrightarrow{c}) \tag{1}$$

where Θ is the rotation angle and $\vec{c}$ and $\vec{a}$ are the center and axis vectors of rotation.

When the camera position is computed, the depth frame can be integrated into TSDF as the case of KinectFusion without need to use ICP method.

4   Experimental Results

In this section, the performance of our method is compared with the original KinectFusion method introduced in [13]. In this context we have used the open-source implementation of KinectFusion called Kinfu, which is available in the Point Cloud Library (PCL). To receive images from Kinect camera, we used a ROS software package called $iai - Kinect$ [23], which bridges the open-source Kinect camera's driver $libreenect2$ with the robot operating system (ROS). Beside bridging the camera driver with ROS, $iai - Kinect$ includes a set of useful functions to calibrate the camera and to register the depth images with the corresponding color images.

In order to quantitatively evaluate our method, we use a display dummy which simulates the human body as shown in Fig. 1(a). For a comparative reference, the dummy was scanned by a laser scanner to generate a 3D model with a precision of 0.1 mm.

To compare our method with the KinectFusion, a Kinect camera is rotated around the dummy and depth images taken in rate of 500 images in full rotation is stored and then a 3D model of the dummy is reconstruct by estimating camera positions at each image frame and merging these images with each other in a common volume (TSDF). The camera positions are estimated by KinectFusion using ICP method, whereas in our method they are directly computed from the scanner set-up parameters (axis and center of rotation) and the measured rotation angle as given in Eq. 1. To measure the rotation angle, an incremental rotary encoder is mounted to the scanner motor and connected to an Arduino micro-controller, which can publish the rotation angle on the ROS network using ROS-Serial package. To get the location of the camera at each depth frame, the ROS synchronizer filter is used to synchronize depth image messages with angle sensor messages to determine the camera locations.

In Fig. 3 we present the results obtained by scanning the dummy. In the odd rows, the meshes obtained using the KinectFusion are presented by images projected from the four sides and the even rows show the corresponding images projected from the meshes obtained by our method. Corresponding meshes are reconstructed from the same depth images and at the same merging parameters (TSDF volume size and truncated threshold).

By comparing meshes at each pair of rows, it is clear how much improvement we have achieved by our method. To illustrate the difference between the meshes we compare them separately with the reference model of the dummy. For this purpose we first register each mesh with the reference model and then calculate the point-to-point distances (distances between each point on the mesh and the nearest point on the reference model). In Fig. 4, these distances are represented

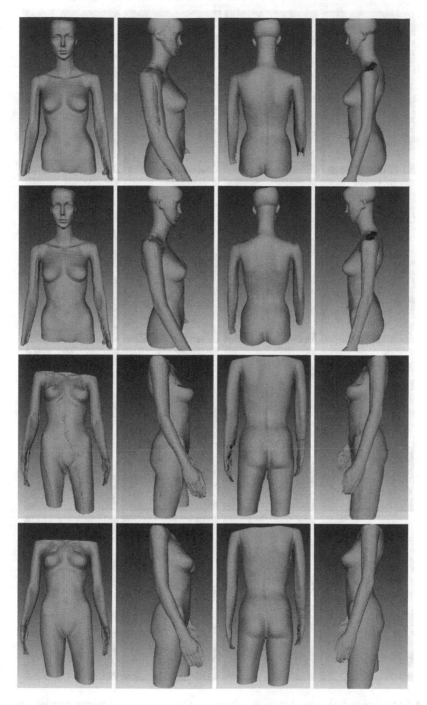

Fig. 3. 3D model of the display dummy obtained by KinectFusion (odd rows) and by our method (even rows).

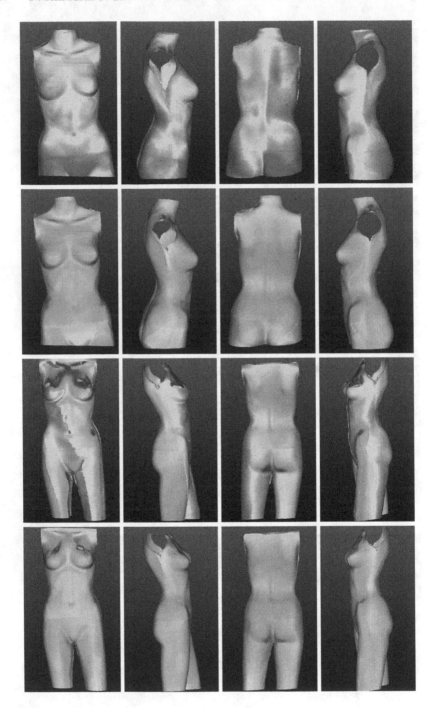

Fig. 4. The point-to-point distances between the dummy reference model and the meshes obtained by KinectFusion (odd rows) and our method (even rows), visualized by color scale. (Color figure online)

by color scale (from blue at negative distances, via green when mesh and reference model are matched and till red at positive distances). As shown from this figure, the improvement we have achieved is more evident. In this experiment we excluded the arms and the head of the dummy from comparison because these parts are movable and we do not know their positions precisely as they are in the 3D model.

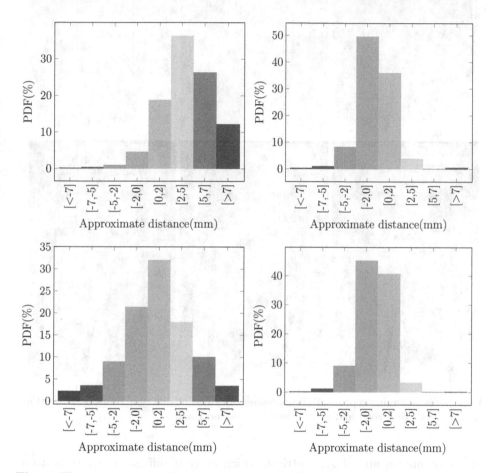

Fig. 5. The point-to-point distances between the dummy reference model and the meshes obtained by KinectFusion (left column) and our method (right column), represented by histograms.

For further explanation, we present these distances by distance histograms as shown in Fig. 5. Through these histograms, we notice that the histograms of the KinectFusion meshes are shifted to the right and this means that the mesh is larger than the reference model. The reason for this is that, while ICP executing, the compared surfaces are slipped on each other because the surface

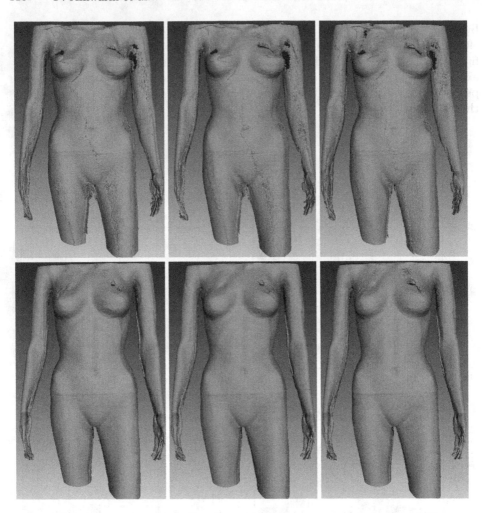

Fig. 6. The scanning reproducibility: Meshes obtained at different times by KinectFusion method (first row) and by our method (second row).

of the dummy is almost symmetrical, which make it difficult to converge to a unique solution. In addition, it is evident that a large percentage of the points have distances greater than a 2 mm. For the meshes obtained by our method, we observe that the histograms are centered around zero (which means no scaling effect is occurred) and the most points have distances of less than 2 mm.

Another advantage gained by our method is the ability to generate models with high reproducibility, unlike KinectFusion method which each time generates different models of the same object. The reason for this is that using KinectFusion, the camera motion tracking is affected by the depth noise, which changes from one frame to another. While using our method, the noise effect on camera motion tracking is neutralized by filtering the depth noise during the

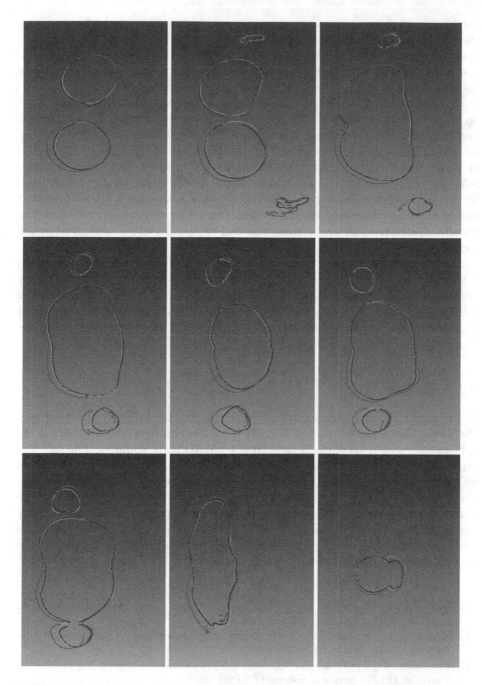

Fig. 7. The 2D views of some slices made along the reference model and meshes to be compared, after registering them together. In each slice (green line comes from reference model while red and blue lines come from KinectFusion and our method respectively. (Color figure online)

calculation of the scanner setup on one hand, and on other hand by replacing the ICP-based camera motion tracking by camera position computation through measuring rotation angle. Figure 6 shows how the model obtained by KinectFusion changes from time to time as it is in the top row, while the bottom row shows the model obtained by our method is fairly constant.

In order to highlight how the model is distorted when using KinectFusion, we do the following experiment. We create models for the dummy by our method and KinectFusion, then we register them with the reference model and then we do a number of cross slices along the model. Some of these slices are shown in Fig. 7. In each slice we get three closed lines. The green line comes from the reference model whereas the blue and red lines come from the meshes constructed by our and KinectFusion respectively. By comparing these lines, it is evident that our method has decreased the distortions caused by depth noise effect on the camera motion tracking and hence enhanced the quality of reconstructed model significantly.

As a future proposal to improve the quality of our method we will design a hardware synchronizer that can synchronize the output signal of the rotary encoder with the image capture mechanism so that we can dispense with the ROS synchronizer filter and compute the camera positions with high accuracy. Therefore we expect to improve the performance of KinectFusion-based scanner significantly.

5   Conclusions

In this paper, we presented a method for optimizing the body scanner that uses the KinectFusion algorithm. The KinectFusion was specified considering that the camera moves on a 3D circle in most (if not all) 3D body scanners. The axis and center of this circle determine the set-up of the scanner and can be estimated offline by averaging many depth frames. This filters out the depth noise and eliminates its effect on these circle parameters. Once the axis and center of the scanner are determined, the camera pose can be computed by measuring only one rotation angle with a rotary encoder. Thanks to this specification, the depth noise impact on the sensor pose estimation was significantly reduced and the quality of reconstructed 3D models was improved.

References

1. Furukawa, Y., Ponce, J.: Accurate, dense, and robust multi-view stereopsis. In: IEEE Computer Society (CVPR) (2007)
2. Hernández, C., Vogiatzis, G., Cipolla, R.: Probabilistic visibility for multi-view stereo. In: IEEE Computer Society (CVPR) (2007)
3. W. Changchang, W.: Towards linear-time incremental structure from motion. In: International Conference 3D Vision, pp. 127–134 (2013)
4. Moulon, P., Monasse, P., Marlet, R.: Global fusion of relative motions for robust, accurate and scalable structure from motion. In: Proceedings of ICCV (2013)

5. Ni, K., Steedly, D., Dellaert, F.: Out-of-core bundle adjustment for large-scale 3D reconstruction (2007)
6. Yu, W., Zhang, H.: 3D reconstruction of indoor scenes based on feature and graph optimization. In: International Conference on Virtual Reality and Visualization (ICVRV) (2016)
7. Schoeps, T., Engel, J., Cremers, D.: Semi-dense visual odometry for AR on a smartphone. In: ISMAR (2014)
8. Davison, A.J., Reid, I.D., Molton, N., Stasse, O.: MonoSLAM: real-time single camera SLAM. IEEE Trans. Pattern Anal. Mach. Intell. **29**, 1052–1067 (2007)
9. Negre, P.L., Bonin-Font, F., Oliver, G.: Cluster-based loop closing detection for underwater SLAM in feature-poor regions. In: IEEE International Conference on Robotics and Automation (ICRA), pp. 2589–2595 (2016)
10. Engel, J., Stückler, J., Cremers, D.: Large-scale direct SLAM with stereo cameras. In: Proceedings of the IEEE International Conference on Intelligent Robots and Systems (IROS) (2015)
11. Kerl, C., Sturm, J., Cremers, D.: Dense visual SLAM for RGB-D cameras. In: Proceedings of the International Conference on Intelligent Robot Systems (IROS) (2013)
12. Fioraio, N., Di Stefano, L.: SlamDunk: affordable real-time RGB-D SLAM. In: Agapito, L., Bronstein, M.M., Rother, C. (eds.) ECCV 2014. LNCS, vol. 8925, pp. 401–414. Springer, Cham (2015). https://doi.org/10.1007/978-3-319-16178-5_28
13. Newcombe, R., et al.: KinectFusion: real-time dense surface mapping and tracking. In: Proceedings of IEEE International Symposium on Mixed and Augmented Reality (2011)
14. Izadi, S., et al.: KinectFusion: real-time 3D reconstruction and interaction using a moving depth camera. In: Proceedings of UIST, pp. 559–568 (2011)
15. Kainz, B., et al.: OmniKinect: real-time dense volumetric data acquisition and applications. In: VRST, pp. 25–32 (2012)
16. Whelan, T., Kaess, M., Fallon, M.F., Johannsson, H., Leonard, J.J., McDonald, J.: Kintinuous: spatially Extended KinectFusion. In: RSS Workshop on RGB-D: Advanced Reasoning with Depth Cameras (2012)
17. Afzal, H., et al.: Kinect deform: enhanced 3D reconstruction of non-rigidly deforming objects. In: 3DV (Workshops), pp. 7–13 (2014)
18. Pagliari, D., Menna, F., Roncella, R., Remondino, F., Pinto, L.: Kinect fusion improvement using depth camera calibration. In: The Technical Commission V Symposium Remote Sensing Spatial and Information Science, pp. 23–25 (2014)
19. Jia, S., Li, B., Zhang, G., Li, X.: Improved KinectFusion based on graph-based optimization and large loop model. In: IEEE International Conference on Information and Automation (ICIA) (2016)
20. Alhwarin, F., Schiffer, S., Ferrein, A., Scholl, I.: Optimized KinectFusion algorithm for 3D scanning applications. In: Proceedings of the 11th International Joint Conference on Biomedical Engineering Systems and Technologies (BIOIMAGING 2018) (2018)
21. Arya, S., Mount, D.M., Netanyahu, N.S., Silverman, R., Wu, A.Y.: Registering multiview range data to create 3D computer objects. IEEE Trans. Pattern Anal. Mach. Intell. (PAMI) **17**, 820–824 (1995)
22. Yang, C., Gerard, M.: Object modelling by registration of multiple range images. Image Vis. Comput. **10**, 145–155 (1992)
23. Wiedemeyer, T.: IAI Kinect2. Institute for Artificial Intelligence, University Bremen (2015). https://github.com/code-iai/iai_kinect2

Going Deeper into Colorectal
Cancer Histopathology

Francesco Ponzio, Enrico Macii, Elisa Ficarra, and Santa Di Cataldo[✉]

Politecnico di Torino, Corso Duca degli Abruzzi 24, 10129 Torino, Italy
{francesco.ponzio,enrico.macii,elisa.ficarra,santa.dicataldo}@polito.it

Abstract. The early diagnosis of colorectal cancer (CRC) traditionally leverages upon the microscopic examination of histological slides by
experienced pathologists, which is very time-consuming and rises many
issues about the reliability of the results. In this paper we propose using
Convolutional Neural Networks (CNNs), a class of deep networks that
are successfully used in many contexts of pattern recognition, to automatically distinguish the cancerous tissues from either healthy or benign
lesions. For this purpose, we designed and compared different CNN-based
classification frameworks, involving either training CNNs from scratch
on three classes of colorectal images, or transfer learning from a different
classification problem. While a CNN trained from scratch obtained very
good (about 90%) classification accuracy in our tests, the same CNN
model pre-trained on the ImageNet dataset obtained even better accuracy (around 96%) on the same testing samples, requiring much lesser
computational resources.

Keywords: Colorectal cancer · Histological image analysis ·
Convolutional Neural Networks · Deep learning · Transfer learning ·
Pattern recognition

1 Introduction

Colorectal carcinoma (CRC) is one of the most diffused cancers worldwide and
one of the leading causes of cancer-related death. Based on most recent epidemiological studies, this type of cancer is particularly frequent in the highly-developed
countries, especially Europe, and it is associated with very high mortality rates
compared to other tumors [9]. Hence, the early diagnosis and differentiation of
CRC is crucial for the survival and well-being of a large number of patients.

The primary diagnosis of CRC is traditionally performed by means of
colonoscopy, that is the endoscopic examination of the large and the distal part
of the small bowel. During this procedure, the surgeon will typically perform a
biopsy on the suspicious colorectal lesions, which implies the resection of a thin
sample of tissue for histopathological evaluation (see Fig. 1).

The samples, fixed and stained by means of Hematoxylin and Eosin (H&E),
are then visually examined by a pathologist, either directly under the microscope,

© Springer Nature Switzerland AG 2019
A. Cliquet jr. et al. (Eds.): BIOSTEC 2018, CCIS 1024, pp. 114–131, 2019.
https://doi.org/10.1007/978-3-030-29196-9_7

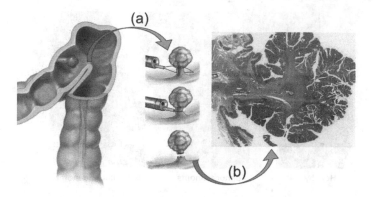

Fig. 1. Primary diagnosis of CRC. (a) Suspicious lesions and polyps are resected during colonoscopy. (b) The bioptic samples are fixated and stained (e.g. by H&E) to highlight tissue architecture.

or on a computer monitor. In the latter case, the physical slide is first digitalised by a scanner in the form of a so-called virtual slide or whole-slide-image (WSI), a very large multi-resolution zoomable image file, and then visualised on a screen by means of specific viewing software.

The presence and level of malignancy is assessed by observing the organisational changes in the tissues, which are highlighted by the two stains. As shown in Fig. 2, normal colon tissues have a well-defined organisation, with the epithelial cells forming glandular structures and the non-epithelial cells (i.e. stroma) lying in between these glands. The main benign precursor of CRC, adenoma, is characterised by enlarged, hyper-chromatic and elongated nuclei arranged in a typically stratified configuration, characterised by either tubular or villous (finger-like) tissue architecture. Adenocarcinomas, on the other hand, produce abnormal glands that infiltrate into the surrounding tissues.

Traditional visual examination has two major drawbacks, that are widely pointed out by literature. First, it is time-consuming, especially for large image datasets. Second, it is highly subjective, which translates into large variability, both inter and intra observer [2]. To solve these drawbacks, there are growing efforts towards the automatisation of the analysis flow and the development of computer-aided diagnostic techniques. The major directions of the research efforts were mainly two in the last few years: (i) automated segmentation, aimed at partitioning the heterogeneous colorectal samples into regions of interest that are homogeneous in terms of tissue architecture. (ii) automated classification, aimed at partitioning the homogeneous tissue regions into a number of histological categories, either normal or malignant, leveraging quantitative features extracted from the image. In both the tasks, the large intra-class image variability is the main challenge to be tackled. This work focuses on the automated classification task, targeting the three histological categories that are most relevant for CRC diagnosis: (i) healthy tissue, (ii) adenocarcinoma, (iii) tubulovillous adenoma (see Fig. 2).

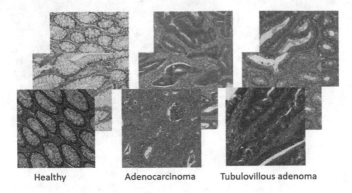

Healthy   Adenocarcinoma   Tubulovillous adenoma

Fig. 2. Examples of histological H&E images of colorectal tissues (cropped patches), respectively from healthy samples, adenocarcinoma and tubulovillous adenoma.

Recent literature on automated classification of histological images has been extensive not only on colon but also on brain, breast, prostate and lungs cancer applications. These works generally propose solutions based on automated texture analysis, where a limited set of local descriptors (for example, statistical features based on grey level co-occurrence matrix, GLCM, local binary patterns, LBP, Gabor and wavelet transforms, etc.) are computed from the input images and then fed into a classifier. The texture descriptors, eventually encoded into a compact dictionary of visual words, are used as input of machine learning techniques such as Support Vector Machines (SVM), Random Forests or Logistic Regression classifiers [4]. In spite of the good level of accuracy obtained by some of these works, the dependence on a fixed set of handcrafted features is a major limitation to the robustness of the classical texture analysis approaches. First, because it leverages upon a priori knowledge about the image characteristics that are best suited for classification, which is not obvious for all types of cancers. Second, because it puts severe constraints to the generalisation and transfer capabilities of the proposed classifiers, especially in the presence of inter-dataset variability.

As an answer to such limitations, deep learning (DL) architectures, and more specifically Convolutional Neural Networks (CNNs), have now become a major trend [6,7]. In CNNs a number of convolutional and pooling layers learn by backpropagation a set of features that are best for classification, thus avoiding the extraction of handcrafted texture descriptors. Nonetheless, the need of computational resources and the necessity of extensively training the networks with a huge number of independent samples are open issues in histopathology, and put limits to the usability of this approach in the everyday clinical setting. Transfer learning techniques (i.e applying CNNs pre-trained on a different type of images, for which large datasets are available) might be a promising solution to this problem [13], which deserves better investigations.

In this work, we apply a CNN-based approach to automatically differentiate healthy tissues and tubulovillous adenomas from cancerous samples, which is a challenging task in histological image analysis. For this purpose, we fully train a CNN on a large set of colorectal samples, and assess its accuracy on a completely independent test set. This technique is experimentally compared with two different transfer learning approaches, both leveraging upon a CNN pre-trained on a completely different classification problem. The first approach uses the pre-trained CNN to extract a set of discriminative features that will be fed into a separate SVM classifier. The second approach fine-tunes on CRC histological images only the last stages of the pre-trained CNN. By doing so, we investigate and discuss the transfer learning capabilities of CNNs in the domain of CRC classification.

This paper revises and extends [10]. In this version we provide a better introduction to histopathological image analysis, ameliorated pictorial representations of the proposed methodologies, as well as a new section on the visualisation and exploitation of the CNN outcome for CRC tissue classification.

2   Materials and Methods

2.1   Image Dataset

The dataset used in this study was extracted from a public repository of H&E stained whole-slide images (WSIs) of colorectal tissues, that can be freely downloaded from [1], together with their anonymised clinical information.

In order to obtain a statistically significant dataset in terms of inter-subjects and inter-class variability, we selected 27 WSIs, obtained from univocal subjects (i.e. one WSI per patient). As a WSI is typically very wide, it may contain different types of tissues (e.g. healthy and cancerous portions). Hence, the original WSI cannot be given a unique histological label. With the supervision of a pathologist, we identified on each WSI large regions of interest (ROIs) that are homogeneous in terms of tissue architecture (see example of Fig. 3). Hence, each ROI can be univocally associated to one out of the three tissue subtypes: (i) adenocarcinoma (AC); (ii) tubuvillous adenoma (TV) and (iii) healthy tissue (H). Then, the obtained ROIs were cropped into a total number of 13500 1089×1089 patches (500 per patient), at a 40x magnification level, without applying any data augmentation.

The original image cohort was randomly split into two disjoint subsets, one for training and one for testing purposes, respectively containing 9000 and 4500 patches. In order to ensure a complete independence of the two sets, the training and testing patches belong to different subjects. More specifically, 18 patients were used to generate the training patches, and 9 for the testing patches.

The random sampling was stratified, so that both the training and the testing set are balanced among the three classes of interest (H, AC and TV). Hence, the accuracy assessment was not affected by class prevalence.

Before being fed into the CNN, each patch was down sampled by a factor five, that was empirically set as a trade-off between computational burden of the processing and architectural detail of the images. To compensate for possible color inconsistencies, all the patches were normalised by mean and standard

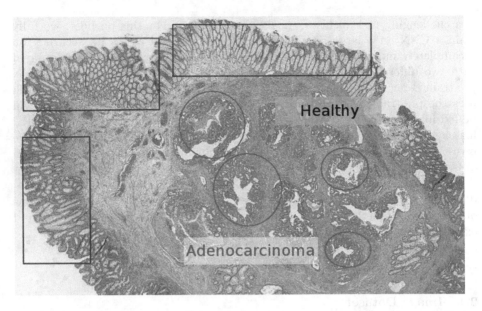

Fig. 3. Identification and annotation of homogeneous ROIs from a colorectal whole slide image (WSI).

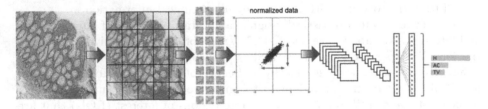

Fig. 4. CRC classification by means of CNN: schematic representation. Homogeneous ROIs are cropped into small non-overlapping patches, that are fed into the CNN after normalisation by mean and standard deviation on the training set. The output of the CNN is a probability map of the input patch into one three tissue classes: healthy, adenocarcinoma or tubulovillous adenoma.

deviation, computed over the whole training dataset. A pictorial representation of the patches preparation and classification process is shown in Fig. 4.

2.2   Convolutional Neural Network: Architecture and Training Paradigm

Convolutional Neural Networks (CNNs) consist of a sequence of multiple locally connected trainable stages, aimed at learning the image representation at a progressively increasing level of abstraction, and of two or more fully-connected layers as the last step, aimed at learning the class partitioning task like a traditional multi-layer perceptron.

The locally connected part of a CNN implements two main types of building blocks:

1. Convolutional (CONV) blocks basically act like kernel filters with trainable parameters, performing a 2D convolution operation on the input image. Based on the value of these parameters, a filter is able to detect different types of local patterns. After convolution, typically the stage applies a non-linear transfer function, such as Rectified Linear Unit (ReLU).
2. Pooling (POOL) blocks perform a non-linear down-sampling of the input, typically applying a max function. Down-sampling has the two-fold effect of reducing the number of parameters of the network that need to be learned (and hence of controlling overfitting), as well as of introducing space invariance into the image representation.

The higher the number of CONV and POOL layers in a CNN, the higher the depth of the network, and the higher the level of detail that can be achieved by the hierarchical representation of the image. Hence, deeper networks are usually able to achieve much better classification performance that their shallow counterparts. Nonetheless, a higher depth also translates into a higher number of parameters that need to be learned, and hence into a much higher computational cost of the training process.

The training paradigm of the CNN is usually a classic backpropagation scheme: that is, an iterative process involving multiple passes of the whole input dataset until convergence of the optimisation algorithm. At each training step, the whole dataset flows from the first to the last layer in order to compute a classification error, quantified by a loss function. Such error flows backward through the net, and at each training step the model parameters (i.e. the weights of the network) are tuned in the direction that minimises the classification error on the training data.

In our work we used a VGG16 CNN model [12], that ensured the best compromise between representation capabilities (and hence, depth) and computational costs of the training. The model is schematically reported in Fig. 5.

VGG16 model was successfully applied to a large number of computer vision tasks. In spite of its large depth (16 layers, including convolutional and fully-connected stages), its architecture is very simple and repetitive. More specifically, the model consists of a linear sequence of 13 3×3 CONV layers, that can be conceptually grouped into 5 macro-blocks, each ending with a 2×2 POOL, and of 3 fully-connected (FC) layers as final classification stage. All the non-linearities are ReLU, except for the last fully-connected layer (FC3), that is a softmax activation function. The convolution stride and the padding are fixed to 1 pixel and the max pooling stride to 2. Differently from the original VGG16 model, we modified the architecture by implementing a final FC3 stage of 3 units, matching the number of categories targeted by our research problem. The output values of this final stage can be interpreted as the probability of the input patch belonging respectively to the healthy, the adenocarcinoma or the tubulovillous adenoma class.

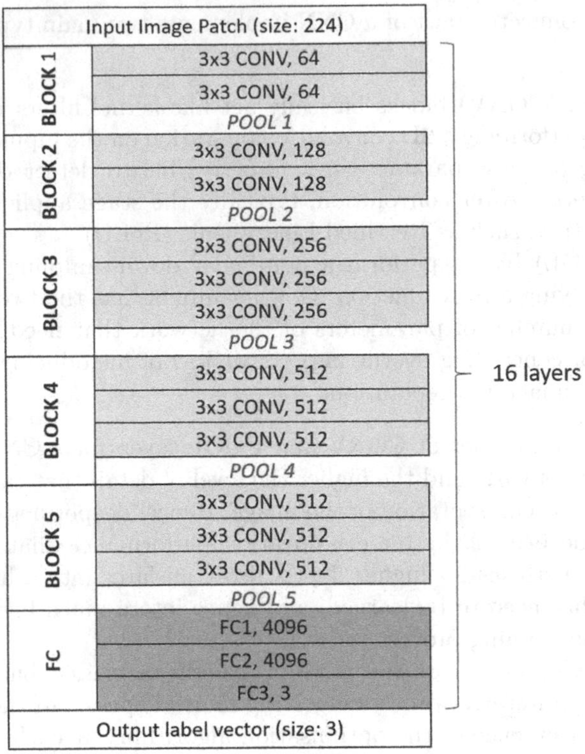

Input Image Patch (size: 224)
BLOCK 1 3x3 CONV, 64
3x3 CONV, 64
POOL 1
BLOCK 2 3x3 CONV, 128
3x3 CONV, 128
POOL 2
BLOCK 3 3x3 CONV, 256
3x3 CONV, 256
3x3 CONV, 256
POOL 3
BLOCK 4 3x3 CONV, 512
3x3 CONV, 512
3x3 CONV, 512
POOL 4
BLOCK 5 3x3 CONV, 512
3x3 CONV, 512
3x3 CONV, 512
POOL 5
FC FC1, 4096
FC2, 4096
FC3, 3
Output label vector (size: 3)

16 layers

Fig. 5. CNN architecture (VGG16 model).

The net was developed within Keras framework [3] and trained with a classic backpropagation paradigm. More specifically, we applied a stochastic gradient descent (SGD), implemented with a momentum update approach [11] as iterative optimisation algorithm to minimise the categorical cross-entropy function between the three classes of interest (H, AC and TV).

The monitoring of the training process and the optimisation of the hyperparameters of the net leverage upon 10% of the training set, that were appointed as independent validation data and excluded from the training per se. This validation set was solely used to compute the validation accuracy metric upon which the training process is optimised. Based on validation, we set the learning rate (LR) to 0.0001, the momentum (M) to 0.9 and the batch size (BS) to 32.

To reduce overfitting, the learning process implemented a *early stopping* strategy (i.e., the training is stopped when validation accuracy does not improve for 10 subsequent epochs), as well as a progressive reduction of LR each time the validation accuracy does not improve for 5 consecutive epochs [14].

The CNN was trained for 30 epochs on the training set, which lasted 8 h on Linux Infiniband-QDR MIMD Distributed Shared-Memory Cluster provided with single GPU (NVIDIA Tesla K40 - 12 GB - 2880 CUDA cores).

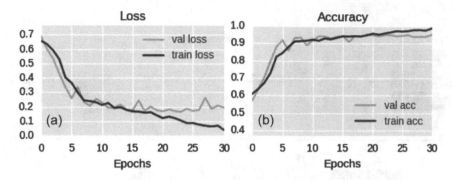

Fig. 6. Training vs validation loss per epoch (a) and training vs validation accuracy per epoch (b). Figure from [10].

As shown by the trend of loss and accuracy curves on both the training and validation datasets (see Fig. 6(a) and (b), respectively), the model converged quite quickly. Indeed, while training accuracy was still increasing, the value of validation accuracy saturated within 15 epochs. The decay speed of the validation loss curve indicates that the learning rate was appropriate. On top of that, validation and training accuracy were fairly similar. This reasonably rules out overfitting.

2.3 Transfer Learning from Pre-trained CNN

CNNs are cascades of trainable filter banks, where the first blocks of filters are devoted to the detection of low-level features (i.e. edges or simple shapes), and the following ones are activated by high-level semantic aggregations of the previous patterns, that are more problem-specific. Hence, while the top-most blocks are generally tailored to a specific classification task, the lower-level features can be ideally generalised to a large number of applications. This concept is at the basis of transfer learning techniques, that leverage CNNs pre-trained on a very large set of examples, with significant variability of image characteristics, to solve a different classification problem.

In our work, we used a pre-trained CNN model with the same architecture and topology of the one used for full training on colorectal cancer images (VGG16, shown in Fig. 5). The model was pre-trained on the ImageNet dataset, from the Large Scale Visual Recognition Challenge 2012 (ILSVRC-2012). This dataset contains 1.2 million photographs depicting 1000 different categories of natural objects. Hence, the training images are completely different from our specific target, in terms of imaging technology, image content as well as of number of categories of the classification problem.

Figure 7 shows two different transfer learning strategies that we implemented and compared:

(a) *CNN as a fixed feature generator.* The CRC patches are given as input to the pre-trained CNN only for inference. The output of the convolutional blocks

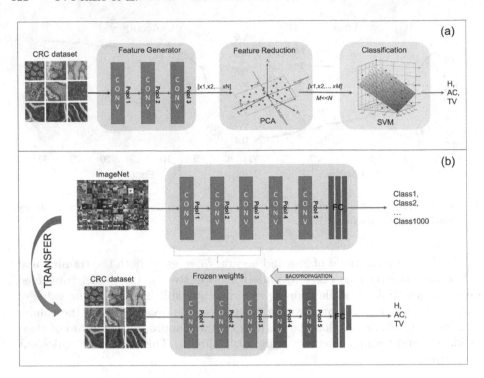

Fig. 7. Transfer learning approaches. (a) Pre-trained CNN as a fixed feature generator. (b) Fine tuning of pre-trained CNN. Figure from [10].

are fed into a separate machine learning framework, consisting of a feature reduction stage and a supervised classifier.

(b) *Fine-tuning the CNN.* The CNN model is re-trained on our training set of histological images, keeping all the parameters of the low-level blocks fixed to their initial value. Hence, only the weights of the top-most layers are fine-tuned for colorectal cancer classification.

As a preliminary step to both the two approaches, we analysed the discriminative capabilities of the features generated by all the major blocks of the pre-trained CNN, as follows. We randomly selected a small subset of the training images (500 per class) and fed them into the pre-trained CNN for inference. The output of each successive macro-block of the CNN was then analysed, to assess the degree of separation of samples belonging to the three different classes. As a trade-off between thoroughness and computational burden of the investigation, we analysed the intermediate output of the CNN only at the end of the pooling layers (i.e. POOL1 to 5, as represented Fig. 8). As POOL layers apply a dimensionality reduction operation, their output are expected to have lower redundancy compared to CONV layers.

The degree of class separation was assessed by means of t-Distributed Stochastic Neighbour Embedding (t-SNE) [8], a non-linear dimensionality reduc-

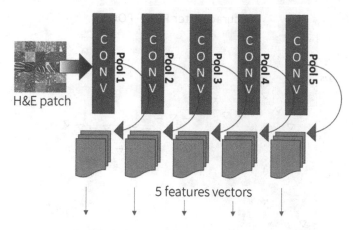

Evaluate class separability by means of t-SNE

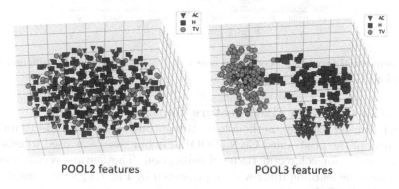

POOL2 features   POOL3 features

Fig. 8. Using the pre-trained CNN to generate discriminative features. The output of the five macro-blocks of the CNN are analysed by means of t-SNE, to assess the class separability obtained by each of the five feature vectors in a reduced 3-dimensional feature space. For example, features extracted from POOL3 (bottom-right) ensure much better class separation than features extracted from POOL2 (bottom-left).

tion algorithm that is used for the visualisation of high-dimensional datasets in a reduced 3-dimensional space. More specifically, t-SNE represents each high-dimensional object (in our case, the feature vector obtained at the output of a POOL layer) by means of a three-dimensional point in a Cartesian space, so that similar feature vectors are represented by nearby points and dissimilar vectors by distant points. The distance between different categories of points in the Cartesian space drawn by t-SNE provides a qualitative measure of class separability in the original feature space. Hence, by repeating the analysis for all the five feature vectors, we were able to establish which of the five POOL blocks ensures the best image representation for our specific classification problem (see the examples at the bottom of Fig. 8). In our experiments, POOL3 outperformed all the other blocks.

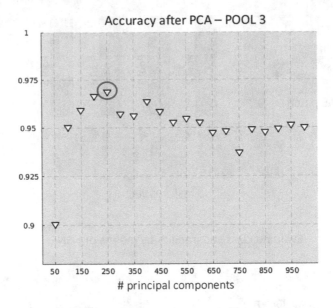

Fig. 9. Sequential forward procedure to select the optimal number of principal components for PCA. Figure from [10].

Pre-trained CNN as a Fixed Feature Generator

As a first transfer learning methodology, the output of the most discriminative POOL layer of the pre-trained CNN (POOL3, in our case) was used to generate a feature vector for colorectal tissue classification. The feature vector was fed into the machine learning framework represented by Fig. 7(a), that consists of a feature reduction followed by a classification step.

(a) *Feature Reduction.* To reduce further the dimensionality and redundancy of the data and prevent overfitting we applied Principal Component Analysis (PCA). PCA applies an orthogonal transformation of the original features into a reduced number of so-called principal components, that are linear combinations of the original characteristics. As PCA works towards the minimisation of the correlation between the features, the new descriptors are expected to be the most representative for the classes of interest. In our work, we empirically set the optimal number of principal component by implementing a sequential forward procedure. More specifically, we computed the mean classification accuracy on the training set at increasing number of principal components (step of 50) and selected the minimum number of principal components after which the classification accuracy had started decreasing. As shown in the graph of Fig. 9, this value was found to be 250).

(b) *Classification.* The final classification into the three categories of interest (H, AC, TV) was performed by a Support Vector Machine (SVM) with Gaussian radial basis function kernel. The hyper-parameters of the kernel were set by means of a Bayesian Optimisation (BO) algorithm [5], implementing a 10-fold cross-validation on the training images. In our preliminary experiments, BO was found to provide much better and faster results compared to classic methods based on grid search or heuristic techniques.

Fine-Tuning of Pre-trained CNN
As a second transfer learning methodology, we adapted the pre-trained VGG16 net to our specific classification task, using it as a standalone feature extractor and classifier. For this purpose, we first initialised all the weights of the network to the values learned on the ImageNet dataset, as represented in Fig. 7(b). Then, we started a backpropagation algorithm on our CRC dataset, keeping the weights of the first blocks of the net frozen. More specifically, we froze all the weights up-to the most discriminative pooling layer (POOL3), as determined by t-SNE. The rationale of this strategy is trying to maintain the low-level features, that are expected to describe the most generic and generalisable details (e.g. edges and simple shapes), as they were learned from the ImageNet. Hence, all the computational efforts can be focused on the top-most layers, which are expected to learn high-level task-specific features for colorectal image classification.

3 Results and Discussion

The classification accuracy was assessed on the colorectal dataset described in Sect. 2.1. As already pointed out, the test dataset is completely independent from the one used for training the network and optimising the classification parameters and it is balanced among the three categories of interest. The accuracy of the system was assessed at two different levels of abstraction (per patch and per patient, respectively). For this purpose, in [10] we introduced the following performance metrics.

(a) *Patch score: (S_P)*, defined as the fraction of patches of the test set that were correctly classified:
$$S_P = \frac{N_C}{N},$$
where N_C is the number of patches correctly classified and N the total number of patches in the test set.

(b) *Patient score: (S_{Pt})*, defined as the fraction of patches of a single patient that were correctly classified (i.e. *per-patient* patch score), averaged over all the patients in the test set:
$$S_{Pt} = \frac{\sum_i S_P(i)}{N_P},$$
where $S_P(i)$ is the patch score of the $i-th$ patient and N_P the total number of patients in the test set.

The patch and patient scores obtained for the three classification frameworks described in Sect. 2 are reported in Table 1. More specifically, in the first row (*full-train-CNN*) we report the values of the CNN fully trained on CRC samples. In the second row (*CNN+SVM*) we refer to the SVM, with pre-trained CNN used as fixed feature generator. Finally, in the last row (*fine-tune-CNN*) we quantify the accuracy of the pre-trained CNN with fine-tuning of the stages after POOL3. The first column of the table reports the patch score S_P, that is a value in $[0, 1]$ range, and the second column the patient score S_{Pt} as mean ± standard deviation.

Table 1. Patch and patient scores on the test set. Table from [10].

	S_P	S_{Pt}
full-train-CNN	0.9037	0.9022 (± 0.0155)
CNN+SVM:	0.9646	0.9667 (± 0.0082)
fine-tune-CNN	0.9682	0.9678 (± 0.00092)

From the values in Table 1 we can observe that all the proposed classification frameworks obtained very good accuracy (above 90%), both in terms of patch and patient scores. Hence, our experiments confirm the promising results obtained by CNNs in other contexts. The patch-wise accuracy (S_P) was very similar to the patient-wise accuracy (S_{Pt}), with a very small standard deviation of the latter value, suggesting a good robustness of the classification frameworks. Hence, the CNN-based classifiers cope well with inter-patient variability, that is a typical challenge of histopathological image analysis.

The same conclusions hold if we analyse the per-class accuracy values, that are reported in the form of 3×3 confusion matrices in Fig. 10. From such results we can easily gather that the performance of the classification frameworks was fairly homogeneous for the three classes of interest (H, AC and TV).

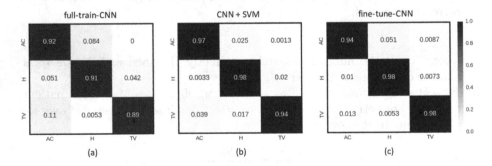

Fig. 10. Patch-wise confusion matrices for (a) CNN fully trained on CRC samples, (b) SVM with pre-trained CNN as fixed features generator, (c) pre-trained CNN with fine-tuning of the stages after POOL3 block. Figure from [10].

The most interesting point arising from our results is that both the transfer learning methodologies overcome the accuracy obtained by the CNN fully trained on colorectal samples by almost 7%. More specifically, the pre-trained CNN with fine-tuning of the blocks following POOL3 obtained the best accuracy values among all the tested methodologies. This is quite surprising, given that the dataset used for the training (i.e. ImageNet) was extremely different from the one used for testing the network.

From this result we can draw the following considerations.

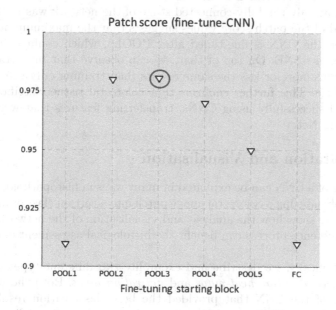

Fig. 11. Mean accuracy in relation to the first block till back-propagation is continued. Figure from [10].

Most probably, even though the full training seemed to converge well and without overfitting on the training images (see the graph in Fig. 6), our CRC training sample is not large enough to burst the generalisation capability of the CNN. The full training methodology works best only with a very large cohort of training examples, especially in the presence of very high inter-class variability. On the other hand, obtaining much larger training dataset is not always viable, especially in a clinical context.

In spite of the fact that the pre-training was performed on a completely different dataset (i.e. the ImageNet, which contains photographs of every-day objects and natural scenes, and not histological samples), the low-level features learned by the first stages of a CNN can be successfully generalised to the context of CRC image classification. Hence, as a matter of fact the CNNs are capable of extracting useful semantic knowledge from totally different domains. This partially avoids the computational problems and overfitting risks associated with full-training. Indeed, fine-tuning a pre-trained CNN took only two hours against the eight taken by full-training on the same hardware.

To investigate further on these findings, we run few additional experiments on fine-tuned CNNs by changing the starting block for the backpropagation algorithm. The results of this experiment are reported in Fig. 11, where we show the patch score obtained on the test set at different configurations of the fine-tuning. More specifically, $POOL$-i in the x-axis means that only the weights after the i-th POOL block were learned on the CRC training set, while all the rest of the parameters were frozen to the values learned on the ImageNet. Likewise, FC means that only the fully-connected stage of the network was re-trained.

The trend of the patch score values suggests that the maximum accuracy is reached when the CNN is fine-tuned after POOL3, which confirms the qualitative results of t-SNE. On top of that, we can observe that fully-training the network obtains more or less the same results than training only the last fully-connected stage. This further confirms that colorectal tissue classification can be performed successfully using CNNs, transferring features that were learned from the ImageNet.

4   Exploitation and Visualisation

The outcome of a CNN can be exploited in many ways in histopathology, that go beyond simply labeling a colorectal image patch into a certain class or another. In this section, we show how the analysis and visualisation of the network response during the inference process can benefit the histological assessment of colorectal images.

More specifically, we describe and exemplify two different types of visualisations, namely *attention heat-maps* and *activation maps*. Both the maps were built on top of the CNN that provided the best classification results in our experiments (i.e. a VGG16 model pre-trained on ImageNet and fine-tuned on colorectal samples).

As the name *attention heat-map* suggests, this map serves the specific purpose of driving the observer's attention towards the areas of the slide that mostly deserve it, i.e. the potentially cancerous ones. As we discussed is Sect. 2, the output layer of our CNN implements a three-dimensional softmax. Hence, when a histological image is given as input to the CNN, the value returned by each of the three output units can be interpreted as the probability of this image being a healthy tissue, adenocarcinoma, or tubulovillous adenoma, respectively. Taking this into consideration, we implemented a visualisation framework that exploits the value of the output unit associated to the adenocarcinoma class to generate the attention heat-map for CRC assessment, as follows. First, the input WSI is cropped into patches, and given as input to the CNN for inference. Then, by aggregating the CNN outcome of each patch, a heat-map of the same size of the input WSI is built, where the saturation of the red color in each pixel is proportional to the likelihood of cancer in that pixel, as predicted by the CNN. Hence, the most intensely red areas are the ones that should catch the pathologist's attention during the slide assessment. In Fig. 12 we show an example of such heat-map, where the input WSI is the same that was shown in Fig. 3.

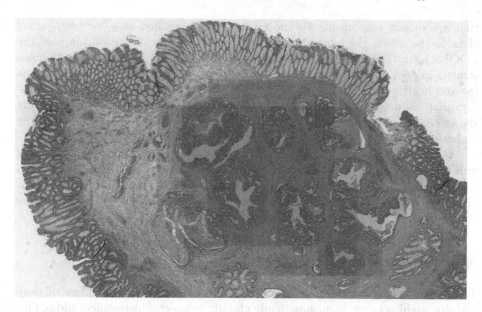

Fig. 12. *Attention heat-map* for colorectal cancer assessment. The intensity of the red color is proportional to cancer probability, as obtained from the CNN output layer.

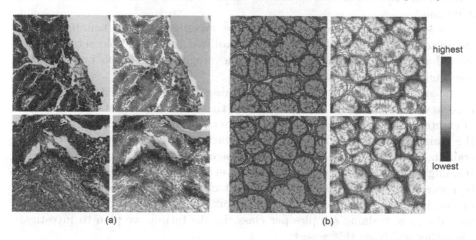

Fig. 13. *Activation maps* for (a) adenocarcinoma and (b) healthy colorectal patches. The colormap is proportional to the level of activation of the POOL3 layer (blue: lowest activation, red: highest activation). (Color figure online)

Besides the output stage of the CNN, even the hidden layers can be a very useful source of information. As discussed in Sect. 2, the hidden layers of the CNN are filter banks that are triggered by local patterns in the image. Hence, visually representing the response of such filters into so-called activation maps can provide interesting insights into the architectural characteristics of a tissue that are mostly responsible for the image being classified into one histological class or the other. For example, in Fig. 13 we show the activation maps of the POOL3 layer (i.e. the most class-discriminative of our CNN model, as demonstrated in Sect. 2), for input patches belonging respectively to adenocarcinoma (a) and healthy (b) class. More specifically, the color of each pixel in the activation maps is proportional to the level of activation of the POOL3 layer during the inference, with blue color associated to the lowest activation and red to the highest.

As we can easily gather from Fig. 13, POOL3 activation maps capture very well the dysplasia of the colonic glands in the adenocarcinomas (a). Very interestingly, the highest activations are actually localised where the dysplasya is more pronounced. On the other hand, the activation maps of the healthy slides (b) highlight the regularity of normal colonic glands.

5   Conclusions

This work leverages Convolutional Neural Networks, a powerful class of deep learning architectures, to automatically classify colorectal histological slides. Our specific target is the primary diagnosis of colorectal cancer. Hence, we address three main histological classes: healthy tissue, adenocarcinoma or tubulovillous adenoma.

To seek a solution to our problem, we investigated both training a CNN from scratch on a large dataset of pre-annotated images of colorectal samples, as well as transfer learning methodologies leveraging upon CNNs pre-trained on the ImageNet.

According to our experiments, full training obtained satisfactory results (i.e. accuracy in the order of 90%). Nonetheless, this solution was costly both in terms of computational resources as well of number of annotated samples required for the training. Quite surprisingly, transfer learning largely outperformed the full training approach, obtaining classification accuracy above 96% with much lesser training time. This proves that the low-level features learned by the CNNs can be successfully generalised to very different classification problems, such as colorectal image classification, and offers a promising solution to cases with limited availability of training samples per class. In the future, we plan to investigate more thoroughly on this aspect.

As we show in our work, besides classifying an input patch into a certain class or another, the outcome of a CNN can be exploited in many ways in clinics. The analysis and visualisation of the filters' response at different depth of the network, as well as of the probability map provided by the final softmax layer, provide useful insights into the patterns that most triggered the classification outcome, possibly guiding the pathologists towards local architectural alterations otherwise difficult to spot.

Acknowledgements. We thank the anonymous reviewers for their helpful suggestions.

References

1. Virtual pathology at the university of leeds (2018). http://www.virtualpathology. leeds.ac.uk/
2. Young, A., Hobbs, R., Kerr, D.: ABC of Colorectal Cancer, 2nd edn. Wiley, Hoboken (2011)
3. Chollet, F., et al.: Keras (2015). https://github.com/fchollet/keras
4. Di Cataldo, S., Ficarra, E.: Mining textural knowledge in biological images: applications, methods and trends. Comput. Struct. Biotechnol. J. **15**, 56–67 (2017). https://doi.org/10.1016/j.csbj.2016.11.002
5. Hastie, T., Tibshirani, R., Friedman, J.: Overview of supervised learning. In: Hastie, T., Tibshirani, R., Friedman, J. (eds.) The Elements of Statistical Learning. SSS, pp. 9–41. Springer, New York (2009). https://doi.org/10.1007/978-0-387-84858-7_2
6. Janowczyk, A., Madabhushi, A.: Deep learning for digital pathology image analysis: a comprehensive tutorial with selected use cases. J. Pathol. Inform. **7**(1), 29 (2016). https://doi.org/10.4103/2153-3539.186902
7. Korbar, B., et al.: Deep learning for classification of colorectal polyps on whole-slide images. J. Pathol. Inform. **8**, 30 (2017). https://doi.org/10.4103/jpi.jpi_34_17
8. Van der Maaten, L., Hinton, G.: Visualizing data using t-SNE. J. Mach. Learn. Res. **9**(Nov), 2579–2605 (2008)
9. Marley, A.R., Nan, H.: Epidemiology of colorectal cancer. Int. J. Mol. Epidemiol. Genet. **7**(3), 105–114 (2016)
10. Ponzio, F., Macii, E., Ficarra, E., Di Cataldo, S.: Colorectal cancer classification using deep convolutional networks - an experimental study. In: Proceedings of the 11th International Joint Conference on Biomedical Engineering Systems and Technologies, BIOIMAGING, vol. 2, pp. 58–66. INSTICC, SciTePress (2018). https://doi.org/10.5220/0006643100580066
11. Qian, N.: On the momentum term in gradient descent learning algorithms. Neural Netw. **12**(1), 145–151 (1999)
12. Simonyan, K., Zisserman, A.: Very deep convolutional networks for large-scale image recognition. arXiv preprint arXiv:1409.1556 (2014)
13. Weiss, K., Khoshgoftaar, T.M., Wang, D.: A survey of transfer learning. J. Big Data **3**(1), 9 (2016). https://doi.org/10.1186/s40537-016-0043-6
14. Yao, Y., Rosasco, L., Caponnetto, A.: On early stopping in gradient descent learning. Constr. Approx. **26**(2), 289–315 (2007)

A Convolutional Neural Network for Spot Detection in Microscopy Images

Matsilele Mabaso[1,3]([✉]), Daniel Withey[1], and Bhekisipho Twala[2]

[1] MDS(MIAS), Council for Scientific and Industrial Research,
Pretoria, South Africa
{MMabaso,DWithey}@csir.co.za
[2] Department of Electrical and Mining Engineering,
University of South Africa, Pretoria, South Africa
Twalab@unisa.ac.za
[3] Department of Electrical and Electronic Engineering Science,
University of Johannesburg, Auckland Park, South Africa

Abstract. This paper developed and evaluated a method for the detection of spots in microscopy images. Spots are subcellular particles formed as a result of biomarkers tagged to biomolecules in a specimen and observed via fluorescence microscopy as bright spots. Various approaches that automatically detect spots have been proposed to improve the analysis of biological images. The proposed spot detection method named, detectSpot includes the following steps: (1) A convolutional neural network is trained on image patches containing single spots. This trained network will act as a classifier to the next step. (2) Apply a sliding-window on images containing multiple spots, classify and accept all windows with a score above a given threshold. (3) Perform post-processing on all accepted windows to extract spot locations, then, (4) finally, suppress overlapping detections which are caused by the sliding window-approach. The proposed method was evaluated on realistic synthetic images with known and reliable ground truth. The proposed approach was compared to two other popular CNNs namely, GoogleNet and AlexNet and three traditional methods namely, Isotropic Undecimated Wavelet Transform, Laplacian of Gaussian and Feature Point Detection, using two types of synthetic images. The experimental results indicate that the proposed methodology provides fast spot detection with precision, recall and F_score values that are comparable to GoogleNet and higher compared to other methods in comparison. Statistical test between detectSpot and GoogleNet shows that the difference in performance between them is insignificant. This implies that one can use either of these two methods for solving the problem of spot detection.

Keywords: Microscopy images · Convolutional neural network · Spot detection

1 Introduction

The ability to accurately detect and monitor sub-cellular structures in the biological environment has potential in addressing open questions in biology, such as understanding the variations between pathological and normal situations in a cell.

© Springer Nature Switzerland AG 2019
A. Cliquet jr. et al. (Eds.): BIOSTEC 2018, CCIS 1024, pp. 132–145, 2019.
https://doi.org/10.1007/978-3-030-29196-9_8

Investigation and study of malaria [2], cancer [3], inflammatory processes and wound healing are examples of biological applications which can be tackled in various ways, ranging from biochemistry to microscopy imaging. Detection of objects in images is one of the fundamental computer vision problems that arises in many real-world applications ranging from surveillance [4], robotics [5] to biology [6]. Object detection involves two main steps: (1), classification (determining objects of interest in a given image and, (2), localization (computing the location of these objects in the image).

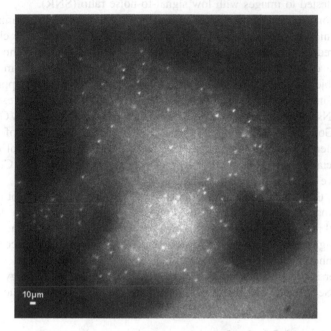

Fig. 1. A sample of real fluorescence image with bright particles obtained using confocal microscopy [1].

However, a lot of existing state-of-the-art methods often treat classification and localization separate with localization regarded as a difficult problem compared to classification.

This work focuses on the detection of small bright particles, referred to as spots, in fluorescence microscopy images. These spots may represent, for example, chromosomes, vesicles or genes in a cell depending on the staining method used. A set of identified spots is shown in Fig. 1. Accurate detection of spots is of significant interests for biomedical researchers as it plays a significant step for further analysis. A number of procedures in biology and medicine require the detection and counting of spots, for example, an individual's health can be deduced based on the number of red and white blood cells. The man goal of spot detection is to find all spots in a given image. There exist several challenges which hinders the performance of spot detection methods, such as noise and inhomogeneity which exist in the background. Besides all these challenges, a lot of applications in bioimage analysis such as spot tracking [7], require high performance and reliable detection results which increases the need for efficiency.

In the past years, several methods were developed for detecting spots in fluorescence microscopy images, some of these methods include Wavelets [8], Mathematical morphology [9]. A review of some of these methods can be found in [10, 11]. According to Smal et al. [10], existing methods for spot detection can be categorized into 'supervised' and 'unsupervised' methods. Supervised methods are methods which require labeled data for training while unsupervised methods refer to methods which do not require training. Smal et al. [10] claimed supervised methods gives better detection results when tested to images with low signal-to-noise ratio (SNR).

Convolutional neural network (CNN) is one of the popular in a family of deep learning techniques which based on the ImageNet2012 classification challenge, it managed to reduce the classification error rate by half. According to the study conducted by He et al. [12] a well-trained CNN technique can outperform humans in identifying objects. The CNNs have since been adopted to various applications in computer vision community [13] and medical image analysis [14]. There exist different forms of CNNs architectures in the literature, such as, AlexNet [15], VGGNet [16], ResNet and GoogLeNet [17] among others. Despite the diverse range of their applications in different fields, the application of these methods to biological data is still lacking, especially for the detection of spots. Recent works suggest that CNNs can be used to resolve some of the existing challenges in biology [18, 19].

Currently, there exist no technique based on CNN developed for spot detection in microscopy images. As such, this work proposes a method based on a deep convolutional neural network with sliding-window approach capable of detecting spots in the presence of high levels of noise and high spot density, and with high accuracy in the presence of inhomogeneity in the background.

This paper is organized as follows: Sect. 2 describes the methodology used in the study, while Sect. 3 presents the results and finally, Sect. 4 concludes the paper.

2 Materials and Methods

2.1 Methodology

Convolutional Neural Network (CNN). Convolutional neural network (CNN) h is defined in [1] and described in Eq. (1) as composition of sequence of L layers $(h_1 \ldots h_L)$ that maps an input vector x to an output vector y, i.e., [1]

$$
\begin{aligned}
y &= f(x; w_1, \ldots, w_L) \\
&= h_L(\cdot\,; w_L) \circ h_{L-1}(\cdot\,; w_{L-1}) \circ \ldots \\
&\circ h_2(\cdot\,; w_2) \circ h_1(x; w_1)
\end{aligned}
\tag{1}
$$

where w_l is the weight and bias vector for the lth layer h_l and h_l is determined to perform one of the following: (a) convolution with a bank of kernels; (b) spatial pooling; and (c) non-linear activation. For any given N training datasets $\{(x^i, y^i)\}_{i=1}^{N}$, we can estimate the weights, $w_1, \ldots, w_L$ by solving the optimization problem:

$$\underset{w_1,\dots,w_L}{\mathrm{augmax}}\frac{1}{N}\sum_{i=1}^{N}\ell\big(f\big(x^i;w_1,\dots,w_L\big)\big) \qquad (2)$$

Where ℓ is defined as the loss function. The numerical optimization of Eq. (2) is often performed via backpropagation and stochastic gradient descent methods [20].

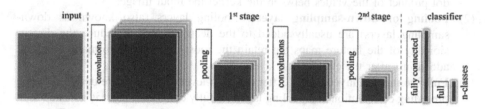

Fig. 2. An illustration of the traditional convolutional neural network which consists of two repeatable stages followed by the classifier.

Table 1. Proposed CNN architecture [1].

Layer	Kernel size, stride	Output $w \times h \times c$
Input	−	$29 \times 29 \times 3$
Convolution	$9 \times 9, 1$	$21 \times 21 \times 32$
ReLu		$21 \times 21 \times 32$
Max-Pool	$2 \times 2, 1$	$20 \times 20 \times 32$
Convolution	$7 \times 7, 1$	$14 \times 14 \times 64$
ReLU		$14 \times 14 \times 64$
Max-Pool	$2 \times 2, 1$	$13 \times 13 \times 64$
Convolution	$5 \times 5, 1$	$9 \times 9 \times 80$
ReLu		$9 \times 9 \times 80$
Max-Pool	$2 \times 2, 1$	$7 \times 7 \times 80$
FC	−	128
ReLu+Dropout	−	128
FC	−	128
ReLu+Dropout	−	128
FC	−	2
Softmax	−	2

Problem Formulation. Consider a labeled grayscale training images patches denoted as $I_i \in R^{w \times h \times 3}$, where i ranges from 1 to N with dimensionality $w \times h \times 3$. The task is to develop a classifier based on CNN to predict if patch, I_i contains a spot or not. Image patches with a full spot contained in the image are labelled as positive, otherwise negative.

Proposed CNN. In general, a CNN architecture can include some of these layers as shown in Fig. 2 described below:

(1) **Convolution layers,** A convolutional layer exploits the local information encoded in the image by computing convolutions between the layer's input (e.g., the original image or the output of a previous convolutional layer) and multiple convolution kernels. A convolution refers to the summation of the elementwise dot product of the values between the kernel the input image.

(2) **Pooling or down-sampling layers.** Pooling layers (also known as down-sampling layers) are usually added to the deep network to reduce the dimensionality of the feature maps but retain the most important information and are added just after the convolution layers.

(3) **Fully connected layers (FC):** After the high-level of features are detected by the preceding convolution and pooling layers, a fully connected layer is attached to at the end of the network with the aim of converting the feature maps to a 1D feature vector. It performs a linear combination of the input vector with a weight matrix.

Given the described building blocks for CNN, we propose CNN architecture for spot detection, named detectSpot as shown in Table 1 detectSpot consists of 5 layers (3 convolution layers and 2 fully connected layers) with learnable weights. Rectified Liner Unit (ReLu) [21] are used as activation function for the first four layers proceeded with softmax for the last layer. To avoid overfitting, dropout with probability of 0.5 for the first two fully connected layers (FC) was introduced. The weights were initialized using truncated random normal. Cross-entropy loss was minimized using Adam optimization with the initial learning rate of 0.001.

Sliding-Window. A sliding window approach is adopted for detecting all spots positions in a given image. A sliding-window is an approach based on moving a rectangular window across an image as illustrated by red and green rectangles in Fig. 3. This is done in order to analyze subpart of the image and extract some information.

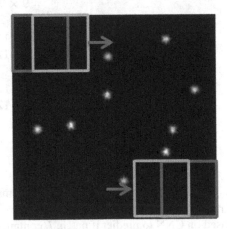

Fig. 3. Illustration of sliding-window approach [1].

Dataset. Image patches of size 29×29 sampled from a synthetic image of size 512×512 were used for training a proposed CNN method. Patches containing spot center were classified as positive while negative patches are those without spot as denoted in Eq. (3). There was a disproportion between negative patches and positive patches, with the number of negative patches being large. In order to make training and validation set more balanced two measure were considered. Firstly, negative patches were randomly discarded so that there is 50* the number of positive patches, and secondly, each positive patch was rotated resulting in 4 extra patches. In total, 21300 patches formed from images with a signal to noise ratio (SNR) in range (20, 10, 5, 2, 1). Then, these image patches were divided as follows:

- 80% for training
- 20% evaluation

Each of the positive patches has >0.6 Jaccard-similarity with any ground truth spot while the negative patches has <0.2 Jaccard-similarity. Jaccard-similarity is denoted as:

$$J\left(X_{patch}, Y_{ground}\right) = \frac{\left|X_{patch} \cap Y_{ground}\right|}{\left|X_{patch} \cup Y_{ground}\right|} \tag{3}$$

Implementation and Training. The proposed CNN was implemented on TFLearn [22], which is a tensorflow [23] wrapper that allows simple implementation and training of deep learning models. Adam [24] was used for the optimization of the algorithm. Linux machine with 16 GB RAM and Nvidia GTX680 running TFLearn (v0.3) and tensorflow (v1.3.0) was used for training the network.

2.2 Detection of Spots in Test Images

The proposed CNN architecture, detectSpot is trained to classify an image patch as containing a spot or not. Figure 4 illustrates the pipeline for the detection of spots using detectSpot method including some post-processing steps. To detect all spots in a given image, a window of size $(w \times h)$ is run through the image. At each iteration, the extracted window is passed onto a detectSpot to compute a probability S, which defines whether a spot is contained in the sub-window. Then, if S is bigger than a given threshold T, the corresponding window is considered to contain spot. All the windows which were classified as containing spots, were subject for further processing to get spot centers (x, y) including the bounding circles marking the spots location in an image. The proposed detectSpot contains two main important parameters, window-size $(w \times h)$ and stride. These parameters influence both speed and detection rate. This approach can only detect spots with fixed size but it can be extended to spots with different sizes by introducing image pyramids. If one select a small stride value, e.g. stride = 1, this will give many overlapping detections of the same spot but at slightly different positions. So, to overcome this challenge, we developed a method that is capable of removing overlapping detections. The proposed approach group all nearby detections so that every spot is detected once. More details about this technique can be found in [1].

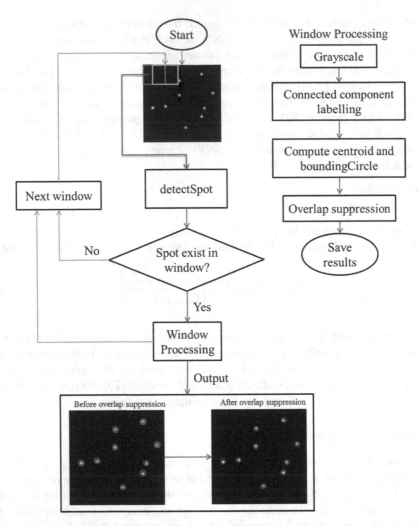

Fig. 4. The proposed architecture for spot detection in microscopy images [1].

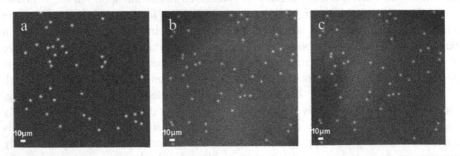

Fig. 5. Examples of synthetic images used for testing with approximately 50 spots per image. (a) Type A, (b) Type B1, and (c) Type B2 [1].

Using Pre-trained Models

Pre-trained Models
The proposed detectSpot method was quantitatively compared to two other CNNs methods, namely, AlexNet and GoogleNet.

AlexNet: This method was proposed by Krizhevsky et al. [15] and won the ImageNet ILSVRC-2012 challenge. The model is made-up of 8 layers (5 convolutional layers and three fully connected layers).

GoogleNet: This method won the ImageNet ILSVRC-2014 challenge and it was proposed by Szegedy et al. [17] from Google. This network has 12X fewer parameters compared to AlexNet yet deeper (22 layers). The main contribution of GoogleNet is the introduction of inception module.

2.3 Synthetic Datasets and Evaluation Criteria

Synthetic Test Datasets. To evaluate the performance of the methods, three kinds of synthetic datasets (Type A and Type B1 and B2) containing spots were used. These images were created using a framework proposed in [25]. Synthetic images are important because they contain ground truth information of each spot in an image, as a result this will demonstrate the effectiveness of the proposed detectSpot model as shown in Fig. 5. Each image contained 50 spots cluttered on the background of size 256×256 pixels. The,, a Gaussian noise was then added to the image dataset was corrupted by white noise. The following signal to noise ratios (SNR) levels was explored $\{10, 8, 6, 4, 2, 1\}$ where the spot intensity was 20 gray levels. The signal to noise ratio is defined as of spot intensity, SP_{max}, divided by the noise standard deviation, σ_{noise},

$$SNR = \frac{SP_{max}}{\sigma_{noise}} \tag{4}$$

The Icy-plugin [26] was used to randomize the spots position in order to mimic properties available in real microscopy images. MATLAB was used to add spots and the OMERO.matlab-5.2.6 toolbox [27] was used to read and save images.

Evaluation Criteria. The well-known measures for evaluating various spot detection methods in microscopy images are F-measure, precision, and recall. Parameters involved in the computations include; TP, FP and FN which denote the number of true positives (number of detected spots that corresponds to the ground-truth), number of false positives (number of detected spots which do not correspond to the ground-truth) and number of false negatives (number of missed ground-truth spots), respectively. A detection result is labelled as TP if the overlap region, O_r between the detection and ground-truth exceeds a predefined threshold T. Explanation of these measures ca be found in [1].

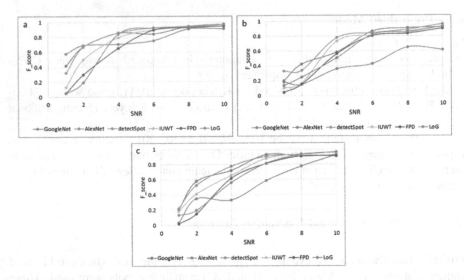

Fig. 6. F_score vs SNR curves for all six methods applied to two kinds of synthetic images (a) Synthetic type A, and (b–c) Synthetic type B.

3 Results

The fully trained CNNs models along with the FPD [28], IUWT [29] and LoG [30], were each applied on two types of synthetic images described in Sect. 0 as shown in Fig. 5 with a signal-to-noise ratio (SNR) in range {10, 8, 6, 4, 2, 1}. Tables 2, 3 and 4 indicates the results for all six methods in terms of average precision, recall and F_score. These values were averaged for all SNR's. Table 2 indicates the results for type A synthetic images. Higher precision value is reported by AlexNet method on type A synthetic images indicating higher accuracy for relevant spots retrieval and less false spots detected. Furthermore, the GoogleNet method recorded larger values for recall rate and F_score followed by detectSpot method. Figure 6(a) summarises the performance of all six methods on type A synthetic images on all SNR values. The results indicate that at high levels of SNR (≈ 8 and 10) the difference in performance of the methods is negligible. However, as SNR drops (< 4) the performance of the methods is reduced and at SNR = 1, deep learning methods reports higher F_score values compared to traditional methods.

Tables 3 and 4 presents the results for type B synthetic images. The results indicate that when the background is introduced into the synthetic images, detectSpot method reports higher precision, recall and F_score values compared to all other methods in comparison. The performance of the AlexNet method is reduced significantly compared to its performance on Type A synthetic images. Figure 6(b–c) gives a clear indication of how each method performs on Type B synthetic images.

Table 2. Evaluation metrics calculated on sythetic images for six detection methods.

Model	Precision	Recall	F_score
GoogleNet	0.833	**0.751**	**0.784**
AlexNet	**0.842**	0.703	0.758
detectSpot	0.836	0.740	0.782
IUWT	0.728	0.689	0.705
FPD	0.717	0.584	0.628
LoG	0.656	0.650	0.652

Table 3. Evaluation metrics calculated on realistic synthetic data. B1.

Method	Precision	Recall	F_score
GoogleNet	0.717	**0.585**	0.633
AlexNet	0.443	0.365	0.397
detectSpot	**0.803**	0.614	**0.675**
IUWT	0.618	0.587	0.598
FPD	0.590	0.534	0.550
LoG	0.647	0.552	0.583

Table 4. Evaluation metrics calculated on realistic synthetic data. B2.

Model	Precision	Recall	F_score
GoogleNet	0.733	**0.699**	0.708
AlexNet	0.567	0.476	0.502
detectSpot	**0.780**	0.675	**0.721**
IUWT	0.740	0.636	0.672
FPD	0.620	0.548	0.571
LoG	0.612	0.533	0.600

The curves for each method in Fig. 6 indicate higher F_score values for all methods for SNR > 6 except for AlexNet method. However, as SNR drops from 4 to 1 most methods start to deteriorate at this point while detectSpot indicates higher F_score value at SNR = 1. According to the curves in Fig. 6(c) for all SNR is the performance of GoogleNet and detectSpot methods show small variability regarding f-score values with both methods having higher F_score values at low SNRs. Traditional spot detection methods also give competitive results at higher SNRs especially the IUWT and LoG methods, and their performance is reduced as SNR decreases. Figure 7 shows the detected spots for each method on Type A synthetic images with SNR = 10.

Fig. 7. Illustrates the performance of each method on Type A synthetic images with SNR = 10. Detected spots by each method are showed in red circles. (a) Original synthetic image. (b) Spots detected by our approach, detectSpot. (c) Detected spots using GoogleNet. (d) Detected spots with AlexNet, and (e–g) represents the detected spots using, IUWT, LoG, and FPD respectively. (Color figure online)

4   Statistical Significant Test

This section implements a comparison of the detection results from detectSpot and GoogleNet methods applied to the same sample, in order to check whether the methods provide similar results or not. The outcome of this test is the acceptance or rejection of the null hypothesis (H_0). To do this significant test, a student t-test will be used which compares the two means between two groups. A paired two tailed t-test was considered to check the statistical significance of the results, with the null hypothesis (H_0) defined as; $\mu_1 - \mu_2 = 0$, with μ being the mean and the subscript $\{1, 2\}$ represents method one and two. The alternate hypothesis (H_a) states the opposite, $\mu_1 - \mu_2 \neq 0$. A Shapiro-Wilk test was used to confirm the normality of the data. The chosen p-value was 0.05. Table 5 indicate the statistical results for two methods, detectSpot and GoogleNet, these two methods provide higher and comparable F_score for all experiments compared to other methods. The p-values for detectSpot and GoogleNet are greater than 0.05 for all experiments, these indicate that the detection results between detectSpot and GoogleNet are statistical insignificant as a result these methods provide similar results.

Table 5. P-values for detectSpot and GoogleNet.

Methods	DATA SET		
	NOBGND	BGND1	BGND2
detectSpot & GoogleNet	>0.05	>0.05	>0.05

5 Conclusions

The detection of spots is an important step towards the analysis of microscopy images. A number of different automated approaches have been developed to perform the task of spot detection. In this study, we have presented an automated approach for the detection and counting of spots in microscopy images, termed detectSpot. The proposed approach is based on a convolutional neural network with a sliding-window based approach to detect multiple spots in images. The comparative experiments demonstrated that the GoogleNet and detectSpot methods achieved comparable performance compared to the AlexNet method and other traditional spot detection methods. We also have shown that rather training a CNN from scratch, knowledge transfer from natural images to microscopy images is possible. A fine-tuned pre-trained CNN can give results which are comparable to fully trained CNN.

Acknowledgements. This work was carried out in financial support from the Council for Scientific and Industrial Research (CSIR) and the Electrical and Electronic Engineering Department at the University of Johannesburg.

References

1. Bashir, A., Mustafa, Z.A., Abdelhameid, I., Ibrahem, R.: Detection of malaria parasites using digital image processing. In: Proceedings of the International Conference on Communication, Control, Computing and Electronics Engineering (ICCCCEE), Khartoum (2017)
2. Verma, A., Khanna, G.: Survey on digital image processing techniques for tumor detection. Indian J. Sci. Technol. **9**(14), 1–15 (2016)
3. Mabaso, M., Withey, D., Twala, B.: Spot detection in microscopy images using convolutional neural network with sliding-window approach. In: Proceedings of the 5th International Conference on Bioimaging, Funchal-Madeira (2018)

4. Varga, D., Szirányi, T.: Detecting pedestrians in surveillance videos based on convolutional neural network and motion. In: 24th European Signal Processing Conference (EUSIPCO), Budapest, Hungary (2016)
5. Wang, Z., Li, Z., Wang, B., Liu, H.: Robot grasp detection using multimodal deep convolutional neural networks. Adv. Mech. Eng. **8**(9), 1–12 (2016)
6. Li, R., et al.: Deep learning based imaging data completion for improved brain disease diagnosis. In: International Conference on Medical Image Computing and Computer-Assisted Intervention, Quebec City (2014)
7. Genovesio, A., Liendl, T., Emiliana, V., Parak, W.J., Coppey-Moisan, M., Olivo-Marin, J.-C.: Multiple particle tracking in 3D+t microscopy: method and application to the tracking of endocytosed quantum dots. IEEE Trans. Image Process. **15**(5), 1062–1070 (2006)
8. Olivo-Marin, J.-C.: Extraction of spots in biological images using multiscale products. Pattern Recogn. **35**(9), 1989–1996 (2002)
9. Kimori, Y., Baba, N., Morone, N.: Extended morphological processing: a practical method for automatic spot detection of biological markers from microscopic images. BMC Bioinf. **11**(373), 1–13 (2010)
10. Smal, I., Loog, M., Niessen, W., Meijering, E.: Quantitative comparison of spot detection methods in fluorescence microscopy. IEEE Trans. Med. Imaging **29**(2), 282–301 (2010)
11. Mabaso, M., Withey, D., Twala, B.: Spot detection methods in fluorescence microscopy imaging: a review. Image Anal. Stereol. **37**(3), 173–190 (2018)
12. He, K., Zhang, X., Ren, S., Sun, J.: Deep residual learning for image recognition. In: arXiv: 1512.03385 (2015)
13. Noh, H., Hong, S., Han, B.: Learning deconvolution network for semantic segmentation. In: IEEE International Conference on Computer Vision (2015)
14. Tajbakhsh, N., et al.: Convolutional neural networks for medical image analysis: full training or fine tuning? IEEE Trans. Med. Imaging **35**(5), 1299–1312 (2016)
15. Krizhevsky, A., Sutskever, I., Hinton, G.E.: Imagenet Classification with deep convolutional neural networks. In: Neural Information Processing Systems (2012)
16. Simonyan, K., Zisserman, A.: Very deep convolutional networks for large-scale image recognition. In: International Conference on Learning Representations (2014)
17. Szegedy, C., et al.: Going deeper with convolutions. In: Computer Vision and Pattern Recognition, Boston (2015)
18. Van Valen, D.A., et al.: Deep learning automates the quantitative analysis of individual cells in live-cell imaging experiments. PLoS Comput. Biol. **12**(11), 1–24 (2016)
19. Mabaso, M., Withey, D., Twala, B. Spot detection in microscopy images using convolutional neural network with sliding-window approach. In: Proceedings of the 5th International Conference on Bioimaging, Funchal (2018)
20. Ruder, S.: An overview of gradient descent optimization algorithms (2017). http://ruder.io/optimizing-gradient-descent/. Accessed 10 Oct 2017
21. Nair, V., Hinton, G.E.: Rectified linear units improve restricted Boltzmann machines. In: Proceedings of the 27th International Conference on Machine Learning (2010)
22. Damien, A.: TFLearn, GitHub (2016)
23. Abadi, M., et al.: TensorFlow: large-scale machine learning on heterogeneous system. In: 12th USENIX Symposium on Operating Systems Design and Implementation (2015)
24. Kingma, D.P., Ba, J.L.: Adam: a method for stochastic optimization. In: 3rd International Conference for Learning Representations, San Diego (2015)
25. Mabaso, M., Withey, D., Twala, B.: A framework for creating realistic synthetic fluorescence microscopy image sequences. In: Bioimaging 2016, Rome (2016)
26. Chenouard, N.: Particle tracking benchmark generator. Institut Pasteur (2015). http://icy.bioimageanalysis.org/plugin/Particle_tracking_benchmark_generator. Accessed 1 Nov 2016

27. The open microscopy environment (2016). http://www.openmicroscopy.org/site/support/ omero5.2/developers/Matlab.html. Accessed 15 Nov 2016
28. Sbalzarini, I.F., Koumoutsakos, P.: Feature point tracking and trajectory analysis for video imaging in cell biology. J. Struct. Biol. **151**(2), 182–195 (2005)
29. Olivo-Marin, J.-C.: Extraction of spots in biological images using multiscale products. Pattern Recognit. **35**(9), 1989–1996 (2002)
30. Raj, A., van den Bogaard, P., Rifkin, S.A., van Oudenaarfen, A., Tyagi, S.: Imaging individual mRNA molecules using multiple singly labeled probes. Nat. Methods **5**(10), 877– 879 (2008)

Bioinformatics Models, Methods and Algorithms

Inferring the Synaptical Weights of Leaky Integrate and Fire Asynchronous Neural Networks: Modelled as Timed Automata

Elisabetta De Maria and Cinzia Di Giusto$^{(\boxtimes)}$

Université Côte d'Azur, CNRS, I3S, Sophia Antipolis, France
cinzia.di-giusto@unice.fr

Abstract. In this work we introduce a new approach to learn the synaptical weights of neural biological networks. At this aim, we consider networks of Leaky Integrate and Fire neurons and model them as timed automata networks. Each neuron receives input spikes through its incoming synapses (modelled as channels) and computes its membrane *potential* value according to the (present and past) received inputs. Whenever the potential value overtakes a given *firing threshold*, the neuron emits a spike (modelled as a broadcast signal over the output channel of the corresponding automaton). After each spike emission, the neuron enters first an *absolute refractory period*, in which signal emission is not allowed, and then a *relative refractory period*, in which the firing threshold is higher than usual. Neural networks are modelled as sets of timed automata running in parallel and sharing channels in compliance with the network structure. Such a formal encoding allows us to propose an algorithm which automatically infers the synaptical weights of neural networks such that a given dynamical behaviour can be displayed. Behaviours are encoded as temporal logic formulae and the algorithm modifies the network weights until un assignment satisfying the specification is found.

Keywords: Neural networks · Parameter learning · Timed automata · Temporal logic · Model checking

1 Introduction

In the last decades, the study of biological neurons and their interactions has become very intensive, especially in the perspective of identifying the circuits involved in the main vital functions, such as breathing or walking, and detecting how they are modified in case of disease. The majority of the approaches aiming at exploring the brain functioning mainly relies on large-scale simulations [9]. In this paper we propose a formal approach based on the use of timed automata [2]. This formalism extends finite state automata with timed behaviours: constraints are allowed to limit the amount of time an automaton can remain within a particular state, or the time interval during which a particular transition may be

© Springer Nature Switzerland AG 2019
A. Cliquet jr. et al. (Eds.): BIOSTEC 2018, CCIS 1024, pp. 149–166, 2019.
https://doi.org/10.1007/978-3-030-29196-9_9

enabled. It is possible to build timed automata networks, where several automata can synchronise over *channel* communications.

As far as the modelling of neuronal networks is concerned, three different and progressive *generations* of networks can be found in the literature [24,26]. *First generation* models handle discrete inputs and outputs and their computational units are threshold-based transfer functions; they include McCulloch and Pitt's threshold gate model [25], the perceptron model [15], Hopfield networks [20], and Boltzmann machines [1]. *Second generation* models exploit real valued activation functions, e.g., the sigmoid function, accepting and producing real values: a well known example is the multi-layer perceptron [8,29]. *Third generation* networks are known as spiking neural networks. They extend second generation models treating time-dependent and real valued signals often composed by *spike trains*. Neurons may fire output spikes according to threshold-based rules which take into account input spike magnitudes and occurrence times [26].

In this work we focus on *spiking neural networks* [16]. Because of the introduction of timing aspects they are considered closer to the actual brain functioning than other generations models. Spiking neurons emit spikes taking into account input impulses strength and their occurrence instants. Models of this sort are of great interest, not only because they are closer to natural neural networks behaviour, but also because the temporal dimension allows to represent information according to various *coding schemes* [26,27]: e.g., the amount of spikes occurred within a given time window (*rate* coding), the reception/absence of spikes over different synapses (*binary* coding), the relative order of spikes occurrences (*rate rank* coding), or the precise time difference between any two successive spikes (*timing* coding).

Several spiking neuron models, with different capabilities and complexities, have been proposed in the literature. In [22], Izhikevich classifies spiking neuron models according to some *behaviour* (i.e., typical responses to an input pattern) that they should exhibit in order to be considered biologically relevant. The leaky integrate & fire (LI&F) model [23], where past inputs relevance exponentially decays with time, is one of the most employed neuron models because it is straightforward and easy to use [22,26]. By contrast, the Hodgkin-Huxley (H-H) model [19] is one of the most complex being composed by four differential equations comparing neurons to electrical circuits. In [22], the H-H model can reproduce all behaviours at issue, but the simulation process is really expensive even for just a few neurons being simulated for a small amount of time. Our aim is to produce a neuron model being meaningful from a biological point of view but also suitable to formal analysis and verification, that could be therefore exploited to detect non-active portions within some network (i.e., the subset of neurons not contributing to the network outcome), to test whether a particular output sequence can be produced or not, to prove that a network may never be able to emit, to assess if a change to the network structure can alter its behaviour, or to investigate (new) learning algorithms which take time into account.

The core of our studies is the *leaky integrate & fire* (LI&F) model originally proposed in [23]. It is a computationally efficient approximation of single-compartment model [22] and is abstracted enough to be able to apply formal verification techniques such as model-checking. Here we work on an extended version of the discretised formulation proposed in [13], which relies on the notion of logical time. Time is considered as a sequence of logical discrete instants, and an instant is a point in time where external input events can be observed, computations can be done, and outputs can be emitted. The variant we introduce here takes into account some new time-related aspects, such as the *refractory period*, a lapse of time in which the neuron cannot emit (or can only emit under some restrictive conditions).

Our modelling of spiking neural networks consists of timed automata networks where each neuron is an automaton. Each neuron receives input spikes through its incoming synapses (modelled as *channels*) and computes its membrane *potential* value according to the (present and past) received inputs. Whenever the potential value overtakes a given *firing threshold*, the neuron emits a spike (modelled as a *broadcast signal* over an output channel of the corresponding automaton).

As a central contribution, we exploit our automata-based modelling to propose a new methodology for parameter inference in spiking neural networks. In particular, our approach allows to find an assignment for the synaptical weights of a given neural network such that it can reproduce a given (expected) behaviour.

This paper is an improved and revised version of the conference paper [10]. In particular, the neuron model we introduce here is substantially different. In [10], neurons need to wait for the end of some specific accumulation periods (during which signals are received) before emitting spikes. Here, accumulation periods are removed and neurons can receive and emit signals in an *asynchronous* way. Furthermore, a unique refractory period is replaced by an *absolute refractory period*, in which signal emission is not allowed, and a *relative refractory period*, in which the firing threshold is higher than usual. This entails a new definition of Leaky Integrate and Fire neuron and a new encoding into timed automata. The examples are adapted to fit to the new model and new consistent parameters are computed. Finally, the algorithm for parameter inference is refined in order to avoid deadlock scenarios and a new simulation-oriented approach to implement this algorithm is briefly introduced (see [11] for a detailed description of this technique).

The rest of the paper is organised as follows: in Sect. 2 we recall definitions of timed automata networks, temporal logics, and model checking; in Sect. 3 we describe our reference model, the LI&F one, and its encoding into timed automata networks; in Sect. 4 we develop the parameter learning approach and we introduce a case study; in Sect. 5 we give an overview of the related work. Finally, Sect. 6 summarises our contribution and presents some future research directions.

2   Preliminaries

In this section we introduce the formalisms we adopt in the rest of the paper, that is, timed automata and temporal logics.

2.1 Timed Automata

Timed automata [2] are a powerful theoretical formalism for modelling and verifying real time systems. A timed automaton is an annotated directed (and connected) graph, with an initial node and provided with a finite set of non-negative real variables called *clocks*. Nodes (called *locations*) are annotated with *invariants* (predicates allowing to enter or stay in a location), arcs with *guards*, *communication labels*, and possibly with some variables upgrades and clock *resets*. Guards are conjunctions of elementary predicates of the form x op c, where $op \in \{>, \geq, =, <, \leq\}$, x is a clock, and c a (possibly parameterised) positive integer constant. As usual, the empty conjunction is interpreted as true. The set of all guards and invariant predicates will be denoted by G.

Definition 1. *A timed automaton TA is a tuple $(L, l^0, X, \Sigma, Arcs, Inv)$, where*

- *L is a set of locations with $l^0 \in L$ the initial one*
- *X is the set of clocks,*
- *Σ is a set of communication labels,*
- *$Arcs \subseteq L \times (G \cup \Sigma \cup U) \times L$ is a set of arcs between locations with a guard in G, a communication label in $\Sigma \cup \{\varepsilon\}$, and a set of variable upgrades (e.g., clock resets);*
- *$Inv : L \to G$ assigns invariants to locations.*

It is possible to define a synchronised product of a set of timed automata that work and synchronise in parallel. The automata are required to have disjoint sets of locations, but may share clocks and communication labels which are used for synchronisation. We restrict communications to be *broadcast* through labels $b!, b? \in \Sigma$, meaning that a set of automata can synchronise if one is emitting; notice that a process can always emit (e.g., $b!$) and the receivers ($b?$) must synchronise if they can.

Locations can be normal, urgent or committed. Urgent locations force the time to freeze, committed ones freeze time and the automaton must leave the location as soon as possible, i.e., they have higher priority.

The synchronous product $TA_1 \parallel \ldots \parallel TA_n$ of timed automata, where $TA_j = (L_j, l_j^0, X_j, \Sigma_j, Arcs_j, Inv_j)$ and L_j are pairwise disjoint sets of locations for each $j \in [1, \ldots, n]$, is the timed automaton

$$TA = (L, l^0, X, \Sigma, Arcs, Inv)$$

such that:

- $L = L_1 \times \ldots \times L_n$ and $l^0 = (l_1^0, \ldots, l_n^0)$, $X = \bigcup_{j=1}^n X_j$, $\Sigma = \bigcup_{j=1}^n \Sigma_j$,
- $\forall l = (l_1, \ldots, l_n) \in L$: $Inv(l) = \bigwedge_j Inv_j(l_j)$,
- $Arcs$ is the set of arcs $(l_1, \ldots, l_n) \xrightarrow{g,a,r} (l_1', \ldots, l_n')$ such that for all $1 \leq j \leq n$ then $l_j' = l_j$.

Its semantics is the one of the underlying timed automaton TA with the following notations. A location is a vector $l = (l_1, \ldots, l_n)$. We write $l[l_j'/l_j, j \in S]$

to denote the location l in which the jth element l_j is replaced by l'_j, for all j in some set S. A valuation is a function ν from the set of clocks to the non-negative reals. Let $\mathbb{V}$ be the set of all clock valuations, and $\nu_0(x) = 0$ for all $x \in X$. We shall denote by $\nu \vDash F$ the fact that the valuation ν satisfies (makes true) the formula F. If r is a clock reset, we shall denote by $\nu[r]$ the valuation obtained after applying the clock reset $r \subseteq X$ to ν; and if $d \in \mathbb{R}_{>0}$ is a delay, $\nu + d$ is the valuation such that, for any clock $x \in X$, $(\nu + d)(x) = \nu(x) + d$.

The semantics of a synchronous product $TA_1 \parallel \ldots \parallel TA_n$ is defined as a timed transition system $(S, s_0, \rightarrow)$, where $S = (L_1 \times, \ldots \times L_n) \times \mathbb{V}$ is the set of states, $s_0 = (l^0, \nu_0)$ is the initial state, and $\rightarrow \subseteq S \times S$ is the transition relation defined by:

- (silent): $(l, \nu) \rightarrow (l', \nu')$ if there exists $l_i \xrightarrow{g,\varepsilon,r} l'_i$, for some i, such that $l' = l[l'_i/l_i]$, $\nu \vDash g$ and $\nu' = \nu[r]$,

- (broadcast): $(\bar{l}, \nu) \rightarrow (\bar{l'}, \nu')$ if there exists an output arc $l_j \xrightarrow{g_j,b!,r_j} l'_j \in Arcs_j$ and a (possibly empty) set of input arcs of the form $l_k \xrightarrow{g_k,b?,r_k} l'_k \in Arcs_k$ such that for all $k \in K = \{k_1, \ldots, k_m\} \subseteq \{l_1, \ldots, l_n\} \setminus \{l_j\}$, the size of K is maximal, $\nu \vDash \bigwedge_{k \in K \cup \{j\}} g_k$, $l' = l[l'_k/l_k, k \in K \cup \{j\}]$ and $\nu' = \nu[r_k, k \in K \cup \{j\}]$;

- (timed): $(l, \nu) \rightarrow (l, \nu + d)$ if $\nu + d \vDash Inv(l)$.

The valuation function ν is extended to handle a set of shared bounded integer variables: predicates concerning such variables can be part of edges guards or locations invariants, moreover variables can be updated on edges firings but they cannot be assigned to or from clocks.

Example 1. In Fig. 1 we consider the network of timed automata TA_1 and TA_2 with broadcast communications, and we give a possible run. TA_1 and TA_2 start in the l_1 and l_3 locations, respectively, so the initial state is $[(l_1, l_3); x = 0]$. A *timed* transition produces a delay of 1 time unit, making the system move to state $[(l_1, l_3); x = 1]$. A *broadcast* transition is now enabled, making the system move to state $[(l_2, l_3); x = 0]$, broadcasting over channel a and resetting the x clock. Two successive *timed* transitions (0.5 time units) followed by a *broadcast* one will eventually lead the system to state $[(l_2, l_4); x = 1]$.   ◇

To model neural networks, we have used the specification and analysis tool **Uppaal** [4], which allows to design and simulate timed automata networks and to validate networks against temporal logic formulae. All figures depicting timed automata follow the graphic conventions of the tool (e.g., initial states are denoted with a double circle).

2.2 Temporal Logics and Model Checking

Model checking is one of the most common approaches to the verification of software and hardware (distributed) systems [7]. It allows to automatically prove whether a system verifies or not a given specification. In order to apply such a

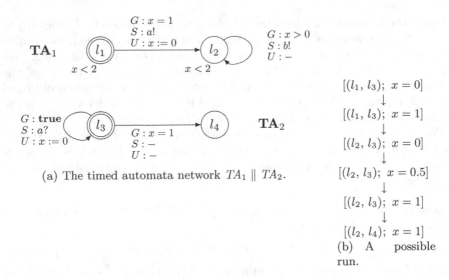

(a) The timed automata network $TA_1 \parallel TA_2$.

$[(l_1, l_3);\ x = 0]$
$\downarrow$
$[(l_1, l_3);\ x = 1]$
$\downarrow$
$[(l_2, l_3);\ x = 0]$
$\downarrow$
$[(l_2, l_3);\ x = 0.5]$
$\downarrow$
$[(l_2, l_3);\ x = 1]$
$\downarrow$
$[(l_2, l_4);\ x = 1]$
(b)   A   possible run.

Fig. 1. A network of timed automata with a possible run.

technique, the system at issue should be encoded as a finite transition system and the specification should be written using propositional temporal logic. Formally, a transition system over a set AP of atomic propositions is a tuple $M = (Q, T, L)$, where Q is a finite set of states, $T \subseteq Q \times Q$ is a total transition relation, and $L : Q \to 2^{AP}$ is a labelling function that maps every state into the set of atomic propositions that hold at that state.

Temporal formulae describe the dynamical evolution of a given system. The computation tree logic CTL* allows to describe properties of computation trees. Its formulas are obtained by (repeatedly) applying boolean connectives ($\wedge$, $\vee$, $\neg$, $\to$), *path quantifiers*, and *state quantifiers* to atomic formulas. The path quantifier $\mathbf{A}$ (resp., $\mathbf{E}$) can be used to state that all the paths (resp., some path) starting from a given state have some property. The state quantifiers are $\mathbf{X}$ (next time), which specifies that a property holds at the next state of a path, $\mathbf{F}$ (sometimes in the future), which requires a property to hold at some state on the path, $\mathbf{G}$ (always in the future), which imposes that a property is true at every state on the path, and $\mathbf{U}$ (until), which holds if there is a state on the path where the second of its argument properties holds and, at every preceding state on the path, the first of its two argument properties holds. Given two formulas φ_1 and φ_2, in the rest of the paper we use the shortcut $\varphi_1 \rightsquigarrow \varphi_2$ to denote the liveness property $AG(\varphi_1 \to AF\varphi_2)$, which can be read as "$\varphi_1$ always leads to φ_2".

The branching time logic CTL is a fragment of CTL* that allows quantification over the paths starting from a given state. Unlike CTL*, it constrains every state quantifier to be immediately preceded by a path quantifier.

Given a transition system $M = (Q, T, L)$, a state $q \in Q$, and a temporal logic formula φ expressing some desirable property of the system, the *model checking problem* consists of establishing whether φ holds at q or not, namely, whether $M, q \models \varphi$.

3 Leaky Integrate and Fire Model and Mapping to Timed Automata

Spiking neural networks [24] have been traditionally modelled as directed graphs, where vertices represent *neurons* and oriented edges are the *synapses*. Each neuron is a computational unit whose evolution depends on time passing by and on the reception of signals through its ingoing synapses. The weight associated to each synapse defines the nature of the signal: excitatory if positive, inhibitory if negative. Input signals are, then, summed up by the neuron in a variable called the *potential*. The potential accumulated decreases as time passes by and its loss is regulated by the *leak factor*. As soon as the potential exceeds the *firing threshold*, the neuron emits a signal called *spike* over all its outgoing synapses. When the neuron fires, its potential is reset to zero and the neuron enters a special state: the *refractory period*. This period is divided into two parts, the absolute and the relative refractory period. During the former, the neuron is completely inhibited: it ignores each incoming spike and it cannot fire. During the latter, the neuron can receive spikes but its firing threshold is much higher than usual. This threshold decreases with time passing by, by a *threshold factor* η, until it reaches the normal value. This entails that, during the relative refractory period, if the neuron is stimulated enough it will fire, thus resetting the potential to zero and restarting a new refractory period (absolute and relative).

In this paper we consider discrete time. Next we give a formal definition of Spiking Integrate and Fire Neural Networks and their dynamics.

Definition 2 (Spiking Integrate and Fire Neural Network). A spiking integrate and fire neural network *is a tuple* (V, A, w), *where:*

- *V are spiking integrate and fire neurons,*
- *$A \subseteq V \times V$ are synapses,*
- *$w : A \to \mathbb{Q} \cap [-1, 1]$ is the synapse weight function associating to each synapse (u, v) a weight $w_{u,v}$.*

Each spiking integrate and fire neuron v *is characterized by a parameter tuple* $(\theta_v, \theta'_v, \tau_v, \eta_v, \lambda_v)$, *where:*

- *$\theta_v, \theta'_v \in \mathbb{N}$ are the* firing threshold *for the normal and relative refractory period respectively,*
- *$\tau_v \in \mathbb{N}^+$ is the duration of the* absolute refractory period,
- *$\eta_v \in \mathbb{Q} \cap [0, 1]$ is the* threshold factor
- *$\lambda_v \in \mathbb{Q} \cap [0, 1]$ is the* leak factor.

The state of each neuron v is described by the tuple (s_v, p_v, f_v, t_v), where

- t_v is a timer;
- $s_v \in \{n, a, r\}$ is the state of v, n for a neuron in a normal state, a for a neuron in the absolute refractory period, and r for the relative one;
- p_v is the potential of v;
- f_v is a boolean value stating whether the neuron has fired or not.

A configuration C is the set of states of all neurons $v \in V$. The semantics of the neural network is given by the set of reachable configurations from an initial one. The initial configuration sets the state of all neurons $v \in V$ to $(n, 0, 0, 0)$. Let $C = \{(s_v, p_v, f_v, t_v) \mid v \in V\}$, then $C \to C'$ if and only if $C' = \{(s'_v, p'_v, f'_v, t'_v) \mid v \in V\}$ and $(s_v, p_v, f_v, t_v) \to_v (s'_v, p'_v, f'_v, t'_v)$ for all $v \in V$ and $\to_v$ is defined as follows:

$$\frac{p'_v < \theta_v}{(n, p_v, 0, t_v) \to_v (n, p'_v, 0, t_v + 1)} \text{ Rule 1}$$

$$\frac{p'_v \geq \theta_v}{(n, p_v, 0, t_v) \to_v (a, 0, 1, 0)} \text{ Rule 2}$$

$$\frac{t_v + 1 < \tau_v}{(a, 0, f_v, t_v) \to_v (a, 0, 0, t_v + 1)} \text{ Rule 3}$$

$$\frac{t_v + 1 \geq \tau_v}{(a, 0, 0, t_v) \to_v (r, 0, 0, 0)} \text{ Rule 4}$$

$$\frac{p'_v < \theta'_v \cdot \eta_v^{t_v+1} \qquad \theta'_v \cdot \eta_v^{t_v+1} > \theta_v}{(r, p_v, 0, t_v) \to_v (r, p'_v, 0, t_v + 1)} \text{ Rule 5}$$

$$\frac{p'_v < \theta'_v \cdot \eta_v^{t_v+1} \qquad \theta'_v \cdot \eta_v^{t_v+1} \leq \theta_v}{(r, p_v, 0, t_v) \to_v (n, p'_v, 0, 0)} \text{ Rule 6}$$

$$\frac{p'_v \geq \theta'_v \cdot \eta_v^{t_v+1}}{(r, p_v, 0, t_v) \to_v (a, 0, 1, 0)} \text{ Rule 7}$$

with $p'_v = \sum_{i=1}^{m} w_{i,v} \cdot f_i + \lambda_v \cdot p_v$ and where i is the ith out of m input neuron of v, $w_{i,v}$ is the weight of the synapse connecting i and v, and f_i is the third component in the state of neuron i in configuration C.

More in detail, Rules 1 and 2 regulate the neuron when it is not in the refractory period (absolute or relative). In this case, at each instant, there are two possibilities:

Rule 1: the new potential (taking into account input spikes and the leak factor) is smaller than the firing threshold, thus the neuron remains in the normal state, it updates its potential and the timer increases of one unit,

Rule 2: the new potential is greater than the firing threshold, thus the neuron fires a spike (setting to 1 the boolean f_v), it changes its state to the absolute refractory period and resets the timer to 0.

During its absolute refractory period, the neuron ignores any received spike. The only visible change is that time passes by and the timer is incremented by one time unit (Rule 3). When the timer is greater than τ_v (the duration of the absolute refractory period), the neuron changes its state moving to the relative refractory state and resetting all the other variables of the state (Rule 4).

Last, as far as the relative refractory period is concerned, we have that its duration is determined by two parameters: θ'_v and η_v. We thus have three possible scenarios:

Rule 5: The neuron can receive spikes from its input neurons but the new potential p'_v does not exceed the firing threshold θ'_v (diminished by the threshold factor η_v) and θ'_v has not yet reached the normal firing threshold $(\theta'_v \cdot \eta_v^{t_v+1} > \theta_v)$. In this case the neuron remains in the relative refractory state, it updates its potential and increases the timer.

Rule 6: In this case the neuron potential has not yet passed the firing threshold but the relative refractory period is terminated since θ'_v has been diminished until reaching θ_v. The neuron then returns in the normal state with the updated potential and the timer is reset.

Rule 7: The new potential is bigger than the firing threshold, then the neuron fires: $f'_v = 1$ and it moves to the absolute refractory state resetting to 0 both the potential and the timer.

In a spiking integrate and fire neural network, we distinguish three disjoint sets of neurons: V_i (input neurons), V_{int} (intermediary neurons), and V_o (output neurons), with $V = V_i \cup V_{int} \cup V_o$. Each input neuron receives as input an external signal. The output of each output neuron is considered as an output for the network. We have given the definition of input generators and output consumer in [11]. For the sake of this paper, it is sufficient to know that input generators are encoded as timed automata that provide trains of spike. Symmetrically, output consumers are timed automata that can in each moment receive spikes from the connected output neurons.

The encoding of neurons is as follows (it generalises the definition given in [10] by introducing the relative refractory period and removing the notion of accumulation period):

Definition 3. *Given a neuron* $v = (\theta_v, \theta'_v, \tau_v, \eta_v, \lambda_v)$ *with* m *input neurons, its encoding into timed automata is* $\mathcal{N} = (L, \mathbf{N}, X, Var, \Sigma, Arcs, Inv)$ *with:*

- $L = \{\mathbf{N}, \mathbf{F}, \mathbf{A}, \mathbf{R}\}$ *with* $\mathbf{F}$ *committed,*
- $X = \{t\}$
- $Var = \{p, f\}$
- $\Sigma = \{x_i \mid i \in [1..m]\} \cup \{x_v\},$
- $Arcs =$
  $\{(\mathbf{N}, p + w_i \geq \theta_v, x_i?, \sim, \mathbf{F}) \mid i \in [1..m]\} \cup$
  $\{(\mathbf{N}, p + w_i < \theta_v, x_i?, \sim, \mathbf{N}) \mid i \in [1..m]\} \cup$
  $\{(\mathbf{R}, p + w_i \geq f, x_i?, \sim, \mathbf{F}) \mid i \in [1..m]\} \cup$
  $\{(\mathbf{R}, p + w_i < f, x_i?, \sim, \mathbf{R}) \mid i \in [1..m]\} \cup$

$\{(\mathbf{N}, t = 1, \sim, \{t := 0, p := p \cdot \lambda_v\}, \mathbf{N}),$
$(\mathbf{F}, \sim, x_v!, \{p := 0, t := 0\}, \mathbf{A})$
$(\mathbf{A}, t = \tau_v, \sim, \{t := 0, f := \theta_v'\}, \mathbf{R})$
$(\mathbf{R}, t = 1, \sim, \{t := 0, p := p \cdot \lambda_v, f := f \cdot \eta_v\}, \mathbf{R}),$
$(\mathbf{R}, \sim, \sim, \{t := 0\}, \mathbf{N})\}$

$- \; Inv(\mathbf{N}) = t < 1, \sim Inv(\mathbf{F}) = \mathbf{true},$
$Inv(\mathbf{A}) = t < \tau_v, Inv(\mathbf{R}) = t < 1 \wedge f > \theta_v.$

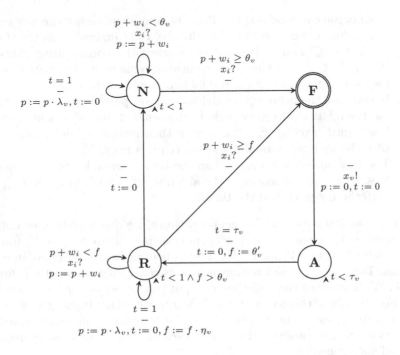

Fig. 2. Encoding of the spiking integrate and fire neuron with absolute and relative refractory period.

The automaton encoding of a neuron v is given in Fig. 2. We comment now on the definition. States $\mathbf{N}, \mathbf{F}, \mathbf{A}, \mathbf{R}$ represent, respectively, the fact that the neuron is in the normal state, it is firing, and it is in the absolute and then relative refractory period. Spikes are communicated through broadcast channels: each neuron $v \in V$ is associated to a channel x_v. The passing of time is explicit in the encoding, it is implemented by the self loop on state $\mathbf{N}$ with guard ($t = 1, -, \{p := p \cdot \lambda_v, t := 0\}$), by the similar self loop on state $\mathbf{R}$ with guard ($t = 1, -, \{p := p \cdot \lambda_v, t := 0, f := f \cdot \eta_v\}$), and by the arc from state $\mathbf{A}$ to state $\mathbf{R}$. All other actions (arcs) are meant to be instantaneous.

The rules above are encoded into arcs in the automata in the following way:

Rule 1: it is encoded by both self loops on state $\mathbf{N}$,
Rule 2: it is encoded by the arcs from $\mathbf{N}$ to $\mathbf{F}$ and from $\mathbf{F}$ to $\mathbf{A}$. Notice that, as state $\mathbf{F}$ is committed, time cannot pass by,

Rule 3: has no counterpart in the arcs, it is represented by the invariant $t < \tau_v$
on state **A**,
Rule 4: it is given by the arc from state **A** to **R**,
Rule 5: it is encoded by both self loops on state **R**,
Rule 6: it is represented by the arc from state **R** to **N**,
Rule 7: similarly as for Rule 2, it is encoded by the arcs from **R** to **F** and from
F to **A**.

4   Parameter Inference

In this section we focus on the *Learning Problem*, which consists in determining
a parameter assignment for a network with a fixed topology and a given input
such that a desired output behaviour is displayed. More precisely, we examine
the estimation of synaptic weights in a given spiking neural network and we leave
the generalisation of our methodology to other parameters for future work.

Our technique takes inspiration from the SpikeProp algorithm [5]; in a similar
way, here, the learning process is led by *supervisors*. Each output neuron $\mathcal{N}$ is
linked to a supervisor. Supervisors compare the expected output behaviour with
the one of the output neuron they are connected to (function EVALUATE($\mathcal{N}$) in
Algorithm 1). Thus either the output neuron behaved consistently or not. In the
second case, and in order to instruct the network, the supervisor back-propagates
advices to the output neuron depending on two possible scenarios:

 (i) the neuron fires a spike, but it was supposed to be quiescent,
(ii) the neuron remains quiescent, but it was supposed to fire a spike.

In the first case the supervisor addresses a *should not have fired* message (SNHF)
and in the second one a *should have fired* (SHF). Then each output neuron
modifies its ingoing synaptic weights and in turn behaves as a supervisor with
respect to its predecessors, back-propagating the proper advice.

The advice back-propagation (ABP), Algorithm 1, is based on a depth-first
visit of the graph topology of the network. Let $\mathcal{N}_i$ be the i-th predecessor of
an automaton $\mathcal{N}$, then we say that $\mathcal{N}_i$ fired, if it emitted a spike during the
current or previous accumulate-fire-wait cycle of $\mathcal{N}$. Thus, upon reception of a
SHF message, $\mathcal{N}$ has to *strengthen* the weight of each ingoing *excitatory* synapse
and *weaken* the weight of each ingoing *inhibitory* synapse. Then, it propagates a
SHF advice to each ingoing *excitatory* synapse (i.e., an arc with weight greater
than 0: WT ≥ 0) corresponding to a neuron which *did not* fire recently ($\neg$F($\mathcal{N}$)),
and symmetrically a SNHF advice to each ingoing *inhibitory* synapse (WT < 0)
corresponding to a neuron which fired recently (see Algorithm 2 for SHF, and
Algorithm 3 for the dual case of SNHF). When the graph visit reaches an input
generator, it will simply ignore any received advice (because input sequences
should not be affected by the learning process). The learning process ends when
all supervisors do not detect any more errors.

There are several possibilities on how to implement supervisors and the ABP
algorithm. We propose here two different techniques: the first one is model checking oriented while the second one is simulation oriented.

Algorithm 1. The advice back-propagation algorithm.

```
1: function ABP
2:     discovered = ∅
3:     for all N ∈ Output do
4:         if N ∉ discovered then
5:             discovered = discovered ∪ N
6:             if EVALUATE(N) = SHF then
7:                 SHF(N)
8:             else if EVALUATE(N) = SNHF then
9:                 SNHF(N)
```

Algorithm 2. Should Have Fired algorithm.

```
1: procedure SHOULD-HAVE-FIRED(N)
2:     if N ∈ discovered ∪ Output then
3:         return
4:     discovered = discovered ∪ N
5:     for all M ∈ PRED(N) do
6:         if M ∉ Input then
7:             if WT(N, M) ≥ 0 ∧ ¬ F(M) then
8:                 SHF(M)
9:             if WT(N, M) < 0 ∧ F(M) then
10:                SNHF(M)
11:            INCREASE-WEIGHT(N, M)
12:    return
```

As far as the first technique is concerned, it consists in iterating the learning process until a desired CTL temporal logic formula concerning the output of the network is verified. At each step of the algorithm, we make an external call to a model checker to test whether the network satisfies the formula or not. If the formula is verified, the learning process ends; otherwise, the model checker provides a trace as a counterexample. Such a trace is exploited to derive the proper corrective action to be applied to each output neuron, that is, the invocation of either the SHF procedure, or the SNHF procedure previously described (or no procedure).

In the second technique, parameters are modified during the simulation of the network. This entails that the encoding of neurons as automata needs to be adjusted in order to take care of the adaptation of such parameters. Algorithm ABP is realised by a dedicated automaton, and the role of supervisor is given to some output consumer automata. The idea is that, if an output neuron misbehaves, then its corresponding output consumer sets whether it has to be treated according to the SHF or the SNHF function. Furthermore, it signals that some adjustments on the network have to be done. Then the functions SHF or SNHF are recursively applied on the predecessors of the output neuron. Once there

---

Algorithm 3. Abstract ABP: Should *Not* Have Fired advice pseudo-code.

1: **procedure** SHOULD-NOT-HAVE-FIRED($neuron$)
2:     **if** $\mathcal{N} \in$ discovered $\cup$ Output **then**
3:         **return**
4:     discovered $=$ discovered $\cup \mathcal{N}$
5:     **for all** $\mathcal{M} \in$ PREDECESSORS($\mathcal{N}$) **do**
6:         **if** $\mathcal{M} \notin$ Input **then**
7:             **if** WT($\mathcal{N}, \mathcal{M}$) $\geq 0 \wedge$ F($\mathcal{M}$) **then**
8:                 SNHF($\mathcal{M}$)
9:             **if** WT($\mathcal{N}, \mathcal{M}$) $< 0 \ \wedge \neg$ F($\mathcal{M}$) **then**
10:                SHF($\mathcal{M}$)
11:            DECREASE-WEIGHT($\mathcal{N}, \mathcal{M}$)
12:     **return**

---

is no more neuron to whom the algorithm should be applied (for instance all neurons in the current run have been visited), the simulation is restarted in the network with the new parameters.

For a detailed description of the aforementioned techniques, the reader can refer to [11].

Example 2 (Turning on and off a diamond network of neurons). This example illustrates how the ABP algorithm can be used to make a neuron emit at least once in a spiking neural network having the *diamond* structure shown in Fig. 3. We assume that $\mathcal{N}_1$ is fed by an input generator $\mathcal{I}$ that continuously emits spikes. The neurons $\mathcal{N}_1$, $\mathcal{N}_2$, and $\mathcal{N}_3$ have the same tuple of parameters:

$$(\theta = 0.35, \theta' = 1.75, \tau = 3, \eta = 1, \lambda = \frac{7}{9})$$

while $\mathcal{N}_4$ has the parameters:

$$(\theta = 0.55, \theta' = 2.75, \tau = 3, \eta = 1, \lambda = \frac{1}{2}).$$

The initial weights are:

$w_{0,1}$	$w_{1,2}$	$w_{1,3}$	$w_{2,4}$	$w_{3,4}$
0.1	0.1	0.1	0.1	0.1

No neuron in the network is able to emit because all the weights of their input synapses are equal to 0.1 and their thresholds are 0.35.

We want the network to learn a weight assignment so that $\mathcal{N}_4$ is able to emit, that is, to produce a spike after an initial pause. At the beginning we expect no activity from neuron $\mathcal{N}_4$. As soon as the initial pause is elapsed, we require a spike but, as all weights are equal to zero, no emission can happen. Thus a SHF advice

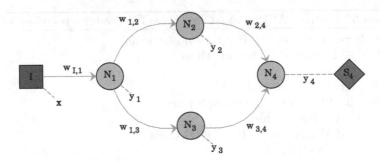

Fig. 3. A neural network with a diamond structure (Fig. 2 in [10]).

is back-propagated to the neurons $\mathcal{N}_2$ and $\mathcal{N}_3$ and consequently to $\mathcal{N}_1$. The process is then iterated until all weights stabilise and the neuron $\mathcal{N}_4$ is able to fire.

As far as the model checking approach is concerned, we want to test whether $\mathcal{N}_4$ can fire every 20 units of time. Notice that, as we cannot write recursive formulae, we only test if the formula is true for the first N times (N = 100 in our tests):

$$EG(((O4.n4 < N) \wedge (O4.O)) \Rightarrow (O4.s \leqslant 20)) \wedge EF(O4.O)$$

where $O4.n4$ is the number of spikes fired by $\mathcal{N}_4$, $O4.O$ states whether $\mathcal{N}_4$ has fired or not, and $O4.s$ is a clock signalling when $\mathcal{N}_4$ has fired. The last part of the formula ensures that the neuron fires at least once.

The next table details the steps of the model checking approach:

Step	Action	Update
1	$\mathcal{N}_4$ falsifies the formula	
2	SHF($\mathcal{N}_4$)	$w_{3,4} = 0.2$
		$w_{2,4} = 0.2$
3	SHF($\mathcal{N}_3$)	$w_{1,3} = 0.2$
4	SHF($\mathcal{N}_1$)	$w_{0,1} = 0.2$
5	SHF($\mathcal{N}_2$)	$w_{1,2} = 0.2$
6	$\mathcal{N}_4$ falsifies the formula	
7	SHF($\mathcal{N}_4$)	$w_{3,4} = 0.3$
		$w_{2,4} = 0.3$
8	SHF($\mathcal{N}_3$)	$w_{1,3} = 0.3$
9	SHF($\mathcal{N}_2$)	$w_{1,2} = 0.3$
10	$\mathcal{N}_4$ falsifies the formula	
11	SHF($\mathcal{N}_4$)	$w_{3,4} = 0.4$
		$w_{2,4} = 0.4$
12	SHF($\mathcal{N}_3$)	$w_{1,3} = 0.4$
13	SHF($\mathcal{N}_2$)	$w_{1,2} = 0.4$
14	The formula is satisfied	

For the simulation approach we obtain a similar sequence of calls to the SHF algorithm (changes in the order of calls are due to a different scheduling). The number of steps is also different as the checks on the validation of the formula are replaced by a simulation of the network. The obtained weights are only visible at the end of the simulation.

Step	Action
14	$\mathcal{N}_4$ does not behave as expected
21	SHF($\mathcal{N}_4$)
21	SHF($\mathcal{N}_2$)
21	SHF($\mathcal{N}_1$)
21	SHF($\mathcal{N}_3$)
39	$\mathcal{N}_4$ does not behave as expected
42	SHF($\mathcal{N}_4$)
42	SHF($\mathcal{N}_2$)
42	SHF($\mathcal{N}_3$)
62	$\mathcal{N}_4$ does not behave as expected
63	SHF($\mathcal{N}_4$)
63	SHF($\mathcal{N}_2$)
63	SHF($\mathcal{N}_3$)
83	$\mathcal{N}_4$ does not behave as expected
84	SHF($\mathcal{N}_4$)
488	$\mathcal{N}_4$ behaves as expected

Summing up, with the two approaches we obtain the following weights:

Method	$w_{0,1}$	$w_{1,2}$	$w_{1,3}$	$w_{2,4}$	$w_{3,4}$
Model checking	0.2	0.4	0.4	0.4	0.4
Simulation	0.2	0.4	0.4	0.5	0.5

Notice that with the simulation method we obtain a set of weights that is slightly different. This is not contradictory as the solution to the learning problem is not necessarily unique.   ◇

5   Related Work

To the best of our knowledge, there are few attempts of giving formal models for LI&F. Apart from the already discussed approach of [13], where the authors model and verify LI&F networks thanks to the synchronous language Lustre, the closest related work we are aware of is [3]. In this work, the authors propose a mapping of spiking neural P systems into timed automata. The modelling is substantially different from ours. They consider neurons as static objects and the dynamics is given in terms of evolution rules while for us the dynamics is intrinsic to the modelling of the neuron. This, for instance, entails that inhibitions are not just negative weights as in our case, but are represented as *forgetting rules*. On top of this, the notion of time is also different: while they consider durations in terms of number of applied rules, we have an explicit notion of duration given in terms of accumulation and refractory period.

As far as our parameter learning approach is concerned, we borrow inspiration from the SpikeProp rule [5], a variant of the well known back-propagation algorithm [29] used for supervised learning in second generation learning. The SpikeProp rule deals with multi-layered cycle-free spiking neural networks and aims at training networks to produce a given output sequence for each class of input sequences. The main difference with respect to our approach is that we are considering here a discrete model and our networks are not multi-layered. We also rest on Hebb's learning rule [18] and its time-dependent generalisation rule, the spike timing dependent plasticity (STDP) rule [30], which aims at adjusting the synaptical weights of a network according to the time occurrences of input and output spikes of neurons. It acts locally, with respect to each neuron, i.e., no prior assumption on the network topology is required in order to compute the weight variations for some neuron input synapses. Differently from the STDP, our approach takes into account not only recent spikes but also some external feedback (*advices*) in order to determine which weights should be modified and whether they must increase or decrease. Moreover, we do not prevent excitatory synapses from becoming inhibitory (or vice versa), which is usually a constraint for STDP implementations. A general overview on spiking neural network learning approaches and open problems in this context can be found in [17].

6   Conclusion

In this paper we formalised the LI&F model of spiking neural networks via timed automata networks. We improved the neuron model proposed in [10] by relaxing some stringent constraints related to spike emission times and by modelling a more realistic refractory period divided into absolute and relative one. We have a complete implementation of the proposed model and examples via the tool `Uppaal`, that can be found at the web pages [6] and [12]. As for future work concerning the modelling aspects, we plan to provide analogous formalisations for more complex spiking neuron models, such as the theta-neuron model [14] or the Izhikevich one [21]. We also intend to extend our model to incorporate propagation delays, which are considered relevant within the scope of spiking neural networks [26]. Our extension is intended to add some locations and clocks to model synapses. We also plan to perform a robustness analysis of the obtained model, in order to detect which neuron parameters influence most the satisfaction of some expected temporal properties.

As a salient contribution, we introduced a technique to learn the synaptical weights of spiking neural networks. At this aim, we adapted machine learning techniques to bio-inspired models, which makes our work original and complementary with respect to the main international projects aiming at understanding the human brain, such as the Human Brain Project [9], which mainly relies on large-scale simulations.

For our learning approach, we have focussed on a simplified type of supervisors: each supervisor describes the output of a single specific neuron. However, the back-propagation algorithm still works for more complex scenarios that specify and compare the behaviour of sets of neurons. As for future work, we intend to formalise more involved supervisors, allowing to compare the output of several neurons. Moreover, to refine our learning algorithm, we could exploit some key results coming from the domain of gene regulatory networks, where some theorems linking the topology of the network and its dynamical behaviour are given [28].

To conclude, we intend to extend our methodology to the inference of other crucial parameters of neural networks, such as the leak factor or the firing threshold. We plan to consider the other parameters first one by one, and then all at the same time.

Acknowledgements. We are grateful to Laetitia Laversa for her preliminary implementation work and for her enthusiasm in collaborating with us.

References

1. Ackley, D.H., Hinton, G.E., Sejnowski, T.J.: A learning algorithm for Boltzmann machines. In: Waltz, D., Feldman, J.A. (eds.) Connectionist Models and Their Implications: Readings from Cognitive Science, pp. 285–307. Ablex Publishing Corporation, Norwood (1988)
2. Alur, R., Dill, D.L.: A theory of timed automata. Theor. Comput. Sci. **126**(2), 183–235 (1994)
3. Aman, B., Ciobanu, G.: Modelling and verification of weighted spiking neural systems. Theor. Comput. Sci. **623**, 92–102 (2016). https://doi.org/10.1016/j.tcs.2015.11.005. http://www.sciencedirect.com/science/article/pii/S0304397515009792
4. Bengtsson, J., Larsen, K., Larsson, F., Pettersson, P., Yi, W.: UPPAAL—a tool suite for automatic verification of real-time systems. In: Alur, R., Henzinger, T.A., Sontag, E.D. (eds.) HS 1995. LNCS, vol. 1066, pp. 232–243. Springer, Heidelberg (1996). https://doi.org/10.1007/BFb0020949
5. Bohte, S.M., Poutré, H.A.L., Kok, J.N., La, H.A., Joost, P., Kok, N.: Error-backpropagation in temporally encoded networks of spiking neurons. Neurocomputing **48**, 17–37 (2002)
6. Ciatto, G., De Maria, E., Di Giusto, C.: Additional material (2016). https://github.com/gciatto/snn_as_ta
7. Clarke Jr., E.M., Grumberg, O., Peled, D.A.: Model Checking. MIT Press, Cambridge (1999)
8. Cybenko, G.: Approximation by superpositions of a sigmoidal function. Math. Control Signals Syst. **2**(4), 303–314 (1989)
9. D'Angelo, E., et al.: The human brain project: high performance computing for brain cells HW/SW simulation and understanding. In: 2015 Euromicro Conference on Digital System Design, DSD 2015, Madeira, Portugal, 26–28 August 2015, pp. 740–747. IEEE Computer Society (2015). https://doi.org/10.1109/DSD.2015.80

10. De Maria, E., Di Giusto, C.: Parameter learning for spiking neural networks modelled as timed automata. In: Anderson, P., Gamboa, H., Fred, A.L.N., i Badia, S.B. (eds.) Proceedings of the 11th International Joint Conference on Biomedical Engineering Systems and Technologies (BIOSTEC 2018). BIOINFORMATICS, Funchal, Madeira, Portugal, 19–21 January 2018, vol. 3, pp. 17–28. SciTePress (2018). https://doi.org/10.5220/0006530300170028

11. De Maria, E., Di Giusto, C.: Spiking neural networks modelled as timed automata with parameter learning. Research report, Université Côte d'Azur, CNRS, I3S, France, June 2018

12. De Maria, E., Di Giusto, C., Laversa, L.: Additional material (2017). https://digiusto.bitbucket.io/

13. De Maria, E., Muzy, A., Gaffé, D., Ressouche, A., Grammont, F.: Verification of temporal properties of neuronal archetypes using synchronous models. In: Fifth International Workshop on Hybrid Systems Biology, Grenoble, France (2016)

14. Ermentrout, G.B., Kopell, N.: Parabolic bursting in an excitable system coupled with a slow oscillation. SIAM J. Appl. Math. **46**(2), 233–253 (1986)

15. Freund, Y., Schapire, R.E.: Large margin classification using the perceptron algorithm. Mach. Learn. **37**(3), 277–296 (1999)

16. Gerstner, W., Kistler, W.: Spiking Neuron Models: An Introduction. Cambridge University Press, New York (2002)

17. Grüning, A., Bohte, S.: Spiking neural networks: principles and challenges (2014)

18. Hebb, D.O.: The Organization of Behavior. Wiley, New York (1949)

19. Hodgkin, A.L., Huxley, A.F.: A quantitative description of membrane current and its application to conduction and excitation in nerve. J. Physiol. **117**(4), 500–544 (1952)

20. Hopfield, J.J.: Neural networks and physical systems with emergent collective computational abilities. In: Anderson, J.A., Rosenfeld, E. (eds.) Neurocomputing: Foundations of Research, pp. 457–464. MIT Press, Cambridge (1988)

21. Izhikevich, E.M.: Simple model of spiking neurons. Trans. Neural Netw. **14**(6), 1569–1572 (2003)

22. Izhikevich, E.M.: Which model to use for cortical spiking neurons? IEEE Trans. Neural Netw. **15**(5), 1063–1070 (2004)

23. Lapicque, L.: Recherches quantitatives sur l'excitation electrique des nerfs traitee comme une polarization. J. Physiol. Pathol. Gen. **9**, 620–635 (1907)

24. Maass, W.: Networks of spiking neurons: the third generation of neural network models. Neural Netw. **10**(9), 1659–1671 (1997)

25. McCulloch, W.S., Pitts, W.: A logical calculus of the ideas immanent in nervous activity. Bull. Math. Biophys. **5**(4), 115–133 (1943)

26. Paugam-Moisy, H., Bohte, S.: Computing with spiking neuron networks. In: Rozenberg, G., Bäck, T., Kok, J.N. (eds.) Handbook of Natural Computing, pp. 335–376. Springer, Heidelberg (2012). https://doi.org/10.1007/978-3-540-92910-9_10

27. Recce, M.: Encoding information in neuronal activity. In: Maass, W., Bishop, C.M. (eds.) Pulsed Neural Networks, pp. 111–131. MIT Press, Cambridge (1999)

28. Richard, A.: Negative circuits and sustained oscillations in asynchronous automata networks. Adv. Appl. Math. **44**(4), 378–392 (2010)

29. Rumelhart, D.E., Hinton, G.E., Williams, R.J.: Learning representations by back-propagating errors. In: Anderson, J.A., Rosenfeld, E. (eds.) Neurocomputing: Foundations of Research, pp. 696–699. MIT Press, Cambridge (1988)

30. Sjöström, J., Gerstner, W.: Spike-timing dependent plasticity. Scholarpedia **5**(2), 1362 (2010)

Formal Neuron Models: Delays Offer a Simplified Dendritic Integration for Free

Ophélie Guinaudeau[1(✉)], Gilles Bernot[1], Alexandre Muzy[1], Daniel Gaffé[2], and Franck Grammont[3]

[1] Université Côte d'Azur, CNRS, I3S - UMR 7271, Sophia-Antipolis, France
`ophelie.guinaudeau@i3s.unice.fr`
[2] Université Côte d'Azur, CNRS, LEAT - UMR 7248, Sophia-Antipolis, France
[3] Université Côte d'Azur, CNRS, LJAD - UMR 7351, Nice, France

Abstract. We firstly define an improved version of the spiking neuron model with dendrites introduced in [8] and we focus here on the fundamental mathematical properties of the framework. Our main result is that, under few simplifications with respect to biology, dendrites can be simply abstracted by delays. Technically, we define a method allowing to reduce neuron shapes and we prove that reduced forms define equivalence classes of dendritic structures sharing the same input/output spiking behaviour. Finally, delays by themselves appear to be a simple and efficient way to perform an abstract dendritic integration into spiking neurons without explicit dendritic trees. This overcomes an explicit morphology representation and allows exploring many equivalent configurations via a single simplified model structure.

Keywords: Spiking neuron models · Dendrites · Formal models · Behavioural equivalence classes · Delays · Leaky integrate-and-fire

1 Introduction

Formal single neuron models can be classified into different generations. First generation is referred to as threshold gates, giving digital output [17] while second generation neurons employ continuous activation functions allowing analogue output [14,15]. The latter generation is more biologically realistic as their output can be interpreted as an instantaneous firing rate. However, experimental evidences question this standard "rate coding" paradigm, and suggest that many neural systems encode information through precise spike timing [23,25–27]. With respect to this temporal interpretation, third generation neurons, called spiking neurons, have thus been investigated [13].

In biological neurons, the input/output (I/O) spiking behaviour is strongly influenced by dendrites acting on information-processing parameters [24,28]. Dendrites alone are the focus of several complex biophysical models [20–22] but they are usually neglected in abstract single neuron models [1,6,13]. Nevertheless, delays are sometimes added to abstract models in order to take into account

© Springer Nature Switzerland AG 2019
A. Cliquet jr. et al. (Eds.): BIOSTEC 2018, CCIS 1024, pp. 167–191, 2019.
https://doi.org/10.1007/978-3-030-29196-9_10

the signal conduction in dendrites or to represent the time for transmitting spikes trough the axon [12, 15].

In this paper, we present a model of spiking neuron with dendrites which we preliminarily introduced in [8] and [9]. We developed this model at an appropriate abstraction level in order to take the best from computer science formal methods while being relevant from the biological point of view. Our motivation was not to define a biophysical model but we aimed at defining a bio-inspired model focusing more on computational capabilities and algebraic properties rather than precise molecular processes.

This framework, with proper discretization, was previously shown to be interesting for simulation [9] and model checking purposes [8]. Here, we define a more elaborated version of the framework and we are interested in its fundamental mathematical properties. We establish a surprising property: Delays and attenuations *are sufficient* to fully capture the impact of passive signal integration into tree-shaped dendrites. Consequently, we mathematically proved that, under specific parameter constraints, neurons with different dendritic structures have the same I/O spiking behaviour. This generalizes the computer-aided proofs on particular neurons performed in [8].

In the next section, we give a static description of our neuron model. Then, in Sect. 3, we focus on its dynamics. We demonstrate in Sect. 4 key theorems about neuron reduction and finally, in Sect. 5, we discuss the open question of "normalization."

2   Static Description of a Neuron

As a reminder and in a simplified way, a biological neuron is made of a cell body, also called *soma* and of two kinds of extensions: *dendrites* on one side with a highly branched structure and a unique *axon* on the other side. A neuron receives electrical impulses (called *action potentials* or *spikes*) at specific locations on dendrites called *synapses*. Spikes trigger movements of ionic charges through the neuron membrane making the potential locally change, this phenomenon is called *post-synaptic potential*. Charges then propagate through the dendrites and finally reach the soma. If the resulting soma potential is strong enough, a spike is emitted by the neuron and transmitted to other neurons through the axon. Usually, in biology as well as in modelling, the variable of interest is the *potential* value. Here, we make the original choice of considering *charges* which greatly simplify our definitions: it is possible to *sum* charges at branching points in dendrites whereas it is not credible to sum voltages. Nevertheless, those two physical quantities are easy to relate.

In this section, we give a strictly static description of our formal neuron even though static parameters are largely driven by dynamics. It certainly makes more sense in the next section which gives a dynamic description of the framework.

Quite naturally in relation to its structure, we model a *neuron* by a tree whose root is labelled by a *soma* (∇), any other internal node is labelled by a *compartment* and any leaf node is labelled by a *synapse* (Fig. 1). The axon is not considered here because at first approximation, it transmits the signal faithfully [2,5,11] and the axon constant transmission time can be easily considered afterwards in networks.

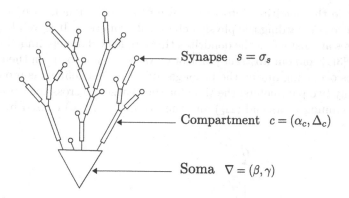

Fig. 1. Schematic representation of our formal neuron model. Parameters attached to the nodes are described further in this section.

We note $Co(N)$ (respectively $Sy(N)$) the set of all compartments (respectively synapses) of a neuron N and we note $Nodes(N)$ the set $Sy(N) \cup Co(N) \cup \{\nabla\}$. Moreover, we call the *dendritic forest* of N the set of sub-trees attached to ∇. Finally, we note $\mathcal{N}$ the set of all neurons.

Here, we consider a *unidirectional* and *passive* propagation of charges [24]. Therefore, charges will go from the leafs to the root of the neuron. In an unusual way for trees, we thus call *predecessor* of a node $x \in Nodes(N)$, any child node of x in N. We note $Pred_N(x)$ the set of the predecessors of x in N and we note $CoPred_N(x)$ (respectively $SyPred_N(x)$) the set of all the compartments (respectively synapses) belonging to $Pred_N(x)$. Definitions 1, 2 and 3 below formalize these ideas.

A synapse is mainly characterized by a function σ defining the shape with respect to time of the post-synaptic potential triggered by each spike received at this specific location (Fig. 2). Let us consider for example an excitatory synapse: When a spike is received at a synapse s, charges accumulate locally due to the capacitive properties of the membrane and after a time $\hat{\tau}_s$ (the *time-to-peak*), they reach a maximal value w_s (the *weight* of s). Then, they leave this location and propagate through the dendrites, making the quantity decrease and return to the resting value after a delay $\check{\tau}_s$ (the *descent delay*). In this framework, the resting value is normalized to 0.

Definition 1 [Synapse]. *A synapse is a symbol s together with a synaptic function σ, that is a continuous function $\sigma : \mathbb{R}^+ \rightarrow \mathbb{R}$ satisfying the following conditions:*

- *There exists $\hat{\tau}_s, \check{\tau}_s \in \mathbb{R}^{*+}$ such that $|\sigma|$ is strictly increasing on $[0, \hat{\tau}_s]$ and strictly decreasing on $[\hat{\tau}_s, \hat{\tau}_s + \check{\tau}_s]$.*
- *$\sigma(0) = 0$ and $\forall t \in [\hat{\tau}_s + \check{\tau}_s, +\infty], \sigma(t) = 0;$*

If $w_s = \sigma_s(\hat{\tau}_s)$ is a positive number, s is said excitatory *otherwise it is said* inhibitory.

We divide the dendrites into *compartments*, small enough to be considered as homogeneous regarding the physico-chemical properties. It is well known that some charges are lost along the dendrites through leak channels embedded in the membrane [3]. From our abstract point of view, we do not focus on the molecular mechanisms occurring during the propagation. We thus define a compartment c by using only two parameters: the time for the charges to cross the compartment from its beginning to its end (Δ_c) and the attenuation (α_c) caused by the leak.

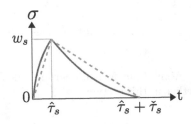

Fig. 2. Examples of synaptic functions σ. The particular case of a piecewise affine function is shown in dashed line.

Definition 2 [Compartment]. *A* compartment *is a symbol c together with a couple $(\alpha_c, \Delta_c) \in]0, 1] \times I\!\!R^{*+}$ where α_c is called the* electric attenuation *at the end of c and Δ_c is called the* delay for electrical charges to cross c.

A *soma* is mainly characterized by a threshold β to be reached for the neuron to emit a spike. β is a function of the time elapsed since the last emitted spike (denoted e). An infinite threshold models the *absolute refractory period* (lasting e_β) during which the neuron cannot emit any spike. Moreover, a *threshold increase* ($\leqslant \hat{p}_\beta$) is added to the *activation threshold* p_β to simulate the *relative refractory period* (lasting $\hat{e}_\beta$). This is illustrated in Fig. 3. A similar approach can be found in [16].

Definition 3 [Soma]. *A* soma *is a symbol ∇, together with a leak factor $\gamma \in I\!\!R^{*+}$ and a nominal function β where $\beta : I\!\!R^+ \cup \{+\infty\} \rightarrow I\!\!R^{*+} \cup \{+\infty\}$ is a function satisfying the following conditions:*

- *There exists $e_\beta \in I\!\!R^{*+}$ such that $\forall e \in [0, e_\beta[, \beta(e) = +\infty$;*
- *β is continuous and decreasing on $[e_\beta, +\infty[$; $p_\beta = \beta(+\infty)$ must belong to $[1, +\infty[$;*
- *There exists $\hat{p}_\beta \in I\!\!R^{*+}$ such that $\beta(e_\beta) = p_\beta + \hat{p}_\beta$ (i.e. $p_\beta < \beta(e_\beta) < +\infty$).*

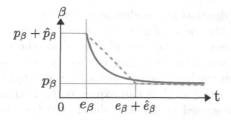

Fig. 3. Examples of nominal functions. The particular case of a piecewise affine function is shown in dashed line. However, all the results presented in this paper holds for the general case.

All the couples (e, p) satisfying $p \leqslant \beta(e)$ are called nominal. *We note* Nominal(β) *the set of all nominal couples. Finally, β is said* normal *if and only if $p_\beta = 1$.*

Within a neuron N, as illustrated in Fig. 1, we use the notations $s = \sigma_s$, $c = (\alpha_c, \Delta_c)$ and $\nabla = (\beta, \gamma)$.

The following classical definition is at the basis of many others. A *segment* is a function defined on a specific time interval.

Definition 4 [Segment]. *Given a set E, a* segment *with values in E is a map $\omega : [t_1, t_2] \to E$ where $(t_2 - t_1) \in \mathbb{R}^+ \cup \{+\infty\}$ is called the* duration. *We admit $t_1 = -\infty$ or $t_2 = +\infty$ with the convention that $[-\infty, +\infty] =]-\infty, +\infty[= \mathbb{R}$. Let $\star$ be a binary operation on E. If ω_1 and ω_2 are segments of the same domain, we note $\omega_1 \star \omega_2 : [t_1, t_2] \to E$ the segment such that $(\omega_1 \star \omega_2)(t) = \omega_1(t) \star \omega_2(t)$ for all $t \in [t_1, t_2]$. When $\star = +$, we accept the notation $\sum_{i=1}^{n} \omega_i$ for $\omega_1 + \omega_2 + ... + \omega_n$. We will often consider families of segments $W = \{\omega_i\}_{i \in F}$ indexed by a family F. If $W = \{\omega_i\}_{i \in F}$ and $W' = \{\omega'_i\}_{i \in F}$ are families of segments with values in E such that for any $i \in F$, the domain of ω_i is equal to the domain of ω'_i, then we note $W \star W' = \{\omega_i \star \omega'_i\}_{i \in F}$.*

The *state* η of a neuron N at a given time t is basically the charge at any of its points. As part of the state of N, we distinguish the state of its synapses $(\{\eta_s\}_{s \in Sy(N)})$, the state of it compartments $(\{\eta_c\}_{c \in Co(N)})$ and the state of its soma $\eta_\nabla = (e, p)$. More precisely:

- The state of a synapse $s(\eta_s)$ simply represents the value of the charge at a given time at this synapse;
- Intuitively, the state of a compartment $c(\eta_c)$ is the value of the charge at any point of it at a given time. Let us consider a compartment c of length L_c and a point located on c at a distance d from its end (Fig. 4). It is possible to define a function which associates a local charge to any d. If we note δ the time to travel the distance d, it is equivalent to define a function which associates a local charge to any δ. As it simplifies our definitions, we chose to define the state of c as a temporal function.

– We call *potential* (denoted p) the charge at the soma. The state of the soma at a given time is the value of p at this time, associated with the positive real number e representing the time elapsed since the last spike emitted by the soma. e is necessary for managing refractory periods (Fig. 3). Biological constraints make unreachable some values for the couple (e, p) (Definition 3, Lemma 1 together with Fig. 6). As an example, if e is greater than the refractory period, p is bounded by the threshold $\beta(e)$ because a spike would be produced before reaching higher values. $Nominal(\beta)$ is the set of possible values for the couple (e, p) (Definition 3).

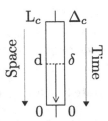

Fig. 4. Abstraction between time and space. We define the state of a compartment c as a segment associating a local charge to each time $\delta \in [0, \Delta_c]$. This is equivalent to consider δ which is the time to go from a given point to the end of c and d which is the distance between those two points.

Definition 5 [State of a Neuron]. *Given a neuron N, the* state *of N is a triple $\eta = (\{\eta_s\}_{s \in Sy(N)}, \{\eta_c\}_{c \in Co(N)}, \eta_\nabla)$ where:*

– $\{\eta_s\}_{s \in Sy(N)}$ *is a $Sy(N)$-indexed family of real numbers; each element $\eta_s \in \mathbb{R}$ is called the* state of the synapse s;
– $\{\eta_c\}_{c \in Co(N)}$ *is a $Co(N)$-indexed family of segments of the form $\eta_c : [0, \Delta_c] \to \mathbb{R}$ where Δ_c is the crossing delay of the compartment c, such that the following continuity condition is satisfied:*

$$\eta_c(\Delta_c) = \left(\sum_{c' \in CoPred_N(c)} \eta_{c'}(0) + \sum_{s \in SyPred_N(c)} \eta_s \right) \times \alpha_c$$

η_c *is called the* state of the compartment c.
– η_∇ *is a couple $(e, p) \in Nominal(\beta)$; η_∇ is called the* state of the soma, *e is the time elapsed since the last spike and p is called the* soma potential.

Finally, we note ζ_N the set of all the possible states of N.

To ensure the consistency of a state, the *continuity condition* of Definition 5 must be satisfied. Intuitively, it is a conservation condition: for example, charges going out of a compartment have to be preserved at the beginning of the next one. More precisely, the value of the charge at the beginning of a compartment must be equal to the sum of the charges coming from the predecessor nodes (compartments and synapses). More details will be given in the next section.

We also define the state of the dendritic forest which includes the state of the synapses together with the state of the compartments. It allows us to ignore the soma in some definitions focusing on the dendritic forest. Formally, given a state $\eta = (\{\eta_s\}_{s \in Sy(N)}, \{\eta_c\}_{c \in Co(N)}, \eta_{\overline{v}})$ of a neuron N, its restriction to the dendritic forest $\partial = (\{\eta_s\}_{s \in Sy(N)}, \{\eta_c\}_{c \in Co(N)})$, is called the *dendritic state*. We note $\mathscr{D}_N$ the set of all the possible dendritic states of N.

3   Neuron Dynamics

The framework defined herein is hybrid: inputs received at synapses and soma output will be discrete spikes whereas the electrical charges within the neuron will be continuously combined in dendrites using real numbers.

For the dynamic part of the framework description, we formalize in Definition 6 and 7, the *input signals* received at synapses. The transition from discrete spikes to a continuous electrical response is modelled here by the *trace* governed by the synaptic functions attached to synapses (Definition 8).

Definition 6 [Signal]. *An elementary* signal *is a segment* $\omega : \mathbb{R} \to \{0, 1\}$ *such that:*

$$\exists r \in \mathbb{R}^{*+}, \forall t \in \mathbb{R}, (\omega(t) = 1 \Rightarrow (\forall t' \in]t, t + r[, \omega(t') = 0))$$

The carrier of ω *is defined by:* $Car(\omega) = \{t \in \mathbb{R} \mid \omega(t) = 1\}$. *An elementary signal such that* $Car(\omega)$ *is a singleton* $\{u\}$ *is called a* spike at time u *(denoted* ω^u*). Obviously, an elementary signal* ω *can be split into a sum of spikes separated by at least* r: $\omega = \sum\limits_{u \in Car(\omega)} \omega^u$.

We define ω as a general notion of *elementary signal*. For clarity, we note I_s (for *Input*) an elementary signal received at a synapse s.

Definition 7 [Input Signal]. *Given a neuron* N, *an* input signal *for* N *is a* $Sy(N)$-*indexed family of signals* $I = \{I_s\}_{s \in Sy(N)}$. *Moreover, given a synapse* $s_0 \in Sy(N)$, *we call* restriction *of* I *to the synapse* s_0, *the input signal* $I_{|s_0} = \{I'_s\}_{s \in Sy(N)}$ *such that* $I'_{s_0} = I_{s_0}$ *and for all* $s \in Sy(N) \setminus \{s_0\}$ *and for any* $t \in \mathbb{R}$, $I'_s(t) = 0$. *Obviously, an input signal can be split according to the set of synapses:* $I = \sum\limits_{s \in Sy(N)} I_{|s}$.

Given a neuron N, an initial state η and an input signal $I = \{I_s\}_{s \in Sy(N)}$, the aim of the following mathematical construction is to build the *output signal* of N (denoted O for *Output*).

Definition 8 [Trace of a Signal]. *Given a synapse* s *of a neuron* N, *the* trace *of a spike* I_s^u *on* s *at time* u *is the segment* $\overline{I}_s^u : \mathbb{R} \to \mathbb{R}$ *defined by:* *If* $t \leqslant u$, *then* $\overline{I}_s^u(t) = 0$, *else* $\overline{I}_s^u(t) = \sigma_s(t - u)$.

Moreover, given an input signal $I = \{I_s\}_{s \in Sy(N)}$ for N, the trace of I_s on s is
$$\bar{I}_s = \sum_{u \in Car(I_s)} \bar{I}_s^u.$$

For consistency, the state of a neuron, at any time, must be in accordance with the spikes received at synapses in the past. A state is *in continuity* with an input signal I at a given time if for each synapse s, the state of s is equal to $\bar{I}_s(0)$. Indeed, input signals and their respective traces are always centred on 0 which represents the present time with negative times representing the past and positive times representing the future.

We firstly define the *extension* of a state in order to unify notations. In fact, we have defined in Definition 5 the state of a synapse as a real number representing the instantaneous charge at this punctual location. In the following definition, we define the extended state of a synapse as a segment, similarly to the state of the compartments. Intuitively, it represents the charge at the synapse from the present time up to a near future.

Definition 9 [Continuity with an Input Signal and State Extension].
Let N be a neuron, let $\eta = (\{\eta_s\}_{s \in Sy(N)}, \{\eta_c\}_{c \in Co(N)}, \eta_\nabla)$ be a state of N, let ∂ be the dendritic restriction of η and let $I = \{I_s\}_{s \in Sy(N)}$ be an input signal. The state η (and similarly ∂) is in continuity with I if and only if for each synapse s, $\eta_s = \bar{I}_s(0)$.
Moreover, given $\varepsilon \in \mathbb{R}^{*+}$, if η is in continuity with I then we define the ε-extension of η (and similarly of ∂) according to I, as the triple $\bar{\eta} = (\{\bar{\eta}_s\}_{s \in Sy(N)}, \{\bar{\eta}_c\}_{c \in Co(N)}, \bar{\eta}_\nabla)$, such that:

- *for all $s \in Sy(N), \bar{\eta}_s = \bar{I}_{s_{|[0,\varepsilon]}}$*
- *for all $c \in Co(N), \bar{\eta}_c = \eta_c$*
- *$\bar{\eta}_\nabla = \eta_\nabla$.*

Extensions of η satisfy $\bar{\eta}_s(0) = \eta_s$, so, extensions conveniently simplify the continuity condition of Definition 5 as $\eta_c(\Delta_c) = \left(\sum_{x \in Pred_N(c)} \bar{\eta}_x(0) \right) \times \alpha_c.$

Coming back to neuron dynamics, the continuous traces generated at synapses then propagate through the dendritic forest, compartment by compartment, towards the soma. As a reminder, we assume in this framework a unidirectional and passive conduction. In a nutshell, the charge at the end of any compartment c at a given time t is equal to the charge at its beginning at time $t - \Delta_c$, multiplied by the attenuation factor α_c. Furthermore, the charge entering c is the sum of the charges coming from its predecessor nodes (compartments and synapses). As formalized in Definition 10 along with Fig. 5, dendritic dynamics is then computed by *shifting* the extended state by a small interval of time. The range of shifting is restricted to a small ε in order to compute the state of any compartment only from the states of its predecessors, avoiding heavy recursive sums. More precisely, ε is chosen such that there is no compartment $c \in Co(N)$ having Δ_c greater than ε.

Definition 10 [Shift of a Dendritic State]. *Given a neuron N, let I be an input signal and let $\varepsilon \in \mathbb{R}^{*+}$ such that $\varepsilon \leqslant inf(\{\Delta_c \mid c \in Co(N)\})$. We define $\varepsilon\text{-shift}^I : \mathcal{D}_N \to \mathcal{D}_N$ as the map that associates to each $\partial = (\{\eta_s\}_{s \in Sy(N)}, \{\eta_c\}_{c \in Co(N)})$, $\varepsilon\text{-shift}^I(\partial) = \partial' = (\{\eta_s'\}_{s \in Sy(N)}, \{\eta_c'\}_{c \in Co(N)})$ where:*

- *For any $s \in Sy(N)$, $\eta_s' = \overline{\eta}_s(\varepsilon)$;*
- *For any $c \in Co(N)$, the segment $\eta_c' : [0, \Delta_c] \to \mathbb{R}$ is defined by:*
  - *$\forall \delta \in [0, \Delta_c - \varepsilon]$, $\eta_c'(\delta) = \eta_c(\delta + \varepsilon)$;*
  - *$\forall \delta \in [\Delta_c - \varepsilon, \Delta_c]$, $\eta_c'(\delta) = \left(\displaystyle\sum_{x \in Pred_N(c)} \overline{\eta}_x(\delta - \Delta_c + \varepsilon) \right) \times \alpha_c.$*

Theorem 1 below shows that from a given dendritic state, a succession of ε-shifts allows to uniquely compute the dendritic state after any delay.

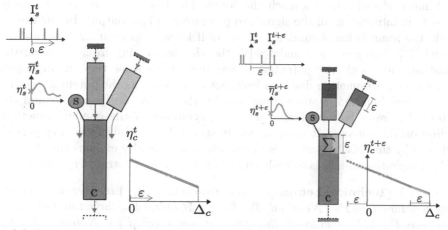

(a) State of a neuron part at time t (b) State of a neuron part at time $t + \varepsilon$

Fig. 5. Dendritic dynamics is computed by a succession of ε-shift. The state $(\eta_c^{t+\varepsilon})$ of a compartment c at time $t + \varepsilon$ is computed from its state (η_c^t) at time t by ε-shift. The charge at the beginning of a compartment c is the sum of the charges coming from its predecessor nodes.

Theorem 1 [Dendritic Dynamics]. *Given a neuron N, let $\partial^0 = (\{\eta_s^0\}_{s \in Sy(N)}, \{\eta_c^0\}_{c \in Co(N)})$ be an initial dendritic state of N in continuity with an input signal I. There exists a unique family $\{\partial^t\}_{t \in \mathbb{R}^+}$ such that for all $t \in \mathbb{R}^+$ and for all $\varepsilon \in [0, inf(\{\Delta_c \mid c \in Co(N)\})]$:*

$$\partial^{t+\varepsilon} = \varepsilon\text{-shift}^I(\partial^t)$$

Sketch of the Proof.

- *The uniqueness of the family $\{\partial^t\}_{t\in \mathbb{R}^+}$ is easy to prove:*
  Because there is a finite number of compartments, $inf(\{\Delta_c \mid c \in Co(N)\})$ is a strictly positive real number. Consequently, there exists a finite sum $t = \sum_{i=1}^{n} \varepsilon_i$ with $\varepsilon_i \leqslant inf(\{\Delta_c \mid c \in Co(N)\})$. Thus, ∂^t must be equal to: $\varepsilon_n\text{-}shift^I(\varepsilon_{n-1}\text{-}shift^I(...(\varepsilon_1\text{-}shift^I(\partial^0))...))$.
- *The existence of the family $\{\partial^t\}_{t\in \mathbb{R}^+}$ amounts to prove that ∂^t does not depend on the choice of the ε_i in the decomposition $t = \sum_{i=1}^{n} \varepsilon_i$. Even if it may seem obvious according to the shift intuition offered by Fig. 5, the formal transformations required for the proof are heavy. See Appendix A.2 (which uses Appendix A.1) for a completely rigorous proof.* $\square$

Finally, electric charges reach the soma. The function of the soma mainly consists in integrating all the signals to produce a unique output. In our framework, the soma behaves similarly to the well known "leaky integrate-and-fire" model [13]: The soma accumulates all the charges coming from the dendritic forest making its electric potential evolve, and at the same time, it undergoes a continuous attenuation due to a leak factor. As soon as the potential reaches the nominal function, a spike is emitted by the neuron on its output and the potential is reset by subtracting p_β (the asymptote of the nominal function, Definition 3). Moreover, it simultaneously starts the absolute refractory period, followed by the relative one. This behaviour which slighlty extends the classical leaky integrate-and-fire, is formalized in Lemma 1 and illustrated by Fig. 6.

Lemma 1 [Technical Lemma]. *Given a soma $\nabla = (\beta, \gamma)$ there exists a unique family of functions $P_F : Nominal(\beta) \times \mathbb{R}^+ \to \mathbb{R}$ indexed by the set of continuous functions $F : \mathbb{R}^+ \to \mathbb{R}$, such that for any couple $(e^0, p^0) \in Nominal(\beta)$, P_F satisfies:*

- $P_F(e^0, p^0, 0) = p^0$;
- *For all $t \in \mathbb{R}^+$ the right derivative $\frac{dP_F(e^0,p^0,t)}{dt}$ exists and is equal to $F(t) - \gamma.P_F(e^0, p^0, t)$; Moreover for all $t \in \mathbb{R}^{+*}$, $\ell = \lim_{h \to t^-}(P_F(e^0, p^0, h))$ exists and: If $(t + e^0, \ell) \in Nominal(\beta)$ then $P_F(e^0, p^0, t)$ is differentiable, therefore $P_F(e^0, p^0, t) = \ell$; Otherwise, for any $h \geqslant t$, $P_F(e^0, p^0, h) = P_G(0, \ell - p^\beta, h - t)$ where G is defined by: $\forall u \in \mathbb{R}^+, G(u) = F(u + t)$.*

Sketch of the Proof. Starting from time e^0, at value p^0, the function $P_F(t)$ is simply the unique integral of $\frac{dP}{dt} = F(t) - \gamma.P$ such that $P_F(e^0) = p^0$. However things are a little bit more complicated:

- *The existence of the integral results from the continuity of F and the Cauchy-Lipschitz theorem.*
- *When $P_F(t)$ reaches the nominal function, one has to reset e^0 to 0 and p^0 to $P_F(t) - p_\beta$. So one has to perform an inductive proof "from reset to reset."*

Figure 6 offers a visualization of these inductive steps, where the nominal function is "translated" at each reset step. The fully rigorous proof is given in Appendix A.3. □

The global neuron dynamics is the dynamics of the dendritic forest (generated by successive shifts) coupled with the soma dynamics (according to Lemma 1). Definition 11 describes how the whole dynamics is computed from an initial state according to an input signal.

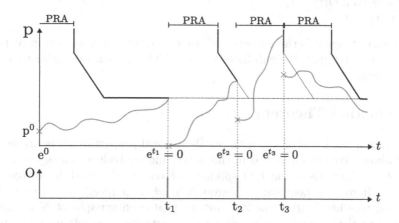

Fig. 6. Soma dynamics of a neuron N. Starting from an initial condition (e^0, p^0), the soma potential p follows its derivative. When the nominal function (represented here as piecewise affine) is reached, a spike is emitted on the output (O, at the bottom of the figure), resetting e to 0, updating p and starting an absolute refractory period (ARP). This is illustrated at successive times t_1, t_2 and t_3. Then p continues to evolve, starting from a new initial condition, depending on the derivative until reaching the threshold again, and so on.

Definition 11 [Dynamics of a Neuron]. *Given a neuron N and a state η^0 in continuity with an input signal $I = \{I_s\}_{s \in Sy(N)}$, the dynamics of N, according to I with η^0 as initial state, is the segment $d_I : \mathbb{R}^+ \to \zeta_N$ defined by:*

- $d_I(0) = \eta^0$;
- $\forall t \in \mathbb{R}^+, d_I(t) = \eta^t = (\{\eta_s^t\}_{s \in Sy(N)}, \{\eta_c^t\}_{c \in Co(N)}, (e^t, p^t))$ *where:*
  - $\partial^t = (\{\eta_s^t\}_{s \in Sy(N)}, \{\eta_c^t\}_{c \in Co(N)})$ *is defined as in Theorem 1;*
  - *Consider beforehand the function $F(t) = \sum\limits_{x \in Pred_N(\nabla)} \overline{\eta}_x^t(0)$; F is continuous (from Definition 10) and according to Lemma 1, there exists a unique function P_F such that $P_F(e^0, p^0, 0) = p^0$ and $\forall t$, $\frac{dP_F(e^0, p^0, t)}{dt} = F(t) - \gamma.P_F(e^0, p^0, t)$; If $P_F(e^0, p^0, t)$ is continuous on the interval $]0, t]$, then $e^t = e^0 + t$; otherwise, let t' be the greatest t such that $P_F(e^0, p^0, t)$ is discontinuous, then $e^t = t - t'$; finally, considering the previous P_F function, $p^t = P_F(e^0, p^0, t)$.*

Lastly, the output signal of the neuron is simply obtained by emitting a spike each time the soma state (e, p) undergoes a discontinuity (i.e. reaches the nominal function).

Definition 12 [Output Signal of a Neuron]. *Given a neuron N and an initial state η_0 in continuity with an input signal I, let $d_I = \{\eta^t\}_{t \in \mathbb{R}^+} = (\{\eta_s^t\}_{s \in Sy(N)}, \{\eta_c^t\}_{c \in Co(N)}, (e^t, p^t))$ be the corresponding dynamics of N. The output signal O of N is the signal such that for all $t \in \mathbb{R}^+$:*

- *if $e^t = 0$ then $O(t) = 1$,*
- *else $O(t) = 0$.*

The output signal is the sequence of spikes emitted by a neuron in response to a given input signal. We will focus on this I/O function throughout the rest of this article.

4   Reduction Theorem

In this section, we focus on the main mathematical properties of the framework defined above. We are interested in characterizing equivalence classes of neuron models that share the same I/O spiking behaviour. We start by introducing what we call *reduced* neurons: A neuron $N \in \mathcal{N}$ is reduced, if and only if the underlying tree has height 1 or 2. It means that each synapse of N is directly connected to the soma or via a unique compartment (see left part of Fig. 7). We note $\mathscr{P}$ the set of all reduced neurons. Given any neuron, we build its corresponding reduced neuron via a *reduction function* $\mathbb{P}$ defined as follows:

Definition 13 [Reduction Function]. *Given a neuron N and two nodes $x, y \in Nodes(N)$ such that y belongs to the path from x to the soma, noted $Path_N(x \to y)$, is the unique sequence of compartments $c_1, ..., c_n$ joining x to y in N where $c_n = y$ and $c_1 = x$ if x is a compartment and the successor of x if x is a synapse. We firstly define:*

- *The cumulative delay from x to y as $\Sigma_N^{x \to y} = \displaystyle\sum_{c_i \in Path_N(x \to y)} \Delta_{c_i}$;*
- *The cumulative attenuation from x to y as $\Pi_N^{x \to y} = \displaystyle\prod_{c_i \in Path_N(x \to y)} \alpha_{c_i}$.*

The reduction function $\mathbb{P} : \mathcal{N} \to \mathscr{P}$ is the map which associates to each neuron $N \in \mathcal{N}$ the reduced neuron of $\mathscr{P}$ built as follows:

- *$\mathbb{P}(N)$ has the same soma (∇) and the same set of synapses than N: $Sy(\mathbb{P}(N)) = Sy(N)$;*
- *For each synapse $s \in Sy(N)$, if $s \in Pred_N(\nabla)$ then s remains directly connected to the soma else, the unique compartment joining s to ∇ in $\mathbb{P}(N)$ is the couple $c_s = (\alpha_s, \Delta_s)$ with $\alpha_s = \Pi_N^{s \to \nabla}$ and $\Delta_s = \Sigma_N^{s \to \nabla}$.*

Given a neuron N and its corresponding reduced neuron P, the following definition describes how to uniquely build (*reconstruct*) the state of N from a state of P (see also Fig. 7).

Definition 14 [State Reconstruction]. *Given a neuron N, $\overleftarrow{\mathbb{P}_N} : \zeta_{\mathbb{P}(N)} \to \zeta_N$ is the map that associates to any state of $\mathbb{P}(N)$, $\eta = (\{\eta_s\}_{s \in Sy(\mathbb{P}(N))}, \{\eta_c\}_{c \in Co(\mathbb{P}(N))}, \eta_\nabla)$, the state of $N\overleftarrow{\mathbb{P}_N}(\eta) = \tilde{\eta} = (\{\tilde{\eta}_s\}_{s \in Sy(N)}, \{\tilde{\eta}_c\}_{c \in Co(N)}, \tilde{\eta}_\nabla)$ defined by:*

- *$\forall s \in Sy(N)$, $\tilde{\eta}_s = \eta_s$ and $\tilde{\eta}_\nabla = \eta_\nabla$;*
- *Given a synapse $s \in \mathbb{P}(N)$, let $c_s \in \mathbb{P}(N)$ be the compartment joining s to the soma in $\mathbb{P}(N)$, we first define the c_s-contribution of η to $\overleftarrow{\mathbb{P}_N}(\eta)$ as the state $\tilde{\eta}_c^{c_s}$ such that for all $c \in Co(N)$:*
  - *If $c \notin Path_N(s \to \nabla)$ then $\forall \delta \in [0, \Delta_c]$, $\tilde{\eta}_c^{c_s}(\delta) = 0$;*
  - *Else, there exists i such that $c = c_i$ where $Path_N(s \to \nabla) = c_1, ..., c_i, ..., c_n$; hence, $\forall \delta \in [0, \Delta_c]$: $\tilde{\eta}_c^{c_s}(\delta) = \left(\eta_{c_s}(\Sigma_N^{c_{i+1} \to c_n} + \delta)\right) / \Pi_N^{c_{i+1} \to c_n}$.*

  Then, we define $\tilde{\eta}_c = \displaystyle\sum_{s \in Sy(\mathbb{P}(N))} \tilde{\eta}_c^{c_s}$.

We define $\overleftarrow{\mathbb{P}_N} : \mathscr{D}_{\mathbb{P}(N)} \to \mathscr{D}_N$ the restriction of $\overleftarrow{\mathbb{P}_N}$ to dendritic states.
Note that if η is in continuity with an input signal I, then $\tilde{\eta}$ is also in continuity with I.

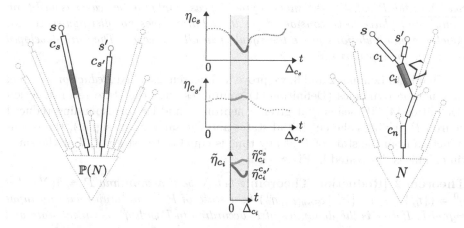

Fig. 7. State reconstruction of a neuron N (on the right) from the state of its corresponding reduced neuron $\mathbb{P}(N)$ (on the left). In the middle is represented the state of c_i ($\tilde{\eta}_{c_i}$), computed from the states of c_s (η_{c_s}) and $c_{s'}$ ($\eta_{c_{s'}}$): $\tilde{\eta}_{c_i}$ is the sum of the c_s and $c_{s'}$-contributions (respectively $\tilde{\eta}_{c_i}^{c_s}$ and $\tilde{\eta}_{c_i}^{c_{s'}}$). The contribution of the dashed compartments to the state of c_i is null.

We show in the following lemmas that shifting commutes with the dendritic reconstruction (Lemma 2) and it also commutes with the sum (Lemma 3).

Lemma 2 [Commutativity $shift \leftrightarrow \overleftarrow{\mathbb{P}_N}$]. *Given a neuron N, let $\partial = (\{\eta_s\}_{s \in Sy(\mathbb{P}(N))}, \{\eta_c\}_{c \in Co(\mathbb{P}(N))})$ be a dendritic state of $\mathbb{P}(N)$ in continuity with* an input signal I and let $\varepsilon \in \mathbb{R}^+$ such that $\varepsilon \leqslant \inf(\{\Delta_c \mid c \in Co(N)\})$. For any $c_s \in Co(\mathbb{P}(N))$ we have:

$$\varepsilon\text{-}shift^{I_{|s}}(\overleftarrow{\mathbb{P}_N}(\{\eta_c\}, c_s)) = \overleftarrow{\mathbb{P}_N}(\varepsilon\text{-}shift^{I_{|s}}(\{\eta_c\}), c_s)$$

Sketch of the Proof. It mainly consists in expanding Definitions 10 and 14. Definition 10 distinguishes two cases and Definition 14 distinguishes two cases with two sub-cases in one of them, so one has basically to properly consider six cases for each side of the equality. Algebraic manipulations show the equality in all cases. The full (rather tedious) proof is given in Appendix A.4. □

Lemma 3 [Commutativity *shift* $\leftrightarrow$ **+].** *Given a neuron N, let $\partial = (\{\eta_s\}_{s \in Sy(N)}, \{\eta_c\}_{c \in Co(N)})$ and $\partial' = (\{\eta'_s\}_{s \in Sy(N)}, \{\eta'_c\}_{c \in Co(N)})$ be two dendritic states of N in continuity with an input signal I. Let A and A' be two disjoint subsets of $Sy(N)$ such that $A \cup A' = Sy(N)$ and let $\varepsilon \in \mathbb{R}^+$ such that $\varepsilon \leqslant \inf(\{\Delta_c \mid c \in Co(N)\})$.*
We have:

$$\varepsilon\text{-}shift^I(\{\eta_c\} + \{\eta'_c\}) = \varepsilon\text{-}shift^{I_{|A}}(\{\eta_c\}) + \varepsilon\text{-}shift^{I_{|A'}}(\{\eta'_c\})$$

Sketch of the Proof. We still make a proof by case, only the two cases issued from Definition 10 have to be considered (as the addition does not distinguish cases). Algebraic manipulations prove the equality in all two cases. They are developed in details in Appendix A.5. □

Thanks to Lemmas 2 and 3, we prove in Theorem 2, called *Reduction theorem* that neuron dynamics (Definition 11) commutes with the state reconstruction (Definition 14). It means that given a neuron N and its corresponding reduced neuron P (having coherent initial states and the same input signal), the reconstruction from the state of P at any time is equal to the state of N at the same time. This is illustrated in Fig. 8.

Theorem 2 [Reduction Theorem]. *Let N be a neuron and $P = \mathbb{P}(N)$. Let $\eta^0 = (\{\eta^0_s\}_{s \in Sy(P)}, \{\eta^0_{c_s}\}_{s \in Sy(P)}, \eta^0_\nabla)$ be a state of P in continuity with an input signal I. If $d_{P,I}$ is the dynamics of P according to I with η^0 as initial state and if $d_{N,I}$ is the dynamics of N according to I with $\overleftarrow{\mathbb{P}_N}(\eta^0)$ as initial state, then for all $t \in \mathbb{R}^+$:*

$$d_{N,I}(t) = \overleftarrow{\mathbb{P}_N}(d_{P,I}(t))$$

Proof. From Theorem 1 and Definition 14, it is sufficient to prove that $\forall \varepsilon \in \mathbb{R}^+$, $\varepsilon\text{-}shift^I(\overleftarrow{\mathbb{P}_N}(\{\eta_{c_s}\})) = \overleftarrow{\mathbb{P}_N}(\varepsilon\text{-}shift^I(\{\eta_{c_s}\}))$.

1. $\varepsilon\text{-}shift^I(\overleftarrow{\mathbb{P}_N}(\{\eta_{c_s}\})) = \varepsilon\text{-}shift^I\left(\sum_{s \in Sy(N)} \overleftarrow{\mathbb{P}_N}(\{\eta_{c_s}\}, c_s)\right)$ *(from Definition 14),*

which is equal to $\sum_{s \in Sy(N)} \varepsilon\text{-}shift^{I_{|s}}\left(\overleftarrow{\mathbb{P}_N}(\{\eta_{c_s}\}, c_s)\right)$ *(from Lemma 3), which is*

equal to $\sum_{s \in Sy(N)} \overleftarrow{\mathbb{P}_N}(\varepsilon\text{-}shift^{I_{|s}}(\{\eta_{c_s}\}), c_s)$ *(from Lemma 2).*

2. Let $\{\eta_{c_s}^{\varepsilon}\} = \varepsilon\text{-}shift^I(\{\eta_{c_s}\})$. We have: $\overleftarrow{\mathbb{P}_N}(\varepsilon\text{-}shift^I(\{\eta_{c_s}\})) = \overleftarrow{\mathbb{P}_N}(\{\eta_{c_s}^{\varepsilon}\}) = $
$\sum_{s \in Sy(N)} \overleftarrow{\mathbb{P}_N}(\{\eta_{c_s}^{\varepsilon}\}, c_s)$ (from Definition 14) which is equal to $\sum_{s \in Sy(N)} \overleftarrow{\mathbb{P}_N}(\varepsilon\text{-}$
$shift^I(\{\eta_{c_s}\}), c_s)$.

From Definition 10, since $CoPred_P(c_s) = \varnothing$ and $SyPred_P(c_s) = \{s\}$, for all
$s \in Sy(P)$, $\varepsilon\text{-}shift^I(\eta_{c_s}) = \varepsilon\text{-}shift^{I_{|s}}(\eta_{c_s})$.

Therefore, we have $\overleftarrow{\mathbb{P}_N}(\varepsilon\text{-}shift^I(\{\eta_{c_s}\}), c_s) = \overleftarrow{\mathbb{P}_N}(\varepsilon\text{-}shift^{I_{|s}}(\{\eta_{c_s}\}), c_s)$. Thus,
$\overleftarrow{\mathbb{P}_N}(\varepsilon\text{-}shift^I(\{\eta_{c_s}\}))$ (computed in 2.) is equal to $\varepsilon\text{-}shift^I(\overleftarrow{\mathbb{P}_N}(\{\eta_{c_s}\}))$ (computed
in 1.). □

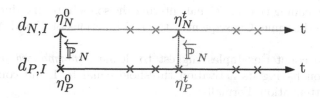

Fig. 8. Reduction theorem. Given a neuron N, its corresponding reduced neuron P
and an input signal I, if the dynamics of N at time 0 is the state reconstruction from
the dynamics of P at time 0 (i.e. $d_{N,I}(0) = \eta_N^0 = \overleftarrow{\mathbb{P}_N}(d_{P,I}(0)) = \overleftarrow{\mathbb{P}_N}(\eta_P^0)$) then, at any
time t, the dynamics of N is equal to the state reconstruction from the dynamics of P
at the same time t (i.e. $d_{N,I}(t) = \eta_N^t = \overleftarrow{\mathbb{P}_N}(d_{P,I}(t)) = \overleftarrow{\mathbb{P}_N}(\eta_P^t)$).

The Reduction theorem states that, for all time t, $d_{N,I}(t) = \overleftarrow{\mathbb{P}_N}(d_{P,I}(t))$.
Yet, we know, from Definition 14, that applying the map $\overleftarrow{\mathbb{P}_N}$ to $d_{P,I}(t)$ (being
the state of P at time t) does not change the state of the soma. It means that
for all t, the state of the soma of P is equal to the state of the soma of N.
Moreover, from Definition 13, the soma of P and the soma of N are the same.
Consequently, the neuron N and its corresponding reduced neuron P (having
coherent initial states) will always have the same output according to any input
signal.

So, we have defined in this section a reduction function (Definition 13) allowing to build for any neuron, its corresponding reduced neuron that preserves
I/O dynamics. Its dendritic-tree structure is basically reduced to a set of couples delay/attenuation. The reduced representation thus greatly simplifies the
neuron structure while preserving the I/O spiking behaviour. This generalizes
the proof of equivalence which was automatically performed in [8] for specific
toy examples.

5   From Reduction to Normalization

A natural continuation of the reduction process would be to obtain "normalized"
neurons such that each neuron would be the unique canonical representative of

a given I/O spiking behaviour. Two different normalized neurons should have at least one input signal that distinguishes their behaviours.

Reduced neuron as defined in the previous section are not "sufficiently reduced." Let us consider a reduced neuron N having a soma $\triangledown$ and only one synapse s connected to $\triangledown$ via a unique compartment c. Let us also consider a second reduced neuron N' having the same compartment c but connecting a synapse s' to a soma $\triangledown'$. If $\sigma_{s'} = 2 \times \sigma_s$ and $\beta_{N'} = 2 \times \beta_N$, then it is obvious that N and N' I/O functions will be the same as the higher weight of the synapse compensates the higher threshold to be reached in N'. As a second example, let us consider a reduced neuron N'' having the same soma $\triangledown$ than N but having a synapse s'' where $\sigma_{s''} = 2 \times \sigma_s$ connected to $\triangledown$ by a compartment c'' where $\alpha_{c''} = \alpha_c/2$. The weight of the synapse is twice higher in N'' but the attenuation is also twice, meaning that the signal entering the soma in both reduced neurons will always be the same. Consequently, the I/O functions of N and N'' will also be the same.

The above counter-examples suggest to define a *normalized neuron* as a reduced neuron having its activation threshold equal to 1 and compartments carrying no attenuation. Formally:

Definition 15 [Normalized Neuron]. *A reduced neuron $N \in \mathscr{P}$ is normalized if and only if:*

- *for all $c \in Co(N)$, $\alpha_c = 1$;*
- *the nominal function for N satisfies $p_\beta = 1$ (with notations of Definition 3).*

This would lead to extend Definition 13 into "Normalization functions" as defined in Fig. 9.

Unfortunately, two different normalized neurons can still have the same I/O function. The counter-examples are quite subtle and some of them are rather complex. The simplest one is obtained by considering a normalized neuron N having only one synapse s connected to a soma $\triangledown$ by a compartment $c = (1, \Delta_c)$. If σ_s is tiny and β_N is high, the threshold will never be reached (due to the leak γ) and the output of N will always be null. Therefore, two such normalized neurons N and N' (with $\Delta_c \neq \Delta_{c'}$ for example) have the same I/O functions while they differ at least by one parameter.

One could believe that it is sufficient to add a "functionality" condition on synapses to ensure that each σ_s is strong enough to make the signals reach the nominal function β along time. Unfortunately, we still encountered counter-examples. Among others: very strong σ_s that always produce a spike at the refractory time e_β, so β does not matter.

Many other more sophisticated examples exist and we are currently making a careful analysis of them. Yet, we fail to find proper restrictive conditions to ensure the bijection between normalized neurons and I/O spiking behaviours. The existence of a satisfactory notion of "normalized neuron" is in fact a very difficult *open question*.

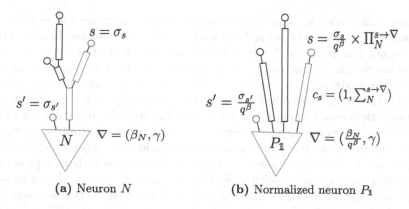

(a) Neuron N (b) Normalized neuron P_1

Fig. 9. Normalized form of a neuron. For any given input signal and given coherent initial states, the neuron N and its corresponding normalized form P_1 have the same output signal. The quotient $q^\beta = \frac{\beta_N}{\beta_1}$, where β_1 is the normal nominal function for P_1, is a constant function whose values belong to $[1, +\infty[$.

6   Conclusion

Although we were not focusing on the precise molecular mechanisms, an important motivation of this work was to preserve the essence of the biological functioning of neurons *with dendrites*, while providing a sufficiently simple framework to take benefit from algebraic properties and computer science formal methods.

We proved that neurons can be reduced while preserving the I/O spiking behaviours. In reduced and normalized neurons, dendrites are reduced to a set of parallel channels with the same properties. Those neurons have no dendritic tree (each synapse is connected to the soma via a unique branch without any attenuation) consequently, we formally proved that tree-shaped dendrites can be simply abstracted by using delays. This is the main result of this work.

However, a normalized neuron is not a "canonical" object since two different normalized neurons can have the same I/O spiking behaviours. Finding hypotheses under which a normalized neuron would be the unique canonical representative of equivalence classes of structures sharing the same I/O function could become an active research field.

With respect to current biological knowledge, our results rely on simplifying assumptions. Let us mention *passive conduction* (as it is now largely admitted that dendrites exhibit active mechanisms) as well as the mutual independence between synapses [7,10,18,19,24]. Technically, we made the original choice to deal with charges instead of voltages in order to manipulate sums at branching points. Indeed, our main theorems mostly relies on the associativity and commutativity of this operation, which would not be satisfied with voltage as all other frameworks do.

Most of neuron modelling work mainly consists of numerical simulations. Dendrites, among others, are complex components making difficult analytical approaches [22]. Formal methods from computer science partly alleviate this lack with the ability to make proofs subsuming an infinity of numerical simulations. A remarkable advantage of our approach which was not developed herein, is that based on our framework and with a proper time discretization, we are able to perform automatic proofs using model checking [8]. It is an encouraging step towards a new strategy to comprehensively understand dendritic integration. Moreover, this framework offers nice algebraic properties: it offers a theoretical foundation that could guide biology research towards the investigation of the features that separate biological neurons from this abstract idealized neuron.

All in all, the major result of this paper is that adding delays is finally a simple way to take into account an abstract dendritic integration without representing the dendritic morphology explicitly. Spiking networks have been shown to be at least as powerful as networks made of first or second generation neurons [15]. Our result shows that including delays in those networks implicitly represents a dendritic integration without requiring additional computing power, as there is no need to compute transfers through the tree-structure.

A   Appendices

A.1   Induction Lemmas and Proofs

Lemma 4 [Interval Induction Principle]. *Let ψ be a property on positive real numbers, we define the* interval induction principle *as follows: If there exists an increasing sequence $\{t_i\}_{I\!N}$ of positive real numbers such that $t_0 = 0$ and $\lim\limits_{n \to +\infty} t_i = +\infty$, and such that $\forall i \in I\!N, (\forall t \in [0, t_i[, \psi(t)) \Rightarrow (\forall t \in [t_i, t_{i+1}[, \psi(t)),$ then $\forall t \in I\!R^+, \psi(t).$*

Proof. Let us prove by induction on i that $\forall i \in I\!N, \forall t \in [0, t_i[, \psi(t)$ is satisfied.

- If $i = 0$ then $[0, t_0[= \emptyset$ so $\forall t \in [0, t_0[, \psi(t)$ is satisfied.
- If $\forall t \in [0, t_i[, \psi(t)$ is satisfied, then from the induction principle of the lemma, $\forall t \in [t_i, t_{i+1}[, \psi(t)$ is satisfied. Therefore, considering the union of the two intervals, it comes $\forall t \in [0, t_{i+1}[, \psi(t)$ is satisfied.

So for any $t \in I\!R^+$, there exists i such that $t_i > t$ because $\lim\limits_{i \to +\infty} t_i = +\infty$ and therefore, $\psi(t)$ is satisfied because $t \in [0, t_i[.$ □

Lemma 5 [Archimedean Induction Principle]. *Let ψ be a property on positive real numbers, we define the* archimedean induction principle *as follows: If there exists $a \in I\!R^{+*}$ such that $\forall t_0 \in I\!R^+, (\forall t \in [0, t_0[, \psi(t)) \Rightarrow (\forall t \in [t_0, t_0 + a[, \psi(t)),$ then $\forall t \in I\!R^+, \psi(t).$*

Proof. Because $I\!R^+$ is archimedean, it is sufficient to apply Lemma 4 with $t_i = i \times a.$

A.2   Proof of Theorem 1

Given a neuron N, let $\partial^0 = (\{\eta_s^0\}_{s \in Sy(N)}, \{\eta_c^0\}_{c \in Co(N)})$ be an initial dendritic state of N in continuity with an input signal I. There exists a unique family $\{\partial^t\}_{t \in \mathbb{R}^+}$ such that for all $t \in \mathbb{R}^+$ and for all $\varepsilon \in [0, inf(\{\Delta_c \mid c \in Co(N)\})]$:
$$\partial^{t+\varepsilon} = \varepsilon\text{-shift}^I(\partial^t).$$

Proof. The **uniqueness** of the family $\{\partial^t\}$ was already proved in the body of this paper. Let us prove the **existence** of the family $\{\partial^t\}_{t \in \mathbb{R}^+} = (\{\eta_s^t\}_{s \in Sy(N)}, \{\eta_c^t\}_{c \in Co(N)})$. It is equivalent to prove that for any t_0 the definition of ∂^{t_0} does not depend on its decomposition. Therefore, assuming $t_0 = t_1 + \varepsilon_1 = t_2 + \varepsilon_2$, one must have $\varepsilon_2\text{-shift}^I(\partial^{t_2}) = \varepsilon_1\text{-shift}^I(\partial^{t_1})$.

One can always assume that $t_1 < t_2$ and hence $t_2 = t_1 + \varepsilon_0$ where $\varepsilon_0 > 0$. We note $\{\overline{\partial}^t\}_{t \in \mathbb{R}^+} = (\{\overline{\eta}_s^t\}_{s \in Sy(N)}, \{\overline{\eta}_c^t\}_{c \in Co(N)})$, the ε_1-extension of $\{\partial^t\}$.

1. ∂^{t_0} as the ε_1-shift of ∂^{t_1}:
   (a) For all synapse $s \in Sy(N)$: $\eta_s^{t_0} = \eta_s^{t_1+\varepsilon_1} = \overline{\eta}_s^{t_1}(\varepsilon_1)$.
   (b) For all compartment $c \in Co(N)$:
      i. $\forall \delta \in [0, \Delta_c - \varepsilon_1]$, $\eta_c^{t_0}(\delta) = \eta_c^{t_1+\varepsilon_1}(\delta) = \eta_c^{t_1}(\delta + \varepsilon_1)$;

      ii. $\forall \delta \in [\Delta_c - \varepsilon_1, \Delta_c]$, $\eta_c^{t_0}(\delta) = \eta_c^{t_1+\varepsilon_1}(\delta) = \left(\sum\limits_{x \in Pred_N(c)} \overline{\eta}_x^{t_1}(\delta - \Delta_c + \varepsilon_1) \right)$
      $\times \alpha_c$.

2. ∂^{t_0} as the ε_2-shift of ∂^{t_2}:
   (a) For all synapse $s \in Sy(N)$: $\eta_s^{t_0} = \eta_s^{t_2+\varepsilon_2} = \overline{\eta}_s^{t_2}(\varepsilon_2) = \overline{\eta}_s^{t_1+\varepsilon_0}(\varepsilon_2) = \overline{\eta}_s^{t_1}(\varepsilon_2 + \varepsilon_0) = \overline{\eta}_s^{t_1}(\varepsilon_1)$ which is equal to $\eta_s^{t_1+\varepsilon_1}$ (computed in 1. (a)). This proves that the definition of $\eta_s^{t_0}$ does not depend on its decomposition.
   (b) For all compartment $c \in Co(N)$, one has to consider 3 cases, the union of which covers all the interval $[0, \Delta_c]$.
      i. If $\delta \in [0, \Delta_c - \varepsilon_1]$ then a fortiori $\delta \in [0, \Delta_c - \varepsilon_2]$ because $\varepsilon_2 < \varepsilon_1$. So: $\eta_c^{t_0}(\delta) = \eta_c^{t_2+\varepsilon_2}(\delta) = \eta_c^{t_2}(\delta + \varepsilon_2)$. Moreover, $\delta + \varepsilon_2 \leqslant \Delta_c - \varepsilon_0$ as $\delta \leqslant \Delta_c - (\varepsilon_0 + \varepsilon_2) = \Delta_c - \varepsilon_1$. So: $\eta_c^{t_2}(\delta + \varepsilon_2) = \eta_c^{t_1+\varepsilon_0}(\delta + \varepsilon_2) = \eta_c^{t_1}(\delta - \varepsilon_2 + \varepsilon_0) = \eta_c^{t_1}(\delta + \varepsilon_1)$ which is equal to $\eta_c^{t_1+\varepsilon_1}(\delta)$ from 1(b).
      ii. If $\delta \in [\Delta_c - \varepsilon_1, \Delta_c - \varepsilon_2]$ then a fortiori $\delta \in [0, \Delta_c - \varepsilon_2]$ because $\varepsilon_1 < \Delta_c$. So: $\eta_c^{t_0}(\delta) = \eta_c^{t_2+\varepsilon_2}(\delta) = \eta_c^{t_2}(\delta + \varepsilon_2)$. Moreover, $\delta + \varepsilon_2 \in [\Delta_c - \varepsilon_0, \Delta_c]$ as $\Delta_c - \varepsilon_1 + \varepsilon_2 = \Delta_c - (\varepsilon_1 - \varepsilon_2) = \Delta_c - \varepsilon_0$. So:

$$\eta_c^{t_2}(\delta + \varepsilon_2) = \eta_c^{t_1+\varepsilon_0}(\delta + \varepsilon_2) = \left(\sum\limits_{x \in Pred_N(c)} \overline{\eta}_x^{t_1}(\delta + \varepsilon_2 - \Delta_c + \varepsilon_0) \right) \times \alpha_c$$

$$= \left(\sum\limits_{x \in Pred_N(c)} \overline{\eta}_x^{t_1}(\delta - \Delta_c + \varepsilon_1) \right) \times \alpha_c$$

which is equal to $\eta_c^{t_1+\varepsilon_1}(t)$ from 1(b).

      iii. If $\delta \in [\Delta_c - \varepsilon_2, \Delta_c]$ then: $\eta_c^{t_2+\varepsilon_2}(\delta) = \left(\sum\limits_{x \in Pred_N(c)} \overline{\eta}_x^{t_2}(\delta - \Delta_c + \varepsilon_2) \right) \times$
      α_c. Moreover, since $\delta \in [\Delta_c - \varepsilon_2, \Delta_c]$, $(\delta - \Delta_c + \varepsilon_2) \in [0, \varepsilon_2] \subset [0, \Delta_c -$

ε_0] because $\varepsilon_1 = \varepsilon_2 + \varepsilon_0 \leqslant \Delta_c$ and hence $\varepsilon_2 < \Delta_c - \varepsilon_0$. Therefore $\overline{\eta}_x^{t_2}(\delta - \Delta_c + \varepsilon_2) = \overline{\eta}_x^{t_1 + \varepsilon_0}(\delta - \Delta_c + \varepsilon_2) = \overline{\eta}_x^{t_1}(\delta - \Delta_c + \varepsilon_2 + \varepsilon_0) = \overline{\eta}_x^{t_1}(\delta -$

$\Delta_c + \varepsilon_1)$. It comes: $\eta_c^{t_2 + \varepsilon_2}(\delta) = \left(\displaystyle\sum_{x \in Pred_N(c)} \overline{\eta}_x^{t_1}(\delta - \Delta_c + \varepsilon_1) \right) \times \alpha_c$

which is equal to $\eta_c^{t_1 + \varepsilon_1}(\delta)$ from 1(b).

Thus, $\forall \delta \in [0, \Delta_c]$, η_c^{to} as the ε_2-shift of $\eta_c^{t_2}$ (computed in 2.) is equal to η_c^{to} as the ε_1-shift of $\eta_c^{t_1}$ (computed in 1.) which proves that the definition of η_c^{to} does not depend on its decomposition.   □

A.3   Proof of Lemma 1

Given a soma $\nabla = (\beta, \gamma)$ there exists a unique family of functions $P_F :$ $Nominal(\beta) \times \mathbb{R}^+ \to \mathbb{R}$ indexed by the set of continuous functions $F : \mathbb{R}^+ \to \mathbb{R}$, such that for any couple $(e^0, p^0) \in Nominal(\beta)$, P_F satisfies:

- $P_F(e^0, p^0, 0) = p^0$;
- For all $t \in \mathbb{R}^+$ the right derivative $\frac{dP_F(e^0, p^0, t)}{dt}$ exists and is equal to $F(t) - \gamma.P_F(e^0, p^0, t)$; Moreover for all $t \in \mathbb{R}^{+*}$, $\ell = \lim_{h \to t^-} (P_F(e^0, p^0, h))$ exists and: If $(t + e^0, \ell) \in Nominal(\beta)$ then $P_F(e^0, p^0, t)$ is differentiable, therefore $P_F(e^0, p^0, t) = \ell$; Otherwise, for any $h \geqslant t$, $P_F(e^0, p^0, h) = P_G(0, \ell - p^\beta, h - t)$ where G is defined by: $\forall u \in \mathbb{R}^+$, $G(u) = F(u + t)$.

Proof. We need to prove the existence of a unique function $P_F(e^0, p^0, t)$. Let us consider the strictly increasing sequence of positive real numbers $t_0...t_n...$ built as follows:

Basic Case:

- From the Cauchy-Lipschitz theorem (also known as Picard-Lindelöf), there exists a unique function $f(t)$ such that $f'(t) = g(t, f(t)) = F(t) - \gamma.f(t)$ and $f(0) = p^0$ because:
  - g is uniformly Lipschitz continuous in f, meaning that the Lipschitz constant (k) is not dependent of t so $\forall t, \exists k \in R^{*+}$ such that $|g(t, x) - g(t, y)| \leqslant k|x - y|$ meaning $|(F(t) - \gamma.x) - (F(t) - \gamma.y)| \leqslant k|x - y|$ meaning $\gamma|y - x| \leqslant k|x - y|$ which is obvious for $k = \gamma$;
  - g is continuous in t because F is continuous in t.
- Let t_0 be the smallest $t \in \mathbb{R}^+ \cup \{+\infty\}$ such that $(e^0 + t, f(t)) \notin Nominal(\beta)$ then $t_0 > 0$ because $(e^0, f(0)) = (e^0, p^0) \in Nominal(\beta)$. If $t_0 = +\infty$ then the lemma is proven. Otherwise, $P_F(e^0, p^0, t_0) = P_G(0, p_1, 0)$. Therefore, there exists a unique function $P_F(e^0, p^0, t)$ on the interval $[0, t_0]$ and since it is differentiable, $\lim_{h \to t^-} (P_F(e^0, p^0, h))$ exists on $]0, t_0]$.

Induction Step:

- Inductively, assume that the existence of a unique function $P_F(e^0, p^0, t)$ is proved on an interval $[0, t_i]$ where $t_i \in \mathbb{R}^+$ and $P_F(e^0, p^0, t_i) = P_{G_i}(0, p_i, 0)$ where $G_i(u) = F(u + t_i)$. Let Δt be the smallest $t \in \mathbb{R}^+ \cup \{+\infty\}$ such that $(e^0 + \Delta t, f(t)) \notin Nominal(\beta)$. If $\Delta t = +\infty$ then the lemma is proven. Otherwise, let $t_{i+1} = t_i + \Delta t$, we have proven that there exists a unique function $P_F(e^0, p^0, t)$ on the interval $[0, t_{i+1}]$ and since it is differentiable on $[t_i, t_{i+1}]$, $\lim_{h \to t^-} (P_F(e^0, p^0, h))$ exists on this interval and therefore it exists on $[0, t_{i+1}]$.
- Finally for any i, Δt is greater than e_β and consequently the sequence of t_i diverges towards $+\infty$ which proves the lemma, according to Lemma 4.   □

A.4   Proof of Commutativity Lemma 2

Given a neuron N, let $\partial = (\{\eta_s\}_{s \in Sy(\mathbb{P}(N))}, \{\eta_c\}_{c \in Co(\mathbb{P}(N))})$ be a dendritic state of $\mathbb{P}(N)$ in continuity with an input signal I and let $\varepsilon \in \mathbb{R}^+$ such that $\varepsilon \leqslant inf(\{\Delta_c \mid c \in Co(N)\})$. For any $c_s \in Co(\mathbb{P}(N))$ we have: ε-shift$^{I_{|s}}(\overleftarrow{\mathbb{P}}_N(\{\eta_c\}, c_s)) = \overleftarrow{\mathbb{P}}_N(\varepsilon\text{-shift}^{I_{|s}}(\{\eta_c\}), c_s)$.

Proof. We need to prove ε-shift$^{I_{|s}}(\overleftarrow{\mathbb{P}}_N(\{\eta_c\}, c_s)) = \overleftarrow{\mathbb{P}}_N(\varepsilon\text{-shift}^{I_{|s}}(\{\eta_c\}), c_s)$. Let us note:

1. $\overleftarrow{\mathbb{P}}_N(\{\eta_c\}, c_s) = \overleftarrow{\eta}_c = \{\overleftarrow{\eta}_c\}_{c \in Co(N)}$
2. ε-shift$^{I_{|s}}(\{\overleftarrow{\eta}_c\}) = \overleftarrow{\eta}_c^\varepsilon = \{\overleftarrow{\eta}_c^\varepsilon\}_{c \in Co(N)}$
3. ε-shift$^{I_{|s}}(\{\eta_c\}) = \eta_{c_s}^\varepsilon = \{\eta_{c_s}^\varepsilon\}_{c_s \in Co(\mathbb{P}(N))}$
4. $\overleftarrow{\mathbb{P}}_N(\{\eta_c^\varepsilon\}, c_s) = \overleftarrow{\eta}_c^\varepsilon = \{\overleftarrow{\eta}_c^\varepsilon\}_{c \in Co(N)}$

We then need to prove $\forall c \in Co(N)$, $\overleftarrow{\eta}_c^\varepsilon = \overleftarrow{\eta_c^\varepsilon}$. For simplicity, we note $\eta_s(x) = \overline{\eta}_s(x)$ since we only consider ε-extended synaptic states in this proof.

1. From Definition 14:
   (a) If $c \notin Path_N(s \to \nabla)$ then $\forall \delta \in [0, \Delta_c]$, $\overleftarrow{\eta}_c(\delta) = 0$;
   (b) If $c \in Path_N(s \to \nabla)$, there exists i such that $c = c_i$ with $Path_N(s \to \nabla) = c_1, ..., c_i, ..., c_n$.
   Therefore, $\forall \delta \in [0, \Delta_c]$, $\overleftarrow{\eta}_c(\delta) = \eta_{c_s} \left(\Sigma_N^{c_{i+1} \to c_n} + \delta \right) / \Pi_N^{c_{i+1} \to c_n}$.
2. From Definition 10:
   (a) If $c \notin Path_N(s \to \nabla)$:
      i. If $\delta \in [0, \Delta_c - \varepsilon]$, $\overleftarrow{\eta}_c^\varepsilon(\delta) = \overleftarrow{\eta}_c(\delta + \varepsilon) = 0$ (because of 1. (a)).

      ii. If $\delta \in [\Delta_c - \varepsilon, \Delta_c]$, $\overleftarrow{\eta}_c^\varepsilon(\delta) = \left(\sum_{x \in Pred_N(c)} \overleftarrow{\eta}_x(\delta - \Delta_c + \varepsilon) \right) \times \alpha_c$.

      For each $x \in CoPred_N(c)$, since $c \notin Path_N(s \to \nabla)$ then $x \notin Path_N(s \to \nabla)$ and therefore $\overleftarrow{\eta}_x = 0$ (because of 1. (a)). Moreover, for each $x \in SyPred_N(c)$ and considering $I_{|s}$, $\overleftarrow{\eta}_x = 0$ because $\forall x \in SyPred_N(c)$, x is different from s as $c \notin Path_N(s \to \nabla)$. We thus have $\overleftarrow{\eta}_c^\varepsilon(\delta) = 0$.

(b) If $c \in Path_N(s \rightarrow \triangledown)$:

    i. If $\delta \in [0, \Delta_c - \varepsilon]$, $\overleftarrow{\eta}_c^\varepsilon(\delta) = \overleftarrow{\eta}_c(\delta + \varepsilon) = \eta_{c_s}\left(\Sigma_N^{c_{i+1} \rightarrow c_n} + \delta + \varepsilon\right) / \Pi_N^{c_{i+1} \rightarrow c_n}$ (because of 1. (b)).

    ii. If $\delta \in [\Delta_c - \varepsilon, \Delta_c]$, $\overleftarrow{\eta}_c^\varepsilon(\delta) = \left(\sum_{x \in Pred_N(c)} \overleftarrow{\eta}_x(\delta - \Delta_c + \varepsilon) \right) \times \alpha_c.$

    Since c has only one predecessor compartment $x \in Path_N(s \rightarrow \triangledown)$ (potentially having $\overleftarrow{\eta}_x \neq 0$), we have $CoPred_N(c) = \{c_{i-1}\}$ (except $CoPred_N(c) = \varnothing$ if $c_i = c_1$). Moreover, $SyPred_N(c) = \{s\}$ if $c_i = c_1$ while if $c_i \neq c_1$ for each $x \in SyPred_N(c)$, $\overleftarrow{\eta}_x = 0$ (considering $I_{|_s}$). Therefore:

    A. if $c_i \neq c_1$, $\overleftarrow{\eta}_c^\varepsilon(\delta) = \overleftarrow{\eta}_{c_{i-1}}(\delta - \Delta_c + \varepsilon) \times \alpha_c$. From 1. (b), $\overleftarrow{\eta}_{c_{i-1}}(\delta) = \eta_{c_s}\left(\Sigma_N^{c_i \rightarrow c_n} + \delta\right) / \Pi_N^{c_i \rightarrow c_n}$.
    Therefore, $\overleftarrow{\eta}_c^\varepsilon(\delta) = (\eta_{c_s}\left(\Sigma_N^{c_i \rightarrow c_n} + \delta - \Delta_c + \varepsilon\right) / \Pi_N^{c_i \rightarrow c_n}) \times \alpha_c = \eta_{c_s}\left(\Sigma_N^{c_{i+1} \rightarrow c_n} + \delta + \varepsilon\right) / \Pi_N^{c_{i+1} \rightarrow c_n}$.
    B. if $c_i = c_1$, $\overleftarrow{\eta}_c^\varepsilon(\delta) = (\overleftarrow{\eta}_s(\delta - \Delta_c + \varepsilon)) \times \alpha_c$ and from the remark of Definition 14, $\overleftarrow{\eta}_c^\varepsilon(\delta) = (\eta_s(\delta - \Delta_c + \varepsilon)) \times \alpha_c$.

3. From Definition 10:

    (a) if $\delta \in [0, \Delta_{c_s} - \varepsilon]$, $\eta_{c_s}^\varepsilon(\delta) = \eta_{c_s}(\delta + \varepsilon)$.

    (b) if $\delta \in [\Delta_{c_s} - \varepsilon, \Delta_{c_s}]$, $\eta_{c_s}^\varepsilon(\delta) = \left(\sum_{x \in Pred_N(c_s)} \eta_x(\delta - \Delta_{c_s} + \varepsilon) \right) \times \alpha_c.$

    Since $c_s \in Co(\mathbb{P}(N))$, $CoPred_N(c_s) = \varnothing$ and $SyPred_N(c_s) = \{s\}$. Therefore, $\eta_{c_s}^\varepsilon(\delta) = (\eta_s(\delta - \Delta_{c_s} + \varepsilon)) \times \alpha_c$.

4. Lastly, from Definition 14:

    (a) If $c \notin Path_N(s \rightarrow \triangledown)$ then $\forall \delta \in [0, \Delta_c]$, $\overleftarrow{v}_c^\varepsilon(\delta) = 0$ <u>which is equal to</u> $\overleftarrow{\eta}_c^\varepsilon(\delta)$ (computed in 2. (a)).

    (b) If $c \in Path_N(s \rightarrow \triangledown)$, there exists i such that $c = c_i$ and $Path_N(s \rightarrow \triangledown) = c_1, ..., c_i, ..., c_n$. Therefore, $\forall \delta \in [0, \Delta_c]$, $\overleftarrow{\eta}_c^\varepsilon(\delta) = \eta_{c_s}^\varepsilon\left(\Sigma_N^{c_{i+1} \rightarrow c_n} + \delta\right) / \Pi_N^{c_{i+1} \rightarrow c_n}$. Since $\eta_{c_s}^\varepsilon = \varepsilon\text{-shift}^{I_{|s}}(\eta_{c_s})$, we have:

      i. If $\delta \in [0, \Delta_c - \varepsilon]$ then $\left(\Sigma_N^{c_{i+1} \rightarrow c_n} + \delta\right) \in [0, \Delta_{c_s} - \varepsilon]$ therefore, $\eta_{c_s}^\varepsilon\left(\Sigma_N^{c_{i+1} \rightarrow c_n} + \delta\right) = \eta_{c_s}\left(\Sigma_N^{c_{i+1} \rightarrow c_n} + \delta + \varepsilon\right)$ and hence, $\overleftarrow{\eta}_c^\varepsilon(\delta) = \eta_{c_s}\left(\Sigma_N^{c_{i+1} \rightarrow c_n} + \delta + \varepsilon\right) / \Pi_N^{c_{i+1} \rightarrow c_n}$ <u>which is equal to</u> $\overleftarrow{\eta}_c^\varepsilon(\delta)$ (computed in 2. (b) i.).

      ii. If $\delta \in [\Delta_c - \varepsilon, \Delta_c]$ then:

        A. If $c_i \neq c_1$, $\left(\Sigma_N^{c_{i+1} \rightarrow c_n} + \delta\right) \in [0, \Delta_{c_s} - \varepsilon]$ therefore, $\eta_{c_s}^\varepsilon\left(\Sigma_N^{c_{i+1} \rightarrow c_n} + \delta\right) = \eta_{c_s}\left(\Sigma_N^{c_{i+1} \rightarrow c_n} + \delta + \varepsilon\right)$ and hence, $\overleftarrow{\eta}_c^\varepsilon(\delta) = \eta_{c_s}\left(\Sigma_N^{c_{i+1} \rightarrow c_n} + \delta + \varepsilon\right) / \Pi_N^{c_{i+1} \rightarrow c_n}$ <u>which is equal to</u> $\overleftarrow{\eta}_c^\varepsilon(\delta)$ (computed in 2. (b) ii. A.).

        B. If $c_i = c_1$, $\left(\Sigma_N^{c_{i+1} \rightarrow c_n} + \delta\right) \in [\Delta_{c_s} - \varepsilon, \Delta_{c_s}]$ thus, $\eta_{c_s}^\varepsilon\left(\Sigma_N^{c_{i+1} \rightarrow c_n} + \delta\right)$
$$= \left(\sum_{x \in Pred_N(c_s)} \eta_x\left(\Sigma_N^{c_{i+1} \rightarrow c_n} + \delta - \Delta_{c_s} + \varepsilon\right) \right) \times \alpha_{c_s} \text{ and hence}$$
$\overleftarrow{\eta}_c^\varepsilon(\delta) = \left(\eta_s\left(\Sigma_N^{c_{i+1} \rightarrow c_n} + \delta - \Delta_{c_s} + \varepsilon\right) \times \alpha_{c_s}\right) / \Pi_N^{c_{i+1} \rightarrow c_n}$ (because $CoPred_N(c_s) = \varnothing$ and $SyPred_N(c_s) = \{s\}$). Since $c_i = c_1$, $\Sigma_N^{c_{i+1} \rightarrow c_n} = \Delta_{c_s} - \Delta_{c_1}$ therefore $\overleftarrow{\eta}_c^\varepsilon(\delta) = (\eta_s(\delta - \Delta_{c_1} + \varepsilon)$

$$\times \alpha_{c_s}) / \Pi_N^{c_{i+1} \to c_n} \text{ and hence } \overleftarrow{\eta_c^\varepsilon}(\delta) = (\eta_s(\delta - \Delta_{c_1} + \varepsilon)) \times \alpha_{c_1}$$

which is equal to $\overleftarrow{\eta}_c^\varepsilon(\delta)$ (computed in 2. (b) ii. B.).

This concludes the proof. In 4., we had to consider two cases (a) and (b). The case (a) was directly solved whereas the case (b) was divided in two sub-cases i. and ii. The case i. was directly solved whereas the case ii. was divided in two sub-sub-cases A. and B. which were both solved. So, owing to this decomposition, the lemma is proved for all the possible conditions. □

A.5   Proof of Commutativity Lemma 3

Given a neuron N, let $\partial = (\{\eta_s\}_{s \in Sy(N)}, \{\eta_c\}_{c \in Co(N)})$ and $\partial' = (\{\eta'_s\}_{s \in Sy(N)}, \{\eta'_c\}_{c \in Co(N)})$ be two dendritic states of N in continuity with an input signal I. Let A and A' be two disjoint subsets of $Sy(N)$ such that $A \cup A' = Sy(N)$ and let $\varepsilon \in \mathbb{R}^+$ such that $\varepsilon \leqslant inf(\{\Delta_c \mid c \in Co(N)\})$.

We have: $\varepsilon\text{-shift}^I(\{\eta_c\} + \{\eta'_c\}) = \varepsilon\text{-shift}^{I_{|A}}(\{\eta_c\}) + \varepsilon\text{-shift}^{I_{|A'}}(\{\eta'_c\})$.

Proof. According to Definition 10, for any $c \in Co(N)$, we note $\eta''_c = \eta_c + \eta'_c$.

1. Let us consider $\varepsilon\text{-shift}^I(\{\eta_c\} + \{\eta'_c\})$:
   - If $\delta \in [0, \Delta_c - \varepsilon]$, $\varepsilon\text{-shift}^I(\eta_c + \eta'_c)(\delta) = \varepsilon\text{-shift}^I(\eta''_c)(\delta) = \eta''_c(\delta + \varepsilon) = (\eta_c + \eta'_c)(\delta + \varepsilon) = \eta_c(\delta + \varepsilon) + \eta'_c(\delta + \varepsilon)$.
   - If $\delta \in [\Delta_c - \varepsilon, \Delta_c]$, $\varepsilon\text{-shift}^I(\eta_c + \eta'_c)(\delta) = \varepsilon\text{-shift}^I(\eta''_c)(\delta)$
$$= (\sum_{x \in Pred_N(c)} (\overline{\eta}''_x(\delta - \Delta_c + \varepsilon))) \times \alpha_c$$
$$= (\sum_{x \in Pred_N(c)} ((\overline{\eta}_x + \overline{\eta}'_x)(\delta - \Delta_c + \varepsilon))) \times \alpha_c$$
$$= (\sum_{x \in Pred_N(c)} (\overline{\eta}_x(\delta - \Delta_c + \varepsilon) + \overline{\eta}'_x(\delta - \Delta_c + \varepsilon))) \times \alpha_c$$

2. Let us consider $\varepsilon\text{-shift}^{I_{|A}}(\{\eta_c\}) + \varepsilon\text{-shift}^{I_{|A'}}(\{\eta'_c\})$:
   - If $\delta \in [0, \Delta_c - \varepsilon]$, $\varepsilon\text{-shift}^{I_{|A}}(\eta_c) + \varepsilon\text{-shift}^{I_{|A'}}(\eta'_c) = \eta_c(\delta + \varepsilon) + \eta'_c(\delta + \varepsilon)$.
   - If $\delta \in [\Delta_c - \varepsilon, \Delta_c]$, $\varepsilon\text{-shift}^{I_{|A}}(\eta_c) + \varepsilon\text{-shift}^{I_{|A'}}(\eta'_c)$
$$= (\sum_{c' \in CoPred_N(c)} \overline{\eta}_{c'}(\delta - \Delta_c + \varepsilon) + \sum_{s \in SyPred_N(c) \cap s \in A} \overline{\eta}_s(\delta - \Delta_c + \varepsilon)) \times \alpha_c$$
$$+ (\sum_{c' \in CoPred_N(c)} \overline{\eta}'_{c'}(\delta - \Delta_c + \varepsilon) + \sum_{s \in SyPred_N(c) \cap s \in A'} \overline{\eta}_s(\delta - \Delta_c + \varepsilon)) \times \alpha_c$$
$$= (\sum_{c' \in CoPred_N(c)} \overline{\eta}_{c'}(\delta - \Delta_c + \varepsilon) + \sum_{s \in SyPred_N(c) \cap s \in A} \overline{\eta}_s(\delta - \Delta_c)$$
$$+ \sum_{c' \in CoPred_N(c)} \overline{\eta}'_{c'}(\delta - \Delta_c + \varepsilon) + \sum_{s \in SyPred_N(c) \cap s \in A'} \overline{\eta}_s(\delta - \Delta_c + \varepsilon)) \times \alpha_c$$
$$= (\sum_{c' \in CoPred_N(c)} (\overline{\eta}_{c'}(\delta - \Delta_c + \varepsilon) + \overline{\eta}'_{c'}(\delta - \Delta_c + \varepsilon))$$
$$+ \sum_{s \in SyPred_N(c)} \overline{\eta}_s(\delta - \Delta_c + \varepsilon)) \times \alpha_c$$
$$= (\sum_{x \in Pred_N(c)} (\overline{\eta}_x(\delta - \Delta_c + \varepsilon) + \overline{\eta}'_x(\delta - \Delta_c + \varepsilon))) \times \alpha_c.$$

Thus, $\varepsilon\text{-shift}^{I_{|A}}(\{\eta_c\}) + \varepsilon\text{-shift}^{I_{|A'}}(\{\eta'_c\}) = \varepsilon\text{-shift}^I(\{\eta_c\} + \{\eta'_c\})$ as the formulas obtained in 1. and 2. are the same. □

References

1. Brette, R., Gerstner, W.: Adaptive exponential integrate-and-fire model as an effective description of neuronal activity. J. Neurophysiol. **94**(5), 3637–3642 (2005)
2. Buchera, D., Goaillard, J.M.: Beyond faithful conduction: short-term dynamics, neuromodulation, and long-term regulation of spike propagation in the axon. Prog. Neurobiol. **94**(4), 307–346 (2011)
3. Byrne, J.H., Roberts, J.L.: From Molecules to Networks. Academic Press, Cambridge (2004)
4. Dayan, P., Abbott, L.F.: Theoretical Neuroscience: Computational and Mathematical Modeling of Neural Systems. Massachusetts Institute of Technology Press, Cambridge (2001)
5. Debanne, D.: Information processing in the axon. Nat. Rev. Neurosci. **5**, 304–316 (2004)
6. Gerstner, W., Naud, R.: How good are neuron models? Science **326**(5951), 379–380 (2009)
7. Gorski, T., Veltz, R., Galtier, M., Fragnaud, H., Telenczuk, B., Destexhe, A.: Inverse correlation processing by neurons with active dendrites. bioRxiv, Forthcoming (2017)
8. Guinaudeau, O., Bernot, G., Muzy, A., Gaffé, D., Grammont, F.: Computer-aided formal proofs about dendritic integration within a neuron. In: BIOINFORMATICS 2018–9th International Conference on Bioinformatics Models, Methods and Algorithms (2018)
9. Guinaudeau, O., Bernot, G., Muzy, A., Grammont, F.: Abstraction of the structure and dynamics of the biological neuron for a formal study of the dendritic integration. In: Advances in Systems and Synthetic Biology (2017)
10. Häusser, M., Mel, B.: Dendrites: bug or feature? Curr. Opin. Neurobiol. **13**(3), 372–383 (2003)
11. Huguenard, J.R.: Reliability of axonal propagation: the spike doesn't stop here. Proc. Natl. Acad. Sci. **97**(17), 9349–9350 (2000)
12. Izhikevich, E.M.: Polychronization: computation with spikes. Neural Comput. **18**(2), 245–282 (2006)
13. Lapicque, L.: Recherches quatitatives sur l'excitation electrique des nerfs traitee comme polarisation. J. Physiol. Pathol. Gen. **9**, 620–635 (1907)
14. Maass, W., Schnitger, G., Sontag, E.D.: On the computational power of sigmoid versus Boolean threshold circuits. In: Proceedings of the 32nd Annual Symposium on Foundations of Computer Science, pp. 767–776. IEEE (1991)
15. Maass, W.: Networks of spiking neurons: the third generation of neural network models. Neural Netw. **10**(9), 1659–1671 (1997)
16. Maass, W.: On the relevance of time in neural computation and learning. Theoret. Comput. Sci. **261**(1), 157–178 (2001)
17. McCulloch, W.S., Pitts, W.: A logical calculus of the ideas immanent in nervous activity. Bull. Math. Biophys. **5**(4), 115–133 (1943)
18. Mel, B.W.: Information processing in dendritic trees. Neural Comput. **6**(6), 1031–1085 (1994)
19. Paulus, W., Rothwell, J.C.: Membrane resistance and shunting inhibition: where biophysics meets satate dependent human neurophysiology. J. Physiol. **594**(10), 2719–2728 (2016)
20. Rall, W.: Branching dendritic trees and motoneuron membrane resistivity. Exp. Neurol. **1**(5), 491–527 (1959)

21. Rall, W.: Theory of physiological properties of dendrites. Ann. N. Y. Acad. Sci. **96**(1), 1071–1092 (1962)
22. Segev, I., London, M.: Untangling dendrites with quantitative models. Science **290**(5492), 744–750 (2000)
23. Stern, E.A., Jaeger, D., Wilson, C.J.: Membrane potential synchrony of simultaneously recorded striatal spiny neurons in vivo. Nature **394**(6692), 475–478 (1998)
24. Stuart, G., Spruston, N., Häusser, M.: Dendrites. Oxford University Press, Oxford (2016)
25. Thorpe, S., Imbert, M.: Biological constraints on connectionist modelling. In: Connectionism in Perspective, pp. 63–92 (1989)
26. Thorpe, S., Delorme, A., Van Rullen, R.: Spike-based strategies for rapid processing. Neural Netw. **14**(6), 715–725 (2001)
27. Van Rullen, R., Thorpe, S.J.: Rate coding versus temporal order coding: what the retinal ganglion cells tell the visual cortex. Neural Comput. **13**(6), 1255–1283 (2001)
28. Williams, S.R., Stuart, G.J.: Dependence of EPSP efficacy on synapse location in neocortical pyramidal neurons. Science **295**(5561), 1907–1910 (2002)

Discovering Trends in Environmental Time-Series with Supervised Classification of Metatranscriptomic Reads and Empirical Mode Decomposition

Enzo Acerbi[1], Caroline Chénard[2], Stephan C. Schuster[1], and Federico M. Lauro[1,2(✉)]

[1] Singapore Centre for Environmental Life Sciences Engineering (SCELSE), Nanyang Technological University, Jurong West, Singapore
flauro@ntu.edu.sg
[2] Asian School of the Environment, Nanyang Technological University, Jurong West, Singapore

Abstract. In metagenomic and metatranscriptomic studies, the assignment of reads to taxonomic bins is typically performed by sequence similarity or phylogeny based approaches. Such methods become less effective if the sequences are closely related and/or of limited length. Here, we propose an approach for multi-class supervised classification of metatranscriptomic reads of short length (100–300 bp) which exploits k-mers frequencies as discriminating features. In addition, we take a first step in addressing the lack of established methods for the analysis of periodic features in environmental time-series by proposing Empirical Mode Decomposition as a way of extracting information on heterogeneity and population dynamics in natural microbial communities. To prove the validity of our computational approach as an effective tool to generate new biological insights, we applied it to investigate the transcriptional dynamics of viral infection in the ocean. We used data extracted from a previously published metatranscriptome profile of a naturally occurring oceanic bacterial assemblage sampled Lagrangially over 3 days. We discovered the existence of light-dark oscillations in the expression patterns of auxiliary metabolic genes in cyanophages which follow the harmonic diel transcription of both oxygenic photoautotrophic and heterotrophic members of the community, in agreement to what other studies have just recently found. Our proposed methodology can be extended to many other datasets opening opportunities for a better understanding of the structure and function of microbial communities in their natural environment.

E. Acerbi and C. Chénard—Contributed equally.

Electronic supplementary material The online version of this chapter (https://doi.org/10.1007/978-3-030-29196-9_11) contains supplementary material, which is available to authorized users.

© Springer Nature Switzerland AG 2019
A. Cliquet jr. et al. (Eds.): BIOSTEC 2018, CCIS 1024, pp. 192–210, 2019.
https://doi.org/10.1007/978-3-030-29196-9_11

Keywords: Empirical mode decomposition · Metatranscriptomics · Metagenomics · Marine microbial ecology · Environmental time-series · Microbial communities · K-mers

1   Introduction

Taxonomical identification of DNA/RNA sequences from metagenomic or metatranscriptomic datasets is typically performed by checking for the existence of similarity by alignment to the genomes of all the known microbial species in a brute force kind of fashion. If matches are found, phylogenetic analysis may subsequently be conducted to unravel the evolutionary relationships among the species. This similarity based identification approach has two main limitations: firstly, the extensive number of comparison to be performed makes the task computationally expensive, which translate in high costs and long processing time. Secondly, NGS technologies can generate sequences of limited length (a typical Illumina read is 250–300 bp long). While this may not represent an issue with distantly related sequences, it can make the discrimination of closely related sequences (high similarity) difficult. This is the case for auxiliary metabolic genes (AMGs) in cyanobacteria and their associated viruses (also referred to as cyanophages). AMGs are encoding key metabolic functions such as photosynthesis, carbon metabolism, etc. Upon infection, viruses take over the control of the bacterial cell and keep it alive expressing the AMGs that they are carrying, for which an high similarity with the bacterial AMGs is required for a successful infection.

Being able to determine whether an AMG short fragment (fragments that does not cover the entire length of the AMG) belongs to a bacterial host or its associated viruses is an extremely valuable resource in microbial ecology. In the past, alternative methods exploiting specific genetic content have been used to characterize the origin of a gene [39]. Recently, Tzahor *et al.* [46] used a multi-class Support Vector Machine (SVM) to rapidly classify core-photosystem-II gene and transcripts fragments coming from marine samples based on their oligonucleotide frequencies. However, Tzahor *et al.* performed the multi-class classification using mostly sequences covering the entire gene of interest, while tests with short fragments (100, 200 and 300 bp) were limited to binary classification.

Here, we applied a SVM-based approach to specifically classify short fragments (length ranging between 150 and 300 bp) of two different AMGs from marine cyanobacteria and their viruses, namely *psbA* and *phoH*, retrieved from a previously published metatranscriptome profiling of multiple naturally occurring oceanic bacterial populations sampled in situ over 3 days [35]. The short *psbA* and *phoH* fragments were initially classified into 5 classes each using GC content, mono-, di-, tri- and tetra-nucleotide frequencies as discriminating features (Fig. 1A, C).

The outputs were further processed using Empirical Mode Decomposition (EMD) to identify the underlying frequency dynamics of transcription during viral infection in environmental cyanobacterial populations. EMD can deconvolve natural time-series data into composing frequencies also known as intrinsic

194   E. Acerbi et al.

mode functions (IMFs). EMD requires no initial assumption on the composition of the signal, which represent a major advantage over other decomposition
methods such as wavelet transform or Fourier transform. EMD has been used
successfully to analyse time series data in other scientific domains including the
detection of periodically expressed genes in microarray data [9], analysis of seismic data [21], electrocardiograms [8] and anomaly in sea-surface height [28].
This represents a first step in addressing the lack of established methods for the
analysis of environmental time-series, from which information on population heterogeneity and structure can potentially be extracted. This study is an extended
version of the one appeared in the Proceedings of BIOSTEC 2018 [1], Figs. 1, 2,
5 and 6 of this document are taken from the earlier version.

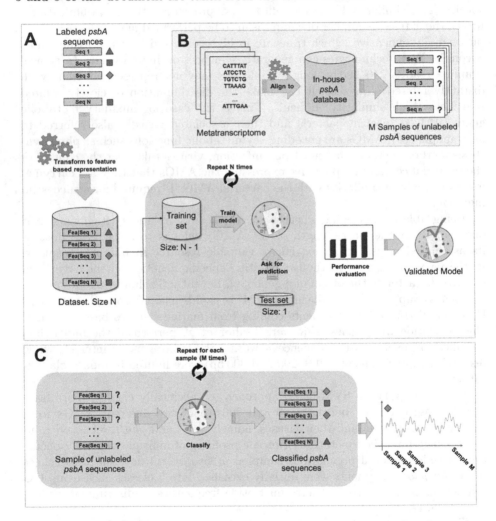

Fig. 1. (A) Training and validation of the SVM-based classifier (B) Extraction of *psbA*
fragments from the metatranscriptome. (C) Classification of new sequences using the
SVM-based classifier. The same procedure was performed for the *phoH* gene.

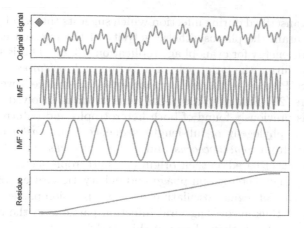

Fig. 2. Example of Empirical Mode Decomposition of a simulated signal. Each IMF represents a different oscillatory component/frequency of the original signal and can be used to identify the different underlying processes that are responsible for generating the original signal. Oscillatory components are extracted in decreasing order of frequency.

2 Biological Problem

Marine picocyanobacteria from the genera *Synechococcus* and *Prochlorococcus* are major primary producers in the ocean at low- and mid-latitude and contribute significantly to the global carbon cycle [22,36]. Given that light represents the main source of energy for cyanobacteria, it also determines the tempo of carbon fixation, metabolic and physiological activity such as the timing of cell division, amino acid uptake, nitrogen fixation, photosynthesis and respiration [17,34]. For example, nearly half of all *Prochlorococcus* population in the North Pacific Subtropical Gyre demonstrated a transcriptional diel cycle [35].

Viral infection in the oceans might also be synchronized with the light cycle. Some studies suggest a diel cycle in the number of infective viruses which could mainly be attributed to UV damage during the peak of sunlight [43,47]. However, the timing of viral replication can also be influenced by the presence and absence of light. For example, a temporal study at a station in the Indian Ocean revealed a strong increase in viral abundance in the middle of the night [12]. Logically, the synchronicity between light and replication is especially important for viruses infecting cyanobacteria, the cyanophages. Indeed, it was shown that light influences viral fitness as light is required for viral infection as it might influence the degradation of host genomic DNA, viral transcription or production of new progeny [44].

In addition, cyanophages harbour AMGs which are usually homologs of host genes involved in photosynthesis and carbon metabolism pathways. These AMGs likely play a role in viral infection [5]. For example, the *psbA* gene which encodes the D1 protein, a key component of the reaction centre of photosystem II (PSII), is prevalent in cyanophage genomes. PSII is particularly sensitive to photodamage causing a high turnover rate for the D1 protein. It was shown that viral *psbA* can highly be transcribed during infection which suggests that viral-*psbA* expression might maintain the photosynthetic activity of the infected host cells and therefore provide energy for cyanophage replication [13,29]. This is supported by the notion that during the lytic cycle of infection of *Prochlorococcus* MED4 by cyanophage P-SSP7 most of the *psbA* transcript in infected cells were from viral origin after 6hrs [29]. Similarly, the *phoH* gene which is involved in phosphate metabolism was previously found of both heterotrophs and autotrophs [18].

Based on the phylogeny of full-length sequences, viral *psbA* can generally be distinguished from *Synechococcus* and *Prochlorococcus* [11,41], while *phoH* genes cluster together based on their origin (i.e. autotroph bacteria, heterotroph bacteria, cyanophage, heterotroph phage and eukaryotic viruses [18,19]). Elucidating the existence of regular oscillations in the expression pattern of AMGs in cyanophages, and thus uncovering viral infection patterns in the North Pacific Subtropical Gyre is the biological aim of this study.

3   Biological Interpretation and Validation

A total of 20,235 *psbA* and 5,008 *phoH* short sequences (length ranging from 150 to 300b) extracted from the high-resolution metatranscriptome time course [35] were classified using the SVM-based classifier. As expected, retrieved *psbA* transcripts were most abundant in samples collected around mid-day and less abundant in samples collected around mid-night (Fig. 3).

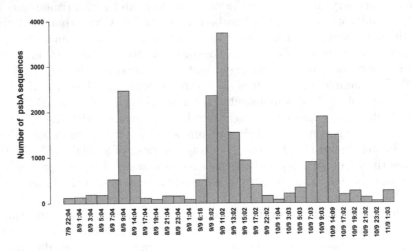

Fig. 3. Number of *psbA* sequences extracted from the metatranscriptome for each time point.

After SVMs-based classification, most of the *psbA* sequences were identified as *Prochlorococcus*, including high light and low light ecotypes (54% and 12% on average respectively and subsequently merged in one category for downstream analysis) while only a minor fraction was classified as *Synechococcus psbA* (1% on average). The remaining sequences were classified as *Synechococcus* virus

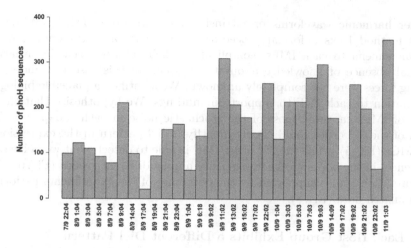

Fig. 4. Number of *phoH* sequences extracted from the metatranscriptome for each time point.

(27% on average) and *Prochlorococcus* virus (6% on average). Given that *Synechococcus* represents only a small fraction of the bacterioplankton in the time series of the North Pacific Subtropical Gyre [35], we hypothesized that the viral-*psbA* clustering into this group were not from *Synechococcus* viruses but instead from viruses that infect both *Prochlorococcus* and *Synechococcus*. Indeed, some cyanophages have shown to have a broad host range and infect strain from both genera [42]. For example, the *psbA* found in the cyanophage P-SSM1, which was isolated using the *Prochlorococcus* strain MIT 9313 clustered with the *Synechococcus* virus group [41]. Consequently, the two virus groups were redefined as Virus Group I (VG1; *Synechococcus* virus) and Virus Group II (VG2; *Prochlorococcus* virus). *Prochlorococcus* and *Synechococcus* are referred to in the figures respectively as Pro Bac and Syn Bac.

PhoH sequences retrieved from the metatranscriptome did not show a change in abundance based on the time of the day (Fig. 4). The lack of variation for the *phoH* gene is probably due to the fact that light has lesser influence on the timing of phosphate uptake. After SVMs-based classification, most *phoH* transcripts were assigned to heterotrophic phages (HP, 31% on average) and autotrophic bacteria host (A Host, 31% on average), followed by heterotrophic bacterial host (H Host, 21% on average) and autotrophic phages (AP, 14% on average). Few *phoH* sequences were classified as eukaryotic phytoplankton viruses (2% on average) in agreement with the notion that most of the primary production in the North Pacific Subtropical was supported by cyanobacteria. As a consequence, the *phoH* group including viruses infecting eukaryotic phytoplankton was removed from downstream analysis.

After classifying the sequences into their respective subgroups, we performed an empirical mode decomposition (EMD) (see Methods) on the transcriptional profiles of each subgroup, from which different diel patterns emerge within *psbA* and *phoH* transcripts. EMD decomposed each profile of classified AMGs into simpler harmonic waveforms or intrinsic mode functions (IMFs). While the EMD method lacks a formal procedure to associate a corresponding meaning/phenomena to each IMFs, complicating their interpretation in situations of total absence of knowledge about the system, in this case the underlying driving forces were not completely unknown. We identified a plausible biological explanation to each IMF to support our findings. We hypothesize that the 1st order of IMFs captured most of the stochastic noise in each time series. The IMFs of the 3rd order could clearly identify a diel pattern in the expression of all AMGs (Fig. 5), while the 2nd order IMF is able to detect what we believe are differences in the population heterogeneity among different groups (Fig. 6). This interpretation is also supported by the outcomes of the experiments performed on simulated data (Fig. 8).

3.1 Each Host Group Exhibits a Different Diel Pattern

The IMFs of the 3rd order identified a diel pattern in the expression of all AMGs (Fig. 5). The peak of expression of *psbA* from *Prochlorococcus* consistently occurred in the morning while a less-pronounced cycling of *Synechococcus psbA* transcripts occurred later in the afternoon (Fig. 5A). This is consistent with a published dataset obtained using real-time PCR [32]. The remarkable difference between the *psbA* expression levels of *Synechococcus* and *Prochlorococcus* is probably caused by the fact that *Prochlorococcus* is not able to withstand solar irradiance as high as *Synechococcus*. Consequently, as *Prochlorococcus* D1 protein is more sensitive to light, *psbA* needs to be highly expressed during the time of the day with the more irradiance [32]. Both VG1 and VG2 peaked during the daytime but the peak for VG2 was precisely matched to the peak in *Prochlorococcus psbA*. On the other hand, maximal expression of VG1 was more variable, possibly as a result of the variable proportions of the infected strains of *Prochlorococcus* and *Synechococcus* hosts.

The timing of the peak expression of the viral *psbA* also provided insights into the timing of cell lysis in the North Pacific Gyre. Based on studies conducted in the laboratory, the viral *psbA* was maximally expressed at the end of the lytic cycle [13] and if replication of viral DNA is delayed until light, viral *psbA* expression should be minimal in the morning and slowly increase throughout the day. Although the slight offset pattern between VG1 and VG2, our findings are consistent with the hypothesis that most of the cell lysis and viral shedding occurs at the end of the day. Using SeaFlow cytometry, which gives real-time continuous observations of cells abundance, Ribalet *et al.* [38] showed that *Prochlorococcus* abundance peaks during the day and sharply decrease at night, suggesting predation (viral and grazing) as the cause of the oscillation. In addition, a recent study using the viral gene transcription in the host cell assemblage also demonstrated an afternoon peak of cyanophage transcriptional activity [2]. Our results further support the hypothesis that viral infection might be a player in the synchronized oscillations of *Prochlorococcus* cell numbers from surface water of a Pacific Gyre [38]. While *psbA* transcripts from viral groups exhibit a very tight coupling with the time of the day, much less diel effect was observed for the viral *phoH* transcripts. The HP transcripts consistently peaked later than the hosts homologs but, in general, the cycling of the viral *phoH* transcripts doesn't show a connection with the daily light cycle (Fig. 5B).

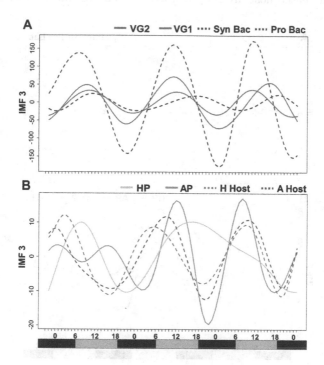

Fig. 5. Intrinsic mode functions of 3rd order of *psbA* and *phoH* groups. X-Axis shows the time of the day, with the colored bar indicating the light-dark cycle. (A) *psbA* groups. (B) *phoH* groups. (Color figure online)

3.2 The Population Structure Shows Different Viral Groups

Underlying the primary diel harmonics of the 3rd order IMF, the 2nd order was able to detect differences in the population heterogeneity among different groups. This was particularly evident during the final 30 h of the time series, when a significant increase in temperature and salinity had been previously associated to a change in the transcriptional profile of SAR324 [35]. Here, the shift in environmental conditions is detected as increased frequency in IMF2 for both *Prochlorococcus* and *Synechococcus* (Fig. 6A), suggesting that the population heterogeneity of the 2 groups has increased to include additional ecotypes.

Differences in population heterogeneity are also observed as differences in IMF2 frequencies in VG1, VG2, AP and HP (Fig. 6B). Interestingly the highest population heterogeneity (i.e. the highest IMF2 frequency) was observed in VG2, which also had the strongest correlation between AMG peak and the time of the day. Taken together, these observations suggest that VG2 includes many viral quasispecies with very narrow host ranges and a very precise control of replication timing as a function of the time of the day. VG1 was less diverse but also appeared to have broader host range and the expression peak shifted in response to increased host diversity towards the end of the time-series.

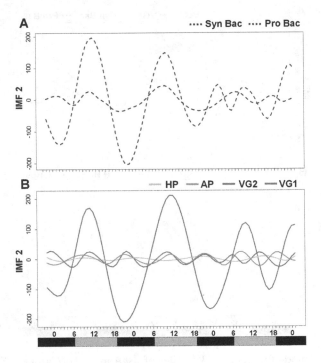

Fig. 6. Intrinsic mode functions of 2nd order of *psbA* and *phoH* groups. X-Axis shows the time of the day, with the colored bar indicating the light-dark cycle. (A) population heterogeneity for *Synechoccocus* and *Prochloroccocus* groups. (B) Differences in population heterogeneity for all viral groups (both *psbA* and *phoH*). (Color figure online)

3.3   Identifying Gene Networks Responsive to Viral Infection

The time-series relative abundance of top 500 most abundant KEGG gene across all the time points were considered and their associated KEGG Orthology (KO) genes were tested for Pearson correlations against the proportion of *psbA* and *phoH* groups (cut off, <-0.5 and >0.5) using lagged correlations (Supplementary Data 3). As shown in Fig. 7, at lag zero most positive correlations observed were with genes involved in chaperones, photosynthesis and KO genes of unknown functions. The expression of chaperones such as *groEL* gene (K04077) correlated with the expression of multiple *psbA* groups. The *groEL* gene encodes a molecular chaperone which helps correct protein folding and rescues partially misfolded proteins. It is not surprising that molecular chaperones may be important during the viral cycle when the host machinery for protein synthesis gets hijacked into making viral proteins. For example, *groEL* expression increases during the infection of the *Thermophilic Geobacillus sp. E263* with its virus GVE 2 [10]. In addition, chaperonin genes have also been found in the genomes of marine viruses [23,26] suggesting that chaperones may have a fundamental role in folding viral capsid proteins. Our results show that different *groEL* genes display different correlation type (positive vs negative) with the viruses and their host (Supplementary Data 3). For example, the expression of *groEL* from the genome of *Prochlorococcus marinus AS9601* showed a negative correlation with VG2, while other *groEL* genes showed a positive correlation. These differences might be the result of the multiple roles that chaperonins play during viral infection. The VG1 expression profile also showed a positive correlation with the expression of the gene *clpC* (K03696). This gene encodes an ATP-dependent Clp protease which is also a chaperone and folding catalysts. Clp ATPases were shown to be involved in stress tolerance [16]. Synchronizing the diel cycles of viral activity, defined as the variation in viral *psbA* relative expression, is triggered by the start of the day and consistently occurred approximately 4 h after dawn, in accordance with previous studies showing that the infection process of the *cyanophage Syn 9* had initiated a lytic cycle of 6 to 8 h prior to the releases of progeny from the infected cells [15].

As shown in Fig. 7, the gene categories that show the highest positive correlation on the −4 shifted time-series belonged to DNA and RNA repair systems of *Prochlorococcus*, suggesting that the first sunlight results in photooxidative stress. Genes involved in ammonium transport also show a positive correlation on the −4 shifted time-series. Ammonium transporter genes from Amt family (K03320) displayed a negative correlation with both VG1 and VG2 at lag 0 and lag +1 while a positive correlation was observed at Lag −4. The main function of Amt protein is to scavenge ammonium and recapture ammonium lost from cells by diffusion. Ammonium is an important nitrogen source in cyanobacteria and the ammonium transporter genes are activated during nitrogen starvation [45]. The ammonium transporter genes from Amt family also showed a peak at the end of the day (Day 1 = 5 pm, Day 2 = 10 pm and Day 3 = 11 pm).

The transcriptional profiles that correlated best with viral AMGs patterns in the 1-h lagged correlations were from heterotrophic bacteria, suggesting that changes in the viral activity elicit a rapid response in the heterotrophic consumers (Fig. 7). This was not observed in the 4-h lagged correlation which mostly included autotrophic transcripts. Most of the positively correlated transcripts were hypothetical proteins belonging to copiotrophic [27] heterotrophs of the community. Other studies have shown that copiotrophic marine bacteria are actively involved in degradation of nutrients released from lysed cells [33]. Based on the sequence analysis of the conserved domains, many of had similarity to cell-wall associated hydrolases, reflecting either the increased in growth rates or a sensory function related to the exit from latency [4,48]. It is possible that the localized increase in nutrients or the partial removal of inhibitory substances produced by cyanobacteria [14] as a result of viral lysis triggers a change in the activity of the heterotrophic community. In fact, Ottesen *et al.* [35] have observed that most pronounced light-dependent transcriptional response in heterotrophs belonged to the Roseobacter clade, which have been previously shown to be active in remineralization of nutrients released from dead phytoplankton cells [20,31]. Cyanophages might therefore be among the most important drivers of synchronicity between the oxygenic photoautotrophic and the heterotrophic marine populations.

4   Methods

4.1   Training Set Generation

Labelled DNA sequences for *psbA* and *phoH* genes are scarce in the literature. In order to generate the *psbA* training set for the SVM-based multiclassificator, we collected 203 *psbA* DNA sequences from NCBI (including those used by Tzahor *et al.* [46]). Sequences in the dataset were labelled as belonging to one of the following five categories: *Synechococcus* bacteria (77), *Synechococcus* virus (42), *Prochlorococcus* bacteria high-light (38), *Prochlorococcus* bacteria low-light (26) and *Prochlorococcus* virus (20). Sequences were long, having different lengths ranging from 720 bp to 1083 bp, with a median of 1080 bp. Analogously, *phoH* training set was created by collecting 84 DNA sequences from NCBI. Sequences in the dataset were labelled as belonging to one of the following five categories: Autotrophic host (i.e. cyanobacteria) (17), cyanophage (29), heterotrophic host (13), heterotrophic phage (14), phytoeukaryotic virus (10). *PhoH* sequences were also long, having different lengths ranging from 603 bp to 1770 bp, with a median of 766.5 bp. In their work, Tzahor *et al.* trained the SVM classifier using full length *psbA* sequences and subsequently used it for classification of other full length *psbA* sequences (Tzahor *et al.* also tested their classifier on short *psbA* fragments, but only limited to binary classification). If the aim is to use the classifier on shorter *psbA* fragments, the approach of Tzahor *et al.* may not always give the best results. In fact, classification accuracy may be low if the training is performed on clean samples (*psbA* full genes, rather than fragments) and the real-world classification is performed on noisy samples (*psbA* fragments. i.e. sequences containing a part of the *psbA* gene and other base pairs not related to the *psbA* gene, as in metagenomic/metatranscriptiomic data). For this reason, *psbA* and *phoH* training sets were generated by randomly extracting sequences of length 300 bp from the original sets. In addition, to deal with the original dataset being slightly unbalanced (not equal number of instances for each class) a combination of undersampling and oversampling was applied to both *psbA* and *phoH* sequences in order to obtain balanced training sets: 100 sequences for each of the five classes (total of 500 sequences) for *psbA* training set and 50 sequences for each of the five classes (total of 250 sequences) for *phoH* training set.

4.2   Feature Generation

GC content, mono-, di-, tri- and tetra-nucleotide frequencies were calculated for each sequence of the training sets (for a total of 341 features per sequence) and used as input feature vector for the SVM classifiers. When including penta- and/or hexa-nucleotide frequencies, no significant improvements in prediction accuracy were observed (data not shown).

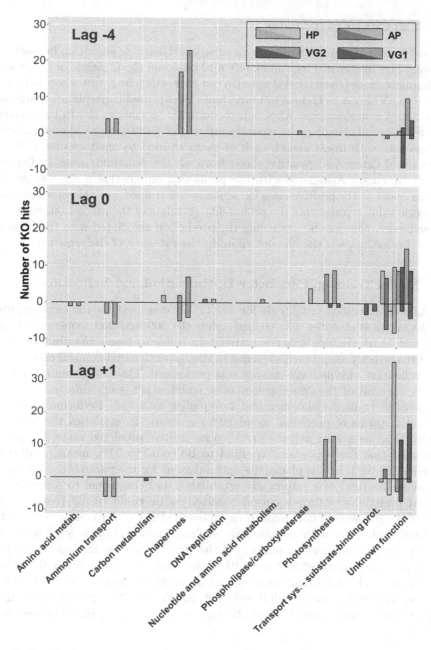

Fig. 7. Correlations among viral groups and time-series relative abundance of different Kegg Orthology (KO) genes. Each bar chart indicates the number of positive or negative correlations of each viral group with KO genes. Light colours are used to denote hits on autotrophs genes, while darker colours are used to denote hits on heterotrophs genes. Lagged correlations at time points −4 and +1 are also shown. (Color figure online)

4.3   The SVM-based Model

Support Vector Machines (SVMs) are a supervised learning algorithm in machine learning, first introduced by Vapnik [40] and based on the principle of structural risk minimization. Given labeled data (in our case, DNA fragment whose origin is known), a SVM can be trained to individuate the optimal hyperplane separating (classifying) new examples. Although through the document it will be referred to as SVM-based classifier, the model composed of 5 different SVM one-against-all classifiers with linear kernel, each of them trained to separate one of the 5 taxonomical categories (positive class) from all the remaining ones (collapsed as negative class). Associated with the prediction on whether a given sequence belongs or not to the positive class for which it was trained, each classifier returns a numeric value representing the probability estimate of the prediction. For each new sequence, the classifier returning the prediction associated with the highest probability estimate is the one determining the category of the sequence.

4.4   Model Training, Parameter Optimization and Validation

The LIBSVM toolbox (v3.22) [7] for MATLAB was used for the experiments. The SVM-based classifier was trained using the 500 and 250 sequences of the *psbA* and *phoH* training sets respectively. In order to assess the ability of the model to correctly assign each sequence to the respective taxonomical category, a cross validation of type leave-one-out was performed. This validating procedure iterates over all of the N sequences of a training set, each time using $N-1$ sequences to train the classifier and 1 sequence as a test. Performances were assessed in terms of precision, recall and f-measure. In statistics the recall is referred to as sensitivity and the precision as positive predicted value. For *psbA*, cross validation mean precision resulted to be equal to 0.95, mean recall 0.92 and mean F_1 0.93. In this phase, the optimal value for the parameter Cost (cost of misclassification) was empirically established as being equal to 8, while the optimal probability estimate cut-off resulted to be equal to 0.3 (resulting in 3.8% of the sequences being marked as unassigned). A direct comparison of the SVM-based classifier with the previous work of Tzahor *et al.* is not feasible as in their study, Tzahor *et al.* performed the multi-class classification using full length *psbA* sequences, while tests with short fragments (100, 200 and 300 bp) were limited to binary classification only. For *phoH*, the mean precision resulted to be equal to 0.98, mean recall 0.98 and mean F_1 0.98. No optimal probability estimate cut-off was applied for *phoH* sequences while the parameter cost was set to 8.

4.5   Classification of Sequences Extracted from the
Metatranscriptome

In order to extract *psbA* and *phoH* fragments from the metatranscriptome data of Ottesen *et al.*, we firstly built in-house *PsbA* and *PhoH* protein databases. The

PsbA database was composed by 11,962 protein sequences retrieved from UniProtKB, while the *PhoH* database was composed by 100,501 protein sequences downloaded from NCBI. Subsequently, metatranscriptome data was screened for homology against these databases using Rapsearch2 [49] (which allows protein similarity search by translating DNA/RNA queries into protein), retaining matches with alignment-length greater than 150 bp and e-value smaller than 0.000001 Fig. 1B). For each time point, *psbA* and *phoH* fragments were then classified using the SVM-based classifier. Counts were normalized using the cumulative sum scaling (CSS) method [37].

4.6   Kegg Orthology (KO) Analysis

Metatranscriptome data was screened for homology against the KEGG genes database (including prokaryotes, addendum, plasmid and viruses categories) using Rapsearch2. Top 500 most abundant KEGG genes across all the time points were retained while the remaining ones were discarded. KEGG genes were grouped by KEGG orthology (KO) category. Different KO categories were then tested for Pearson correlations against *psbA* and *phoH* groups (cut off, < -0.5 and > 0.5). See Fig. 7.

4.7   Empirical Mode Decomposition

Empirical mode decomposition [24], is a data-driven method for analysing of non linear and non stationary time frequency data, such as natural signals. The EMD process iteratively decomposes the original signal into a finite number of intrinsic mode functions (IMF), that is, functions with a single mode/frequency Fig. 2. Each IMF represents a different component/frequency of the original signal and can be used to identify the different underlying processes that are responsible for generating the original signal (Fig. 2). The EMD procedure works as follows: first, all the time serie's local minima and maxima are identified. Interpolation then is applied to connect the local minima among them, generating the lower envelope of the data. The same is performed on the local maxima, generating the upper envelope. Subsequently, the mean value of the envelope is calculated and subtracted from the original signal. This procedure takes the name of sifting and produces an IMF. To be considered valid, an IMF needs to satisfy the following conditions: (i) the number of extrema and of zero-crossings must differ by no more than one (ii) both lower and upper envelopes must have a mean equal to zero. The sifting procedure is repeated until no further IMF can be extracted from the original signal or the specified terminating criterion is met. IMFs are extracted in decreasing frequencies levels. EMD is a relatively recent approach that still holds some drawbacks. For instance, EMD may be prone to suffer from sampling errors as those could lead to incorrect placement of extema and therefore lead to inaccurate IMFs. Similarly, the usage of different interpolation methods can also lead to slight differences in the algorithm results, particularly in terms of flexibly and smoothness of the IMFs [3]. IMFs are also challenging to interpret in absence of knowledge about the underlying system, and IMFs of different orders on different time series may not be capturing the same phenomena. In addition, analogous information may end up being contained in multiple IMFs and there can sometimes be lower-order IMFs that are just spurious fluctuations (which have the purpose of correct errors on other IMFs, so that they can sum up to the original signal) [6]. In this work EMD was run using the EMD R package [25], allowing a maximum number of sift iterations equal to 50, with a periodic type of boundary and constructing the envelops by interpolation. No meaningful changes in the results were observed when different boundaries and interpolation methods were tested.

4.8   Empirical Mode Decomposition Validation

In order to prove the effectiveness of EMD, we generated simulated time course abundances for three assemblages characterized by different amplitudes and frequencies but having similar phases (Fig. 8). This is aimed at simulating the existence of multiple sub-populations within a single taxonomic group. Subsequently, the three signals were merged into a composite signal and some random

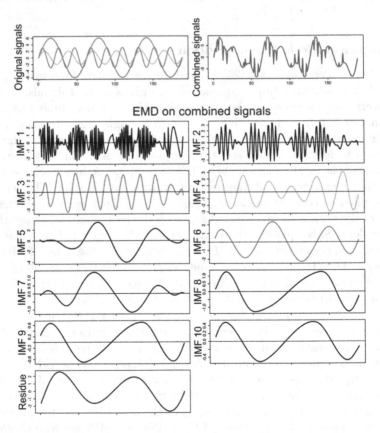

Fig. 8. Empirical Mode Decomposition of a simulated composite noisy signal.

noise was added. The EMD procedure was then run on the noisy composite signal. All of the three original component were successfully extracted by the EMD procedure, with the highest frequency signal being extracted first and the lowest frequency one being extracted last.

5   Conclusions

Using our proposed methodology, we observed the presence of light-dark cycle in the viral infection of cyanobacterial populations in the North Pacific Subtropical Gyre. We separated the viral assemblages based on *psbA* and *phoH* genes which identified major viral groups differing in their response to light-dark cycles, population structure and host range. As other studies using larger datasets [2, 30], our approach showed transcriptional dynamics of viral infection in the ocean. By correlating these dynamics to the transcriptional profiles of functional genes we also posit that the synchronous release of nutrients from autotrophic populations of cyanobacteria, following viral lysis, might provide the mechanism that couples the diel oscillations of the autotrophic and heterotrophic members of the microbial community.

Aside from the derived ecological insights, the proposed k-mers based multiclass supervised classification methods can be used to accurately discriminate short AMGs fragments (or any other group of closely related sequences) coming from metagenomics and/or metatranscriptomic studies. In addition, we have shown how EMD decomposition of environmental time series data uncovers fundamental frequencies of natural processes that otherwise would be overlooked.

6   Data Availability

The Data used in this study and some additional results have been made available at the following URL: https://gitlab.com/enzoace/SequenceClassification. git

- Supplementary_data_1.fasta: *PsbA* sequences used for training the classifier.
- Supplementary_data_2.fasta: *PhoH* sequences used for training the classifier.
- Supplementary_data_3.xlsx: Correlation values among KEGG genes and microbial groups at different time lags.

Acknowledgements. The authors would like to acknowledge financial support from Singapore's Ministry of Education Academic Research Fund Tier 3 under the research grant MOE2013-T3-1-013, Singapore's National Research Foundation under its Marine Science Research and Development Programme (Award No. MSRDP-P13) and the Singapore Centre for Environmental Life Sciences Engineering (SCELSE), whose research is supported by the National Research Foundation Singapore, Ministry of Education, Nanyang Technological University and National University of Singapore, under its Research Centre of Excellence Program. The authors would like to thank Fabio Stella, Rohan Williams and James Houghton for their valuable feedbacks.

References

1. Acerbi, E., Chenard, C., Schuster, S.C., Lauro, F.M.: Supervised classification of metatranscriptomic reads reveals the existence of light-dark oscillations during infection of phytoplankton by viruses. In: Proceedings of the 11th International Joint Conference on Biomedical Engineering Systems and Technologies (BIOSTEC 2018) - Volume 3: BIOINFORMATICS, Funchal, Madeira, Portugal, 19–21 January 2018, pp. 69–77 (2018). https://doi.org/10.5220/0006763200690077
2. Aylward, F.O., et al.: Diel cycling and long-term persistence of viruses in the Ocean's euphotic zone. Proc. Natl. Acad. Sci. **114**(43), 11446–11451 (2017)
3. Bagherzadeh, S.A., Sabzehparvar, M.: A local and online sifting process for the empirical mode decomposition and its application in aircraft damage detection. Mech. Syst. Signal Process. **54**, 68–83 (2015)
4. de Bashan, L.E., Trejo, A., Huss, V.A., Hernandez, J.P., Bashan, Y.: Chlorella sorokiniana utex 2805, a heat and intense, sunlight-tolerant microalga with potential for removing ammonium from wastewater. Bioresour. Technol. **99**(11), 4980–4989 (2008)
5. Breitbart, M., Thompson, L.R., Suttle, C.A., Sullivan, M.: Exploring the vast diversity of marine viruses. Oceanography **20**(SPL. ISS. 2), 135–139 (2007)
6. Chambers, D.P.: Evaluation of empirical mode decomposition for quantifying multi-decadal variations and acceleration in sea level records. Nonlinear Process. Geophys. **22**(2), 157–166 (2015)
7. Chang, C.C., Lin, C.J.: LIBSVM: a library for support vector machines. ACM Trans. Intell. Syst. Technol. **2**, 27:1–27:27 (2011)
8. Chang, K.M.: Ensemble empirical mode decomposition for high frequency ECG noise reduction. Biomed. Tech./Biomed. Eng. **55**(4), 193–201 (2010)
9. Chen, C.R., Shu, W.Y., Chang, C.W., Hsu, I.C.: Identification of under-detected periodicity in time-series microarray data by using empirical mode decomposition. PLoS ONE **9**(11), e111719 (2014)
10. Chen, Y., Wei, D., Wang, Y., Zhang, X.: The role of interactions between bacterial chaperone, aspartate aminotransferase, and viral protein during virus infection in high temperature environment: the interactions between bacterium and virus proteins. BMC Microbiol. **13**(1), 48 (2013)
11. Chenard, C., Suttle, C.A.: Phylogenetic diversity of sequences of cyanophage photosynthetic gene psbA in marine and freshwaters. Appl. Environ. Microbiol. **74**(17), 5317–5324 (2008)
12. Clokie, M.R., Millard, A.D., Mehta, J.Y., Mann, N.H.: Virus isolation studies suggest short-term variations in abundance in natural cyanophage populations of the indian ocean. J. Mar. Biol. Assoc. U. K. **86**(03), 499–505 (2006)
13. Clokie, M.R., et al.: Transcription of a 'photosynthetic' T4-type phage during infection of a marine cyanobacterium. Environ. Microbiol. **8**(5), 827–835 (2006)
14. Cole, J.J.: Interactions between bacteria and algae in aquatic ecosystems. Annu. Rev. Ecol. Syst. **13**(1), 291–314 (1982)
15. Doron, S., et al.: Transcriptome dynamics of a broad host-range cyanophage and its hosts. The ISME J. **10**(6), 1437 (2016)
16. Frees, D., et al.: CLP atpases are required for stress tolerance, intracellular replication and biofilm formation in staphylococcus aureus. Mol. Microbiol. **54**(5), 1445–1462 (2004)
17. Golden, S.S., Ishiura, M., Johnson, C.H., Kondo, T.: Cyanobacterial circadian rhythms. Annu. Rev. Plant Biol. **48**(1), 327–354 (1997)

18. Goldsmith, D.B., et al.: Development of phoh as a novel signature gene for assessing marine phage diversity. Appl. Environ. Microbiol. **77**(21), 7730–7739 (2011)

19. Goldsmith, D.B., Parsons, R.J., Beyene, D., Salamon, P., Breitbart, M.: Deep sequencing of the viral phoH gene reveals temporal variation, depth-specific composition, and persistent dominance of the same viral phoh genes in the sargasso sea. PeerJ **3**, e997 (2015)

20. Hahnke, S., Brock, N.L., Zell, C., Simon, M., Dickschat, J.S., Brinkhoff, T.: Physiological diversity of roseobacter clade bacteria co-occurring during a phytoplankton bloom in the north sea. Syst. Appl. Microbiol. **36**(1), 39–48 (2013)

21. Han, J., van der Baan, M.: Empirical mode decomposition for seismic time-frequency analysis. Geophysics **78**(2), O9–O19 (2013)

22. Hess, W.R.: Genome analysis of marine photosynthetic microbes and their global role. Curr. Opin. Biotechnol. **15**(3), 191–198 (2004)

23. Holmfeldt, K., et al.: Twelve previously unknown phage genera are ubiquitous in global oceans. Proc. Natl. Acad. Sci. **110**(31), 12798–12803 (2013)

24. Huang, N.E., et al.: The empirical mode decomposition and the Hilbert spectrum for nonlinear and non-stationary time series analysis. In: Proceedings of the Royal Society of London A: Mathematical, Physical and Engineering Sciences, vol. 454, pp. 903–995. The Royal Society (1998)

25. Kim, D., Oh, H.S.: EMD: a package for empirical mode decomposition and Hilbert spectrum. R J. **1**(1), 40–46 (2009)

26. Kurochkina, L.P., Semenyuk, P.I., Orlov, V.N., Robben, J., Sykilinda, N.N., Mesyanzhinov, V.V.: Expression and functional characterization of the first bacteriophage-encoded chaperonin. J. Virol. **86**(18), 10103–10111 (2012)

27. Lauro, F.M., et al.: The genomic basis of trophic strategy in marine bacteria. Proc. Natl. Acad. Sci. **106**(37), 15527–15533 (2009)

28. Li, F., Jo, Y.H., Liu, W.T., Yan, X.H.: A dipole pattern of the sea surface height anomaly in the north Atlantic: 1990s–2000s. Geophys. Res. Lett. **39**(15) (2012)

29. Lindell, D., et al.: Genome-wide expression dynamics of a marine virus and host reveal features of co-evolution. Nature **449**(7158), 83–86 (2007)

30. Liu, R., Chen, Y., Zhang, R., Liu, Y., Jiao, N., Zeng, Q.: Cyanophages exhibit rhythmic infection patterns under light-dark cycles. bioRxiv p. 167650 (2017)

31. Mayali, X., Franks, P.J., Azam, F.: Cultivation and ecosystem role of a marine roseobacter clade-affiliated cluster bacterium. Appl. Environ. Microbiol. **74**(9), 2595–2603 (2008)

32. Mella-Flores, D., et al.: Prochlorococcus and synechococcus have evolved different adaptive mechanisms to cope with light and UV stress (2012)

33. Mourino-Pérez, R.R., Worden, A.Z., Azam, F.: Growth of vibrio cholerae o1 in red tide waters off california. Appl. Environ. Microbiol. **69**(11), 6923–6931 (2003)

34. Ni, T., Zeng, Q.: Diel infection of cyanobacteria by cyanophages. Front. Mar. Sci. **2**, 123 (2016)

35. Ottesen, E.A., et al.: Multispecies diel transcriptional oscillations in open ocean heterotrophic bacterial assemblages. Science **345**(6193), 207–212 (2014)

36. Partensky, F., Hess, W.R., Vaulot, D.: Prochlorococcus, a marine photosynthetic prokaryote of global significance. Microbiol. Mol. Biol. Rev. **63**(1), 106–127 (1999)

37. Paulson, J.N., Stine, O.C., Bravo, H.C., Pop, M.: Differential abundance analysis for microbial marker-gene surveys. Nat. Methods **10**(12), 1200–1202 (2013)

38. Ribalet, F., et al.: Light-driven synchrony of prochlorococcus growth and mortality in the subtropical Pacific gyre. Proc. Natl. Acad. Sci. **112**(26), 8008–8012 (2015)

39. Sandberg, R., Winberg, G., Bränden, C.I., Kaske, A., Ernberg, I., Cöster, J.: Capturing whole-genome characteristics in short sequences using a Naive Bayesian classifier. Genome Res. **11**(8), 1404–1409 (2001)

40. Stitson, M., Weston, J., Gammerman, A., Vovk, V., Vapnik, V.: Theory of support vector machines. Technical report, CSD-TR-96-17, Computational Intelligence Group, University of London (1996)

41. Sullivan, M.B., Lindell, D., Lee, J.A., Thompson, L.R., Bielawski, J.P., Chisholm, S.W.: Prevalence and evolution of core photosystem II genes in marine cyanobacterial viruses and their hosts. PLoS Biol. **4**(8), e234 (2006)

42. Sullivan, M.B., Waterbury, J.B., Chisholm, S.W.: Cyanophages infecting the oceanic cyanobacterium prochlorococcus. Nature **424**(6952), 1047–1051 (2003)

43. Suttle, C.A., Chen, F.: Mechanisms and rates of decay of marine viruses in seawater. Appl. Environ. Microbiol. **58**(11), 3721–3729 (1992)

44. Thompson, L.R., et al.: Phage auxiliary metabolic genes and the redirection of cyanobacterial host carbon metabolism. Proc. Natl. Acad. Sci. **108**(39), E757–E764 (2011)

45. Tolonen, A.C., et al.: Global gene expression of prochlorococcus ecotypes in response to changes in nitrogen availability. Mol. Syst. Biol. **2**(1), 53 (2006)

46. Tzahor, S., et al.: A supervised learning approach for taxonomic classification of core-photosystem-II genes and transcripts in the marine environment. BMC Genom. **10**(1), 229 (2009)

47. Wilhelm, S.W., Weinbauer, M.G., Suttle, C.A., Jeffrey, W.H.: The role of sunlight in the removal and repair of viruses in the sea. Limnol. Ocean. **43**(4), 586–592 (1998)

48. Wyckoff, T.J., Taylor, J.A., Salama, N.R.: Beyond growth: novel functions for bacterial cell wall hydrolases. Trends Microbiol. **20**(11), 540–547 (2012)

49. Zhao, Y., Tang, H., Ye, Y.: RAPSearch2: a fast and memory-efficient protein similarity search tool for next-generation sequencing data. Bioinformatics **28**(1), 125–126 (2011)

Health Informatics

How to Realize Device Interoperability and Information Security in mHealth Applications

Christoph Stach[(✉)] [iD], Frank Steimle, and Bernhard Mitschang

Institute for Parallel and Distributed Systems, University of Stuttgart,
Universitätsstraße 38, 70569 Stuttgart, Germany
{stachch,steimlfk,mitsch}@ipvs.uni-stuttgart.de

Abstract. More and more people suffer from chronic diseases such as the chronic obstructive pulmonary disease (COPD). This leads to very high treatment costs every year, as such patients require a periodic screening of their condition. However, many of these checks can be performed at home by the patients themselves. This enables physicians to focus on actual emergencies. Modern smart devices such as Smartphones contribute to the success of these telemedical approaches. So-called mHealth apps combine the usability and versatility of Smartphones with the high accuracy and reliability of medical devices for home use. However, patients often face the problem of how to connect medical devices to their Smartphones (the **device interoperability** problem). Moreover, many patients reject mHealth apps due to the lack of control over their sensitive health data (the **information security** problem).

In our work, we discuss the usage of the **Privacy Management Platform** (*PMP*) to solve these problems. So, we describe the structure of mHealth apps and present a real-world COPD application. From this application we derive relevant functions of an mHealth app, in which device interoperability or information security is an issue. We extend the PMP in order to provide support for these recurring functions. Finally, we evaluate the utility of these PMP extensions based on the real-world mHealth app.

Keywords: mHealth · Device interoperability · Information security · COPD

1 Introduction

Due to long stand-by times and multiple built-in sensors, the Smartphone became our ubiquitous companion. New use cases are constantly emerging. Especially in the health sector, the use of Smartphones can be highly beneficial to save treatment costs and help patients who cannot visit their physicians regularly [33]. The usability of Smartphone apps in the health sector—the so-called mHealth apps—is limitless. There is an app for almost any situation [32].

© Springer Nature Switzerland AG 2019
A. Cliquet jr. et al. (Eds.): BIOSTEC 2018, CCIS 1024, pp. 213–237, 2019.
https://doi.org/10.1007/978-3-030-29196-9_12

While there are some mHealth apps for medical reference (that is, apps providing information about diseases) as well as hospital workflow management apps (i.e., apps supporting physicians in their everyday duties), mHealth apps are mainly from the health management domain [23]. The latter includes cardio fitness, medication adherence, and chronic disease management. To this end, these apps support two essential features: self-observation and feedback [21]. That is, the patient performs health measurements instructed by the app, transmits the measured values to the app and the app performs analyses on these values. Based on the results, the app gives the user medical recommendations.

Since mHealth apps involve the patient actively into the treatment and monitoring process, s/he gets more aware of his or her condition. So, mHealth apps change the physician patient relationship especially for patients with a chronic disease. These patients have to visit their physician periodically in order to check certain health values. However, such a metering can be performed by the patients autonomously, if they receive a proper guidance tailored to their knowhow. That is, with the help of an mHealth app they are able to do the monitoring in a telemedical manner. This take the load off both, patients as well as physicians. Patients benefit from the freedom to do the metering at any arbitrary place and time while physicians are able to concentrate on emergencies. This is not just a huge saving potential but also improves the quality of healthcare at the same time [30].

To capture health data, mHealth apps make use of various sensors. In addition to the already broad spectrum of sensors built into modern Smartphones that can be used for healthcare (e.g., a heart rate sensor, a camera, or a microphone), even medical devices for home-use can be connected to a Smartphone. The *Vitalograph copd-6 bt* is an example for such medical device.

Yet, the data interchange between medical devices and Smartphones often fails because of non-uniform communication protocols. The **device interoperability** of Smartphones and medical devices is a key challenge for the success of mHealth apps [6]. Also the assurance of **information security** is vital for mHealth, as patients have to trust their apps [1]. Thus, we address these two challenges in our work. Therefore, we come up with a concept for an enabler for device interoperability and information security in mHealth apps. To achieve this objective, we proceed as follows: (I) We analyze a real-world mHealth app regarding the collected data and used devices. (II) We deduce a generic data model for mHealth apps. Due to this data model, our approach is applicable for any kind of mHealth app. (III) We identify five recurring tasks within mHealth apps for which device interoperability and information security are key requirements, namely login, metering, localization, data storage and analytics, and data transmission. For each of these tasks, we introduce an extension for the **P**rivacy **M**anagement **P**latform (*PMP*) [37], to ensure interoperability and information security. (IV) We use these extensions to revise the analyzed mHealth app in terms of sensor support and the patients' privacy. With this revised app, we assess the practical effect of our approach.

This paper is the extended and revised version of the paper entitled "The Privacy Management Platform: An Enabler for Device Interoperability and Information Security in mHealth Applications" [41] presented at the 11th International Conference on Health Informatics (HEALTHINF) 2018.

The remainder of this paper is as follows: The layer architecture of mHealth systems is introduced in Sect. 2. Section 3 discusses a real-world application scenario from the mHealth domain, namely *ChronicOnline*, an mHealth app for COPD patients. Then, Sect. 4 takes a look at related work concerning connection techniques used by medical device as well as information security mechanisms in mHealth apps. Based on these findings, we introduce a generic interchange data model for mHealth apps and induct briefly in the PMP, the foundation platform for our solution approach in Sect. 5. Then, Sect. 6 details on the key components of our approach and demonstrates their applicability, using the example of a COPD app. In Sect. 7 we assess how our approach contributes to solve information security and interoperability problems for mHealth apps. Section 8 concludes this work and gives an outlook on some future work.

2   Design of an mHealth system

Typically, mHealth systems consist of three layers [18]. The *Sensor Layer* manages the access to any sensor required by mHealth apps, i.e., it collects the sensors' raw data and provides it to subsequent layers. In the *Smartphone Layer*, this data is collected, assessed, and processed. The processing step transforms the raw data to information. An optional analysis phase can derive events from the information, e.g., to detect a seizure automatically. The data can also be stored on the Smartphone, e.g., to monitor the progress of the disease. Additionally, the data is forwarded to on-line servers managed by the *Back-End Layer*. While the Smartphone Layer holds health data of a single patient, in the Back-End Layer the data of multiple patients is assembled (e.g., to derive new insights into the course of a disease or to prepare the data for subsequent in-depth analyses). Via this layer physicians are able to perform analyses and receive diagnosis support for each of their patients. For this purpose, there is sometimes an additional *Presentation Layer*. This fourth layer preprocesses the health data stored in the back-end and presents the relevant data in a user-friendly manner. So, physicians are able to interpret the results.

Figure 1 shows the interaction of these four layers. A metering device can be connected to a Smartphone via Bluetooth. A patient can install an mHealth app on his or her Smartphone and use the medical data recorded by the external metering device. This data can be enriched by data from the Smartphone's built-in sensors (e.g., location data). The app sends the gathered data to an mHealth back-end for thorough analyses and to store the data at a central repository. Physicians can access the repository via their diagnosis tools to find an adequate method of treatment.

Concerning the two key issues addressed in this paper, namely device interoperability and information security, several components have to be taken into consideration. Any data interchange between two layers is a problem, since there are

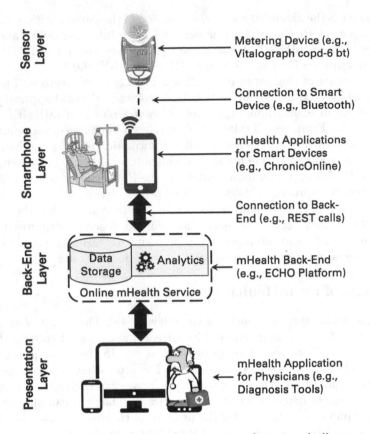

Sensor Layer → Metering Device (e.g., Vitalograph copd-6 bt)

Connection to Smart Device (e.g., Bluetooth)

Smartphone Layer → mHealth Applications for Smart Devices (e.g., ChronicOnline)

Connection to Back-End (e.g., REST calls)

Back-End Layer → Data Storage · Analytics · Online mHealth Service → mHealth Back-End (e.g., ECHO Platform)

Presentation Layer → mHealth Application for Physicians (e.g., Diagnosis Tools)

Fig. 1. Design of an mHealth system [based on [41]].

heterogeneous interchange formats and multiple connection standard. This concerns especially the data interchange between Smartphones and medical devices, since these devices commonly define proprietary communication protocols. Yet, the harmonization of the medical data formats used by mHealth apps and back-ends has to be considered as well. While there are several approaches towards a server-sided unified data model for health data (e.g., in the *HealthVault* [2]), there are no such approaches for apps.

Information security has to be considered at any layer. However, as users cannot influence the security mechanisms implemented in sensors, data protection has to be assured mainly on the Smartphone Layer. While there are approaches to protect sensitive data on the Back-End Layer (e.g., [15]), an adequate solution for the Smartphone Layer is missing. The Presentation Layer does not create any sensitive data.

We focus on the Sensor Layer and the Smartphone Layer in our work regarding device interoperability and information security, as there are solutions for the other layers to solve theses issues. Yet, the usability and security of an mHealth system is impaired by its weakest component. That is, the existing usability and security solutions for the Back-End Layer and the Presentation Layer are worthless with respect to the whole system, as long as there are no appropriate approaches for the Sensor Layer and the Smartphone Layer as well [34].

3 Application Scenario

The chronic obstructive pulmonary disease or short COPD is an obstructive lung disease. COPD patients suffer from a poor airflow which worsens over time. According to the World Health Organization, approximately 6% of all deaths in 2012 resulted directly from COPD [51]. Even though COPD is not curable, a fast and persistent therapy can slow the progression of the disease significantly down. For this purpose telemedicine is very appropriate, since the required measurements can be carried out very easily with affordable medical measuring devices [46].

In the following, we introduce a real-world mHealth app for COPD patients which is based on the *ECHO* project[1]. This example covers all four mHealth layers introduced in the previous section: Patients get an app for Smartphones (see Sect. 3.2) which gathers various health data from medical devices (see Sect. 3.1). The app sends health data to a data analysis back-end and receives medical outcomes from it likewise. Physicians can also access their patients data via the back-end, e.g., via diagnosis tools running in the Presentation Layer (see Sect. 3.3).

3.1 The Vitalograph COPD-6 BT

The Vitalograph copd-6 bt[2] is used to screen the pulmonary function. So, patients with respiratory conditions can perform the metering by themselves. It records various lung function parameters including the Peak Expiratory Flow (PEF) and the Forced Expiratory Volume (FEV) among others. PEF and FEV are key readings for the diagnosis of COPD. The measurement results are transmitted via Bluetooth LE. As today's Smartphones support this battery-saving connection standard, the Vitalograph copd-6 bt provides a sound hardware foundation for telemedical mHealth apps.

For data interchange the proprietary *Terminal I/O* protocol [45] is used which operates on top of Bluetooth LE GATT [5,11]. The basic idea behind this protocol is that a client (e.g., a Smartphone) has to request credits from the server (i.e., the Vitalograph copd-6 bt). Following this, the client can retrieve data from the server (e.g., health data); for each message the client has to pay one credit. Hereby it is ensured that the client is able to make a specific number of requests without having to wait for a response from the server. However, as soon as the client runs out of credits, it has to wait for the server's response

---

[1] See http://chroniconline.eu.
[2] See https://vitalograph.com/product/162427.

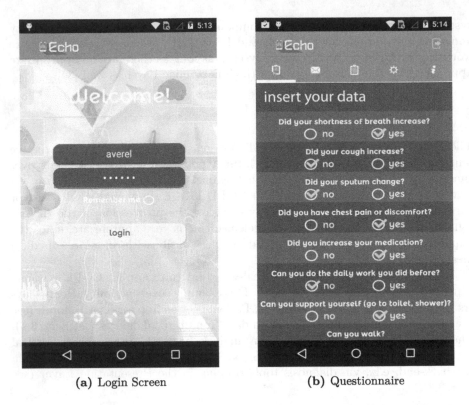

(a) Login Screen   **(b)** Questionnaire

Fig. 2. The ChronicOnline app's key functionality [41].

in order to get additional credits. For more information on the Terminal I/O protocol, please refer to the literature [45]. The application of such proprietary protocols impedes the development of mHealth apps since only a limited number of device types supports the respective protocol. As a common communication standard is not in sight, app developers are in great need of other approaches with which the device interoperability is enhanced.

3.2   The ChronicOnline App

mHealth apps are good for regularly recording various parameters but they are insufficient for a comprehensive COPD screening. For this reason, the University of Stuttgart, the University of Crete, and OpenIT launched the ECHO project in 2013. Within the scope of this project several mHealth apps collect various health data and gather the data in a Cloud infrastructure [3]. Online services are available for physicians enabling various data analytic functions and giving them an holistic overview of their patients' condition. In addition to it, the patients and the physicians remain in contact with each other whereby the physicians can give their patients advices by sending them messages via their mHealth app.

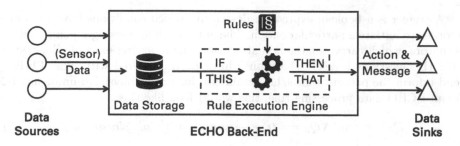

Fig. 3. The operation principle of the ECHO rule execution engine.

The ChronicOnline app [4] is a mobile front-end for the ECHO project. Its key functions (access control and a COPD questionnaire) are shown in Fig. 2.

Initially, the user has to log in his or her account (see Fig. 2a). The app differentiates two user groups, patients who have only access to their personal account and physicians who monitor several patients. The login process as well as any other communication between the app and the ECHO back-end is realized by REST calls.

After authorization is complete, the patient has access to several tabs. The most significant tab is the questionnaire tab (see Fig. 2b). Here the user has to answer five questions about his or her condition. Each question can be answered with 'yes' or 'no'. Depending on the given answers up to six subquestions appear to refine the medical finding. Afterwards, the results are transferred to the back-end as a JSON object. More details on the data format are given in Sect. 5.1.

This app is a representative sample for the innumerable COPD apps available in various app stores. We could use any of them without a loss of argument.

3.3 The ECHO Back-End

After the patient has submitted his or her answers, the back-end performs analyses and preprocesses the data for physicians. The incoming data—i.e., the answers to the questionnaire as well as health data from metering devices such as the Vitalograph copd-6 bt—is processed by the ECHO back-end using a rule execution engine. This strategy is loosely based on the *If This Then That* (*IFTTT*) approach[3]. That approach allows users to define the behavior of their IoT devices in a simple but yet highly versatile manner [22]. Via this so-called trigger-action approach, it is also possible for non-IT experts (e.g., physicians or medical experts) to configure the rule execution engine [47].

Figure 3 shows how the ECHO back-end operates. All incoming data from data sources such as apps (queries) or sensors (medical data) is initially stored as raw data for documentation and subsequent analyses. Then, the data is forwarded to the rule execution engine. All defined rules have a simple IFTTT-like structure:

$$Trigger \rightarrow Action \tag{1}$$

---

[3] See https://ifttt.com.

A trigger is a boolean expression describing which conditions have to apply in order to initiate a particular action. The action defines messages being sent to actuators, which carry out the actual action. The following example illustrates this: **IF** Questions 1 **AND** Question 3 have been answered with 'yes' **THEN** send inform the patient, that s/he should call his or her physician immediately. As an ECHO data processing rule, this would look like this:

$$Q_1 == true \land Q_3 == true \to send\_mail('Call\ physician') \qquad (2)$$

Since the results obtained from the questionnaire are only indicators for a possible aggravation, the discussion of the medical findings still has to take place in a personal meeting with the physician. If the app has also access to data from medical devices, the rules for the analysis could be adapted to get more useful information about the patients' condition. In case of COPD, examples for important measurements to monitor the patients condition would be Peak Expiratory Flow (PEF) or the Forced Expiratory Volume (FEV). Using these values, it could be even possible to skip the personal meeting with the physician while getting a more detailed diagnosis of the patients health condition. This diagnosis could the be used to cope with the disease in a personalized manner. In order to enable the physician to create personalized rules for his or her patients, concepts for editing the rules for the analysis are needed. In the domain of manufacturing, such concepts are already being developed to promote digitalization [49]. The goal is to enable every worker in manufacturing environments to create easy-to-use rules similar to the ones described above to link events to corresponding actions [50]. These concepts can easily be transferred to mHealth apps, such that a physician can define monitoring rules for special groups of patients or even personalized rules for individual patients.

As the definition of the triggers gets complex when more data sources are involved, domain experts can define reusable patterns:

$$Critical\_Condition :== Q_1 == true \land Q_3 == true \qquad (3)$$

Then, this pattern can be used in Eq. (2) in order to simplify the left part of the rule ($Critical\_Condition \to send\_mail('Call\ physician')$).

Obviously, the action can also be used to control apps on the Presentation Layer. Thereby history data from the back-end loaded into the app, e.g., to display former questionnaire answers. Detailed analysis results and history charts can also be preprocessed to include them in web-based dashboards for physicians [43]. Thus, we cover all four layers of an mHealth system with this example, starting with the Sensor Layer up to actuators, i.e., the Presentation Layer.

Please note that the back-end is out of this paper's scope. More information about the back-end can be found in [44]. However, we give a brief outlook about $PATRON^4$ (see [35,36]), a data privacy mechanism for the processing of sensitive data in such a back-end in Sect. 8.

4 Related Work

In the context of device interoperability in mHealth apps, a lot of work is done concerning the back-end systems. For this purpose, these systems introduced harmonized data models for health data and provide generic interfaces so that any kind of mHealth app can use them to collect and share heath data. One of the biggest systems is the HealthVault [2]. It supports various health-related data types ranging from fitness data to entire personal health records. The HealthVault acts as a middleman between the data producers—i.e., the mHealth apps—and the data consumers—i.e., analysis systems. Concerning app-sided device interoperability and information security, such a system provides no help. *Google Fit* [24] is another back-end for storing and processing health data. Google's system deals with fitness data (e.g., the heart rate), only. Google Fit provides interfaces for app developers which enhance the device interoperability and facilitate the reading of sensors in third-party devices—at least for devices that are supported by Google Wear[5]. As especially medical devices are not supported by Google Wear, [29] discuss, how Smartphones can be connected with these devices. However, their solution aims for physical connections and not for harmonized communication standards. [17] recommend to use IoT techniques to solve this problem. In their proposal all sensors are connected to the Internet and send their data to a Cloud-based database which is also accessible for mHealth apps. Even though there are secure transfer protocols for health data (e.g., [20]), a permanent and unrestricted transmission of such sensitive data to an unknown server is ineligible for most users. For that reason, [10] introduce an approach with which the patient stays in total control over his or her data; the mHealth app has full access to the health data while external services (e.g., apps for physicians) only get access as long as the patient grants it. In [27] an mHealth app is introduced which relies on a full encryption of the health data when the data is stored or transmitted. Yet, both approaches assume that only external entities constitute a threat for the security of health data. However, as studies prove, two out of three apps handle their data either carelessly or even maliciously [9]. Thus, none of these approaches solves the device interoperability and information security issues of mHealth apps. Despite the benefit of mHealth apps especially the device incompatibility and the mistrust in app developers repel patients from using such apps [28]. For this reason, we introduce a general approach dealing with both issues in the following sections.

---

[4] PATRON is an acronym for "**Privacy in Stream Processing**".
[5] See https://www.android.com/wear.

5   Interoperability and Security Reflections

In order to come up with a design methodology for interoperable and secure mHealth apps, a secure data management, data input techniques, and defined data access conditions are required. Our solution to this is built upon the PMP. When looking at the ChronicOnline app, it does not take advantage of the full potential of the ECHO back-end and the prevailing hardware. With its analytic functions and notification services, the back-end is able to process more complex data such as location data or respiratory data in addition to the replies to the disease-specific questionnaire. By the integration of medical devices, the ChronicOnline app becomes a full-fledged telemedicine solution.

Therefore we extend the ChronicOnline app by adding location services[6]. Studies show that the location can have a relevant influence on the progression of a disease [16]. Moreover, we provide support for various third-party Bluetooth respiratory monitors. The measurement results are added to the electronic health record (see Sect. 5.1 for its data model) and transferred to the ECHO back-end. There, the data can be automatically pre-analyzed which not only unburdens the physicians in charge, but also results in a faster feedback for the patients. As a consequence this enhanced app has to deal with increasing interoperability and security issues.

Amulet, a tiny Smart Device operating as an information hub, tries to solve both problems [12]. It confirms the user's identity and identifies any available devices in the surrounding belonging to him or her. Then, Amulet ascertains that only trusted third-party devices can be used for the metering and ensures a secure connection to these devices. Moreover, Amulet provides mechanisms to protect the health data against external attackers. In order to transfer the data to (trusted) servers for further processing, Amulet is able to connect to a Smartphone and use it for transmission. Unfortunately, this approach has a severe drawback: The user has to possess another device in addition to his or her Smartphone and the actual medical device. This causes further costs and it is unpractical since the user has to carry the Amulet all the time. The PMP (see Sect. 5.2) is a middleware for application platforms which provides similar features.

5.1   The Internal Data Model

The ChronicOnline app sends up to eleven boolean values, representing the answers to the questionnaire, to the ECHO back-end. For this reason, its data model for the data exchange is quite plain (see Listing 1). In addition to the questionnaire answers, a daily report entails an ID for the patient and for the report itself as well as the submission date. Please note that authorization data to confirm the identity of the submitter is not part of this data model. The authorization is managed via the authorization header of the HTTP protocol.

---

[6] Location based services in general constitute a severe threat to a user's privacy [19].

```
 1 DailyReport {
 2   patientId (integer): Unique Identifier of the Patient,
 3   recordId  (integer): Unique Identifier of this Record,
 4   date (string): Date of Report,
 5   q1  (boolean): Answer to Question 1,
 6   q1a (boolean): Answer to Question 1a,
 7   q1b (boolean): Answer to Question 1b,
 8   q1c (boolean): Answer to Question 1c,
 9   q2  (boolean): Answer to Question 2,
10   ...
11   q5  (boolean): Answer to Question 5
12 }
```

Listing 1. The ChronicOnline Data Model (Excerpt) [based on 41].

We add latitude and longitude to this basic schema to support location data as well as entries for the most relevant COPD readings, including the Peak Expiratory Flow and the Forced Expiratory Volume among others (see Listing 2).

```
 1 DailyReport {
 2   patientId (integer): Unique Identifier of the Patient,
 3   ...
 4   q5 (boolean): Answer to Question 5,
 5   lat (number): Latitude of GPS Location.,
 6   lon (number): Longitude of GPS Location,
 7   pef (integer): Peak Expiratory Flow,
 8   fev1 (number): Forced Expiratory Volume (First Second),
 9   fev10 (number): Forced Expiratory Volume (Ten Seconds),
10   fef2575 (number): Mid-Breath Forced Expiratory Flow,
11   ...
12 }
```

Listing 2. The Extended Data Model (Excerpt) [based on 41].

Since the JSON format is well-suited for the data exchange between the app and the back-end, but not for the data processing within the app, we apply wrapper classes for the conversion of such JSON files to Java objects and vice versa.

5.2 Overview of the PMP

We use the PMP in order to realize interoperability and security features as needed by mHealth apps. We give a brief overview of the PMP at first and describe in detail the new components, which are developed in this work in the next section. The PMP is an intermediate layer between apps and the operating system. It prevents any (potentially malicious) app from accessing sensitive data.

When an app needs access to such data, it has to ask the PMP for permission. The PMP operates several data provisioning services, the so-called *Resources*.

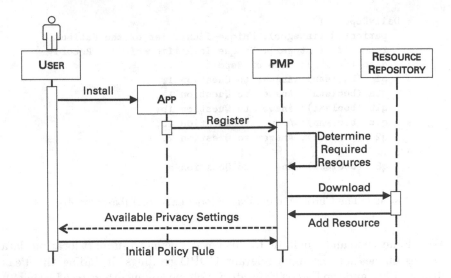

Fig. 4. The registration of an app at the PMP [41].

Each Resource is responsible for a certain type of data but it is not committed to a certain technology; e.g., the Location Resource is able to provide location data from a GPS provider or from a network provider. Thereby it can adapt its functionality to the available hardware. In addition to it, the user can define how accurate the data should be in order to obfuscate his or her private data. Further Resources can be hooked into the PMP at runtime need-based.

A Resource defines *Privacy Settings* which restrict the usage of the corresponding Resource. By default, there is a Privacy Setting for granting or permitting the usage of a Resource. Furthermore, a Privacy Setting can be more specific depending on the type of Resource. For instance, the Location Resource can reduce the location's accuracy.

At installation time an app has to register at the PMP. The PMP identifies which Resources are required and installs missing Resources if necessary. The user then postulates an initial policy rule for this app defining, which data should be given to the app and how accurate this data should be. This registration process is shown in Fig. 4.

Since the user is able to deny that an app gets access to a certain Resource, the app model of the PMP encapsulates logically coherent parts of the app in so-called *Service Features*. So, the withdrawal of access rights simply deactivates the affected Service Features but the app itself can still be executed. Moreover, the user can modify access rights of individual Service Features at runtime. The permission allocation is shown in Fig. 5.

The PMP is primary a fine-grained permission system with additional privacy features (e.g., data obfuscation). However, in the context of interoperability and uncertainty of available hardware, the PMP serves a dual purpose. Each Resource is abstracted from a certain technology and can have several implementations. As

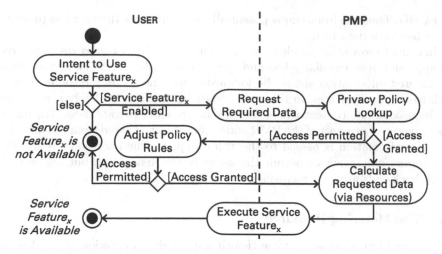

Fig. 5. The PMP's permission allocation process [41].

a consequence, the app developer only has to request a certain type of data (e.g., respiratory data) and the dedicated Resource ensures that it gets this data from the available hardware (e.g., a Vitalograph copd-6 bt). If no hardware providing this kind of data is available—which is similar to a user-defined prohibition to use the hardware via the PMP—then the app gets informed and adapts to this condition by deactivating affected Service Features.

The PMP is able to degrade an app's functionality when it cannot access all of its requested data. Certain Services Features can be deactivate instead of feeding an app with random data. Especially, in the context of mHealth apps, the usage of random medical values is inappropriate. For this reason, the PMP's data obfuscation for health data is severely restricted. For further details on the PMP, please refer to the literature [37,38].

6   Design of mHealth PMP Resources

In the following we introduce five PMP Resources which are developed for mHealth apps, namely a secure **authentication** Resource, a **metering** Resource, a **localization** Resource, a **data storage** Resource, and a **connection** Resource. In addition, a Resource for health data **encryption** is introduced. Finally, we revise the ChronicOnline app with the help of these Resources.

6.1   The Dialog Box Resource

In the ChronicOnline app a user has to enter credential information which is forwarded to an ECHO server for verification. While the back-end is operated by a trusted organization (e.g., a hospital), any developer can implement apps for ECHO. Thus the front-end is potentially insecure—yet the user has to reveal his or her login data to it.

In order to solve this problem, we introduce an isolated *Dialog Box Resource*. An app can invoke the dialog box and specify the displayed text as well as where the entered information should be forwarded to. The server's response is sent back to the invoking app. In this way, the dialog box is completely generic and can be used in any context where the user has to enter private data. The dialog box is executed as a part of the PMP and is completely isolated from the invoking app. No information is passed to the app except for the back-end's reply. The user cannot only grant or permit the usage of the dialog box, but also specify which back-ends are legit recipients.

6.2   The Metering Resource

One of the biggest problems for mHealth apps is the integration of third-party medical devices as there is currently no uniform standard for intercommunication with such devices. This is why most of the currently available apps support some hand-picked medical device only.

That is why we introduce a *Metering Resource* with a simple, yet generic interface (see Listing 3). In order to support as many use-cases as possible, we designed a new data type for health data, called *HealthRecord*. A HealthRecord consists of an id, the answers to the questionnaire, the health data itself, location data, and a timestamp (see Listing 2). The HealthRecord is able to maintain any kind of health data via the generic attributes that can be made up of any (i.e., unspecified or schema-less) JSON object. As a consequence, the Metering Resource defines no fixed schema for the health data, but processes this data as a JSON object. Currently, we adhere to the data schema which is defined by the particular data source and use the same schema for the JSON object. However, as soon as a common standard for electronic health records is defined, we can switch to this standard internally without having to revise any app using the Metering Resource.

```
1  interface IMetering {
2      SealedHealthRecord performMetering();
3  }
```

Listing 3. Interface of the Metering Resource.

Since most modern medical devices exchange their data with Smartphones via a Bluetooth connection, we focus our work on this kind of connection. As there is no common Bluetooth transmission protocol, the Metering Resource has to be able to support several protocols. Currently, we implemented interfaces for the ISO/IEEE 11073 Personal Health Data (PHD) standards [14] as well as the Terminal I/O protocol [45] of the Vitalograph Lung Monitor. Further protocols (e.g., Android Wear) or other connection standards (e.g., USB) can also be supported in the future due to the modular expandability of PMP Resources

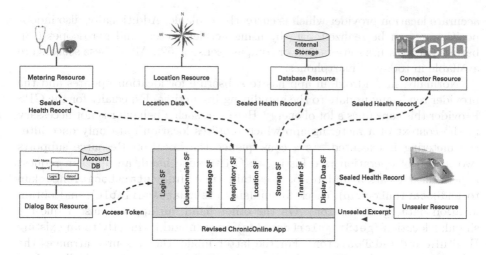

Fig. 6. Service features of the COPD app and their applied PMP resources [41].

(see [42]). The Metering Resource defines no fixed schema for health data, but processes this data as a JSON object with an attribute for every measured value.

As the Metering Resource autonomously connects to any available device, an app developer simply has to request the health record from the Resource. However, concerning information security, the app should not be able to read the health record. Thus, the PMP encrypts the JSON object containing the health data. As a consequence, authorized Resources can process the health data while (potentially malicious) apps cannot access the data. Nevertheless, sometimes an app needs access to certain values of the health data, e.g., in order to display the data. For this purpose, the *Unsealer Resource* (see Sect. 6.6) can be used in order to decrypt certain excerpts of the record.

Moreover, the user is able to restrict which devices are allowed to provide health data for a certain app via a Privacy Setting of the Metering Resource. For instance, s/he can permit an app to use the Metering Resource, but only a certain kind of data from a specific smart watch such as the heart rate is sent back by the Resource. A manipulation or randomization of the health data for privacy reasons is disregarded, since this kind of data has to be as accurate as possible in order to be useful.

6.3   The Location Resource

Since it is relevant for some medical outcomes to know the location where a reading has been recorded in order to detect potential relationships between a patient's condition and his or her whereabouts, we provide a special *Location Resource* for mHealth apps. Android supports different location providers— mainly the *Network Location Provider* for cell tower and Wi-Fi based location and the more accurate *GPS Provider*—which periodically report on the geographical location of the device. Our Location Resource always requests the most accurate location provider which is currently available. Additionally, also indoor positioning can be realized, e.g., by using accelerometers and gyroscopes [13], barometric pressure sensors [53], or compass sensors [52]. All of these sensors are available in today's Smartphones.

Normally, in Android an app has to subscribe for location updates and the provider sends any update to the app during its lifetime. Especially for the GPS Provider this consumes a lot of energy. However, such a behavior is not necessary in the context of a metering app which requires location data only once after the metering is executed. As a consequence the Location Resource supports two modes of operation (see Listing 4): On the one hand, an app can request a periodical location update for a certain time (from `startLocationLookup` to `endLocationLookup`), check for updates (`isUpdateAvailable`), and obtain location data (`getLocation`). On the other hand, an app can also request a singular location (`getSingularLocation`) or even add it directly to an existing HealthRecord (`addPosition`). For the latter mode, the Resource arranges the subscription to and unsubscription from a location provider automatically—since a Resource can be used mutually by several apps, already existing results from another app's location request are utilized for this purpose.

```
1 interface ILocation {
2     void startLocationLookup();
3     void endLocationLookup();
4     boolean isUpdateAvailable();
5     Location getLocation();
6     Location getSingularLocation();
7     void addPosition(inout SealedHealthRecord record);
8 }
```

Listing 4. Interface of the Location Resource.

In order to respect the user's privacy, the Location Resource provides a Privacy Setting to reduce the accuracy of the location data. The user is able to stipulate a maximal accuracy in meters. If the provided location data is more accurate then the Resource adds a random factor depending on the user settings to the latitude and longitude in order to reduce the accuracy. The user is also allowed to use completely random location data, so that his or her location remains unknown to the app.

6.4   The Secure Database Resource

Since Android stores its data in a clear-text readable form, attackers may harvest all stored data. The in Android 5.0 introduced file system encryption functions are no solution for this threat, since the encryption is not kept up during operation, i.e., as soon as the system is fully booted. So, sensitive data such as health data requires additional security features. For this very reason, additional security features are required in order to ensure information security for sensitive data. The **S**ecure **D**ata **C**ontainer (*SDC*) is a *Secure Database Resource* for the PMP [39]. It encrypts the stored data with AES-256 encryption and only the PMP has the key. The SDC has a fine-grained access control to share the stored data with selected apps. Performance measurements show that the thereby caused overhead is within reasonable limits.

We tailor the SDC slightly to our requirements: The database's internal data model is comparable to a key-value store. In accordance with *CURATOR* [40], the Secure Database Resource operates with JSON objects and adopts the therein defined keys and values directly. As several stored JSON objects can use a common key, an internal id is applied to each object. The database's primary key consists of this id and the key. The Secure Database Resource partitions the stored data in several SQLite tables internally (one per app) for performance and security reasons.

The Secure Database Resource's interface (see Listing 5) is minimalistic, yet demand-actuated. A JSON object can be stored (`store`), obtained (`get`), and deleted (`delete`) via its id. In addition to it, the Secure Database Resource supports the usage of HealthRecords which can be passed as a total and the Resource arranges the decryption of the health data and the decomposition into key-value pairs. Obtaining complete HealthRecords operates analog.

```
1 interface IDatabase {
2   int store(in JSONObject data);
3   JSONObject get(in int id);
4   boolean delete(in int id);
5   boolean storeRecord(in SealedHealthRecord record);
6   boolean storeAll(in List<SealedHealthRecord> records);
7   SealedHealthRecord getRecord(in int id);
8   List<SealedHealthRecord> getAllRecords();
9 }
```

Listing 5. Interface of the Secure Database Resource.

The most important contribution of the Secure Database Resource concerning information security is indeed its full encryption. Shmueli et al. [31] describe various attack models against databases and assess different database encryption schemata that should prevent these attacks. The result of their study is quite simple: Only by encrypting the whole database as a total, information leakage as well as unauthorized modifications can be prevented reliably. Therefore, each SQLite file is encrypted in the Secure Database Resource with an AES-256 encryption and only the PMP has the key. This encryption causes an overhead. However, by the partitioning of the data this overhead is within reasonable limits and the fact that the Resource is meant for sensitive data such as health data, any overhead is justified. Moreover, modern Smartphones possess sufficient computing power, whereby this overhead becomes negligible.

6.5   The Connector Resource

Nowadays, most apps do not only operate locally on a single Smartphone, but include various external services. This is why almost every app requests the permission to establish a network connection. The user is not even informed about this request. However, an app having this permission is able to upload sensitive data to any server. To use external services in a secured way, we introduce the *Connector Resource*.

Within the Connector Resource various trusted external services can be included. An app is able to either upload data to or retrieve data from one of these services (e.g., the ECHO back-end or Amazon's SNS). Additional domain-specific information protection policies can be applied within the Connector Resource (such as the *Mobile access to Health Documents* profile [26] or the *Audit Trail and Node Authentication* profile [25]), if they are supported by the back-end.

Currently, only the basic functionality for the ECHO back-end is supported. Hence, the current Resource's interface (see Listing 6) comprises three functions: Analog to the Secure Database Resource, HealthRecords can be stored (storeRecord), obtained (getRecord), and deleted (deleteRecord). Certainly, this interface needs to be extended, when further services are added.

```
1 interface IConnector {
2     boolean storeRecord(in SealedHealthRecord record);
3     SealedHealthRecord getRecord(in int id);
4     boolean deleteRecord(in int id);
5 }
```

Listing 6. Interface of the Connector Resource.

Concerning interoperability, the Connector Resource handles any interface changes of the external services for the apps. i.e., adjustments have to be done only once at the Resource and not for every app. Additionally, it has protective function. Since an app can only pass sensitive data to the Connector Resource and has no further connectivity it is guaranteed that the data is only sent to the appointed service—only connections to trusted services are provided by the Resource. Additionally, the user can remove any service s/he does not trust via the Resource's Privacy Settings.

6.6   The Unsealer Resource

As mentioned above, the health data within the HealthRecord gets encrypted as soon as it is passed from any Resource to any app by the PMP. As a consequence, the app does not have access to this sensitive data. Basically, the health data is only processed in Resources and therefore the encryption represents no constraint for the user (cf. [48]). However, in rare cases it might be necessary for an app to get access to excerpts of the health data, e.g., to display it. For this very reason, we introduce the *Unsealer Resource*. Its interface consists of a single function which converts a SealedHealthRecord into a HealthRecord (see Listing 7).

```
1 interface IUnsealer {
2   HealthRecord unseal(in SealedHealthRecord sealedRecord);
3 }
```

Listing 7. Interface of the Unsealer Resource.

However, the user is not only able to grant or permit the usage of the Unsealer Resource, but s/he can also define via a Privacy Setting which excerpt of the data should be revealed. To that end, the Resource provides a multi-state selection (e.g., general information, lung-related content only, etc.) in order to facilitate the configuration. Since the health data is stored as a JSON object, any unrevealed data is simply cut out of it. For the user's safety also the Unsealer does not provide falsified values, as such an approach is disregarded for the processing of health data.

6.7   Revised ChronicOnline App

Based on these Resources, we revise the ChronicOnline app by including sensor data (e.g., respiratory meters or location sensors) while regarding device interoperability and information security.

After the user has answered the questionnaire, the revised app expects respiratory data from a connected device via the Metering Resource. The user only has to push the *"Lung Monitor"* button and the connection and data transfer is arranged automatically by the PMP. When the measured data is available, the results of the questionnaire are applied to the DailyReport (see Listing 2) and the location data is inquired. Then, the complete DailyReport object is stored internally (e.g., if the data cannot be transmitted immediately) and is transferred subsequently to the ECHO back-end (see Fig. 7a). Please note, that for this capture any data is unsealed for demonstration purpose. The user is informed in each step about the collected data. So, s/he is in total control over the data. The effect of a deactivated Unsealer Resource is shown in Fig. 7b. Without the Unsealer Resource only data which are not related to any health issues are known to the app.

In order to react properly to the restriction of a Resource, an app needs to define Service Features. Figure 6 shows the 8 Service Features of the revised ChronicOnline App (denoted as SF) and which Resources are required for each of them. Not every Service Feature necessarily requires data from a Resource (e.g., the *Questionnaire SF*). The Service Features have a modular design and can be plugged in and out at runtime (e.g., when the corresponding Resource is deactivated). In the app's program flow these features are skipped. However, since the authentication of the user is mandatory, the *Login SF* and therewith the Dialog Box Resource cannot be deactivated or else any other Service Feature is also deactivated.

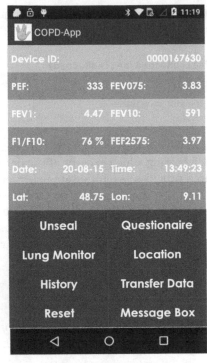
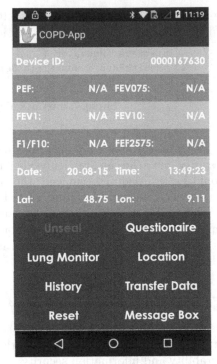

(a) Unsealed Data Screen   **(b)** Sealed Data Screen

Fig. 7. The ChronicOnline privacy-driven app [41].

7   Assessment

Concerning information security, the literature speaks of 7 key protective goals, namely *auditability, authenticity, availability, confidentiality, integrity, non-repudiation,* and *privacy* [7,8]. The original ChronicOnline app only fulfills the authenticity goal and the confidentiality goal directly due to its login mechanism and the auditability goal, the integrity goal, and the non-repudiation server-sided due to the security mechanism of the ECHO back-end. However, as soon as real health data is processed by the app, the user cannot rely on the prevailing mechanisms. Our revised app supports all 7 protective goals due to the used Resources. The auditability as well as the non-repudiation is guaranteed, since the PMP logs any Resource access of an app. The authenticity is given via the login mechanism and since the login data is not shared with the app, it cannot commit an identity theft. The availability is given, as all data is stored on the device using mature database technologies. The confidentiality is ensured, since any app functionality is only usable after the login process is completed. The integrity is guaranteed since any relevant data is encrypted and therefore cannot be manipulated by third-parties. Privacy is retained, as the user decides, which data can be used by an app and s/he can specify for any non-health data how accurate or even randomized it should be provided. As an app cannot access any data without using the PMP, data access is strictly constrained by the Resources' interfaces. Thus, from an information security's point of view the revised app satisfies all requirements.

Concerning device interoperability, the modular expandability of the Resources turns out to be beneficial. For instance, support for additional devices can be added to the Metering Resource need-based at runtime. An app developer only has to code against a Resource's interface, no matter which hardware is actually available. Therefore, complex and labor-intensive coding is required only once (for the Resource) and it can be reused many times (in the apps). Additionally, due to their generic design the Resources are usable in many different application scenarios even for non-mHealth apps. Thus, from an interoperability's point of view the PMP Resources satisfy all requirements regarding compatibility and reusability. Table 1 lists the key contributions of the introduced Resources.

Table 1. Feature summary of the implemented PMP resources [based on [41]].

PMP resource	Device interoperability	Information security
Dialog Box	• Tailoring of dialog text • Tailoring of data processing	• App has no access to data
Metering	• Support of different devices	• Device restriction
Location	• Different location sensors • Different modes of operation	• Restriction of accuracy • Randomized location data
Secure Database	• Generic data model	• Full database encryption
Connector	• Support of different services	• No direct network access • Restriction of usable services
Unsealer		• Limited access to health data

8   Conclusion and Outlook

Today's medical devices for home use can often be connected to Smartphones via Bluetooth. On the one hand, health data can be sent from the medical device to the Smartphone for processing or presentation. On the other hand, the Smartphone can be used to control the medical device. By connecting to several medical devices, the Smartphone virtually becomes a health hub for the pants pocket. This provides entirely new possibilities for telemedicine. This is particularly beneficial for the treatment of chronic diseases such as COPD. The treatment of such a disease makes it necessary for patients to undergo regular screenings. This results in increasing treatment costs as well as overburdened physicians. However, mHealth Apps can drastically reduce the number of visits to the physician. Yet, the patients' confidence in mHealth apps is impaired due to device interoperability and information security issues.

We address these problems in our work. For this purpose, we describe the multilayered architecture of mHealth apps and analyze one particular mHealth app for COPD patients. Based on this analysis, we create a generic data model for mHealth apps. Furthermore, we derive relevant functions of an mHealth app, in which device interoperability or information security is an issue. We design and implement Resources for the PMP (a privacy-aware data provisioning system) which support each of these mHealth functions. To evaluate the practical effect of these PMP extensions, we re-engineer the analyzed COPD app and integrate our Resources into it. Based on this revised app, we assess whether our approach contributes to solve the device interoperability and information security issues.

While our approach is a solution to the device interoperability issue, further comprehensive measures have to be taken regarding information security. As the analysis of the multilayered architecture of mHealth apps shows (see Sect. 2), the health data is preprocessed on the Smartphone, only. Most of the data processing takes place on external servers. A large number of different data sources are combined on these servers. Thus an immense amount of data is available for this external data processing, from which a lot of knowledge about the patients can be derived. Therefore, information security measures for Smartphones, as presented in this paper, are not sufficient. If a user has control over the data on his or her Smartphone, the back-end might still be able to obtain the same data from other sources. Thus, an holistic information security approach has to be applied to both, the Smartphone Layer as well as the Back-End Layer. Therefore, future work has to determine, how a information security system for back-ends such as PATRON [35,36] can be integrated in our PMP-based approach [34].

Acknowledgments. This paper is part of the PATRON research project which is commissioned by the Baden-Württemberg Stiftung gGmbH. The authors would like to thank the BW-Stiftung for the funding of this research.

References

1. Bai, Y., Dai, L., Li, J.: Issues and challenges in securing eHealth systems. Int. J. E-Health Med. Commun. **5**(1), 1–19 (2014)
2. Bhandari, V.: Enabling Programmable Self with HealthVault. O'Reilly Media Inc., Beijing (2012)
3. Bitsaki, M., et al.: An integrated mHealth solution for enhancing patients' health online. In: Lacković, I., Vasic, D. (eds.) MBEC 2014. IP, vol. 45, pp. 695–698. Springer, Cham (2015). https://doi.org/10.1007/978-3-319-11128-5_173
4. Bitsaki, M., et al.: ChronicOnline: implementing a mHealth solution for monitoring and early alerting in chronic obstructive pulmonary disease. Health Inform. J. **23**(3), 197–207 (2016)
5. Bluetooth SIG Inc.: GATT specifications. Technical report (2017). https://www.bluetooth.com/specifications/gatt

6. Chan, M., Estève, D., Fourniols, J.Y., Escriba, C., Campo, E.: Smart wearable systems: current status and future challenges. Artif. Intell. Med. **56**(3), 137–156 (2012)
7. Cherdantseva, Y., Hilton, J.: A reference model of information assurance & security. In: Proceedings of the 2013 International Conference on Availability, Reliability and Security, ARES 2013, pp. 546–555 (2013)
8. Dhillon, G., Backhouse, J.: Technical opinion: information system security management in the new millennium. Commun. ACM **43**(7), 125–128 (2000)
9. Enck, W., et al.: TaintDroid: an information-flow tracking system for realtime privacy monitoring on smartphones. In: Proceedings of the 9th USENIX Conference on Operating Systems Design and Implementation, OSDI 2010, pp. 393–407 (2010)
10. Gardner, R.W., Garera, S., Pagano, M.W., Green, M., Rubin, A.D.: Securing medical records on smart phones. In: Proceedings of the First ACM Workshop on Security and Privacy in Medical and Home-Care Systems, SPIMACS 2009, pp. 31–40 (2009)
11. Gupta, N.: Inside Bluetooth Low Energy. Artech House Publishers, Boston (2013)
12. Hester, J., et al.: Amulet: an energy-efficient, multi-application wearable platform. In: Proceedings of the 14th ACM Conference on Embedded Network Sensor Systems, SenSys 2016, pp. 216–229 (2016)
13. Hsu, H.H., Peng, W.J., Shih, T.K., Pai, T.W., Man, K.L.: Smartphone indoor localization with accelerometer and gyroscope. In: Proceedings of the 2014 17th International Conference on Network-Based Information Systems. NBiS 2014, pp. 465–469 (2014)
14. IEEE 11073 Standards Committee: ISO/IEC/IEEE health informatics-Personal health device communication-Part 20601: application profile-Optimized exchange protocol. ISO/IEEE 11073–20601:2014 (2014)
15. Jafari, M., Safavi-Naini, R., Sheppard, N.P.: A rights management approach to protection of privacy in a cloud of electronic health records. In: Proceedings of the 11th Annual ACM Workshop on Digital Rights Management, DRM 2011, pp. 23–30 (2011)
16. Knöll, M., Moar, M.: On the importance of locations in therapeutic serious games: review on current health games and how they make use of the urban landscape. In: Proceedings of the 2011 5th International Conference on Pervasive Computing Technologies for Healthcare and Workshops. PervasiveHealth 2011, pp. 538–545 (2011)
17. Kouris, I., Koutsouris, D.: Identifying risky environments for COPD patients using smartphones and Internet of Things objects. Int. J. Comput. Intell. Stud. **3**(1), 1–17 (2014)
18. Kumar, S., Nilsen, W., Pavel, M., Srivastava, M.: Mobile health: revolutionizing healthcare through transdisciplinary research. Computer **46**(1), 28–35 (2013)
19. Marcelino, L., Silva, C.: Location privacy concerns in mobile applications. In: Rocha, Á., Reis, L.P. (eds.) Developments and Advances in Intelligent Systems and Applications. SCI, vol. 718, pp. 241–249. Springer, Cham (2018). https://doi.org/10.1007/978-3-319-58965-7_17
20. Mare, S., Sorber, J., Shin, M., Cornelius, C., Kotz, D.: Hide-n-Sense: preserving privacy efficiently in wireless mHealth. Mob. Netw. Appl. **19**(3), 331–344 (2014)
21. Mattila, E., et al.: Empowering citizens for well-being and chronic disease management with wellness diary. IEEE Trans. Inf Technol. Biomed. **14**(2), 456–463 (2010)

22. Mi, X., Qian, F., Zhang, Y., Wang, X.F.: An empirical characterization of IFTTT: ecosystem, usage, and performance. In: Proceedings of the 2017 Internet Measurement Conference, IMC 2017, pp. 398–404 (2017)
23. Milošević, M., Shrove, M.T., Jovanov, E.: Applications of smartphones for ubiquitous health monitoring and wellbeing management. J. Inf. Technol. Appl. 1(1), 7–15 (2011)
24. Mishra, S.M.: Wearable Android: Android Wear and Google FIT App Development. Wiley, Hoboken (2015)
25. Moehrke, J.: Audit trail and node authentication. Techical report, IHE International, August 2017. https://wiki.ihe.net/index.php/Audit_Trail_and_Node_Authentication
26. Moehrke, J.: Mobile access to health documents (MHD). Technical report, IHE International, October 2017. https://wiki.ihe.net/index.php/Mobile_access_to_Health_Documents_(MHD)
27. Murad, A., Schooley, B., Abed, Y.: A secure mHealth application for EMS: design and implementation. In: Proceedings of the 4th Conference on Wireless Health, WH 2013, pp. 15:1–15:2 (2013)
28. Murnane, E.L., Huffaker, D., Kossinets, G.: Mobile health apps: adoption, adherence, and abandonment. In: Adjunct Proceedings of the 2015 ACM International Joint Conference on Pervasive and Ubiquitous Computing and Proceedings of the 2015 ACM International Symposium on Wearable Computers, UbiComp/ISWC 2015 Adjunct, pp. 261–264 (2015)
29. O'Donoghue, J., Herbert, J.: Data management within mHealth environments: patient sensors, mobile devices, and databases. J. Data Inf. Qual. 4(1), 5:1–5:20 (2012)
30. Schweitzer, J., Synowiec, C.: The economics of eHealth and mHealth. J. Health Commun. 17(Supplement 1), 73–81 (2012)
31. Shmueli, E., Vaisenberg, R., Elovici, Y., Glezer, C.: Database encryption: an overview of contemporary challenges and design considerations. ACM SIGMOD Rec. 38(3), 29–34 (2010)
32. Siewiorek, D.: Generation smartphone. IEEE Spectr. 49(9), 54–58 (2012)
33. Silva, B.M., Rodrigues, J.J., de la Torre Díez, I., López-Coronado, M., Saleem, K.: Mobile-health: a review of current state in 2015. J. Biomed. Inform. 56(C), 265–272 (2015)
34. Stach, C., et al.: The AVARE PATRON: a holistic privacy approach for the Internet of Things. In: Proceedings of the 15th International Conference on Security and Cryptography, SECRYPT 2018, pp. 372–379 (2018)
35. Stach, C., et al.: PATRON – Datenschutz in Datenstromverarbeitungssystemen. In: Informatik 2017: Digitale Kulturen, Tagungsband der 47. Jahrestagung der Gesellschaft für Informatik e.V. (GI), 25–29 September 2017, Chemnitz. LNI, vol. 275, pp. 1085–1096 (2017). (in German)
36. Stach, C., Dürr, F., Mindermann, K., Palanisamy, S.M., Wagner, S.: How a pattern-based privacy system contributes to improve context recognition. In: Proceedings of the 2018 IEEE International Conference on Pervasive Computing and Communications Workshops, CoMoRea 2018, pp. 238–243 (2018)
37. Stach, C., Mitschang, B.: Privacy management for mobile platforms - a review of concepts and approaches. In: Proceedings of the 2013 IEEE 14th International Conference on Mobile Data Management, MDM 2013, pp. 305–313 (2013)
38. Stach, C., Mitschang, B.: Design and implementation of the Privacy Management Platform. In: Proceedings of the 2014 IEEE 15th International Conference on Mobile Data Management. MDM 2014, pp. 69–72 (2014)

39. Stach, C., Mitschang, B.: Secure Candy Castle – a prototype for privacy-aware mHealth apps. In: Proceedings of the 2016 IEEE 17th International Conference on Mobile Data Management, MDM 2016, pp. 361–364 (2016)

40. Stach, C., Mitschang, B.: CURATOR–a secure shared object store: design, implementation, and evaluation of a manageable, secure, and performant data exchange mechanism for smart devices. In: Proceedings of the 33rd ACM/SIGAPP Symposium On Applied Computing, DTTA 2018, pp. 533–540 (2018)

41. Stach, C., Steimle, F., Mitschang, B.: The Privacy Management Platform: an enabler for device interoperability and information security in mHealth applications. In: Proceedings of the 11th International Conference on Health Informatics, HEALTHINF 2018, pp. 27–38 (2018)

42. Stach, C., Steimle, F., Franco da Silva, A.C.: TIROL: the extensible interconnectivity layer for mHealth applications. In: Damaševičius, R., Mikašytė, V. (eds.) ICIST 2017. CCIS, vol. 756, pp. 190–202. Springer, Cham (2017). https://doi.org/10.1007/978-3-319-67642-5_16

43. Steimle, F., Wieland, M.: ECHO – an mHealth solution to support treatment of chronic patients. In: Proceedings of the 8th ZEUS Workshop, ZEUS 2016, pp. 64–67 (2016)

44. Steimle, F., Wieland, M., Mitschang, B., Wagner, S., Leymann, F.: Extended provisioning, security and analysis techniques for the ECHO health data management system. Computing **99**(2), 183–201 (2017)

45. Stollmann Entwicklungs- und Vertriebs-GmbH: Terminal I/O Profile: Client implementation guide. Technical report, Telit (2014)

46. de Toledo, P., Jimenez, S., del Pozo, F., Roca, J., Alonso, A., Hernandez, C.: Telemedicine experience for chronic care in COPD. IEEE Trans. Inf Technol. Biomed. **10**(3), 567–573 (2006)

47. Ur, B., McManus, E., Pak Yong Ho, M., Littman, M.L.: Practical trigger-action programming in the smart home. In: Proceedings of the SIGCHI Conference on Human Factors in Computing Systems, CHI 2014, pp. 803–812 (2014)

48. Weerasinghe, D., Rajarajan, M., Rakocevic, V.: Device data protection in mobile healthcare applications. In: Weerasinghe, D. (ed.) eHealth 2008. LNICST, vol. 0001, pp. 82–89. Springer, Heidelberg (2009). https://doi.org/10.1007/978-3-642-00413-1_10

49. Wieland, M., et al.: Towards a rule-based manufacturing integration assistant. Procedia CIRP **57**(1), 213–218 (2016)

50. Wieland, M., et al.: Rule-based integration of smart services using the manufacturing service bus. In: Proceedings of the 2017 IEEE 14th International Conference on Ubiquitous Intelligence and Computing, UIC 2017, pp. 22:1–22:8 (2017)

51. World Health Organization: Chronic Obstructive Pulmonary Disease (COPD). Technical report, WHO Media Centre (2015)

52. Xie, H., Gu, T., Tao, X., Lu, J.: A reliability-augmented particle filter for magnetic fingerprinting based indoor localization on smartphone. IEEE Trans. Mob. Comput. **15**(8), 1877–1892 (2016)

53. Ye, H., Gu, T., Tao, X., Lu, J.: Scalable floor localization using barometer on smartphone. Wirel. Commun. Mob. Comput. **16**(16), 2557–2571 (2016)

Evaluation of Power-Based Stair Climb Performance via Inertial Measurement Units

Sandra Hellmers[1]([✉]), Sandra Lau[1], Rebecca Diekmann[1], Lena Dasenbrock[1,2], Tobias Kromke[1], Jürgen M. Bauer[3], Sebastian Fudickar[1], and Andreas Hein[1]

[1] Carl von Ossietzky University Oldenburg, Oldenburg, Germany
{sandra.hellmers,sandra.lau,rebecca.diekmann,lena.dasenbrock,
tobias.kromke,sebastian.fudickar,andreas.hein}@uni-oldenburg.de
[2] Peter L. Reichertz Institute for Medical Informatics, Hannover, Germany
lena.dasenbrock@plri.de
[3] Heidelberg University, Agaplesion Bethanien Krankenhaus Heidelberg,
Heidelberg, Germany
juergen.bauer@bethanien-heidelberg.de

Abstract. The stair climbing test (SCT) is a standard geriatric assessment to measure lower-limb strength being one of the essential components of physical function. To detect functional decline as early as possible, regular assessments of mobility, balance, and strength are necessary. Inertial measurement units (IMU) are a promising technology for flexible and unobtrusive measurements of the SCTs. We introduce an automated assessment via IMUs in a study of 83 participants aged 70–87 ($75.64 \pm 4,17$) years. The activity of stair ascending has been automatically classified via a k-nearest-neighbor classifier and the performance was evaluated regarding the power. Therefore, we considered both, stair climb average power and peak power. Stair ascending was correctly classified in 93% of the cases with a mean deviation of 2.35% of the average power value in comparison to conventional measurements. Additionally, we showed the medical sensitivity of our system regarding the detection of transitions towards the frail status in controlled conditions and also confirmed the general suitability of automated stair climb analyses in unsupervised home-assessments.

Keywords: Stair climb power ·
Inertial Measurement Unit (IMU) · Power ·
Peak power · Stair ascending · Machine learning · Clinical assessment ·
Unsupervised · Wearable sensors · Stair climbing · kNN

1 Introduction

Functional ability is important for an independent life. But with age functional decline can occur. The functional decline can be slowed down through timely

---

S. Fudickar, A. Hein—Contributed equally.

preventive interventions [1]. For this purpose, an early detection of functional changes is crucial. Usually, the functional status is evaluated via geriatric assessments, covering "strength", "mobility" and "balance" as essential parameters for the physical function [2].

Figure 1 shows an assumed qualitative progress of the functional ability throughout the lifespan. Even a high and continuous status of functional ability can suddenly decline when different health problems appear. According to [3] a minor stressor event such as an infection or a new medication often causes a larger deterioration of function in frail older persons without recovering back to baseline homeostasis; therefore the physical function may decrease (Δa).

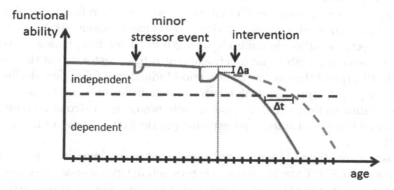

Fig. 1. Qualitative progress of functional ability over time and the progress of ability after a minor stressor event according to [3]. Regularly performed assessments (lines on the horizontal axis) enable the possibility to detect early changes in the ability Δa to start interventions and slow the functional decline and extend the time Δt of independent living. This Figure is an extended version of Fig. 1 in [4]. (Color figure online)

A regular assessment (e.g. monthly) would enable an early detection of functional decline and the initiation of interventions when they are necessary. It is important to detect performance changes Δa as soon as possible because interventions can then be started at an early stage. Since interventions can slow the functional decline (green line in Fig. 1), the time Δt of independent living can be extended. But guided assessments require a lot of effort by health professionals (and hold a significant financial burden to healthcare systems). Thus, they can only be conducted on an occasional basis.

A promising approach to overcome conventional time-intensive and high-effort supervised assessments are technology-supported unsupervised and self-guided home-assessments, where the evaluation takes place during daily life activities. Frenken et al. [5] pointed out that there is a clear need for technical support for implementing unsupervised mobility assessments in home environments in order to objectively measure capacity and performance of patients.

Among balance and mobility, strength is one of the essential components for physical function. A decline in muscle strength and muscle power is a sign for sarcopenia, whereby sarcopenia is defined as the age-related loss of muscle mass, muscle strength and muscle function [6]. Therefore, muscle function has a special importance for screening and diagnosing of sarcopenia [6].

Bean et al. have shown that the muscular strength correlates with the determined stair climb power in the stair climb power test (SCPT) [7] and timed stair tests are considered as an objective measure of functional abilities [8]. Especially the SCPT and the sit-to-stand (STS) test require little technique and physical efforts. Therefore, they can be easily performed and are often possible even with a beginning functional decline. Additionally, the SCPT is suitable for home-assessments, as long as older persons are able to climb stairs in their daily living. Whereby, wearable technologies offer a good approach for unobtrusive and flexible measurements.

It makes sense to focus on the muscle power, which reflects the ability to perform muscular work per unit of time, in (home-)assessments because muscle power declines earlier than muscle strength [9]. Therefore, muscle power can explain variance in mobility and functional status to a greater extent than muscle strength [10,11] and thus, seems to be a good indicator of functional decline [12]. Among the power, especially peak power is a significant measure for power analyses. According to Foldvari et al. peak muscle power has a strong correlation to self-reported functional status and explains physical function as an independent factor [11].

Thus, we investigate an automated assessment of the (muscular) power based on the common SCPT via 3D-accelerometers and 3D gyroscopes - so-called inertial measurement units (IMUs)- integrated into belts. For an automated evaluation of the stair climbing performance two steps are necessary:

1. Classification of phases of stair climbing,
2. Calculation of the stair climb (peak) power.

The rest of the paper is structured as follows: We discuss related work in Sect. 2 and the biomechanics of stair climbing in Sect. 3. The study design is classified in Sect. 4. Section 5 provides insights into the signal interpretation of acceleration data for the activity of stair climbing. The method for the detection of stair climbing is presented in Sect. 6 and the method for (peak) power calculation in Sect. 7. The results and the evaluation are described in Sect. 8 and we discuss the suitability for home-assessments in Sect. 9. Finally, we discuss our findings in Sect. 10 and describe our conclusions and future work in Sect. 11.

2   State of the Art

2.1   Classification of Stair Climbing - Machine Learning

Regarding the suitability to classify climbing stairs, various combinations and placements of IMU-sensors have been shown to be practical. Table 1 shows a selection of studies and the applied sensors and positioning as well as the study size and the age of the participants. It is to mention that these studies do not only concentrate on ascending or descending stairs but on the general recognition of several activities such as walking, sitting, standing, lying, running or cycling.

The first four examples show the influence of the sensor placements on the accuracy: Zheng et al. [13] applied three IMUs positioned at one thigh, shank and foot and pressure sensors at the feet to achieve an accuracy of 99.03% with a linear discriminant analysis (LDA) classifier. Khan et al. [14] used one accelerometer at the chest and artificial neural nets (ANNs) as well as autoregressive (AR) modeling to get an accuracy of 99.0% in stair climbing recognition. Fida et al. [15] achieved an accuracy of 97.2% with a Support Vector Machine (SVM) as classifier and a 3D accelerometer and gyroscope attached to the shank of the dominant leg.

Table 1. Studies investigating classification of stair climbing via machine learning. The type of applied sensors (accelerometer (acc.), gyroscope (gyro.), magnetometer (magn), barometer (baro) and sensor positioning, as well as the sample size and the age of the study population are listed. The classification method with the best accuracy is written in bold. The abbreviations of the methods are: Linear Discriminant Analysis (LDA), Artificial Neural Networks (ANN), Autoregressive (AR) Modeling, Decision Trees (DT), Bayesian Networks (BN), Naive Bayes (NB), Support Vector Machine (SVM), Multiclass-(Hardware Friendly)-SVM (MC-(HF-)SVM), K Nearest Neighbor (kNN), Rule-Based Classifiers (RBC), Logistic Regression (LR), Static Classifier (SC), Hidden Markov Model (HMM). This Table was already presented in [4].

Accuracy	Sensor	Position	Classification method	Size	Age (±SD)	Reference
99.03%	3D acc & gyro & magn; pressure	thigh, foot, shank	**LDA**	5	24.8(±1.3)	[13]
99.0%	3D acc	chest	**ANN, AR**	6	27 (mean)	[14]
97.2%	3D acc & gyro	shank	**SVM**	9	29(±5)	[15]
>95.0 %	3D acc & gyro	waist	SVM, **kNN**, RBC, LR, DT, BN, NB,	10	25–30	[16]
93.8 %	3D acc	waist	**SVM**	7	25–46	[17]
93.2 %	3D acc & gyro	waist	DT, NB, **kNN**, SVM	N/A	N/A	[18]
87.2 %	3D acc	waist	**MC-SVM**, MC-HF-SVM	30	19–48	[19]
84.6 %	acc, baro, ...	waist	**SC**, HMM	12	20–30	[20]

In the other studies mentioned in Table 1, the sensor was positioned at the waist. These studies show a lower precision, but the placement at the waist is less obtrusively and more suitable for unsupervised attachments by the participants.

Shoaib et al. [16] applied an IMU and achieved an accuracy of >95% with a K-Nearest Neighbor (kNN) classifier and Fareed [18] achieved 93.8% with a similar setting. A Support Vector Machine (SVM) as classification method was applied by Sun et al. [17] and the accuracy was 93.8 %. The selection shows that the used classification method also varies within different studies. It has been shown, that the type of classifier affects the accuracies, but the accuracies also vary within one method due to the influences of different data sets and their complexity. Besides the sensor placement and the applied classifier, the derived features and the specifications of the sliding window are important parameters. Therefore, we investigate and describe these parameters in Sect. 6.

It should be pointed out that the mentioned studies have been conducted with rather young participants, which clearly do not represent the intended primary user group to benefit from such systems. Thus, only a small variety of stair climbing patterns might be covered in the discussed works. For this reason, research for recognition of stair ascending in larger studies and especially for older adults is important because their movements can deviate from movements of younger adults. For example, Stacoff et al. [21] found in their study that younger participants walked faster and produced larger vertical ground reaction force (GRF) maxima during level walking and on stair climb than the older age group. Considering this point, we carried out a larger study, which design is described in Sect. 4.

2.2 Power Calculation

An investigation of the suitability of IMU-based power estimations for SCPT has not been conducted yet. Among the conventional calculation of power, mainly two approaches are prominent, which we will discuss in the following.

Average Power. According to Bean et al. [22], power is a physiological attribute related to strength and reflects the ability to perform muscular work per unit of time. Power P can be calculated by the following equation [4]

$$P = Fv = mgv = mg\frac{h}{t} \qquad \left[\frac{kg \cdot m^2}{s^3} = W \right], \tag{1}$$

where F is the force, v the velocity, m the participant's weight, g the gravity, h the covered height and t the test duration. Compared to different other muscle strength and power calculations that focus on single muscle activities, this equation is used for an average power based on IMU data.

Usually, the time for the SCPT is measured by medical professionals via stopwatches. Regarding Eq. 1, the parameters "stair climbing duration" and "covered height" must be determined in the detected phases of stair ascending.

Peak Power. Since Eq. 1 calculates an average power value over the total stair climbing activity, our hypothesis is that the peak power might be a more sensitive parameter for functional decline. In addition, determining the peak power instead of the average power does not require the knowledge of the exact height of the flight of stairs, which might be unknown especially in unsupervised settings. Thus, it supports a more flexible applicability of the system. According to the method of peak power determination for chair risings of [23] the peak power can be calculated by

$$P_{max} = max(P(t)) = max(m \cdot a(t) \cdot v(t)), \tag{2}$$

where a is the acceleration in relation to time t. To take all three dimensions of the movement into account the normalized acceleration is used:

$$a_{norm}(t) = \sqrt{a_{vertical}(t)^2 + a_{ML}(t)^2 + a_{AP}(t)^2}. \tag{3}$$

$a_{vert}(t)$ describes the acceleration in vertical direction (lift), $a_{AP}(t)$ the forward movement in anterior-posterior direction and $a_{ML}(t)$ movements in the mediolateral direction. The velocity can be estimated by a numerical integration of the acceleration:

$$v(t) = v(t - 1) + a(t)/f, \qquad (4)$$

where f is the sampling rate of the sensor unit and the initial speed is $v(t_0) = 0$, since the test starts from a rest position (still standing).

Literature which includes IMU based peak power analysis couldn't be found and seems to be a new topic in the research field. In other studies, peak power analysis were done by pneumatic resistance machines [11] or isokinetic dynamometers [24].

3   Biomechanics of Stair Climbing

Ascending a flight of stairs requires more strength and joint mobility than walking on level ground because the stance limb must lift the body mass in addition to preserve weight-bearing stability, while the swing limb flexes to advance from the stair below to the stair above the stance limb [25]. According to walking gait cycles, the motion of ascending stairs can be also described by different phases. The gait cycle for ascent stair climbing is divided into a stance phase and a swing phase. Whereby, a significantly longer mean cycle duration and a shorter proportion of time in stance was obtained for stair climbing as compared to level walking [33]. The stance phase includes three sub-phases. After the Initial Contact (IC) starting with a footstep on the first step the first sub-phase Weight Acceptance (WA) occurs. In this phase, the body is shifted into an optimal position to start the Pull-Up (PU) phase following a Forward Continuance (FCo) with a full extended stance leg on the step. The cycle ends with a swing phase where the former stance leg now leaves the step to start a new cycle of stair climbing. These last two phases are described as Foot Clearance (FC) and Foot Placement (FP) [26]. Comparing stance leg and swing leg there is a difference in the transition of stance to swing and vice versa. For the stance leg ends the stance phase through FCo before starting the swing phase with FC and FP. For the swing leg ends the swing phase with an extra phase - Push-off (PS) - where the swing leg is pushed off the below step before starting FC and FP. Figure 2 shows double and single support phases of the swing leg and the stance leg during stair ascending.

Regarding the range of motion, the IC occurs with the forefoot and a hip flexion of 50°–60° and a knee flexion of 50°–70°. Then the hip and knee extend throughout PU and FC. A minimum flexion of the hip (10°–15°) and knee (5°–15°) is reached at the end of WA until prior toe-off starts the PU. Ankle joint movement varies among 5–15° dorsiflexion and 10°–20° plantarflexion in all phases. 10° to 20° additional range of motion in each lower limb joint is needed in stair climbing compared to walking [25, 26].

Besides the ability of joint movement, stair negotiating requires a sufficient trunk stability and lower limb muscle activity. Accordingly, ascending a flight of stairs also depends on the power of concentric contractions to lift a body's mass forward and upward against gravity. Therefore, muscle power is more relevant in stair climbing than in walking. Extensor muscles provide stability during stance and flexor muscles provide initially rapid movement during swing. In the context of agonist and antagonist muscle activity, major extensor and flexor muscles can affect both joints, hip and knee. Extensor muscles can extend the knee and flex the hip at the same time while flexor muscles can flex the knee and extend the hip. Muscle power may vary between individuals according to health restrictions e.g. knee osteoarthritis. Important muscles for WA are M. gluteus maximus and medius, M. adductor magnus and M. quadriceps. For PU, Hamstrings, M. gastrocnemius and M. soleus show the highest activity. The swing phase initially starts with a decreasing power of M. gastrocnemius and M. soleus and more re-activity in hamstrings and M. tibialis anterior in preparation of the next step [25,27].

Compared to ground level walking differences in a stair climbing sequence between the first two steps and the last steps can be seen. This phenomenon exists due to the biomechanical deviation in both gait cycles. A walking sequence (gait cycle) starts with an extended knee and almost constant stance and swing phases in an upright position. Alternating stair climbing starts with knee flexion combined with weight lift and a slightly flexed torso. At the end of the first step, the contralateral leg initially starts with a swing phase over the first step ahead to the second step. After the second step the stair gait cycle shows consistency and steady power until the body posture prepares to continue for level walking with an decreasing peak power on the last steps.

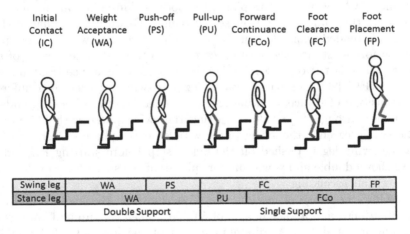

Fig. 2. Double and single support phases of the swing leg (Weight Acceptance (WA), Push-off (PS), Foot Clearance (FC) and Foot Placement (FP)) and the stance leg (Weight Acceptance (WA), Pull-Up (PU) and Forward Continuance (FCo)) during stair ascending.

4 Study Design

In order to develop an inertial-based system to measure the stair-climb power test and to evaluate its sensitivity and specificity, we conducted the following laboratory study. IMUs integrated into belts were used due to their easy applicability, flexibility and suitability for measuring daily life activities. In this study, the SCPT was measured conventional via manual stopwatch measurements (assumed as gold standard) and IMU-based sensor belt recordings. Overall, 83 participants aged 70–87 years (75.64 ± 4.17 years) performed the SCPT twice.

Initially, the examiner stands with each participant at the base of the flight of stairs with eleven steps. The participants were instructed to safely climb the stair as fast as they could and to stop on the 10th step. In accordance with the proceedings introduced by [7], participants were allowed to use the handrail if necessary. Figure 3 shows the used stairway with eleven steps. The white footprints mark the start positions, whereby the participants can choose their preferred side. The first white line is for safety issues and the reduction of the risk of stumbling. The participants should stop on the step before the second white line because the SCPT is usually performed on 10 steps. The yellow dashed lines mark the position of the light barriers. It is to mention that the light barriers measure if the participants cross the lines. Therefore, the measured time is not equal to typical stopwatch measurements, because timing begins on the signal to start and terminates when the participant returns with both feet to the ground level on the 10th step.

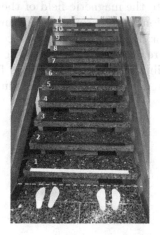

Fig. 3. The flight of stairs used in the study: The participants start at the white footprints and should stop before the second white line at the 10th step. The yellow dashed lines mark the position of the light barriers. The first white line is for safety issues. (Color figure online)

Besides the SCPT, other geriatric tests such as the Short Physical Performance Battery (SPPB), Frailty Criteria, de Morton Mobility Index (DEMMI), 6 min Walk Test (6MWT), and Counter Movement Jumps (CMJ) were performed. After these assessments, the participants wore the sensor belts continuously for one week in their daily life and wrote an activity diary. The study and the utilized technologies for each assessment item were summarized in [28].

Besides the stair climb recognition and average power calculation, we also analyzed the data of a randomly selected subgroup of 40 participants for peak power evaluations. Table 2 lists the characteristics of this group.

Table 2. Characteristics of the subgroup for peak power evaluations.

	Mean	SD	Min	Max
Age	75.8	3.48	70	86
Height	167.96	8.22	153.2	184.7
Weight	79.04	16.37	52.25	123.4

Sensor Belt

The sensor system integrated into the belt includes four sensors: A Bosch BMA180 triaxial accelerometer, which measures the acceleration force in $g \approx 9.81\,\mathrm{ms}^{-2}$ applied to the device on all three physical axes. The accelerometer has the following parameters: Sensitivity ranges from 1G up to 16G and the chip supports sampling rates up to 1200 Hz. The STMicroelectronics L3GD20H gyroscope measures the device's rate of rotation in $deg \cdot s^{-2}$ around each of the three physical axes. A magnetometer measures the ambient geomagnetic field for all three physical axes in μT. This sensor can be used for sensor orientation determinations in relation to the magnetic field of the earth or for indoor navigation purposes [29]. Additionally, a barometer measures the air pressure in hPa and can be used for (outdoor) height estimations, since the atmospheric pressure decreases when altitude increases [30]. The coordinate orientation of the sensors is shown in Fig. 4. A sampling rate of 100 Hz is used for all four sensors in this study, since the parameter settings have a significant influence on the recognition accuracies [31].

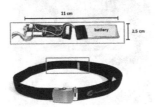

Fig. 4. The sensor belt includes a 3D accelerometer, gyroscope and magnetometer, as well as a barometer. The sampling rates of the sensors are 100 Hz.

5 Signal Interpretation

Figure 5 shows the acceleration data in vertical (top), anterior-posterior AP (middle) and mediolateral ML direction (bottom) during a stride (left and right step). Three strides of the same subject and same walk are illustrated in the diagram. The first and last stride of the eleven steps high stairs of flight were not included due to their diverging process since preparation for stair ascending at the start and preparation for on ground level walking at the end influence the signal pattern (see Sect. 3). Between the three strides, similar patterns with minor intra-personal variability can be observed. The correlation coefficient for the acceleration in vertical direction is $r_{vertical} > 0.92$ and in anterior-posterior direction $r = {}_{AP} > 0.95$. The variability in mediolateral direction is higher. Differences between left and right or rather dominant and non-dominant leg are recognizable by the slight deviations in acceleration between the steps and the step duration.

Analogous to Sect. 3 we identified the different phases of a stride and marked them in Fig. 5. The initial contact (IC) is characterized by a minimum in AP acceleration. Followed by weight acceptance (WA) with a peak in vertical acceleration. Next, the phase of push-off (PS) starts and ends at the inflection point of vertical acceleration. At this point the double support changes in a single support. The phase of pull-up (PU) ends with a minimum in vertical acceleration. After that, the phase of foot clearance (FC) starts. The last phase is the foot placement (FP), which is hard to identify within the signal.

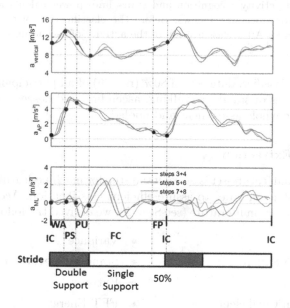

Fig. 5. Acceleration in vertical, anterior-posterior (AP) and mediolateral (ML) direction during the activity of stair ascending.

6 Stair Climb Detection

Figure 6 shows the general processing work-flow of activity recognition via the applied machine learning approach and stair-climb power calculation. The data collection during the different geriatric tests within the assessment (see Sect. 4), is followed by pre-processing and feature extraction for the classification of the activities. The stair climb power is calculated for the time spans, classified as stair ascending.

In order to describe our algorithm, we focus on the extracted features, the sliding window and the used classifiers in the following sections.

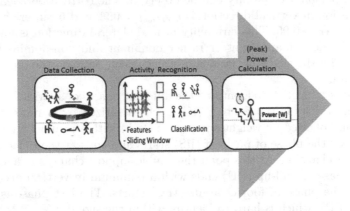

Fig. 6. Process of activity recognition and stair-climb power calculation. After data collection, data pre-processing follows. Before the classification of activities, feature sets must be selected. After classification of the activity of ascending stairs, the power can be calculated.

To train the classifier, data sets of 80% (n = 66) of all participants are considered. The activities of standing, walking, ascending and descending stairs were selected from the whole assessment and pooled.

6.1   Feature Extraction

Deriving a minimal feature-set is an essential step for machine-learning based classification algorithms in order to assure efficient classification. According to frequently used features in literature (see Sect. 2), we derived the following features:

- Mean
- Root Mean Square
- Median
- Correlation Coefficient

- Variance
- Standard Deviation
- Entropy
- FFT Energy

These eight features are considered per axis of accelerometer and gyroscope, resulting in an overall set of 48 features. The data of the magnetometer was excluded due to its high influence to environmental noise. Including the magnetometer data would result in an over-fit for this specific stairway. Figure 7 shows, as an example, the standard deviation (SD) in comparison to the root mean square (RMS) in AP-direction of the activities ascending and descending stairs, walking and standing.

As expected, the SD for a static activity is quite small and therefore, a good feature to detect static activities. The values for the dynamic activities show a high overlap in SD and RMS. Therefore, these features are not alone sufficient to distinguish between the activities. However, there is only a relatively low scattering of the walking activity, whereas the values for ascending and descending stairs scatter significantly broader.

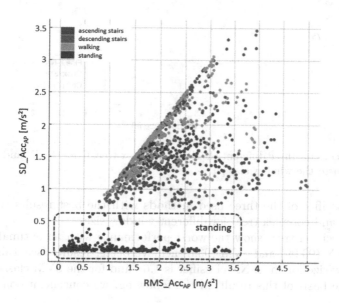

Fig. 7. Scatterplot of Standard Deviation (SD) and Root Mean Square (RMS) of the accelerometer data in AP-direction (straight forward). The SD seems to be a good feature to detect static activities. This Figure was already presented in [4].

6.2 Sliding Window and Classifier

Besides the features, the sliding window parameters and the used classifier are also crucial factors. Since Shoaib et al. [16] have shown that an overlap of 50% of the sliding windows produces reasonable results, we considered a sliding window approach with a 50% overlap.

In accordance with the related work, we used the following classifiers, due to their high sensitivity. All of them are available in Mathworks' MATLAB (version R2015a):

- Decision tree (complex, medium, simple),
- Support vector machine (linear, quadratic, cubic, fine Gaussian, medium Gaussian, coarse Gaussian),
- K-Nearest-Neighbor (fine, medium, coarse, cosine, cubic, weighted).

The F1-Score was used for the evaluation to consider both, precision and recall. Figure 8 shows the F1-Scores for the recognition of the activity "ascending stairs"

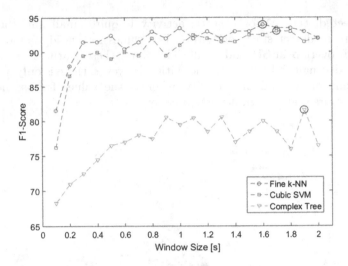

Fig. 8. F1-Score for three different classifiers complex tree, Cubic SVW and Fine k-NN in correlation to the window size [4].

for each classifier of the three used methods with the best results (fine k-NN, cubic SVM and complex tree) for different window sizes.

While decision trees show the worst performance with an optimal F1-Score of 81.5, k-NN (93.99) and SVM (93.0) achieve better results (see Table 3). The best window size for the k-NN classifier is 1.6 s and for the SVM classifier about 1.7 s. At the basis of this result, in the following, we concentrate on the k-NN classifier.

Table 3. Best results of F1-Scores by optimized window sizes and an overlap of 50% of the sliding windows for the three used classifiers. This Table was already presented in [4].

Classifier	Window size [s]	F1 score
Decision Tree	1.9	81.50
SVM	1.7	93.00
k-NN	1.6	93.99

6.3 Post-Filtering of Classified Activities

To remove incorrectly detected stair climbing activities, a minimum duration of 3 s for this activity was defined in a post-filtering step. Shorter phases of ascending stairs were ignored. This threshold value is based on stopwatch measurements over all participants, who generally took over 3 s. The majority of SCPT-studies use a stairway of 10 to 12 stairs for testing, which is likely to be the average staircase length available in buildings and therefore a practical length for testing [8]. But in those studies, which are looking at medical conditions involving the heart and lungs, longer stairways are used to elicit a more cardiovascular response. Therefore, stair ascending activities with fewer stairs than 10 are less meaningful for the SCPT.

7   Calculation of Stair Climb Power

7.1   Average Power

In order to calculate the power in accordance with Eq. 1, the covered height and the duration for the SCPT are measured. While the duration is determined by the sequence of the recognized activity, the height was evaluated by counting the steps within this sequence of ascending stairs. As an example, Fig. 9 shows the acceleration of a sequence of climbing 10 steps. The activity of climbing stairs or other rhythmic activities usually show repetitive patterns. In cases of walking or ascending stairs, the impact of the foot on the floor causes a peak in acceleration data. These peaks were counted and assumed as steps. On the basis of the step number n the covered height h can be calculated by $h = n * 16.5$, where 16.5 is the height of one step in cm. In most European countries the height of steps is standardized by building regulations. Barometers can also be used for elevation measurements. But due to the low accuracy of the barometer in our study (± 10 cm), we decided to use the peak detection algorithm based on the acceleration data for height estimations.

The participant's weight was measured via a stadiometer (seca 285) and the gravity is assumed to be $g = 9.81\,\mathrm{ms^{-2}}$.

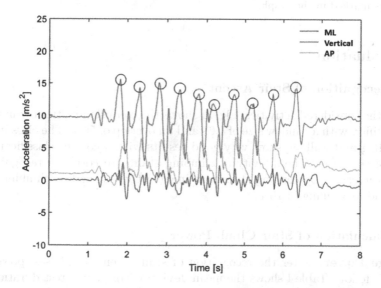

Fig. 9. Acceleration in vertical, anterior-posterior(AP) and mediolateral (ML) direction during a phase of ascending stairs in a laboratory setting. The single steps can be recognized by characteristic peaks. This Figure was already presented in [4].

7.2   Peak Power

The peak power is calculated by multiplying the normalized acceleration, the weight of the participant and the velocity (cf. Eq. 2). Figure 10 shows the acceleration, velocity, and power over one stride (third and fourth step). The peak power is defined as the maximum power value within one step and is marked in the Figure. The point of maximum power lies typically behind the maximum in acceleration and in the phase of the push-off within the gait cycle (cf. Figure 5 in Sect. 5). It can also be seen that the dominant leg reaches higher peak values than the non-dominant leg.

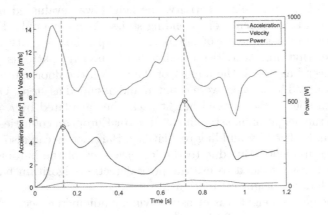

Fig. 10. Normalized acceleration, velocity and power over one stride. The peak-power values are marked in the graph.

8   Evaluation

8.1   Recognition of Stair Ascent

Among the considered activities, Fig. 11 shows the confusion matrix of our fine k-NN classifier, with a window size of 1.6 s and an overlap of 50%. The classification of standing and walking show very good results with a correct classification in >98% of the cases. The activity of climbing stairs are correctly recognized in 93% of the cases. Descending stairs was incorrectly assigned as climbing stairs in 6% and as walking in 10%.

8.2   Calculation of Stair Climb Power

Average Power. After the recognition of stair ascending phases, power calculations follow. Table 4 shows the mean deviations of power, test duration and covered height of the sensor-based measurements with the already presented k-NN classifier to stop watch measurements. The weight and the gravity values are same in both calculations and therefore not further considered. While the k-NN classifier achieves quite good power values with a mean deviation of 2.35 %

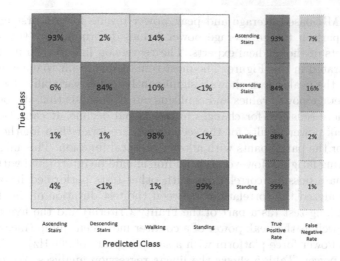

Fig. 11. Confusion matrix of activity recognition with a kNN classifier [4].

Table 4. Mean deviations of sensor-based power measurements to stopwatch measurements [4].

	Mean deviation [%]	Median [%]
Power	2.35	4.71
Duration	14.49	6.46
Height	15.00	15.00

to the gold standard, the deviation of the estimated height and durations are with respectively ≤15% very high. As already described in Sect. 4 the duration of climbing ten stairs will be measured by the stop watch in the SCPT and is assumed as gold standard. But the technically detected number of stairs is not exactly 10 in all cases. In our assessments, the number of passed steps varied among users between 10 and 11 stair due to the following reasons: The setting consists of an 11 step stair flight, but some participants forget to stop at the 10th step, as instructed. In addition, a step might be not recognized due to the transition from standing to climbing stairs. However, this isn't a problem due to the fact that according to Eq. 1 the ratio of height and duration influences the power ($v = h/t$). Thus, the difference in the power of the gold standard measurement (ten stairs) is small, due to the low effect on the participants' fatigue or the fluency of the test sequence (acceleration and deceleration) of climbing one additional or less stair. But of course, the accurate detection of the beginning and end of the activity is a major task and needs further investigations.

Peak Power. We calculated the peak power for a randomly selected subgroup of 40 participants. The characteristics of this group are listed in Table 2. Figure 12 shows the IMU-based average and peak power results for the first and second run in comparison to the average power values determined by the stopwatch measurements of the medical experts. The regression line of each measurement is also illustrated in this Figure. The most remarkable result to emerge from the data is that the peak power shows a significantly higher variability (see Table 5) than the average power values and confirms our hypothesis that the peak power might be more sensitive for changes in functional decline. It can also be seen, that the peak power results for the second run are lower than for the first run, especially for the participants with a lower physical function. This might be due to an occurring fatigue. However, this finding should be interpreted with caution.

To evaluate possible correlations with other tests performed in our assessment, we analyzed the correlations between the test duration of the TUG test, a 4.57 m walking test (as a part of the Frailty Criteria) and the five time chair rise test, as well as the peak power of a counter movement jump (measured by a AMTI AccuPower force platform with a sampling rate of 200 Hz) with the stair climb peak power. Table 5 shows the linear regression analyses. We could only find a significant relation between stair climb peak power and stair climb average power.

Table 5. Results of the regression analysis: Stair Climb Peak Power versus TUG, walking and chair-rise test duration as well as jump peak power. Significant results are marked by an asterisk.

	Estimate	Std.	Error	t
Tug test duration	−80.40	63.73	1.29	0.21
Walking test duration	117.12	161.45	0.725	0.47
Chair rise test duration	−13.84	0.21	−0.43	0.67
Jump peak power	−0.09	0.21	−0.43	0.67
Stair climb average power	3.82	1.7	2.254	0.03*

Additionally, we made regression analyses for the average stair climbing power and the other considered tests and could find a significant relationship between stair climbing average power and jump power (Table 6).

Table 6. Results of the regression analysis: Stair Climb Average Power versus TUG, walking and chair-rise test duration as well as jump peak power. Significant results are marked by an asterisk.

	Estimate	Std.	Error	t
Tug test duration	−2.28	6.93	−0.329	0.74
Walking test duration	9.70	17.15	0.566	0.57
Chair rise test duration	−1.17	2.83	−0.414	0.68
Jump peak power	0.06212	0.018	3.401	<0.005**
Stair climb peak power	0.04278	0.018	2.254	0.03*

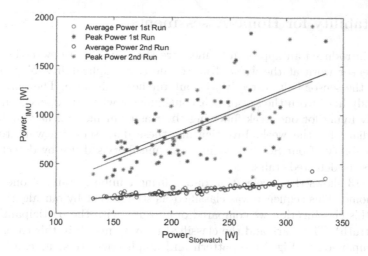

Fig. 12. Peak and average power during the Stair Climb Power Test. The x-axis shows the values calculated by the measured time by stopwatch and the y-axis the power values based on IMU measurements.

8.3   Medical Sensitivity

In order to clarify the medical sensitivity of our system, we compared its error to the medically required sensitivity to detect the transition to functional decline (as covered by the frailty status). Table 7 summarizes the power values of our participants at baseline (t0) and after 6 month (t1). They were categorized in groups of frail and non-frail according to the Frailty Criteria of Fried et al. [32].

The mean deviation in power between these groups is about 14% and therefore, significantly higher than our system's deviation from the gold standard measurements of about 2%. Thus, we conclude that our system's sensitivity is sufficient for detection of transitions towards the frail status under controlled conditions. Regarding the mean deviation in peak power, we observed a difference of 3.5%, which is also higher than the system's sensitivity (right side of Table 7).

Table 7. Stair climb average power (P) of participants in our study at baseline (t0) and after 6 month (t1) and stair climb peak power (PP) of our subgroup categorized in groups of frail and non-frail according to the classification of the Frailty Criteria of Fried et al. [32].

	Average power			Peak power	
	Subjects	P_{t0} [W]	P_{t1} [W]	Number	PP_{t0} [W]
Non-frail	56	2302	2298.0	28	878.03
Frail	27	1979.5	1968.1	12	847,72
Δ		322.5 (14.0%)	329.9 (14.0%)		30.32 (3.5%)

9   Suitability for Home-Assessments

We have introduced an approach to measure the stair climb power via a single inertial sensor worn at the waist. Due to the easy applicability, older persons can wear the sensor belt correctly without further assistance. The participants of our study have worn the sensor belt continuously without supervision during their daily living for one week following their assessments and have written an activity diary for the week. Investigating these data sets, we want to study the applicability of our SCPT system to an unsupervised use by detecting the correctness of detected stairs.

Figure 13 shows the acceleration data during climbing stairs of one participant at home. This sequence was classified as stair ascent by our algorithm. To validate this classification we compared our results with the participant's diary (ground truth). The diary and the classified activity match in this case.

In comparison to Fig. 9 the pattern and amplitudes are significantly different from the acceleration data measured during the assessment (test situation) although it shows the activity of the same participant. Thus, we could confirm, that phases of climbing stairs could also be recognized during these home-assessments.

Furthermore, to clarify the degree of variations in stair-climbing patterns for different environments by investigating it in the participant's daily life. Therefore, the one-week measurements of the sensors will be analyzed concerning the frequency, the covered steps and the estimated stair climb power of the activity stair climbing.

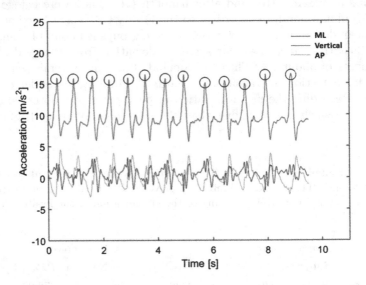

Fig. 13. Acceleration in vertical anterior-posterior and mediolateral direction during a phase of climbing stairs in daily life. This Figure was already presented in [4].

Table 8. Comparison of power results for stair climbing in an assessment and in daily life.

	Average power	Peak power
Assessment	228.7	797.1
Daily life	129.2	511.2
Differences	99.5 (43%)	285.9 (36%)

To analyze the medical significance of unsupervised power measurements at home, we compare exemplarily the average and peak power results of stair climbing in the laboratory setting with results at home. The power calculations are listed in Table 8. As expected, the applied power at home is significantly lower than in a test situation. Due to the unknown step height of the stairs at the home of the participant, the average power value at home should be interpreted with caution, because it was assumed to be the same height as in our laboratory setting. The differences of peak power in laboratory and daily-life environments are slightly lower than for the average power. This could be an indicator, that peak power is a more suitable parameter for comparing supervised and unsupervised performances of stair ascending. However, further investigations are necessary. Besides this point, the influence of diverging conditions such as step number or the absence of a test situation will be examined in a next step. For further validation of our stair climbing detection in domestic environments, it is planned to install ambient sensors at the stairways in the homes of a subgroup of our participants.

10   Discussion

The main purpose of the present study was to develop an automated assessment of the SCPT based on inertial measurement units (IMU), which automatically classifies the activity of climbing stairs via machine learning and evaluates the performance on the basis of power analyses of the lower extremities. Therefore, we conducted a prospective study with 80 participants aged 70 and above and used the data to identify a suitable classifier. The evaluation of the automatically calculated average and peak power was done for a subgroup of 40 participants. The activity of ascending stairs has been correctly classified in 93% of the cases. In comparison to other studies, these results are satisfactory, especially regarding the so far rarely considered study population of older adults, whose movement patterns are more complicated to differentiate. For average power calculations, we achieved good results in comparison to conventional measurements with a mean deviation of 2.35%. This underlines the suitability of our system to analyze stair climb power in laboratory settings. Additionally, we introduced the peak power, which might be more sensitive for changes in the physical function. The system's sensitivity to detect the transition towards frailty has been confirmed, since the system's deviation is significantly higher than the mean deviation in power between the group of frail and non-frail subjects.

The peak power has a high variability and is not more sensitive for detection of frail and non-frail states (based on the Frailty Criteria) than average power. Further analyses are required to find evidence of the hypothesis that the peak power is more sensitive to changes in the physical function.

The evaluation of the automatically calculated average and peak power shows a significant linear correlation. In addition, a higher variability of the peak power values was found. This confirms our hypothesis that the peak power might be more sensitive to changes in functional decline. Linear regression analyses with other geriatric tests (TUG, chair rise, walking, and jump test) could reveal the expected qualitative relationship between these tests, but no significant correlation was found (Table 5). This apparent lack of correlation is attributed to the differences between the dynamic movement processes and the used muscles. Furthermore, the other tests, except the jump, assess also an overall performance and not a peak performance. These findings are consistent with the regression analysis of the average peak power, which shows also only a significant correlation with the jump power and not with the other tests.

Additionally, we showed the general suitability of sensor belt measurements at home and confirmed, that phases of climbing stairs could be also recognized during home-assessments. Whereby the movement patterns differ from the pattern in the laboratory setting. The comparison of the performed power confirmed the expected result that participants climb stairs with a lower power in non-test situations. Further analyses are necessary to find a possibly existing correlation between (peak) power in laboratory settings and in daily life.

In summary, our system is applicable for a flexible measurement of stair climbing performance in laboratory settings as well as in home-assessments. The average power calculations achieved good results in comparison to calculations on stopwatch measurements by medical experts. Peak power might be a worthwhile enhancement of power analyses but needs further investigations.

11   Conclusion

Stair climbing tests are well-suited to measure the strength of the lower limbs. Due to the less requirement of technique and physical demands, the SCT is also applicable for unsupervised home-assessments. IMUs are a promising technology for flexible and unobtrusive measurements of the physical function within SCTs.

In this paper, we have presented a system for automated assessment of the SCPT based on inertial measurement units (IMU), which automatically classifies the activity of climbing stairs via machine learning and evaluates the performance on the basis of power analyses of the lower extremities. The findings of our conducted study with 83 participants (aged 70–87 years) confirmed the suitability of our system for the correct classification of the activity of stair ascending in 93% of the cases and correct average power measurements in laboratory settings (with a mean deviation of 2.35% in comparison to conventional measurements).

We also showed the general suitability for home-assessments. Additionally, we found a significant correlation between the average power and the introduced peak power, whereby the peak power measure shows a higher variability than average power. But, further investigations regarding the medical significance and especially for the possible higher sensitivity of peak power for changes in the functional status are necessary. In conclusion, a promising system for flexible and automated stair climb performance evaluations was presented and confirmed in an initial evaluation study.

Acknowledgements. The study is funded by the German Federal Ministry of Education and Research (Project No. 01EL1422D). The study has been approved by the appropriate ethics committee (ethical vote: Hannover Medical School No. 6948) and conducted in accordance with the Declaration of Helsinki.

References

1. Gill, T.M., Baker, D.I., Gottschalk, M., Peduzzi, P.N., Allore, H., Byers, A.: A program to prevent functional decline in physically frail, elderly persons who live at home. N. Engl. J. Med. **347**(14), 1068–1074 (2002)
2. Hellmers, S., et al.: Towards a minimized unsupervised technical assessment of physical performance in domestic environments. In: Pervasive Health (2017)
3. Clegg, A., Young, J., Iliffe, S., Rikkert, M.O., Rockwood, K.: Frailty in elderly people. Lancet **381**(9868), 752–762 (2013)
4. Hellmers, S., et al.: Stair climb power measurements via inertial measurement units - towards an unsupervised assessment of strength in domestic environments. In: Proceedings of the 11th International Joint Conference on Biomedical Engineering Systems and Technologies, HEALTHINF, INSTICC, vol. 5, pp. 39–47. SciTePress (2018)
5. Frenken, T., et al.: Novel approach to unsupervised mobility assessment tests: field trial for aTUG. In: 2012 6th International Conference on Pervasive Computing Technologies for Healthcare (PervasiveHealth), pp. 131–138. IEEE (2012)
6. Cruz-Jentoft, A.J., et al.: Sarcopenia: European consensus on definition and diagnosisreport of the european working group on sarcopenia in older people. Age Ageing **39**(4), 412–423 (2010)
7. Bean, J.F., Kiely, D.K., LaRose, S., Alian, J., Frontera, W.R.: Is stair climb power a clinically relevant measure of leg power impairments in at-risk older adults? Arch. Phys. Med. Rehabil. **88**(5), 604–609 (2007)
8. Nightingale, E.J., Pourkazemi, F., Hiller, C.E.: Systematic review of timed stair tests. J. Rehabil. Res. Dev. **51**(3), 335–50 (2014)
9. Klass, M., Baudry, S., Duchateau, J.: Age-related decline in rate of torque development is accompanied by lower maximal motor unit discharge frequency during fast contractions. J. Appl. Physiol. **104**(3), 739–746 (2008)
10. Kidde, J., Marcus, R., Dibble, L., Smith, S., LaStayo, P.: Regional muscle and whole-body composition factors related to mobility in older individuals: a review. Physiotherapy Canada **61**(4), 197–209 (2009)
11. Foldvari, M., et al.: Association of muscle power with functional status in community-dwelling elderly women. J. Gerontol. Ser. A: Biol. Sci. Med. Sci. **55**(4), M192–M199 (2000)

12. Reid, K.F., Fielding, R.A.: Skeletal muscle power: a critical determinant of physical functioning in older adults. Exerc. Sport Sci. Rev. **40**(1), 4 (2012)
13. Zheng, E., Chen, B., Wang, X., Huang, Y., Wang, Q.: On the design of a wearable multi-sensor system for recognizing motion modes and sit-to-stand transition. Int. J. Adv. Robot. Syst. **11**(2), 30 (2014)
14. Khan, A.M., Lee, Y.K., Lee, S.Y., Kim, T.S.: A triaxial accelerometer-based physical-activity recognition via augmented-signal features and a hierarchical recognizer. IEEE Trans. Inf Technol. Biomed. **14**(5), 1166–1172 (2010)
15. Fida, B., Bernabucci, I., Bibbo, D., Conforto, S., Schmid, M.: Pre-processing effect on the accuracy of event-based activity segmentation and classification through inertial sensors. Sensors **15**(9), 23095–23109 (2015)
16. Shoaib, M., Bosch, S., Incel, O.D., Scholten, H., Havinga, P.J.: Fusion of smartphone motion sensors for physical activity recognition. Sensors **14**(6), 10146–10176 (2014)
17. Sun, L., Zhang, D., Li, B., Guo, B., Li, S.: Activity recognition on an accelerometer embedded mobile phone with varying positions and orientations. In: Yu, Z., Liscano, R., Chen, G., Zhang, D., Zhou, X. (eds.) UIC 2010. LNCS, vol. 6406, pp. 548–562. Springer, Heidelberg (2010). https://doi.org/10.1007/978-3-642-16355-5_42
18. Fareed, U.: Smartphone sensor fusion based activity recognition system for elderly healthcare. In: Proceedings of the 2015 Workshop on Pervasive Wireless Healthcare, pp. 29–34. ACM (2015)
19. Anguita, D., Ghio, A., Oneto, L., Parra, X., Reyes-Ortiz, J.L.: Human activity recognition on smartphones using a multiclass hardware-friendly support vector machine. In: Bravo, J., Hervás, R., Rodríguez, M. (eds.) IWAAL 2012. LNCS, vol. 7657, pp. 216–223. Springer, Heidelberg (2012). https://doi.org/10.1007/978-3-642-35395-6_30
20. Lester, J., Choudhury, T., Borriello, G.: A practical approach to recognizing physical activities. In: Fishkin, K.P., Schiele, B., Nixon, P., Quigley, A. (eds.) Pervasive 2006. LNCS, vol. 3968, pp. 1–16. Springer, Heidelberg (2006). https://doi.org/10.1007/11748625_1
21. Stacoff, A., Diezi, C., Luder, G., Stüssi, E., Kramers-de Quervain, I.A.: Ground reaction forces on stairs: effects of stair inclination and age. Gait Posture **21**(1), 24–38 (2005)
22. Bean, J., et al.: Weighted stair climbing in mobility-limited older people: a pilot study. J. Am. Geriatr. Soc. **50**(4), 663–670 (2002)
23. Regterschot, G.R.H., Folkersma, M., Zhang, W., Baldus, H., Stevens, M., Zijlstra, W.: Sensitivity of sensor-based sit-to-stand peak power to the effects of training leg strength, leg power and balance in older adults. Gait Posture **39**(1), 303–307 (2014)
24. Suzuki, T., Bean, J.F., Fielding, R.A.: Muscle power of the ankle flexors predicts functional performance in community-dwelling older women. J. Am. Geriatr. Soc. **49**(9), 1161–1167 (2001)
25. Perry, J., Burnfield, J.M.: Gait Analysis: Normal and Pathological Function, 2nd edn. SLACK Incorporated (2010)
26. Novak, A.C., Reid, S.M., Costigan, P.A., Brouwer, B.: Stair negotiation alters stability in older adults. Lower Extremity Rev. **2**(10), 47–51 (2010)
27. Dietz, B.: PNF in Lokomotion: Let's Sprint, Let's Skate. Springer, Heidelberg (2017). https://doi.org/10.1007/978-3-642-27666-8. ISBN 9783642276668

28. Hellmers, S., et al.: Technology supported geriatric assessment. In: Wichert, R., Mand, B. (eds.) Ambient Assisted Living. ATSC, pp. 85–100. Springer, Cham (2017). https://doi.org/10.1007/978-3-319-52322-4_6

29. Gozick, B., Subbu, K.P., Dantu, R., Maeshiro, T.: Magnetic maps for indoor navigation. IEEE Trans. Instrum. Meas. **60**(12), 3883–3891 (2011)

30. Li, B., Harvey, B., Gallagher, T.: Using barometers to determine the height for indoor positioning. In: 2013 International Conference on Indoor Positioning and Indoor Navigation (IPIN), pp. 1–7. IEEE (2013)

31. Fudickar, S., Lindemann, A., Schnor, B.: Threshold-based fall detection on smart phones. In: Proceedings of HEALTHINF 2014–7th International Conference on Health Informatics, Part of 7th International Joint Conference on Biomedical Engineering Systems and Technologies, BIOSTEC, pp. 303–309 (2014)

32. Fried, L.P., et al.: Frailty in older adults: evidence for a phenotype. J. Gerontol. Ser. A: Biol. Sci. Med. Sci. **56**(3), M146–M157 (2001)

33. Nadeau, S., McFadyen, B.J., Malouin, F.: Frontal and sagittal plane analyses of the stair climbing task in healthy adults aged over 40 years: what are the challenges compared to level walking? Clin. Biomech. **18**(10), 950–959 (2003)

Considerations on the Usability of SClínico

João Pavão[1] , Rute Bastardo[2] , Luís Torres Pereira[1] ,
Paula Oliveira[3] , Victor Costa[4] , Ana Isabel Martins[5] ,
Alexandra Queirós[6] , and Nelson Pacheco Rocha[7(✉)]

[1] Science and Technology School, INESC-TEC,
University of Trás-os-Montes and Alto Douro, Quinta de Prados,
5000-801 Vila Real, Portugal
{jpavao, tpereira}@utad.pt
[2] Science and Technology School, University of Trás-os-Montes
and Alto Douro, Quinta de Prados, 5000-801 Vila Real, Portugal
rbpinto@utad.pt
[3] Centre for the Research and Technology of Agro-Environmental
and Biological Sciences, CITAB, University of Trás-os-Montes and Alto Douro,
Quinta de Prados, 5000-801 Vila Real, Portugal
poliveira@utad.pt
[4] Centro Hospitalar of Trás-os-Montes e Alto Douro,
Av. da Noruega, Lordelo, 5000-508 Vila Real, Portugal
vcosta@chtmad.min-saude.pt
[5] IEETA, University of Aveiro, Campo Universitário de Santiago,
3810-193 Aveiro, Portugal
anaisabel@ua.pt
[6] Health Sciences School, IEETA, University of Aveiro,
Campo Universitário de Santiago, 3810-193 Aveiro, Portugal
alexandra@ua.pt
[7] Department of Medical Sciences, IEETA, University of Aveiro,
Campo Universitário de Santiago, 3810-193 Aveiro, Portugal
npr@ua.pt

Abstract. To increase the quality of the health care services and, at the same time, to control their costs, the use of Electronic Health Records (EHR) has substantially increased during the last years. Usability of EHR systems is a key factor to increase their efficiency. The SClínico is an EHR system widely used in public hospitals and primary care centres of the Portuguese National Health Service and the present article reports the assessment of its usability. This usability assessment consisted in three stages: in the first stage, an exploratory assessment was carried out, while in the second stage a quantitative assessment was performed using a validated usability assessment instrument, and, finally, in the third stage a focus group involving clinicians and usability experts was conducted. The results showed that SClínico presents important usability issues and, therefore, recommendations are suggested to overcome the identified issues.

Keywords: Usability · Electronic health record · SClínico

A. Cliquet jr. et al. (Eds.): BIOSTEC 2018, CCIS 1024, pp. 262–278, 2019.
https://doi.org/10.1007/978-3-030-29196-9_14

1   Introduction

In the Portuguese public hospitals, clinical records have been carried out in electronic format since 1988, using two Electronic Health Records (EHR) systems for physicians and nurses, respectively the Sistema de Apoio ao Médico (Medical Support Service), known as SAM, and the Sistema de Apoio à Prática de Enfermagem (Nursing Practice Support System), known as SAPE. In 2014, the system known as SClínico replaced the previous two systems, by integrating in a single system the physician and nurse profiles.

According to the organization responsible for the development of SClínico, the Serviços Partilhados do Ministério da Saúde (Shared Services of the Ministry of Health), known as SPMS, SClínico is part of the strategy defined by the Portuguese health Ministry to introduce information technologies in the Serviço Nacional de Saúde (National Health Service), the SNS [1, 2].

The SClínico has two versions: the SClínico Hospital and the SClínico Primary Health Care [1, 2]. The first, SClínico Hospital, is present in more than 50 public hospitals and has more than 60.000 registered clinicians [1]. In turn, SClínico Primary Health Care is present in more than 300 primary care centers and has more than 13.000 registered clinicians [2].

The scientific literature (e.g. [3]) reports that some of the problems with the implementation of EHR systems may be related to the usability of the respective user interfaces, such as poor readability, poor alarm identification or insufficient feedback on the actions being taken. Considering that EHR systems are fundamental tools for the health care delivery, it is important to assess their usability [4]. Therefore, the study reported in this paper, that complements the study reported in [5], aimed to assess the usability of SClínico, namely the usability of the SClínico Hospital version.

The experimental study was performed in several clinical services of the Centro Hospitalar de Trás-os-Montes e Alto Douro (Trás-os-Montes and Alto Douro Hospital Centre), known as CHTMAD, composed by four hospitals of the Portuguese SNS: Vila Real, Lamego, Chaves and Peso da Régua.

In addition to this introductory section, the present article comprises five more sections: Related Work, Methods, Results, Discussion and Conclusion.

2   Related Work

Health information systems such as the ones supporting EHR allow the clinical report, as well as the access, exchange and share of the required clinical information for preventing and treating the disease [6]. In terms of health care delivery, EHR systems represent a benefit to both the patient and organizations, since they enable secure, accessible and efficient clinical information reporting and retrieving.

Internationally, during the last two decades, the adoption of EHR system has been recognized as a priority. For instance, in the United States the Health Information Technology for Economic and Clinical Health (HITECH) Act of 2009.2 had accelerated the rate of EHR adoption [7].

EHR support highly collaborative and demanding processes, involving large number of clinicians with distinct profiles (e.g. physicians, nurses or therapists), social workers, managers and administrative personnel [8]. In addition, the context of health care delivery can strongly influence the capabilities of the clinicians and put them permanently under stress. In fact, the considerable amount of continuous working hours, as well as the rotating work shifts, promote sleep disturbances, fatigue and deficits of attention [9]. Therefore, the deployment of EHR systems requires organizational changes at different levels, not only in terms of the clinical workflow, but also in terms of how the clinicians interact with the patients [10].

The literature reports various factors that facilitate the deployment of EHR (e.g. efficiency, quality, access to data, perceived value, and ability to transfer information [11]), but also a set of barriers, including initial cost, technical support, eligibility criteria, technical infrastructure, physician attitude, effort needed to select systems, degree of integration, staff shortages, agility to make changes, external factors, and interoperability, among others [12].

It is not always easy to define what to report, or how to report, mainly because the clinical information must be conveniently contextualized, which is not easy to achieve with the existing EHR systems. Moreover, adequate and efficient mechanisms must be made available to allow the visualization of the needed information, whenever and wherever required [3]. The adaptability of EHR systems to different situations might influence the way the clinical information is reported and retrieved, which, necessarily, impacts the benefits expected from EHRs. These included advanced functions such as using EHR data for performance measurement (e.g. performance feedback via dashboards and other approaches to identify domains of suboptimal performance), and engaging patients through better access to their data as well as supporting other patient-centric care activities (e.g. to ensure that patients can be active participants in their care and to facilitate engagement in self-management) [13]. For that, aspects such as user acceptance, perceived usefulness or ability to easily input historical medical record data assume a great importance [12], which means that usability of EHR systems should be a major concern.

In 1998, the International Organization for Standardization (ISO) defined usability as being the "extent to which a product can be used by specified users to achieve specified goals with effectiveness, efficiency, and satisfaction in a specified context of use" [14].

Internationally, there are many usability studies of EHR systems, targeting different clinical domains [3, 15–20]. There are also efforts to standardize the usability assessment methods attempting to find a common ground, which is fundamental to perform comparative studies [21, 22].

According to Saitwal and colleagues [23], some EHR systems do not have user-friendly interfaces, as they often do not take in consideration the user centric development. The EHR user interfaces may be improved, making them easier to use, easier to learn and more resistant to errors. In the referred study of Saitwal and colleagues [23], a cognitive analysis method was applied to assess the usability of EHR systems, which made possible the identification of issues that could be improved, namely the reduction of the number of steps to perform certain tasks, together with the minimization of the cognitive effort required to execute them.

Edward and colleagues [24] argue that the usability of EHR systems is crucial to ensure safety and to enable clinicians to focus more on patients and less on technology. These authors used a heuristic assessment method to identify points of possible usability improvements of an EHR system supporting a pediatrics service. The results of this usability assessment allowed immediate improvements in the EHR system configuration and training materials.

Since there is a worldwide trend to consider usability as one of the important factors of the implementation of EHR systems, the American Medical Informatics Association (AMIA) has defined a working group to propose relevant recommendations [25]. Moreover, the National Institute of Standards and Technology (NIST) describes a set of procedures for design evaluation and user performance testing of EHR systems by defining an EHR usability protocol (EUP) [26]. The purpose of this protocol is to provide methods to measure and validate user performance prior to deployment and it comprises a three-step process: EHR application analysis, EHR user interface expert review, and EHR user interface validation testing [26].

3 Methods

The primary objective of the experimental study reported in this paper was to assess the usability of the SClínico, particularly the SClínico Hospital version, as well as the level of satisfaction of its users. As a secondary objective, it was intended to identify, in terms of usability, improvements that should be implemented.

Considering these objectives, a research study was planned, taking into consideration assessment instruments and methods to be used [27], the participants in the study and the regulatory, ethical and data protection aspects.

3.1 Research Plan

Several clinical services of CHTMAD were considered for data collection. The protocol of the experimental study comprised three stages. In each of them, a specific usability assessment method was used: (i) in the first stage, an exploratory assessment was carried out; (ii) while in the second stage, a quantitative assessment was performed using a validated usability assessment instrument, the Portuguese version [28] of Post-Study System Usability Questionnaire (PSSUQ) [29]; and (iii) finally, in the third stage, a focus group was performed. The focus group included both clinicians and usability experts.

The first stage of usability assessment of SClínico was planned to take place few weeks after it has been introduced in the clinical services of CHTMAD (i.e. May and June 2014). In turn, the second step was planned to be performed eighteen months after the first assessment, when all potential users were already familiar with SClínico. The focus group was planned to take place after the analysis of the results of the second stage.

3.2   Assessment Instruments and Methods

The exploratory assessment for the first stage was performed by a specially prepared questionnaire [30]. The development of this questionnaire was based on a literature research related to relevant questions that should be considered when assessing the usability of EHR systems [30]. The questionnaire is composed of two sections, the first one dealing with demographic aspects and the second one dealing with the interaction with SClínico. This second section has 45 questions, and if an inquired clinician was allocated to the emergency service, he/she would have to answer four more questions. Most of the questions are closed answer questions, being seven of them open answer questions aimed to detail some of the closed answer questions.

The questions that constitute the second section were grouped in the following classes, accordingly to the recommendations of other studies [30]:

- System performance (10 questions).
- Clarity of information (12 questions).
- Quality of the graphical interface (12 questions).
- Adequacy of the system's functions to the tasks performed (11 generic questions plus four questions specifically related to the emergency service).

In turn, the second stage consisted in a quantitative self-reported assessment of the SClínico usability (user opinion) using the PSSUQ [29]. Specifically, after using SClínico the clinicians were invited to participate in the study and to complete the PSSUQ [5].

The PSSUQ was developed by the International Business Machines (IBM) and was later translated and adapted from the cultural and linguistic point of view to the European Portuguese [28]. It consists of 19 items rated on a seven-point likert scale (from "strongly agree" - 1, to "strongly disagree" - 7) [29]. The PSSUQ addresses five usability characteristics of a system: (i) rapid completion of the task; (ii) ease of learning; (iii) high quality documentation; (iv) online information; and (v) functional adequacy [29].

According to the authors of the original version, the score of the PSSUQ can be specified by three sub-scores, system utility (SysUse), information quality (InfoQual), and interface quality (IntQual), that can be obtained as follows [29]:

- The mean value related to the system utility (SysUse) - items 1 to 8.
- The mean value related to the quality of information (InfoQual) - items 9 to 15.
- The mean value related to the quality of the interface (IntQual) - items 16 to 18.

The final score of PSSUQ is the average of the scores of its items. If a participant fails to respond to an item or classify it as N/A (not applicable), then that item should be scored with the average score of the remaining items. Finally, higher scores indicate lower usability and vice-versa.

The objective of the third stage was two-fold:

- To see how the previously detected usability problems could affect the overall performance of the clinicians.
- To find possible new usability problems, previously undetected.

For this purpose, a focus group was conducted. Focus group is a qualitative data collection technique involving a small number of participants in an informal discussion group, focused on a specific subject [31], including usability assessment [32]. Based on the presentation of several functions of the SClínico, a moderator guided the discussion aiming to extract perceptions, feelings, attitudes and ideas from the participants. Finally, the team made a brainstorm about their findings and built a report on the subject.

3.3   Participants

All physicians and nurses of CHTMAD using SClínico in their clinical practice were eligible to participate in two first stages if they previously gave a written informed consent accepting to participate in the study, whereby the available population covered by the two first stage was composed of 1253 elements, out of which 426 were physicians and 827 were nurses. As the SClínico interface is different for physicians and nurses, the data analysis was performed separately.

In turn, two clinicians with a long experience using SClínico and four usability experts with years of experience in evaluating healthcare applications composed the focus groups.

3.4   Regulatory, Ethical and Data Protection Aspects

To address the ethical issues, a request of approval was directed to the administration and ethical committee of the CHTMAD.

Additionally, in the different phases of the study, all the involved subjects received all the information regarding the study and their participation. This whole study considered all ethical principles underlying the Helsinki Declaration [33], the Good Epidemiological Practice Guidelines [34], and the applicable legislation and regulations.

All necessary steps were taken to protect the participant's privacy and all relevant guidelines on data privacy were followed: information that may allow the identification of participants was not stored in the study database; participants were identified in all study documents by a unique identification number; and the only document linking the identification number to personal information (e.g. names, addresses or telephone numbers) was stored in a safe that could only be accessed by the principal investigator.

4   Results

4.1   Results of the Exploratory Assessment

The exploratory assessment involved a convenience sample of 22 physicians and 47 nurses from the following clinical services of CHTMAD: medicine, surgery, intensive care, oncology, gastroenterology, pediatrics and emergency [35]

The sample presented the following characteristics:

- Gender: most participants were female in both groups, being 75% female and 25% male.

- Age: the participant's age varied between 26 and 58 years for the physicians group, while in the nurses group, the participant's age varied between 27 and 55 years. The mean age was 43 years (SD = 11.8) for the physicians group and 38 years (SD = 8.3) for the nurses group.

Table 1. Appropriateness of SClínico as a clinical information reporting and retrieving tool, as facilitator of the clinical practice, and appropriateness of its graphic environment is favorable after consecutive working hours.

	Yes	No	Not answered
Do you consider the SClínico appropriate tool for the reporting and retrieving of clinical information?			
Physicians	44%	39%	17%
Nurses	59%	28%	13%
Do you consider that SClínico facilitates your clinical practice?			
Physicians	43%	22%	35%
Nurses	66%	23%	11%
Do you consider that the graphical environment SClínico facilitate your clinical practice, after hours of consecutive work?			
Physicians	52%	31%	17%
Nurses	34%	66%	0%

Table 1 reports the opinion of the participants about SClínico. Most nurses (59%) and 44% of physicians think SClínico is an appropriate EHR system. The results are similar when participants where asked if SClínico facilitates the clinical practice (66% of positive answers from the nurses group and 43% of positive answers from the physician group). The main concern, in the case of physicians, is related to the organization of information that seems to be inadequate to the needs of these clinicians. In the case of the nurses, the ambiguity of some information fields together with the low contrast of the colors selected for the user interface (e.g. in the initial menu, the design of the icons is ambiguous with colors difficult to differentiate, which does not facilitate the user interaction).

However, the results are quite different when participants were asked about the graphic environment: most of the nurses consider that the graphic environment is not favorable after consecutive working hours, while most physicians (52%) have a positive impression about the SClínico environment after consecutive working hours.

Regarding the clinicians allocated to the emergency service, specifically when it is required to rapidly access to a comprehensive perspective of the clinical history of the patient (Table 2), most of the participants referred SClínico is not adequate, since 57% of physicians and 53% of nurses answered accordingly. Most clinicians think that it is very important, or even decisive, to have a direct access to relevant patient information in cases of urgency, to speed up and facilitate the evaluation of the clinical history of the patients. Nevertheless, the participants have expressed disappointment with SClínico in this regard. The main reason given is related to the slowness of the system, and it is unclear whether this is due to issues related to the communication network of the CHTMAD or related to usability issues of SClínico (e.g. the need for many tasks using the pointing device or a deficient organization of the information).

Table 2. Adequacy of SClínico for the clinical evaluation of the patient in the emergency service.

	Yes	No	Not answered
Do you consider SClínico adequate for the clinical evaluation of the patient?			
Physicians	39%	57%	4%
Nurses	41%	53%	6%

One of the most desired features for all clinicians is the ability to view patient's information in a comprehensive way to cover the entire clinical situation in a glance. This form of visualization would allow a rapid assessment and correlation of different clinical aspects of a patient. This question was asked in the questionnaire and 100% of the participants of both groups considered important the existence of this type of functions.

4.2   Usability Assessment Using PSSUQ

For the quantitative assessment using the PSSUQ, the sample consisted of 33 physicians and 21 nurses of all the clinical services of one of the three hospital that constitute the CHTMAD: Hospital of Lamego.

The sample presented the following characteristics:

- Gender: most participants were female in both groups, being 52% female and 48% male.
- Age: the participant's age varied between 25 and 66 years for the physicians group, while in the nurses group, the participant's age varied between 24 and 57 years. The mean age was 39 years (SD = 11.5) for the physicians group and 38 years (SD = 9.3) for the nurses group.

The average score of PSSUQ for all nurses was 4,83 out of 7 (SD = 1,21), and for all physicians was 4,10 out of 7 (SD = 1,35). These results indicate a medium low degree of usability and satisfaction.

For the physicians group, the results of the subscales associated with PSSUQ were:

- System Utility (SysUse): average of the responses from items 1 to 8 = 3,75 (SD = 1,48).
- Quality of information (InfoQual): average of the responses from items 9 to 15 = 4,47 (SD = 1,47).

- Interface Quality (IntQual): average of the responses from items 16 to 18 = 4,00 (SD = 1,60).

In turn, for the nurses group, the results of the subscales associated with PSSUQ were:

- System Utility (SysUse): average of the responses from items 1 to 8 = 4,83 (SD = 1,38).
- Quality of information (InfoQual): average of the responses from items 9 to 15 = 4,84 (SD = 1,40).
- Interface Quality (IntQual): average of the responses from items 16 to 18 = 4,67 (SD = 1,32).

In a more detailed analysis, for the physicians group, the questions that obtained better results were "I felt comfortable using this system" (3,20 out of 7) and "it was easy to learn to use this system" (3,30 out of 7,00). Both questions are related to the System Utility (SysUse) subscale. Moreover, the questions that obtained worse results were "the system gave error messages that clearly told me how to fix problems" (5,20 out of 7,00) and "whenever I made a mistake using the system, I could recover easily and quickly" (5,03 out of 7,00). Both questions are part of the quality of information (IfoQual) subscale related to the ability to recover from errors and the availability of support when recovering from errors.

When looking in more detail for the results of the nurses group, the questions that obtained better results were "I felt comfortable using this system" (4,38 out of 7,00) and "the interface of this system was pleasant" (4,43 out of 7,00). In opposite, the questions that obtained worse results were "overall, I am satisfied with this system" (5,38 out of 7,00) and "I believe I could become productive quickly using this system" (5,33 out of 7,00).

4.3   Results of the Focus Group

The focus group was composed by six elements (i.e. two clinicians and four usability experts) and took place in May 2018. In terms of analysis, the relevant results of the focus group where extracted and were classified according to their positive or negative aspects.

Considering the positive aspects, the overall evaluation of SClínico was very positive in terms of the impact of the system on the daily tasks of the clinicians. Although the system presents some debilities, in general it is a good tool to report and retrieve clinical information.

In turn, several negative aspects were highlighted by the focus group, namely:

- The lack of formal training programs related to the usage of SClínico, leading to the knowledge share between clinicians.
- Unavailability of good manuals to help the users to get acquainted with the several functionalities being offered. These might not be used because they are out of the strict learning paths transmitted by the more experienced users, with their own routines and ways of interacting with SClínico. The manuals included in the

SClínico are not up to date, and an integrated digital help, other than rudimental, is not also available to cover pressing doubts or actions.

- Although the SClínico presents a fresh look over its antecedents, it is an old system made of many modules, showing themselves as developed at different points in time, with different principles for the graphical user interfaces. That causes an idea of non-unity in the whole of SClínico.
- The organization of the interface presents several drawbacks.

The negative aspects related with the organization of the interface were further detailed into: (i) inconsistencies and discordances; and (ii) functionality issues.

Interface metaphors should be simple, familiar, and logical. These should be constructed according to a coherent standard that shares the same basic diagramming: layout, graphic elements, conventions, information hierarchies and organization, thus making the layout coherent and predictable. In some instances, these principles were not followed when developing the SClínico interface which lead to some inconsistencies and discordances. Therefore, when analyzing the SClínico Hospitalar (both physician and nurse profile), the focus group reported inconsistencies in the layout design regarding the use of color, the consistency of communication (acronyms), the design and positioning of icons, the positioning of graphic elements and in the own hierarchy of information and organization.

Color is a complex and variable phenomenon, both in physical terms because our perception of color depends not only on the pigmentation of the surfaces themselves, but also on the intensity and type of ambient light, as well as on cultural terms. In order that the color could be described and understood, a precise vocabulary was established over time so that the color could communicate with some degree of clarity. Based on the color one can express an atmosphere, create relations of belonging or even encode information. Thus, the color is used to unite or differentiate, point out or hide information. SClínico uses several color codes to encode information, but they lack effectiveness due to lack of consistency. An example is the same color to be used to represent different situations. For instance, as stated on the help menu for color codes, the color blue is used to represent a "non-urgent" situation but at the same time it represents the patients that are selected. Furthermore, the blue color also has a different meaning when it is used in the calendar

In SClínico one can find lack of coherence in the acronyms used. For example, the use of the abbreviation N for the codification of "Enfermeiro" (the Portuguese word for "nurse") is not expected, opposing the letter M for the designation of "Médico" (the Portuguese word for physician), that fits the Portuguese vocabulary. Another example of inconsistency in acronyms is in the case of the Medical Agenda screen (Medical version) in the scheduled appointments. The abbreviations available on the board are: U – Urgente (urgent); S – Sem agendamento (no appointment); R – Rotina (Routine) and E – Além vagas (Extra appointment). The acronym E escapes the logic of using the initial letter as an abbreviation, concerning the Portuguese vocabulary, which is the language in use.

There is an effort to promote the graphical unit in the design of SClínico icons, giving them the same style or graphical nature. However, it is possible to verify that some icons are totally inconsistent with the expressed contents, proving incapable of expressing their meaning and function.

The poor differentiation between the design of the icons compromises its recognition as well as its immediate decoding and consequently its memorization. For instance, SClínico has icons that, when visualized in their actual size, become very similar promoting the error. In several situations, the icons are practically impossible to decode without the respective label.

Another point to note is the fact that certain icons have a different color but that does not represent any state of the button (e.g. active or deactivated), rather it refers to a different area with content available for consult. However not all icons have this particularity, becoming prone to error.

Another category of inconsistences is related to the grouping of elements, which is an important issue in visual messages. The icons in the initial menu of SClínico are not always grouped in the same way, varying their location in space. In some cases, there is an attempt to join icons, however there is a lack of logic in the groups and consistency throughout the interface, appearing these grouped in different ways.

In SClínico one can observe that there are functions after others at the same level. At this same level we have two icons to mark and unmark actions on the same calendar. These should be options of a sub-level of the calendar. The hierarchy can be simple or complex, rigorous or flexible, shallow or extremely articulate. Whatever the approach, the hierarchy employs clear marks of separation to signal the change from one level to another.

In the field of functionality, the issues we found can be categorized as feedback, notification, registration, flexibility, forms submission and processing delays and performance degradation.

The questions about feedback are mainly concerned about situations where there are fields that are considered mandatory in the context of a local hospital policy but are not treated as such by SClínico. In fact, the user may not fill those fields and not be alerted for the fact. Another situation happens when a physician or a nurse must complete a form that another clinician initiated previously. Some fields may be blank, because they were not applicable at the time, or they might be blank because the user just forgot to fill them. This is not possible to know. Some feedback about a more objective way to look at those fields would be important.

There is a lack of a consistent system for notifications. The focus group reported some situations where a physician needs a certain patient to be observed by a colleague and generates a request for that matter in the SClínico. That request sits on the system waiting for the requested physician to collect it. Those kind of situations call for a more aggressive notification system, which eventually cross the boundary of the SClínico and send, for example, an SMS, or any sort of similar message to the professional that is requested to see a notification in the SClínico.

In the registration practice there are some flows that are not very intuitive (such as in the case of the creation of a new therapy) where the path to conclude the action is too long.

Some of the above situations could be mitigated if there were a more flexible, parametrized mechanisms, which SClínico do not allow. A situation where flexibility works is in the integration of third party applications, for example to call complementary diagnostic services. There is a central point, a right click of the mouse over a patient's name, where there is a list of available external applications integrating SClínico information. This possibility has, however its own drawbacks. First, an entire list of applications appears, all with the same aspect. That list could be big, depending on the hospital. There are applications that are not of concern of a particular user but still appear. Finally, although not SClínico' s concern, this flexibility comes with a cost: delegating the responsibility to other applications, which means that any interface policy of SClínico is completely loss and are the exclusive responsibility of the third part applications and the local hospitals.

A personal administrative interface to allow some small settings in the interfaces is inexistent and this fact makes the system less efficient because all functionality is present whether the user use it or not. In hospitals that do not have certain specialties they still have access to the related aspects of those specialties, although they will never use them. Facilitator settings that might improve usability, hence the efficiency, are not possible in SClínico on a per user basis.

The nurse profile sometimes has over parametrization, whereas in physician profile sometimes there is too much freedom even when some parametrization would be good. Some flexibility should be possible to adjust processual requirements that usually change from hospital to hospital. An example is the patient discharge on the situations of ambulatory surgery that is based on the same process of internship, so, it must accomplish internship processual issues that are not adequate to ambulatory surgery, causing delays in the patient flow. Another example is that sometimes in the nurse profile the parametrization is so tight that it does not fully apply to reality. It should be possible to parametrize some forms to meet the needs of some hospital procedures.

The forms submission would benefit from a capability of separating the "save" state from the "submit" state. This should be completed with a stronger notification/feedback system so no open forms would be admissible at the intended end of the process.

Still in terms of flexibility, most participants considered difficult, especially in the context of emergency services, the rapid access to the clinical history of the patients, which was considered a fundamental requirement.

Some problems of delays in the processing of the forms were also reported that causes some inefficiency in the normal flow of the hospital. These periods are well characterized in terms of the period that occur, and, therefore, it seems to be mainly related to the server capacity rather to network faults or delays.

5 Discussion

The analysis of the results related to the exploratory assessment identified several usability problems that were addressed in more detail in the subsequent phases of the study (i.e. the quantitative assessment and the focus group).

Looking at the subscales scores of the PSSUQ, the best-performing score was the system utility (SysUse). The second best-performance score was the quality of interface (IntQual) and the worst-performance score of the information quality (InfoQual).

These results seem to suggest that clinicians consider that a system such as SClínico benefits their clinical practice. However, the clinicians are unsatisfied with the mode the information is presented and the general usability of the system. This means that the usability problems of SClínico are reflected in the perception that clinicians have of the information quality that SClínico provides, which must be deeply studied since the quality of the health care delivery relies on the quality of the information.

The nurses group classified the usability of SClínico even lower than the physicians group. One of the reasons that may explain this result is the fact that nurses spend more time reporting and retrieving clinical information using SClínico than physicians. This fact may justify a greater frustration of the nurses group in terms of the SClínico usability. The overall functioning of the system and the ability to use it productively were the most critical aspects for the nurses group.

Additionally, the focus group study found several problems at different levels. There were found other sorts of questions that were considered usability issues. One group of questions was related with inconsistencies and discordances among the different parts of SClínico. These had to do with colors, acronyms, icons, spatial distribution of the components in the interface and some architectural issues that do not respect a hierarchy. These factors play against usability and have a negative impact on the care given service.

Globally speaking, SClínico is incoherent in terms of the colors being used, the design of the icons and their grouping. The lack of consistency in the metaphors used or even the scarcity of differentiation in the design of the icons may compromise their meaning and function. Some icons are complex in their design and carry too many details. As stated by Yan [36], icons should be used to facilitate the perception, understanding and memorization, and not only with the purpose of the design beauty.

Although an effort is being made to promote the graphical unity in the design of the icons in SClínico, by giving them the same style and graphical nature, it is possible to verify that some of them are totally inconsistent with the expressed contents, proving to be incapable of expressing their meaning and function. The poor differentiation between the design of the icons compromises its recognition as well as its immediate decoding and consequently its memorization.

A coherent approach to communication (whether graphically or textual) through titles, subtitles, navigation links and acronyms should be used to reinforce the sense of context in the user, making the environment more integrated, consistent and, therefore, easier to decode. This way the cognitive load is reduced during operation due to visual experience and familiarity, which might prevent the information overload that appears when the ability to perceive and understand is exceeded by the amount of information presented by a user interface, to the point of facilitating information processing errors [3].

One aspect worthen to be noted is the SClínico interaction when the clinicians have a considerable amount of continuous working hours. This is a very usual situation in the health care sector, particularly in the hospital environment, since physicians and nurses often do long shifts. There is a large percentage of unsatisfied participants due to decreased cognitive ability or attention related to fatigue and stress as already shown by Marquié and colleagues [9]. In this aspect, the group of nurses seems to be the most affected. It was this group of clinicians that emphasizes problems related to the cognitive capacity even in normal operation, which seems to have more impact after considerable amount of continuous working hours.

During the experimental study it was also noticed that some work about spatial organization of the information should be made, namely to improve grouping related issues. Grouping allows an element of the interface to have an immediate visual relationship with another near element. Kimberly Elam refer that it is important to create visual order, which can be achieved by grouping elements that are related and with white spaces, or negative spaces [37]. Moreover, the lack of visual and functional continuity in the spatial organization can compromise usability, makes the navigation more difficult, increases errors and set the information and application resources more difficult to access for users. According to the Gestalt theory, in visual perception the elements close to each other tend to be seen together, that is, to constitute units. The shorter the distance between the elements, the closer and unified it seems to be.

Some architectural aspects emerged as well through the study that are important to change to improve usability. About this kind of issues, Ellen Lupton says the hierarchy should be employed to clearly mark a change level [38].

Therefore, the organization of the contents according to several hierarchical levels in complex systems, help to create order, relation of belonging favouring the understanding of the entire navigation structure of the interface. Inconsistencies in the navigation structure may compromise the understanding of functionalities, making interaction difficult.

The functionality problems also play a major role in the daily lives of the clinicians and have a real impact on patient flows and in the quality of the service. A good feedback system would be very helpful to ensure the correctness in filling the forms. A notification system that would alert the professional in a very effective way is advisable so that the several requests are dully executed. Some ambiguity in the blank form fields could also be avoided, for instance, by separating "non-applicable" from the absence of answer. Moreover, a reflexion should be made about the excess of parametrization or too much freedom even when some parametrization would be good.

These issues have several different causes, however the most important is the poor interaction efficiency/presentation of ineffective information.

The lack of flexibility was also an important issue that came out during the several phases of the study, in the overall interface, namely, in the case of clinicians allocated to the emergency service, where most participants considered difficult the rapid access to the clinical history of the patients. This is an important issue, known and discussed in information visualization [39], and is related to the user interface adaptability and flexibility, allowing not only the comprehensive visualization of a patient's clinical information but also the clinical details when required.

Finally, we can say that, as in any other case, the expertise in the use of SClínico is earned during years of practice. However, it is necessary for the young professionals to get going fast with the health records of their patients and this leads to a kind of a narrow learnability very limited to what are the paths transmitted by the elder professionals. The absence of clear manuals with an easy access and an effective help system leads to a defective learning of the SClínico because users do not fill secure in doing things differently than what they learned from others.

6 Conclusion

The study reported in this article showed that SClínico has many detailed conceptual and practical issues. The SClínico would clearly benefit from alternative forms of information visualization, as well as a better organization of the interfaces. Another important aspect is the comprehensive visualization of the relevant patient clinical information to correlate possible past situations with the current episode, particularly during an urgency situation. Moreover, it is also intended that, in urgent situations, the retrieving of relevant information should be as direct as possible. Although not the majority, many clinicians felt that prolonged exposure to SClínico increases the usability issues due to fatigue. This aspect, together with criticisms pointed to the color scheme, the flat typology of the interface design, and the way information is presented refer the need for a new approach to the graphic design.

One aspect that should be highlighted is related to the fact that the knowledge related to the use of SClínico is transmitted between professionals, since there is the lack of formal training programs, as well as the lack of comprehensive user manuals.

The results of the present study are in line with other studies evaluating EHRs systems. For instance, Robert Behler in his assessment of the new Military Health System Genesis program states "MHS GENESIS is not operationally suitable because of poor system usability, insufficient training, and inadequate help desk support" [40].

Although the present study has limitations, particularly the small sample size, it precludes the need to improve the usability of SClínico. Given the widespread use of SClínico in the Portuguese SNS (i.e. there are tens of thousands of clinicians who use SClínico daily to support their clinical practices), a small improvement in its usability might be translated, overall, into considerable efficiency gains. Moreover, the methods considered for the present experimental study, particularly the usability assessment using the PSSUQ and the focus group, proved to be efficient to detect the usability issues and aspects that lead to the dissatisfaction of the SClínico users. Therefore, the authors strongly recommend that these methods should be used before the deployment of new releases of SClínico.

Acknowledgments. The authors thank the administration board of CHTMAD for all the support provided, as well as all the clinicians of this hospital center who have accepted to participate in the study reported in this article.

References

1. SPMS: Serviços Partilhados do Ministério da Saúde - SPMS - SClinico Hospitalar. http://spms.min-saude.pt/product/sclinicohospitalar/. Accessed 17 July 2017
2. SPMS: Serviços Partilhados do Ministério da Saúde - SPMS - SClinico Cuidados Primários. http://spms.min-saude.pt/product/sclinicocsp/. Accessed 17 July 2017
3. Zahabi, M., Kaber, D.B., Swangnetr, M.: Usability and safety in electronic medical records interface design: a review of recent literature and guideline formulation. Hum. Factors **57**, 805–834 (2015). https://doi.org/10.1177/0018720815576827

4. Bhutkar, G., Konkani, A., Katre, D., Ray, G.G.: A review: healthcare usability evaluation methods. Biomed. Instrum. Technol. Suppl. 45–53 (2013). https://doi.org/10.2345/0899-8205-47.s2.45
5. Pavão, J., et al.: SClinico: usability study. In: Proceedings of the 11th International Joint Conference on Biomedical Engineering Systems and Technologies, pp. 48–56. SCITE-PRESS - Science and Technology Publications (2018)
6. Rouleau, G., Gagnon, M.-P., Côté, J.: Impacts of information and communication technologies on nursing care: an overview of systematic reviews (protocol). Syst Rev. **4**, 75 (2015). https://doi.org/10.1186/s13643-015-0062-y
7. Furukawa, M.F., King, J., Patel, V., Hsiao, C.-J., Adler-Milstein, J., Jha, A.K.: Despite substantial progress in EHR adoption, health information exchange and patient engagement remain low in office settings. Health Aff. **33**, 1672–1679 (2014). https://doi.org/10.1377/hlthaff.2014.0445
8. Marin, H.D.F.: Sistemas de informação em saúde: considerações gerais. J. Health Inform. **2**, 20–24 (2010). https://doi.org/10.1590/S0102-311X2012000800014
9. Marquié, J.-C.C., Tucker, P., Folkard, S., Gentil, C., Ansiau, D.: Chronic effects of shift work on cognition: findings from the VISAT longitudinal study. Occup Env. Med. **72**, 258–264 (2015). https://doi.org/10.1136/oemed-2013-101993
10. Mair, F.S., May, C., O'Donnell, C., Finch, T., Sullivan, F., Murray, E.: Factors that promote or inhibit the implementation of e-health systems: an explanatory systematic review. Bull. World Health Organ. **90**, 357–364 (2012). https://doi.org/10.2471/BLT.11.099424
11. Kruse, C.S., Kothman, K., Anerobi, K., Abanaka, L.: Adoption factors of the electronic health record: a systematic review. JMIR Med. Inform. **4**, e19 (2016). https://doi.org/10.2196/medinform.5525
12. Kruse, C.S., Kristof, C., Jones, B., Mitchell, E., Martinez, A.: Barriers to electronic health record adoption: a systematic literature review. J. Med. Syst. **40**, 252 (2016). https://doi.org/10.1007/s10916-016-0628-9
13. Adler-Milstein, J., Holmgren, A.J., Kralovec, P., Worzala, C., Searcy, T., Patel, V.: Electronic health record adoption in US hospitals: the emergence of a digital "advanced use" divide. J. Am. Med. Inform. Assoc. **24**, 1142–1148 (2017). https://doi.org/10.1093/jamia/ocx080
14. ISO/IEC 9241-14: ISO/IEC 9241-14: 1998 (E) Ergonomic requirements for office work with visual display terminals (VDT)s – Part 14 Menu dialogue (1998). https://www.iso.org/obp/ui/#iso:std:16886:en
15. American Medical Association: Improving Care: Priorities to Improve Electronic Health Record Usability (2014)
16. Feng, R.-C., Chang, P.: Usability of the clinical care classification system for representing nursing practice according to specialty. Comput. Inform. Nurs. **33**, 448–455 (2015)
17. Villa, L.B., Cabezas, I.: A review on usability features for designing electronic health records. In: 2014 IEEE 16th International Conference on e-Health Networking, Applications and Services, HealthCom 2014, pp. 49–54 (2015)
18. Choi, M., Lee, H.S., Park, J.H.: Usability of academic electronic medical record application for nursing students' clinical practicum. Health Inf. Res. **21**, 191–195 (2015). https://doi.org/10.4258/hir.2015.21.3.191
19. Czaja, S.J., Zarcadoolas, C., Vaughon, W.L., Lee, C.C., Rockoff, M.L., Levy, J.: The usability of electronic personal health record systems for an underserved adult population. Hum. Factors **57**, 491–506 (2015). https://doi.org/10.1177/0018720814549238
20. Clarke, M.A., Belden, J.L., Kim, M.S.: Determining differences in user performance between expert and novice primary care doctors when using an electronic health record (EHR). J Eval Clin Pr. **20**, 1153–1161 (2014). https://doi.org/10.1111/jep.12277

21. Johnston, D., Crowle, P.K.: EHR usability toolkit: a background report on usability and electronic health records. Agency for Healthcare Research and Quality, Rockville (2011)
22. Zhang, J., Walji, M. (eds.): Better EHR: Usability, Workflow and Cognitive Support in Electronic Health Records. National Center for Cognitive Informatics & Decision Making in Healthcare (2014). ISBN: 978-0-692-26296-2
23. Saitwal, H., Feng, X., Walji, M., Patel, V., Zhang, J.: Assessing performance of an electronic health record (EHR) using cognitive task analysis. Int J Med Inf. **79**, 501–506 (2010). https://doi.org/10.1016/j.ijmedinf.2010.04.001
24. Edwards, P.J., Moloney, K.P., Jacko, J.A., Sainfort, F.: Evaluating usability of a commercial electronic health record: a case study. Int. J. Hum Comput Stud. **66**, 718–728 (2008). https://doi.org/10.1016/j.ijhcs.2008.06.002
25. Middleton, B., et al.: Enhancing patient safety and quality of care by improving the usability of electronic health record systems: recommendations from AMIA. J. Am. Med. Inform. Assoc. **20**, e2–e8 (2013). https://doi.org/10.1136/amiajnl-2012-001458
26. Lowry, S.Z., et al.: Technical Evaluation, Testing, and Validation of the Usability of Electronic Health Records (2012)
27. Martins, A.I.., Queirós, A.., Silva, A.G.., Rocha, N.P.: Usability evaluation methods: a systematic review. In: Human Factors in Software Development and Design, pp. 250–273 (2014)
28. Rosa, A., Martins, A., Costa, V., Queiros, A., Silva, A., Rocha, N.: European Portuguese validation of the post-study system usability questionnaire (PSSUQ). In: 2015 10th Iberian Conference on Information Systems and Technologies (CISTI), pp. 1–5 (2015)
29. Lewis, J.: Psychometric evaluation of the PSSUQ using data from five years of usability studies. Int. J. Hum. Comput. Interact. **14**, 463–488 (2002). https://doi.org/10.1207/S15327590IJHC143&4_11
30. Covêlo, M.: Interface para Aplicação Informática de Suporte Clínico em Ambiente Hospitalar (2016). http://hdl.handle.net/10348/5694
31. Wilkinson, S.: A practical guide to research methods. In: Smith, J. (ed.) Qualitative Psychology: A Practical Guide to Research Methods. SAGE Publications (2003)
32. Caplan, S.: Using focus group methodology for ergonomic design. Ergonomics **33**, 527–533 (1990). https://doi.org/10.1080/00140139008927160
33. World Medical Association: Declaration of Helsinki - Ethical Principles for Medical Research Involving Human Subjects (2013)
34. International Epidemiological Association: Good Epidemiological Practice (GEP). IEA Guidelines for Proper Conduct in Epidemiologic Research. http://ieaweb.org/good-epidemiological-practice-gep/. Accessed 13 June 2018
35. Pavão, J., et al.: Usability study of SClinico. In: 2016 11th Iberian Conference on Information Systems and Technologies (CISTI), pp. 1–6 (2016)
36. Yan, R.: Icon design study in computer interface. Procedia Eng. **15**, 3134–3138 (2011). https://doi.org/10.1016/J.PROENG.2011.08.588
37. Elam, K.: Grid Systems: Principles of Organizing Type. Princeton Architectural Press, New York (2004)
38. Lupton, E., Phillips, J.C.: Graphic Design: The New Basics. Princeton Architectural Press, New York (2008)
39. Hansen, D., Shneiderman, B., Smith, M.A.: Analyzing Social Media Networks with NodeXL: Insights from a Connected World (2010)
40. Behler, R.: Military Healthcare System (MHS) GENESIS Initial Operational test and Evaluation (IOT&E) Report (2018). https://www.nextgov.com/media/gbc/docs/pdfs_edit/051118letterng.pdf. Accessed 17 July 2018

Interoperability in Pervasive Health: A Systematic Review

Ana Dias[1] , Ana Isabel Martins[2] , Alexandra Queirós[3] ,
and Nelson Pacheco Rocha[4(✉)]

[1] Department of Economics, Management, Industrial Engineering and Tourism,
GOVCOPP, University of Aveiro, Campus Universitário de Santiago,
3810-193 Aveiro, Portugal
anadias@ua.pt
[2] Department of Electronics, Telecommunications and Informatics,
University of Aveiro, Campus Universitário de Santiago,
3810-193 Aveiro, Portugal
anaisabelmartins@ua.pt
[3] Health Sciences School, IEETA, University of Aveiro,
Campus Universitário de Santiago, 3810-193 Aveiro, Portugal
alexandra@ua.pt
[4] Department of Medical Sciences, IEETA, University of Aveiro,
Campus Universitário de Santiago, 3810-193 Aveiro, Portugal
npr@ua.pt

Abstract. Smart components highly integrated and miniaturized facilitate the development of wearable devices to support home monitoring of patients with chronic diseases and that should be interoperable with existing electronic health records. Objective: This study aimed to systematize current evidence of how interoperability is considered during the development of new applications to gather patients' information in their home environments. Methods: A systematic review was performed based on a search of the literature. Results: A total of 37 articles were retrieved from the 4141 articles that result from the initial search. Conclusion: From the 4141 initial references only 81 references explicitly mentioned interoperability issues and, within these 81 references, only eight reported end-to-end solutions that can be integrated and usable in care service provision.

Keywords: eHealth · Pervasive health · Interoperability · Home monitoring

1 Background

During the last two decades, there was a considerable increase in the capacity to develop and manufacture systems that employ smart components highly integrated and miniaturized [1]. Because of this remarkable development, ubiquitous computing is nowadays part of our everyday and social life and impacts our surrounding environments.

According to the vision of Weiser [2], ubiquitous computing aims the enhancement of the computer use by bringing computing devices into everyday life (e.g. integration

© Springer Nature Switzerland AG 2019
A. Cliquet jr. et al. (Eds.): BIOSTEC 2018, CCIS 1024, pp. 279–297, 2019.
https://doi.org/10.1007/978-3-030-29196-9_15

of computing power and sensing features into anything, including everyday objects like white goods, toys or furniture), making them available throughout the physical environment in such a way that the users would not notice their presence. In turn, ubiquitous communication comprises multiple technologies to allow the interaction among multiple devices anytime and anywhere.

Pervasive health has emerged as a specialization of eHealth and deals with the application of ubiquitous computing [3, 4] for health and wellness management, aiming to make health care more seamlessly to our everyday life [5]. Pervasive health can contribute, with different roles, to personalize health and wellness services promoting an evolution from a medical approach to individual-centric operational models, in which the individual becomes an active partner in the care process [5].

Health care services are highly mobile in nature [6] and involve multiple locations (e.g. clinics, outpatients' services or patients' homes), particularly when dealing with older adults and their respective major diseases [7]: cardiovascular disease, hypertension, stroke, diabetes, cancer, chronic obstructive pulmonary disease, musculoskeletal conditions, mental health conditions or visual impairment and blindness. Therefore, the pervasive health landscape includes mobile health (mHealth) application. For that smartphones are fairly robust, truly pervasive and accessible - they are accessible to over 90% of the global population [1] - and they provide ubiquitous user interfaces and have the ability to collect, store and communicate information [1]. Furthermore, an interesting feature of smartphone devices is the availability of short-distance wireless data transmission, such as Bluetooth [6]. This enables the smartphone applications to work with a wide range of hardware devices (e.g. glucose meters, pulse oximeter or thermometers) from different vendors.

Meeting the specific individual needs, namely providing care services at individuals' home together with intelligent applications, is one of the main strategies to guarantee independent living of older people [8]. Considering this context, important goals are to promote personal assistance (e.g. medication reminder) and distance support (e.g. telerehabilitation programs) or to provide the caregiver with accurate and up-to-date information in order to be delivered the right care at the right time (e.g. continuous monitoring of physiological parameters or behaviors, emotions and activities), which can contribute to the overall effort to provide personalized and affordable access to essential services with efficacy and efficiency [9–11]. Therefore, a typical pervasive health application consists in monitoring health conditions or the progress of some chronic diseases.

For monitoring applications, sensors are required to collect relevant physiological data. A wide range of sensors, including pressure and thermal sensors, might be used to measure blood pressure, body temperature, blood glucose, heart sound, heart rate, respiration, respiratory rate, blood oxygen saturation or perspiration. Some sensors are non-invasive, but various biological signals require invasive sensors such as electrodes. Non-invasive wearable and textile devices present a considerable potential, and, for instance, they allow measuring physiological parameters through the use of techniques such as infrared or optical sensing [12].

In health care delivery, there is significant amount of information available, so the problem is less the volume and more the value that is created with the available information. Major difficulties are related to the aggregation of information from different sources, with different formats and meanings, as well as the lack of tools to identify, within all the available information, the one that is relevant for each particular situation and to make it useful rather than just being visible [13].

The information is no longer stored and exclusively managed by the Electronic Health Records (EHR) of the health care institutions [14–17]. Although EHR are adequate for the presentation of information from patients, collected and aggregated in local healthcare information systems, the reality is that the provision of health care is not restricted to an institution or even to a single care provision system. All caregivers need comprehensive, up-to-date, safe and congruent information from the patient, immediately accessible at the place of care, to ensure the highest levels of clinical quality. For instance, when considering the home monitoring of a patient with a chronic disease (e.g. diabetes, heart failure or chronic obstructive pulmonary disease), the resulting monitoring information should be distributed within an information network ranging from clinicians, social care network, and family members to the patients themselves. These requirements promote the emergence of new technological approaches such as Personal Health Record (PHR) [18] that aimed at electronic management of information between the patients and their formal and informal health care providers, and that might contribute to the availability of the patients' clinical information that is collected throughout their lives [13].

However, the implementation of this vision is bounded by a set of problems: for instance, clinical information is blocked in healthcare information systems silos, generated and stored in different systems that either do not communicate with one another or are unable to synthesize information to make it meaningful and usable. Therefore, interoperability must be ensured, in terms of communications protocols and semantic normalization, between a wide range of information sources and eHealth applications. Hence, efforts carried out by international institutions such as the Continua Health Alliance, the Health Care Information and Management Systems Society (HIMSS), the National Institute of Standards and Technology (NIST) and the Integrating the Healthcare Enterprise (IHE), have been crucial to overcome interoperability difficulties and to promote a homogeneous eHealth ecosystem [19].

According to the European Commission [20], interoperability is a key precondition for ensuring more and better coordination and integration in health care delivery, which includes health information sharing.

The need to ensure technological and semantic interoperability in the European context is reinforced, with a set of objectives such as: defining guidelines for the type of data to be included in patient summaries, developing standards and specifications (e.g. for technological and semantic interoperability) and the promotion of systems for testing and certifying the interoperability of solutions. The Commission therefore proposes a greater effort in the development and validation of specifications and components. This effort should be extended to the pervasive health developments [21, 22].

There are also two other dimensions of interoperability mentioned in the European Commission's report [20], which should be stated, given the importance they are assumed to have in achieving the objectives of the health services. These are organizational and legal interoperability. Organizational interoperability is directly related to the integration of processes (and conditions of information sharing between organizations) in order not to compromise collaborative work. Concerning the legal framework, there are a number of legal issues related to the issue of interoperability, such as those relating to data protection rules for patients and citizens, as well as regulatory issues (e.g. lack of definition of the roles of the various actors in the system) around mHealth applications, which offer more possibilities for self-administration of care.

Given this background, the main purpose of the systematic review reported in the present article was to explore if interoperability is a real concern when developing concrete pervasive solutions (e.g. telehealth, mHealth or ambient assisted living applications) to gather patients' information, both clinical and contextual information.

2 Methods

The purpose of this systematic review was to identify and analyse in more detail articles related to home monitoring, which reveal an explicit concern with interoperability requirements. The general goals of this systematic review, that extends the results present in [23] were to identify, within the selected references, how interoperability is addressed in the solutions being proposed, how they are validated and if there is effective technological and semantic interoperability. The goal of this analysis was to assess if, in addition to allowing information sharing, the solutions proposed are able to produce meaningful and contextualized information that can be integrated into EHR, that is, if the information they collect is qualified to be integrated and usable in the care service provision. Moreover, if this is the case, it is important to identify the healthcare interoperability standards that are most commonly used.

2.1 Study Design

Considered the aforementioned purposes, the systematic review of the present study was informed by the following research question: Is there an explicit concern related to interoperability during the development of new eHealth applications to gather patients' information in their home environments?

Within references selected as expressing an effective concern related to interoperability, some sub-questions were raised:

- What are the target users being considered?
- What interoperability solutions are being proposed?
- What healthcare interoperability standards are being used?
- Which methods are being used to validate the proposed interoperability implementations?

To achieve these goals, initially, a systematic review of literature published between 2011 and 2017 was performed.

Exclusively the references that had the keywords "interoperability" or "interoperable" in title or abstract were considered for further assessment and classification, being excluded the first group of references.

Subsequently, the references included for analysis were assessed and some more were excluded reflecting specified criteria, which is described below. The remaining references were then categorized according to the degree of significance to answer the questions posed within this research, that is to say, the option was to analyse in greater depth the references that proposed solutions in which it was assumed as relevant that the information produced could be integrated into the health care service provision.

The methods used to conduct this systematic review of literature as well as the subsequent categorization of search results is described in the following subsections.

2.2 Data Sources and Searches

The research was carried out using the Scopus, Web of Science and IEEE Xplore Digital Library databases, in the publications titles, abstracts and keywords.

The keywords used in the search, simultaneously, were: "monitoring" and "pervasive health", since these are the topics around which it is important to evaluate the centrality of the interoperability issue. Pervasive health is seen as a contribution to a more personalized model of care allowing individuals to be more actively involved in their care process. A classic pervasive health care application is home monitoring of health conditions, particularly patients with chronic diseases. However, it is important to note that pervasive health is more than monitoring applications as it can also include preventive applications (e.g. elderly people to live independently) [24].

The remaining keywords were: "mobile health", "mhealth" and "ambient assisted living". These keywords were combined so that at least one of them corresponded to the subject of the search.

2.3 Inclusion and Exclusion Criteria

References with no author, no abstract, not written in English, duplicates and editorials were excluded. References selected for review were all written in English and all who had a date of publication between 2011 and 2017. Then, all the references that did not explicitly mention the "interoperability" or "interoperable" keywords in tittle and/or in abstract were also rejected.

Subsequently, within the references' full texts revised, those that corresponded to items out of ambit of this systematic review were also excluded. Then, in the group of references within the scope of this systematic review, were also identified and excluded those references that corresponded to categories to be rejected in view of the objectives of this analysis, specifically: overviews, political perspectives, position papers, reviews and systematic reviews.

Then, the remaining references were clustered in ascending order of importance for this study: connection between devices; intermediate components between the devices and the client applications for handling the storage and sharing of the information being gathered (e.g. architectures, gateways, middleware or data hubs); intermediate components but incorporating medical devices specificities; and end-to-end solutions.

2.4   Study Selection

After the first screening, one author assessed all titles for relevance. Those clearly not meeting the inclusion criteria were removed.

Afterwards, the abstracts of the retrieved articles were assessed against the inclusion and exclusion criteria, by two authors. Any disagreements were discussed with a third reviewer and resolved by consensus. Abstracts were then subject to a first classification and grouping.

Finally, the references that were selected by the superior interest for this study were gathered and analysed in more detail. Two authors, according to the outlines criteria, then assessed again these full texts thought to be of relevance, and any divergences were also discussed with a third reviewer and agreed by consensus.

3   Results

This systematic review followed the guidelines of the Preferred Reporting Items for Systematic Reviews and Meta-Analyses (PRISMA) [25], as described in Fig. 1.

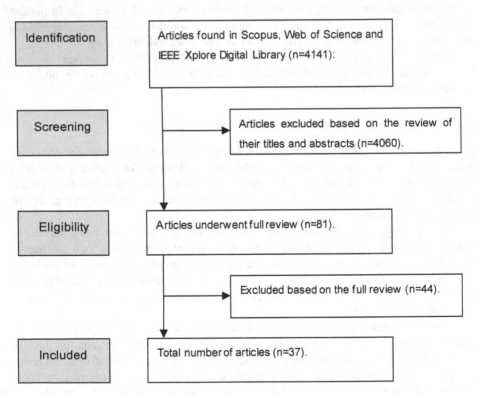

Fig. 1.   PRISMA flowchart (extended from [23]).

After the initial database search, 4141 references were considered for the next phase. Then, 4060 of these references were rejected because they did not explicitly mention "interoperability" or "interoperable" in the tittle and/or in the abstract.

Afterwards, by reviewing these 81 references' full-texts, 44 were excluded: the first 30 references grouped and classified are articles assumed as out of the scope of this study; other cluster (n = 14) are references that, although within the ambit of the present analysis, were also excluded because they correspond to position papers (n = 5), systematic reviews (n = 3), reviews (n = 1), overviews (n = 2) and political standpoints (n = 3).

The remaining 37 references were first clustered in ascending order of importance for this study.

3.1 Characteristics of the Studies

The purpose of the 37 references selected for this systematic review is presented in Table 1. The studies were categorized according to different aspects of interoperability:

- Sensors aggregation: four references [26–29] describe solutions providing communication protocols to network a large number of sensors.
- Data aggregation: 23 references report solutions to aggregate data from various sources to provide it in an integrated way to client applications [30–52]. These articles, though being related to health care applications, they do not allude to interoperability standards used in health care, inhibiting the information that is produced from being integrated into the health care service provision. However, what is described in the type of solutions proposed in three references [31, 33, 39], explicitly refer the use of health care standards, considering the specificity of medical devices (e.g. the already established ISO/IEEE 11073 standards-based Continua personal health ecosystem - X73 protocol [33]).
- End-to-end solutions: ten references [53–62] propose interoperability solutions to ensure that the information produced could be integrated into the health care provision.

Table 1. Scope of the included articles.

ID	Year	Aim	Categorization
[30]	2011	To present the design and implementation of a distributed information infrastructure using intelligent agent paradigm to perform continuous health monitoring	Data aggregation
[26]	2012	To present the design, implementation and test of a framework aimed at supporting Ambient Assisted Living applications, allowing for monitoring and remote-control purposes	Sensors aggregation
[31]	2012	To present a unified interoperable open ambient assisted living platform that incorporates existing ambient assisted living platform concepts and includes the already established ISO/IEEE 11073 standards-based Continua Personal Health ecosystem	Data aggregation
[32]	2013	To present a modular, extensible and scalable sensor middleware, from the design and implementation perspective	Data aggregation

(*continued*)

Table 1. (*continued*)

ID	Year	Aim	Categorization
[33]	2013	To present a system to offer plug-and-play connectivity of ambient assisted living devices	Data aggregation
[34]	2013	To report an interoperable health-assistive platform designed to meet the requirements of the current health services to support the elderly population in their own environment	Data aggregation
[35]	2013	To present the design and development of a basic ambient assisted living application devoted to physical activity monitoring by exploiting open platform and tools	Data aggregation
[53]	2013	To propose a mobile vital sign measurement and data collection system for chronic disease management based on a middleware platform that transmits patient clinical data for services and a messaging interface for interoperability of clinical data exchange were implemented	End-to-end solution
[36]	2013	To present a universal platform for both ambient assisted living and personal health applications	Data aggregation
[37]	2013	To present an extensible, scalable, and customizable platform able to operate in the cloud	Data aggregation
[57]	2014	To present the design of a platform that enables the integration of heterogeneous health related information, the orchestration services and deployment of mobile services independent of mobile device, operating system or network	End-to-end solution
[38]	2014	To present a collaborative network of services and devices aiming to build a heterogeneous ecosystem	Data aggregation
[55]	2014	To present an architecture able to capture, store, merge and process data from various sensor systems at people's home and to provide it integrated into a regional health information system	End-to-end solution
[56]	2014	To present a mobile healthcare application to provide self-diabetes management and able to synchronize data with hospital's EHRs	End-to-end solution
[39]	2014	To present a service-oriented middleware to integrate existing devices or applications in a residential setting	Data aggregation
[40]	2014	To present a platform for ambient assisted living that includes smart objects to monitor activities of daily living and detect any abnormal behaviour that may represent a danger or highlight symptoms of some incipient disease features of home automation	Data aggregation
[41]	2015	To present a conceptual home sensing architecture and a modular device gateway to combine multiple sources and clients of perceptual and actuator devices	Data aggregation
[27]	2015	To present a data format suitable for collection of multiple sensor data	Sensors aggregation
[54]	2015	To present a safe therapy mobile system to support intravenous chemotherapy, and a home monitoring system for monitoring and managing toxicity and improving adherence in patients receiving oral anticancer therapies at home	End-to-end solution

(continued)

Table 1. (*continued*)

ID	Year	Aim	Categorization
[58]	2015	To present a platform that supports personalized smart services to primary users, using advised sensing, context-aware and cloud-based lifestyle reasoning in its design	End-to-end solution
[42]	2015	To present a sensor observation service, able to be executed in low resources devices and allowing interoperability and scalability	Data aggregation
[43]	2015	To present a multi-modal system architecture for ambient assisted living remote healthcare monitoring in the home, able to collect information from multiple (sensor) data sources	Data aggregation
[44]	2016	To present an integrated access gateway, which provides standard interfaces for supporting various applications in home environments, ranging from on-site configuration to node and service access	Data aggregation
[28]	2016	To present an assisted living solution for elderly people based on wireless sensors networking technology	Sensors aggregation
[29]	2016	To present a system able to promote interoperability in ambient assisted living environments, supported in a wireless sensor network, based on IPv6 IP protocol	Sensors aggregation
[59]	2016	To present the development and evaluation of a mobile health application to ensure the interoperability of various personal health devices (PHDs) and electronic medical record systems (EHRs) for continuous self-management of chronic disease patients	End-to-end solution
[45]	2016	To present two platforms addressing two problems: the lack of appropriate user interfaces for the heterogeneous user group of future smart homes and the low interoperability between different smart home systems	Data aggregation
[60]	2016	To present a technological solution of a tele-assistance process for stroke patients in acute phase, which aims to reduce time from symptom onset to treatment of acute phase stroke patients	End-to-end solution
[46]	2016	To present a platform to globally locate and retrieve sensors and actuators respectively adhering to the attributes and behaviours of integral mirrors in the virtual world; to enable the interoperability between virtual and real worlds	Data aggregation
[47]	2017	To allow the use of different smart objects, able to communicate among each other, in a cloud base infrastructure, for the development of services to assist elderly people and their caregivers	Data aggregation
[48]	2017	To provide a framework for home monitoring systems based on a cloud computing platform	Data aggregation
[49]	2017	To improve the feasibility of reference architectures in developing systems of systems	Data aggregation

(*continued*)

Table 1. (*continued*)

ID	Year	Aim	Categorization
[50]	2017	To provide service continuity within the living environment, both indoor and outdoor, by combining technological aids and mobile technologies to facilitate independent living for all in the home or in temporary living environments	Data aggregation
[51]	2017	To propose a smart IoT gateway as a key component to enable the interoperability from several heterogeneous devices over different communication protocols and technologies	Data aggregation
[52]	2017	To present the design, implementation, deployment and evaluation of a human activity detection application	Data aggregation
[61]	2017	To present a prototype implementing a HL7 compatible personal health record system	End-to-end solution
[62]	2017	To provide patients with a unified view of their scattered health records, and healthcare providers access up-to-date data regarding their patients	End-to-end solution

Moreover, Fig. 2 presents the temporal distribution of the selected studies.

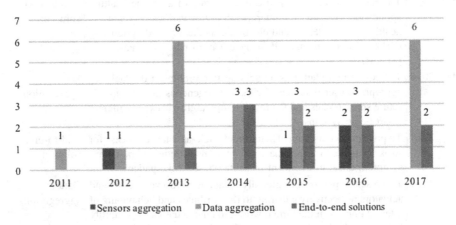

■Sensors aggregation   ■Data aggregation   ■End-to-end solutions

Fig. 2. Evolution of the number of articles per year between 2011 and 2017.

3.2 Target Users

Among the included articles, 19 report studies aiming to develop solutions to support elderly people in their residential environment [29, 31, 33–36, 38–41, 43, 45–47, 49, 51, 52, 55, 58], four articles report studies targeting patients with chronic conditions (i.e. diabetes [56], cardiovascular diseases [60, 62] and cancer [54]) and the remainder articles do not refer the target users or refer that the target users are patients, without specifying their pathologies.

3.3   Interoperability

The main problem being addressed here is the lack of interoperability among different levels of available technologies which restricts a wider deployment among intermediate and end-users [39], therefore the demand for interoperability among devices is emphasized as most commercially available devices include their own software and communication protocols, which cause serious problems and hinder the application of a standard [33]. Therefore, the shortfalls of dominating insulated available products are highlighted [31].

Concerning the type of interoperability computational support, different solutions' designations are reported although they pursue the same objective, which is the aggregation of data from multiple sources to provide them in an integrated way to client applications, namely: architectures [36–38, 43, 44, 46], gateways [38, 41, 44, 45], middleware [32, 35] or data hub [43].

To address interoperability, the references reported different communication protocols, including Bluetooth Health Device Profile (HDP) [39] and Open Services Gateway initiative (OSGi), a framework for modular systems that simplifies building, deploying, and managing complex applications. OSGi is complemented with the X73 standard data model, which allowed, for instance, the modelling of the information being gathered [33] so that the information resulting from different ambient assisted living systems might be integrated [31].

Next, it will be referred the ten articles (within the 81 references assessed for inclusion) that have been highlighted by this systematic review. These ten articles correspond to end-to-end solutions and they report an effective concern related to the interoperability issue, proposing concrete solutions to ensure that the information produced could be integrated into the health care provision, as summarized in Table 2.

Considering these references [53–62], which were subject to a depth analysis, in all the solutions reported the focus is on guaranteeing integration of information, being reported in every case that the resulting information is ready to be integrated in the health care service provision. However, concerning this issue, in some cases more details are given than others.

The integration of information from existing eHealth applications to provide integrated data analysis is a central concern [57]. In particular the demand to ensure interoperability of various Personal Health Devices (PHDs) and EHR for continuous monitoring and self-management of patients with chronic diseases [53–56, 58–60]. The need to provide sensor data in proven standard form is denoted, as the existing coding systems do not appear to be sufficient to encode the data resulting from a variety of sensors [55]. Thus, current solutions are considered to lack interoperability and obstruct the establishment of a remote patient monitoring solution market [58]. Three references are particularly focused on the need to find more advanced solutions to guarantee interconnection with the EHR as well as to improve, optimize and reduce the time in care in particular pathologies, specifically diabetes [56], cancer [54] and stroke [60].

Table 2. Problem addressed, solution and computational support (extended from [23]).

ID	Problem addressed	Interoperability computational support	Proposed solution
[57]	The need to integrate data from existing eHealth applications to provide integrated analysis	Technological engine to integrate data from existing eHealth applications on a service and information level	An Integrated eHealth Platform that consists of two sub-platforms: the health integration and analysis platform and a communications platform composed by a mobile messaging module and a mobile applications gateway
[54]	Allow oncological patients to alert health care professionals automatically in real time when necessary	Web-based, multi-tier architecture	A safe therapy mobile (STM) system for the safe delivery of intravenous chemotherapy, and a home monitoring system for monitoring and managing toxicity and improving adherence in patients receiving oral anticancer therapies at home
[55]	To surpass the inappropriate clinical documents representation	An architectural approach with a centralized registration of placeholder-documents and a decentralized data storage at peoples' home	Open Services Gateway initiative (OSGi)-framework, which runs in a Java virtual machine and the lightweight MQTT protocol for internal communication
[56]	Interconnection of PHR-EHR interconnection	A mHealth application that interfaces with hospital EHR	A PHR service, interconnected with a mHealth application, able to synchronize with EHR system from tertiary hospitals
[53]	Difficulties in identifying and filtering specific patients' data among the data coming from personal devices, to be sent to care providers	A self-organized software platform based	A middleware using Multi-Agent platform in SOS (Self-Organizing System) platform that transmits patient clinical data for services based on interoperability standards
[58]	The need to provide sensor data in standardized formats	A cloud gateway be deployed under predefined guidelines	Interoperable caring home system offering personalized context-aware applications

(continued)

Table 2. (*continued*)

ID	Problem addressed	Interoperability computational support	Proposed solution
[59]	The need to ensure the interoperability of various PHDs and EHR for continuous self-management of chronic disease patients	Definition of an end-to-end architecture to connect EHRs and PHD	Communication of PHD data (e.g. blood pressure monitor, weight scale, glucometer, pulse oximeter) using healthcare interoperability standards
[60]	Critical factors that difficult the access to better therapies and advanced medical devices within the first 4–5 h (from the onset of symptoms) of patients with stroke	A technological platform that supports the defined process following an interoperability model based on standards and on a service-oriented architecture	Integration between mobile EHR system from public companies for healthcare emergencies and EHR systems of the reference hospitals
[61]	The need of communication between PHR and EHR	A FHIR client to communicate with other systems equipped by an FHIR server	Standard information exchange between a PHR system used by patients and the healthcare information system used by physicians
[62]	The need of the patients to have a unified view of their scattered health records, as well as the need of the healthcare providers access up-to-date data regarding their patients	A distributed architecture model to integrate personal health records	A distributed model to integrate PHRs

In order to address interoperability, the reported solutions include, for instance: an application, the self-management mobile PHR that communicates with PHDs (e.g. blood pressure monitor or pulse oximeter) that have implemented standard protocols so that stored vital signs are converted to HL7 and are transmitted to PHR [59]; a PHR service, interconnected with mHealth applications that use clinical information from the EHR system from a tertiary hospital to provide services to support patients with chronic diseases, such as diabetes patients [56]; an architectural approach to integrate Home-Centred Health-Enabling Technology into Regional Health Information Systems; and a centralized registration of placeholder-documents and a decentralized data storage at patients' home, using the Systematic Nomenclature for Contexts, Analysis methods and Problems in Health Enabling Technologies (SNOCAP-HET), which is a nomenclature to describe the context of sensor-based measurements in health-enabling technologies [55].

3.4 Interoperability Standards

Regarding the healthcare interoperability standards applied in the proposed solutions, the choice of HL7 was made in most of the solutions in which standardized solutions are reported [53, 55, 58, 59, 61, 62]. X73 Standard Data Model was used in four cases [31, 33, 58, 59] and X73 with HL7 V2.6 was used in two cases [58, 59]. Other standards were stated such as: Bluetooth Health Device Profile [39], Continuity of Care Document (CCD) and Continuity of Care Record (CCR) [59], the standards based on Continua Personal Health ecosystem [31], openEHR [62], LOINC [62], SNOMED-CT [62], DICOM [62], CEN/ISO 13606, which has been designed to support the semantic interoperability of the communications between EHR [60], and FHIR [61, 62].

3.5 Validation

Finally, concerning the methods used to validate the proposed interoperability solutions (Table 3), in one of the cases the evaluation was carried out by meaningful use [53], in another case, after laboratory tested, it was adopted as a routine in two hospitals, having also been investigated its usability and acceptance within professionals using the system [54], and in other cases the options were the proof of concept [38, 58], prototype [28, 29, 33, 37, 44, 46, 57], simulation [48, 50, 60, 62], case study [35, 42], scenarios implementation [30], and clinical trial [59]. In the remaining cases, the validation methods were not reported.

As an example, a clinical trial was carried out to evaluate the transmission error rate for the measured vital signs transmitted from PHD to an mHealth application and from this to PHR Systems [59]. Another case was the technological platform that was tested with clinician staff, researchers, electronic support staff and actors playing patients role, having been defined several scenarios to test the technological structure, being stated that, after this phase, the platform would be tested with patients suffering from clinical suspicion of stroke [60].

Table 3. Validation (extended from [23]).

ID	Validation
[35, 42]	Case study
[47, 49, 51, 52, 54]	Laboratory tests
[28, 29, 33, 37, 44, 46, 57]	Prototype
[55]	Future work
[30]	Scenarios implementation
[53]	Meaningful use
[38, 58]	Proof of concept
[59]	Clinical trial
[48, 50, 60, 62]	Simulation

4 Conclusion

Considering the target users of the applications being reported, surprisingly in most articles the specifications are quite vague (i.e. elderly or patients, in general). Only four articles do specifically refer which are the target users (i.e. patients suffering from diabetes, cardiovascular diseases or cancer).

A central challenge for healthcare applications is how to handle the complexity and variability caused by the specificities of the healthcare processes. Deeper analyses of the healthcare process reveal the intricacy and the changeability of the clinical information and, therefore, the difficulties in dealing with information interoperability. The vague description of the target users and the respective health conditions precludes that additional elicitations of requirements are needed, which will increase the costs and the density of the resulting implementations.

The design and implementation of pervasive health applications has not yet reached its potential in terms of impact it can have on health care provision, and interoperability is assumed as being an essential requirement. In this respect, the included articles reporting end-to-end solutions aimed to turn possible PHD connected in conjunction with institutional EHR systems. For that, the studies propose interoperability platforms able to gather and distribute the clinical information [53–55, 57, 58, 60], or applications able to guarantee a common understanding between PHD and EHRs, using a diversity of standards (e.g. HL7, CEN/ISO 13606 or X73). In all the solutions reported the focus is on guaranteeing integration of information, being stated in every case that the resulting information is ready to be integrated in the health care service provision, although in only half of the cases the details concerning this issue, are given more objectively. The integration of information from pervasive health applications to provide integrated data analysis should be a concern. Current solutions lacking interoperability might obstruct the establishment of a remote patient monitoring solution market.

In terms of the validation of the solutions being proposed, only one study [59] included a clinical trial. However, evidence-based medicine is supported on statistical significance and the new developments must be conveniently evaluated in real world conditions. It is necessary to go behind studies aiming the design, development and evaluation of prototypes (i.e. proof-of-concept).

The results of the systematic review presented in this article show that interoperability is not the major concern of a significant number of current technological developments related to pervasive health. Indeed, it should be emphasized that of the 4141 initial references only 81 references explicitly mentioned the issue of interoperability. Moreover, within these 81 references assessed for inclusion, only ten corresponded to end-to-end solutions, since the information produced could be integrated into the health care service provision, where interoperability was considered an effective concern. Finally, within these ten references only three refer standards specifically related to semantic interoperability, used in a system whose validation is not yet reported.

Therefore, large-scale collaboration among technology developers, companies, policy makers, patient's organizations and health professionals are essential for pervasive health surpass the interoperability challenge.

References

1. Cook, D.J., Das, S.K.: Pervasive computing at scale: transforming the state of the art. Pervasive Mob. Comput. **8**(1), 22–35 (2012)
2. Weiser, M.: Hot topics: ubiquitous computing. IEEE Comput. **26**(10), 71–72 (1993)
3. Cook, D.J., Augusto, J.C., Jakkula, V.R.: Ambient intelligence, applications, and opportunities. Pervasive Mob. Comput. **5**(4), 277–298 (2009)
4. Connelly, K., et al.: The future of pervasive health. IEEE Pervasive Comput. **16**(1), 16–20 (2017)
5. Korhonen, I., Barddram, J.: Guest editorial introduction to the special section on pervasive healthcare. IEEE Trans. Inf. Technol. Biomed. **8**(3), 229 (2004)
6. Mosa, A., Yoo, I., Sheets, L.: A systematic review of healthcare applications for smartphones. BMC Med. Inform. Decis. Mak. **12**(1), 67 (2012)
7. Heath, I.: Never had it so good? BMJ **336**(7650), 950–951 (2008)
8. Kleinberger, T., Becker, M., Ras, E., Holzinger, A., Müller, P.: Ambient intelligence in assisted living: enable elderly people to handle future interfaces. In: Stephanidis, C. (ed.) UAHCI 2007. LNCS, vol. 4555, pp. 103–112. Springer, Heidelberg (2007). https://doi.org/10.1007/978-3-540-73281-5_11
9. Kapoor, A.: New frontiers in machine learning for predictive user modeling. In: Human-Centric Interfaces for Ambient Intelligence. Academic Press, Oxford (2010)
10. Mirarmandehi, N.: An asynchronous dynamic bayesian network for activity recognition in an Ambient Intelligent environment. In: Pervasive Computing and Applications (ICPCA) (2010)
11. Queirós, A., Carvalho, S., Pavão, J., Rocha, N.: AAL information based services and care integration. In: Healthinf 2013 - Proceedings of the International Conference on Health Informatics. SciTePress (2013)
12. Rashidi, P., Mihailidis, A.: A survey on ambient-assisted living tools for older adults. IEEE J. Biomed. Health Inform. **17**(3), 579–590 (2013)
13. Halevy, A.: Game-changing interoperability for healthcare: bringing semantically harmonized clinical information into provider workflows from disparate health information technologies. In: 8th International Conference and Expo on Emerging Technologies for a Smarter World, CEWIT 2011 (2011). https://doi.org/10.1109/cewit.2011.6135863
14. Emery, D., Heyes, B.J., Cowan, A.M.: Telecare delivery of health and social care information. Health Inform. J. **8**(1), 29–33 (2002)
15. Eysenbach, G.: What is e-health? J. Med. Internet Res. **3**(2), E20 (2001). https://doi.org/10.2196/jmir.3.2.e20 [Medline: 11720962]
16. Kvedar, J., Coye, M.J., Everett, W.: Connected health: a review of technologies and strategies to improve patient care with telemedicine and telehealth. Health Aff. (Millwood) **33**(2), 194–199 (2014). https://doi.org/10.1377/hlthaff.2013.0992 [Medline: 24493760]
17. Rossi, M.A., Mazzeo, M., Mercurio, G., Verbicaro, R.: Holistic health: predicting our data future (from inter-operability among systems to co-operability among people). Int. J. Med. Inform. **82**(4), e14–e28 (2013). https://doi.org/10.1016/j.ijmedinf.2012.09.003 [Medline: 23122923]
18. Krukowski, A., et al.: Personal health record. In: Voros, N.S., Antonopoulos, C.P. (eds.) Cyberphysical Systems for Epilepsy and Related Brain Disorders, pp. 205–238. Springer, Cham (2015). https://doi.org/10.1007/978-3-319-20049-1_11

19. Aragüés, A., et al.: Trends and challenges of the emerging technologies toward interoperability and standardization in e-Health communications. IEEE Commun. Mag. **49** (11), 182–188 (2011). https://doi.org/10.1109/MCOM.2011.6069727

20. European Commission Communication from the Commission to the European Parliament, the Council, the European Economic and Social Committee and the Committee of the Regions: eHealth Action Plan 2012–2020 - Innovative healthcare for the 21st century. European Commission, Brussels (2012). https://ec.europa.eu/digital-single-market/en/news/ehealth-action-plan-2012-2020-innovative-healthcare-21st-century. Accessed 06 June 2018

21. Kuziemsky, C.E., Peyton, L.A.: framework for understanding process interoperability and health information technology. Health Policy Technol. **5**(2), 196–203 (2016). https://doi.org/10.1016/j.hlpt.2016.02.007

22. Perlin, J.B.: Health information technology interoperability and use for better care and evidence. JAMA – J. Am. Med. Assoc. **316**(16), 1667–1668 (2016). https://doi.org/10.1001/jama.2016.12337

23. Dias, A., Martins, A., Queirós, A., Pacheco, R.N.: Interoperability in pervasive health: is it tackled as a priority? In: Proceedings of the 11th International Joint Conference on Biomedical Engineering Systems and Technologies – HEALTHINF, vol. 5, pp. 57–65 (2018). ISBN 978-989-758-281-3. https://doi.org/10.5220/0006545400570065

24. Queirós, A., et al.: Pervasive health and regulatory frameworks. In: Verdier, C., Bienkiewicz, M., Fred, A., Gamboa, H., Elias, D. (eds.) BIOSTEC 2015, Proceedings of the International Joint Conference on Biomedical Engineering Systems and Technologies, vol. 5, pp. 494–501 (2015). https://doi.org/10.5220/0005249204940501

25. Moher, D., Liberati, A., Tetzlaff, J., Altman, D.G.: Preferred reporting items for systematic reviews and meta-analyses: the PRISMA statement. PLoS Med. **6**(7), e1000097 (2009). https://doi.org/10.1371/journal.pmed.1000097

26. Grossi, F., Bianchi, V., Losardo, A., Matrella, G., De Munari, I., Ciampolini, P.: A flexible framework for ambient assisted living applications. In: IASTED International Conference on Assistive Technologies Proceedings, AT 2012, pp. 817–824 (2012). https://doi.org/10.2316/p.2012.766-007

27. Escobar, R., Akopian, D., Boppana, R.: A sensor data format incorporating battery charge information for smartphone-based mHealth applications. In: SPIE - The International Society for Optical Engineering Proceedings, vol. 9411 (2015). https://doi.org/10.1117/12.2083758

28. Elsaadi, R., Shafik, M.: Deployment of assisted living technology using intelligent body sensors platform for elderly people health monitoring. Adv. Transdisc. Eng. **3**, 219–224 (2016). https://doi.org/10.3233/978-1-61499-668-2-219

29. Palma, L., Pernini, L., Belli, A., Valenti, S., Maurizi, L., Pierleoni, P.: IPv6 WSN solution for integration and interoperation between smart home and AAL systems. In: SAS 2016 - Sensors Applications Symposium Proceedings, pp. 171–175 (2016). https://doi.org/10.1109/sas.2016.7479840

30. Su, C., Wu, C.: JADE implemented mobile multi-agent based, distributed information platform for pervasive health care monitoring. Appl. Soft Comput. J. **11**(1), 315–325 (2011). https://doi.org/10.1016/j.asoc.2009.11.022

31. Norgall, T., Wichert, R.: Towards interoperability and integration of personal health and AAL ecosystems. Stud. Health Technol. Inform. **177**, 272–282 (2012). https://doi.org/10.3233/978-1-61499-069-7-272

32. Carr, D., O'Grady, M.J., O'Hare, G.M.P., Collier, R.: SIXTH: a middleware for supporting ubiquitous sensing in personal health monitoring (2013). https://doi.org/10.1007/978-3-642-37893-5_47_e

33. Damas, M., Pomares, H., Gonzalez, S., Olivares, A., Rojas, I.: Ambient assisted living devices interoperability based on OSGi and the X73 standard. Telemed. e-Health **19**(1), 54–60 (2013). https://doi.org/10.1089/tmj.2012.0052

34. Ferreira, L., Ambrósio, P.: Towards an interoperable health-assistive environment: the eHealthCom platform. In: IEEE-EMBS International Conference on Biomedical and Health Informatics Proceedings: Global Grand Challenge of Health Informatics, BHI 2012, pp. 930–932 (2012). https://doi.org/10.1109/bhi.2012.6211740

35. Kilintzis, V., Moulos, I., Koutkias, V., Maglaveras, N.: Exploiting the universAAL platform for the design and development of a physical activity monitoring application. In: ACM International Conference Proceeding Series (2013). https://doi.org/10.1145/2504335.2504351

36. Norgall, T., Wichert, R.: Personalized use of ICT-from telemonitoring to ambient assisted living. Stud. Health Technol. Inform. **187**, 145–151 (2013). https://doi.org/10.3233/978-1-61499-256-1-145

37. Ruiz-Zafra, Á., Benghazi, K., Noguera, M., Garrido, J.L.: Zappa: an open mobile platform to build cloud-based m-Health systems. In: van Berlo, A., Hallenborg, K., Rodríguez, J., Tapia, D., Novais, P. (eds.) Ambient Intelligence - Software and Applications. AISC, vol. 219, pp. 87–94. Springer, Heidelberg (2013). https://doi.org/10.1007/978-3-319-00566-9_12

38. Costa, A., Novais, P., Simoes, R.: An AAL collaborative system: the AAL4ALL and a mobile assistant case study. In: Camarinha-Matos, L.M., Afsarmanesh, H. (eds.) PRO-VE 2014. IAICT, vol. 434, pp. 699–709. Springer, Heidelberg (2014). https://doi.org/10.1007/978-3-662-44745-1_69

39. Pereira, R., Barros, C., Pereira, S., Mendes, P.M., Silva, C.A.: A middleware for intelligent environments in ambient assisted living. In: Annual International Conference of the IEEE Engineering in Medicine and Biology Society, IEEE Engineering in Medicine and Biology Society. Annual Conference, pp. 5924–5927 (2014). https://doi.org/10.1109/embc.2014.6944977

40. Rossi, L., et al.: Interoperability issues among smart home technological frameworks. In: MESA 2014 – 10th IEEE/ASME International Conference on Mechatronic and Embedded Systems and Applications, Conference Proceedings (2014). https://doi.org/10.1109/mesa.2014.6935626

41. Denkovski, D., Atanasovski, V., Gavrilovska, L.: Device gateway design for ambient assisted living. In: Atanasovski, V., Leon-Garcia, A. (eds.) FABULOUS 2015. LNICST, vol. 159, pp. 100–107. Springer, Cham (2015). https://doi.org/10.1007/978-3-319-27072-2_13

42. Pradilla, J., Palau, C., Esteve, M.: SOSLITE: lightweight sensor observation service (SOS) for the internet of things (IOT). In: 2015 ITU Kaleidoscope: Trust in the Information Society (K-2015), Barcelona, pp. 1–7 (2015). https://doi.org/10.1109/kaleidoscope.2015.7383625

43. Woznowski, P., et al.: A multi-modal sensor infrastructure for healthcare in a residential environment. In: 2015 IEEE International Conference on Communication Workshop Proceedings, ICCW 2015, pp. 271–277 (2015). https://doi.org/10.1109/iccw.2015.7247190

44. Ding, F., Song, A., Tong, E., Li, J.: A smart gateway architecture for improving efficiency of home network applications. J. Sens. **216**, 10 p. (2016). https://doi.org/10.1155/2016/2197237

45. Smirek, L., Zimmermann, G., Beigl, M.: Just a smart home or your smart home - a framework for personalized user interfaces based on eclipse smart home and universal remote console. Procedia Comput. Sci. **58**, 107–116 (2016). https://doi.org/10.1016/j.procs.2016.09.018

46. Xiao, B., Kanter, T., Rahmani, R.: Logical interactions for heterogeneous IoT entities via virtual world mirrors in support of ambient assisted living. J. Ambient Intell. Smart Environ. **8**(5), 565–580 (2016). https://doi.org/10.3233/AIS-160398

47. Frontoni, E., Pollini, R., Russo, P., Zingaretti, P., Cerri, G.: HDOMO: smart sensor integration for an active and independent longevity of the elderly. Sensors **17**(11), 2610 (2017)

48. Xu, B., Xu, L., Cai, H., Jiang, L., Luo, Y., Gu, Y.: The design of an m-Health monitoring system based on a cloud computing platform. Enterp. Inf. Syst. **11**(1), 17–36 (2017)

49. Costa, A., Julián, V., Novais, P.: Advances and trends for the development of ambient-assisted living platforms. Expert Syst. **34**(2), e12163 (2017)

50. Garcés, L., Nakagawa, E.Y.: A process to establish, model and validate missions of systems-of-systems in reference architectures. In: the Symposium on Applied Computing Proceedings, pp. 1765–1772. ACM (2017)

51. Yacchirema, D.C., Palau, C.E., Esteve, M.: Enable IoT interoperability in ambient assisted living: Active and healthy aging scenarios. In: Proceedings of 2017 14th IEEE Annual Consumer Communications & Networking Conference (CCNC), pp. 53–58. IEEE (2017)

52. Zgheib, R., De Nicola, A., Villani, M.L., Conchon, E., Bastide, R.: A flexible architecture for cognitive sensing of activities in ambient assisted living. In: Proceedings of Enabling Technologies: Infrastructure for Collaborative Enterprises (WETICE), pp. 284–289. IEEE (2017)

53. Lee, D., Bae, S., Song, J.H., Yi, B., Kim, I.K.: Improving chronic disease management with mobile health platform. In: Annual International Conference of the IEEE Engineering in Medicine and Biology Society Proceedings, EMBS, pp. 2275–2278 (2013). https://doi.org/10.1109/embc.2013.6609991

54. Galligioni, E., et al.: Integrating mHealth in oncology: experience in the province of trento. J. Med. Internet Res. **17**(5), e114 (2015). https://doi.org/10.2196/jmir.3743

55. Gietzelt, M., et al.: Home-centered health-enabling technologies and regional health information systems an integration approach based on international standards. Methods Inf. Med. **53**(3), 160–166 (2014). https://doi.org/10.3414/ME13-02-0008

56. Jung, E., Kim, J., Chung, K., Park, D.K.: Mobile healthcare application with EMR interoperability for diabetes patients. Clust. Comput. **17**(3), 871–880 (2014). https://doi.org/10.1007/s10586-013-0315-2

57. Alberts, R., Fogwill, T., Botra, A., Cretty, M.: An integrative ICT platform for eHealth. In: 2014 IST-Africa Conference and Exhibition Proceedings, IST-Africa 2014 (2014). https://doi.org/10.1109/istafrica.2014.6880650

58. Mihaylov, M., Mihovska, A., Kyriazakos, S., Prasad, R.: Interoperable eHealth platform for personalized smart services. In: 2015 IEEE International Conference on Communication Workshop Proceedings, ICCW 2015, pp. 240–245 (2015). https://doi.org/10.1109/iccw.2015.7247185

59. Park, H.S., Cho, H., Kim, H.S.: Development of a multi-agent m-health application based on various protocols for chronic disease self-management. J. Med. Syst. **40**(1), 36 (2016). https://doi.org/10.1007/s10916-015-0401-5

60. Torres Zenteno, A.H., et al.: Mobile platform for treatment of stroke: a case study of tele-assistance. Health Inform. J. **22**(3), 676–690 (2016). https://doi.org/10.1177/1460458215572925

61. Aliakbarpoor, Y., Comai, S., Pozzi, G.: Designing a HL7 compatible personal health record for mobile devices. In: 2017 IEEE 3rd International Forum Research and Technologies for Society and Industry (RTSI) Proceedings, pp. 1–6. IEEE (2017)

62. Roehrs, A., da Costa, C.A., da Rosa Righi, R.: OmniPHR: a distributed architecture model to integrate personal health records. J. Biomed. Inform. **71**, 70–81 (2016)

Coping with "Exceptional" Patients in META-GLARE

Alessio Bottrighi, Luca Piovesan$^{(\boxtimes)}$, and Paolo Terenziani

Institute Computer Science, DISIT, University of Eastern Piedmont,
Alessandria, Italy
{alessio.bottrighi, luca.piovesan,
paolo.terenziani}@uniupo.it

Abstract. Many different computer-assisted management systems for Computer Interpretable Guidelines (CIGs) have been developed. While CIGs propose evidence-based treatments of "typical" patients, exceptions may arise, as well the need to cope with comorbidities. Though the treatment of both phenomena involves a deviation from the "standard" execution of CIGs, until now they have been managed as different problems, and no homogeneous approach to cope with both of them has been devised. In this paper we present the extensions to META-GLARE to overcome such a limitation. To achieve such a goal, we propose a modular architecture supporting the concurrent execution of multiple guidelines, integrated with an ontological knowledge base and with several reasoning mechanisms, including temporal reasoning and goal-based planning.

Keywords: Computer Interpretable Guideline (CIG) ·
Concurrent execution of multiple CIGs · CIG-exception handler ·
System architecture

1 Introduction

Clinical Practice Guidelines (CPGs) represent the current understanding of the best clinical practice, as identified by the *evidence-based* medicine. They are "*systematically developed statements to assist practitioner and patient decisions about appropriate healthcare under specific clinical circumstances*" [1]. CPGs provide *evidence-based* recommendations to suggest to physicians the set of diagnostic/therapeutic actions to be executed to cope with a specific disease, supporting their decision-making activity. In such a way, CPGs promote the quality of healthcare services, as well as their standardization and optimization. Therefore, CPGs are gaining a major role in the clinical practice. For instance, the Guideline International Network (http://www.g-i-n.net) groups 103 organizations representing 47 countries from all continents, and provides a library of more than 6400 CPGs. Recent research has shown that the adoption of ***computer-interpretable clinical guidelines*** (**CIGs** henceforth) and computerized approaches to acquire, represent, execute and reason with CIGs can further increase the advantages of CPGs. Many different systems have been developed to manage CIGs. Surveys about the state-of-the-art of the main approaches can be found in [2–4].

© Springer Nature Switzerland AG 2019
A. Cliquet jr. et al. (Eds.): BIOSTEC 2018, CCIS 1024, pp. 298–325, 2019.
https://doi.org/10.1007/978-3-030-29196-9_16

Although it is system-independent, the work reported in this paper is based on META-GLARE [5, 6], a recent evolution of GLARE. GLARE (Guideline Acquisition, Representation and Execution) is the result of a long-term cooperation started in 1997 between the Department of Computer Science of the University of Eastern Piedmont and the Azienda Ospedaliera San Giovanni Battista (one of the largest hospitals in Italy). Besides supporting CIG acquisition, representation, storage and execution, GLARE is characterized by the adoption of advanced Artificial Intelligence and Temporal Database formal techniques to provide advanced supports for different tasks, including reasoning about temporal constraints [7], the treatment of periodic data [8], guideline versioning [9], model-checking verification [10], decision support [11, 12] and CIG contextualization [13].

CPGs and CIGs capture medical evidence and put it into the medical practice. However, in its own nature, *evidence* is a form of statistical knowledge. Indeed, CIGs aims at capturing the generalities of patients, providing evidence-based recommendations for "classes" of patients. It is out of the scope of CIGs to consider the peculiarities of specific patients. Indeed, evidence can be gathered only for "general" cases, and demanding to expert committees the elicitation of all possible executions of a CIG on any possible specific patient in any possible clinical condition is an infeasible task. Thus, while identifying an evidence-based CIG, expert always assume an "ideal" situation, in which: (i) patients are not comorbid (i.e., they have only one disease, the disease treated by the CIG); (ii) patients are "statistically relevant", in that they do not present rare peculiarities/side-effects; (iii) CIGs are executed in an ideal context, in which all necessary resources are available, and no fault occurs. However, when a specific physician applies a given CIG to a specific patient, unexpected conditions may show up. Such situations are unexpected, and, as such, they cannot be specified a priory in the CIGs. When such unexpected conditions/problems arise while treating a patient, the physician has usually to face them soon (this is certainly the situation in case of unexpected life-threatening problems), possibly suspending or ending the "standard" execution of the current CIG, or coping with the new problem concurrently with the execution of the CIG. Such problems, within the CIG community, have been usually indicated with the term "*exceptions*", since they are exceptions with respect to the "standard" execution of a CIG.

Besides the treatment of exceptions, also the treatment of comorbid patients usually involves deviations from the standard execution of CIGs. By definition, a CIG addresses specific clinical circumstances (i.e., a specific disease). However, comorbid patients are affected by more than one disease and, unfortunately, in most cases simply executing concurrently all the CIGs (one for each one of her/his diseases) on a patient is not an acceptable option, since the interaction between the treatments in different CIGs may cause dangerous effects. On the other hand, the approach of proposing ad-hoc "combined" CIGs to cope with each possible comorbidity does not scale up [14]. For these reasons, new methodologies have been recently introduced to manage multiple CIGs on comorbid patients (see, e.g., the surveys in [15, 16]).

1.1   Goals and Original Contributions

Until now, within the CIG literature, exceptions and comorbidities have been treated as *separate* phenomena[1], so that current approaches cope either with exceptions, or with comorbidities (see Sect. 2). This is a clear limitation of the state-of-the-art, since both phenomena may co-occur on specific patients. In this paper, we first propose a CIG approach facing both phenomena, thus overcoming such a relevant limitation of the current literature. Additionally, unlike many current approaches to comorbidities (see, e.g., [18, 19]), that "merge" the different CIGs into a new one, we aim at coping with the interactions between CIGs still maintaining the distinction between them, which can be executed separately by different agents (as it usually happens in the clinical practice).

The starting point of our approach is the consideration that the management of patients affected by multiple problems requires

(1) A support for the *concurrent* and *distributed* (i.e., carried on by different agents) *execution of CIGs*, and for their synchronization. In the case of comorbid patients, it will support the execution of one CIG for each one of the patient's diseases; in the case of an "exception", it will support the execution of the original CIG plus the plan (which can be formalized as a CIG) to manage the exception.
(2) A support for *detecting* the possible *interactions* between such concurrent CIGs.
(3) A support for *detecting new patient's problems* (i.e., changes in the status of the patient that require new treatments – thus, new CIGs).
(4) Knowledge-based supports for the management of interactions between CIGs and of the exceptions.

In the rest of the paper, we propose the first CIG framework providing all such supports, in an integrated way. In our previous work in the area, we have already developed the supports for issues (2), and (3).

As regards CIG interactions (issue (2)), we have provided a framework (see the Interaction Analysis module in Fig. 1) for (i) supporting physicians in the focusing on specific parts of the CIGs[2] [20], (ii) automatically detecting (based on CIG-independent ontological knowledge) the interactions between the focused actions [21], and studying the interactions from the temporal point of view [22].

As regards issue (3), in [17] we have distinguished different types of exceptions, and proposed a treatment of exceptions based on a triggering mechanism (to activate the treatment of exceptions), and of a library of context-and-guideline-dependent plans to cope with them.

---

[1] This choice is, in our opinion, quite surprising, since there does not seem to be a clear cut between the two phenomena. Just as one prototypical example, in [17] heart failure is considered as an "exception" for a patient treated with a CIG for trauma. But, when a patient with a trauma manifests a heart failure, s\he becomes a comorbid patient, and attention must be paid to avoid dangerous interactions between the treatment (CIG) for the trauma and the treatment (CIG) for the hearth failure.

[2] CIGs may consist of hundreds of actions and\or alternative paths. An extensive check of all interactions could provide a combinatorial number of cases, most of which are not interesting for the patient at hand. Physician-driven focusing is an essential step to avoid an unnecessary combinatorial explosion of the computation and of the number of the identified interactions.

The work in this paper extends our Healthinf 2018 publication [23], in which we first took into account issue (1) above, to consider also issue (4). Indeed, in Sect. 4 of this paper, we identify and design several knowledge-based reasoning techniques that we homogeneously use to manage both exceptions and comorbidities, and in Sects. 3 (informally) and 5 (with a more technical treatment) we show how such reasoning mechanisms are integrated in a whole architecture, supporting the distributed execution of multiple CIGs and the treatment of exceptions and comorbidities through the activation of a trigger manager. Another major extension, with respect to the Healthinf publication, is that fact that, in this paper, we also manage a different, important type of exceptions: "external" exceptions (see the discussion in Sect. 3.1), which are not considered in our previous publication.

While the development of an integrated approach supporting issues (1)–(4) above in a homogeneous way is the main goal of our work, it is worth mentioning that we also have a more "technical" goal. In order to cope with exceptions and comorbidities, we have to radically change the "standard" execution of CIGs. Thus, a possible solution could be to develop from scratch a totally new execution engine. However, we think that such a solution would be a real waste from the software engineering point of view, since very good CIG execution engines have been already built by different approaches (including our GLARE and META-GLARE implementations).

Therefore, an additional main goal of our work is that of devising a *modular* approach for the concurrent execution, in which the execution engine for a CIG in isolation is maintained, and it is extended and integrated in a general framework supporting synchronization and concurrency. Notably, although we are building our framework on top of META-GLARE (each "Exec" module – see Fig. 4 below – is an instantiation of META-GLARE execution module), our methodology is general and can be adapted for similar CIG systems (such as, e.g., [24, 25]).

1.2 Summary of the Paper

The paper is organized as follows. Section 2 discusses the other CIG approaches to exceptions and comorbidities in the literature. In Sect. 3, we start to present "top-down" our approach, showing the general behaviour of our approach in a non-technical way, and introducing a running example. In Sect. 4, we introduce the ontological knowledge and the knowledge-based facilities (specifically: Goal-based planning, CIG navigation facilities, Temporal Reasoning) that are at the core of our homogeneous management of exceptions and comorbidities. In Sect. 5, we describe the facilities we provide to manage exceptions and comorbidities. In Sect. 6, we discuss our overall approach, integrating the management above within a general framework for the distributed execution of multiple CIGs, and including a triggering mechanism to activate the treatment of exceptions and interactions between CIGs. Section 7 exemplifies the behaviour of our approach considering the running example. Finally, Sect. 8 proposes some concluding remarks.

2   Related Works

Until now, the phenomena of "exceptions" and "comorbidities" have been considered separately by the approaches in the CIG literature. In particular, several frameworks have been already proposed to cope with "exceptions".

The PROforma language [26] supports the specification of exceptions. The system sets an Exception flag when an abnormal event has occurred in the processing of a CIG operation. Tu and Musen [27] differentiate between normal flow and exceptional flow and contemplate the specification of scenario-based exceptions handlers. Tu and Musen only consider exceptions regarding the execution of actions in a CIG. In their approach, only the current action(s) can generate exceptions, while they do not consider exceptions arising from a change in the patient state. The approach by [28] manages hierarchies of exceptions. They distinguish between "hazards" and "obstacles". They take into account several modalities of interactions between CIGs and exceptions (parallel execution, suspension, abortion). Quaglini et al. [29] managed the flexibility of their guideline-based careflow system introducing a classification of exceptions similar to the one we will consider in this paper. Exceptions can be expected or unexpected, synchronous or asynchronous and CIG-related or unrelated. However, in [29] the treatment of exceptions is directly triggered by the physicians. Peleg, Somekh and Dori [30] propose a methodology for eliciting and modelling exceptions. They describe a conceptual model in which exceptions can be expected or unexpected, and are triggered as asynchronous events. Triggers start a synchronous exception management branch during the CIG execution. Peleg et al. [30] define two types of exception causes: (1) HumanCause, e.g. human errors, malicious actions or non-compliance, and (2) Non-humanCause, e.g. organizational causes, work item failures, deadline expirations. Their management of exceptions is goal driven. First, they suspend the execution of the current CIG. After the execution of the corrective actions to manage an exception, a set of goals should be fulfilled to resume the CIG normal execution otherwise the CIG is aborted.

Considering comorbidities, several CIG approaches have been recently proposed. Among them, the approach in [31] is the most similar to ours. It provides an ontological model of medical actions and their goals and effects. Interactions are detected by first order logic (FOL) rules operating on such a model. However, the approach in [31], differently from our one, does not consider time. Other approaches, exploits constraints logic programming. In particular, [14] and [32] exploit constraint logic programming to identify and treat interactions between actions. In such approaches, the combination of logical models that represent the CIGs provides a constraint logic programming (CLP) model. After that, they apply a mitigation algorithm to detect and mitigate interactions. However, in such approaches, interactions and their managements must be defined a priori by physicians. Sánchez-Garzón et al. [19] propose an agent-based approach to guideline merging. Each CIG is represented by an agent with hierarchical planning capabilities. The result is obtained through the coordination of all the agents. Riaño et al. represent CIGs as sets of clinical actions that are modelled into an ontology [18]. Treatments are first merged into a unique treatment; then they apply a set of "combination rules" to detect and avoid possible interactions. The approach in [33] proposes to achieve a model-based automatic merge of CIGs through the definition of a combining operator. Jafarpour and Abidi [34] introduce semantic-web rules and an ontology to cope with the merging criteria. Such criteria are used by an Execution Engine to dynamically merge several CIGs. The approaches in [35, 36] are based on answer set programming (ASP). They transform CIGs, patient's information and a set of mitigation operators into an ASP program. Each solution of the ASP program corresponds to a possible execution of the merged CIGs. Notably, [35] supports preferences between treatments. GLINDA proposes a wide ontology of cross-guideline interactions (http://glindaproject.stanford.edu/guidelineinteractionontology.html). In GLINDA, one can express "timing interactions", representing scheduling inconsistencies. We have proposed an approach supporting user-driven and interactive interaction detection over different levels of abstractions [21], and we have recently extended it with temporal reasoning capabilities, so that the approach can detect those interaction that actually can occur in time, given the current patient status, execution status of the CIGs, and the temporal constraints in the CIGs [22].

The approach we propose in this paper is, to the best of our knowledge, the first one coping with exceptions and comorbidities in a homogeneous way. Indeed, the core idea of our approach is that, in both cases, a distributed execution of multiple CIGs (we regard as CIGs also the treatments of specific exceptions) is required, as well as supports for handling triggers (monitoring both the status of the patient, and the status of the execution of the CIGs). Notably, such an idea distinguishes our approach from most of the current approaches to cope with comorbidities, which achieved a unified merged CIG, and then treat it as a unique new plan for the patient. Indeed, in the clinical practice the interactions between CIGs are managed, but physicians do not look at the solution as a single "merged" CIG: they still look at the treatment of a comorbid patient as the concurrent execution of multiple CIGs. Our proposal supports such a "distributed" view of CIGs for comorbid patients, and for patients "with exceptions".

3 A General View of the Behavior of Our Framework

While the architecture of our framework is proposed in Sect. 6, here we informally discuss the basic data\knowledge sources (ovals in Fig. 1) managed by our framework, and its general behaviour (see Fig. 1). However, as a preliminary step, we briefly discuss the notion of "exception", divided (from an operational point of view) into two main types of exceptions, and we briefly comment the main operational differences between the treatment of exceptions and of CIG interactions.

3.1 Exceptions and Interactions

Different types of exceptions have been identified by the CIG literature (see the references in Sect. 2). A first fundamental distinction regards the "origin" of the exceptions: exceptions may be related to the state of the execution of the actions in a CIG, or to the state of the patient. The first type (*external exceptions* henceforth) arises whenever, for any contextual reason, the execution of the current action fails (e.g., because of the absence of a resource needed to carry on the action – typically, an instrument, or when the deadline for the execution of the current action expires). The second type of exceptions (*patient exceptions* henceforth) arises when the standard execution of a CIG cannot be carried on due to an unexpected condition in the status of the patient. Such exceptions may be related to a specific action in the CIG (not considered, for the sake of brevity, in this paper), but, in general, they are totally unpredictable, in the sense that can occur at any time during the execution of CIGs. For instance, an ischemic stroke may occur, requiring an immediate treatment, regardless of what is the CIG and the specific action in the CIG currently in execution.

The distinction between *external* and *patient exceptions* is important from the operational point of view:

(1) External exceptions are "pre-locable", in the sense that they can be directly triggered by the (failure of the) execution of a specific action in the CIG, but they are not "pre-plannable", in the sense that the corrective actions are not usually known a priori, but must be planned if and when the exception arises.

(2) *patient* exceptions are not "pre-locable": they can occur at any time, and independently of the specific action being executed in the CIG. Therefore, an external manager triggering the status of the patient is necessary to cope with them. On the other hand, they are usually "pre-plannable", in the sense that the procedure to cope with such exception is usually known "a priory" (and can be stored a library of specialized "procedures", stored as CIGs).

As a final preliminary step, it is important to clarify that there is a main "operational" difference between the management of exceptions and the one of interactions (e.g., the interactions that may arise between actions of different CIGs operating on the same patient). Exceptions cannot be avoided. In the case of patient exceptions, the status of the patient has already changed, and an exception arises because of such a change (i.e., it is *triggered* by the new status of the patient). In the case of external exceptions, a failure in the execution of a CIG action has occurred. On the other hand, undesired interactions should be detected a-priori and must be avoided (through some management operation).

3.2   Management Strategy

In our approach, the treatment of *patient* exceptions is modeled by a knowledge base (called "**Patient Exceptions**"; see Fig. 1) consisting of triggering rules of the form <Condition, Manag>, where "*Condition*" indicates a Boolean condition (called "triggering" conditions) on the **status of the patient**, and "*Manag*" represents the actions to cope with such a condition (representable as a new CIG) plus constraints about how such new actions should be synchronized with the execution of the current CIG(s). Notably, in our approach, the *Patient Exceptions* knowledge base is static, in the sense that the rules it contains are patient-independent, and are permanently stored.

On the other hand, *external* exceptions are directly associated with the execution of CIG actions (i.e., they are directly triggered by the failure of the execution of an action in the CIG). However, since they are not "pre-plannable", they are not directly associated with a plan to treat them. The plan has to be elaborated at the time when the exception arises. This operation is performed by exploiting a knowledge base of CIG-independent ontological medical knowledge, and using a dedicated module (*External Exceptions Manager* in Fig. 1) to determine (on the basis of the medical knowledge) a plan which achieves the same goal of the action that failed. Such a plan is stored in the **"External Exceptions"** knowledge base.

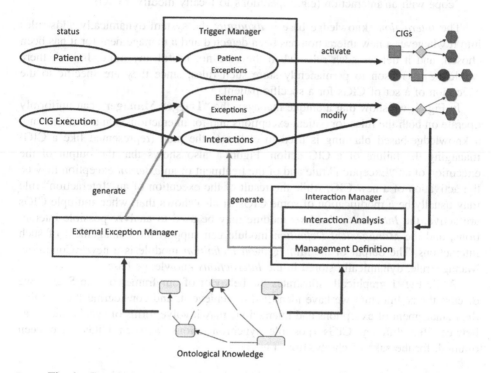

Fig. 1. Graphical representation of our treatment of exceptions and interactions.

On the contrary, (undesired) interactions should be detected a-priori and avoided (through some management operation). This goal involves the identification of possible interactions (see the *Interaction Analysis* module in Fig. 1; rectangles represent computational modules) for (i) supporting physicians in the focusing on specific parts of the CIGs [20], (ii) automatically detecting (based on CIG-independent ontological knowledge) the interactions between the focused action [21].

Once detected, the interactions must be managed, through a set of alternative management options, whose enactment requires different forms of reasoning (see the *Management Definition* module in Fig. 1, and the description in Sect. 5.2). Although the analysis of interaction should be performed *a priori*, generally the management option chosen by physicians has not to be enacted soon. Indeed, it had to be enacted only when, during the execution of the CIGs, the conditions identifying the onset of the interactions arise[3]. Therefore, the treatment of interactions may be modelled by a knowledge base (called "**Interactions**"; see Fig. 1) containing <Condition, Manag> pairs. However, differently from the rules for external exceptions discussed above, here:

(i) triggering conditions have as input the *status of execution* of the *CIG*s
(ii) "Manag" indicates the operations to implement the management option chosen to cope with an interaction (e.g., operations to locally modify a CIG)

The *Interactions* knowledge base is *dynamic*: the system dynamically adds rules into it whenever a new interaction has been detected and a management for it has been chosen, and it deletes such rules when they are not useful any more. Indeed, there would be no reason to permanently store such rules, since they are specific to the execution of a set of CIGs for a specific patient.

In Fig. 1, we show that a unique manager, the "**Trigger Manager**" can uniformly operate on both the rules for patient exceptions and for interactions. On the other hand, a knowledge-based planning is used to elaborate the plan (represented like a CIG) managing the failure of a CIG action. Figure 1 also shows that the output of the execution of an "Exception" rule and of the treatment of an *external* exception may be the activation of a new CIG, while the result of the execution of an "Interaction" rule may usually be a modification of some CIGs. It also shows that, when multiple CIGs are active, the *Interaction Analysis* module may be used to analyze possible interactions, and the *Management Definition* module can support the management of such interactions. The output of the *Management Definition* module is a new <Condition, Manag> rule, dynamically stored in the *Interactions* knowledge base.

While Fig. 1 graphically illustrates the behavior of our framework, in Sect. 6 we discuss the architecture we have identified to achieve it, and considering the fact that the management of exceptions and interactions may involve forms of synchronizations between the different CIGs (possible synchronizations between CIGs have been omitted, for the sake of clarity, from Fig. 1).

3.3 Case Study

In this section, we present a "synthesized" case study, which has been created with the help of some physicians of Azienda Ospedaliera "San Giovanni Battista" in Turin to exemplify the main features of our approach. We consider a comorbid patient, who is treated for Peptic Ulcer (PU) and for deep Venous Thrombosis (VT). To exemplify how our approach works with the two different kinds of exceptions, we also assume that the (invasive) test for H. pylori fails (i.e., an external exception) and, at a certain point of execution, the patient has a heart failure (i.e., a patient exception) during the execution of these CIGs. The two diseases are managed by two specific CIGs (the

---

[3] As an example, a possible undesired interaction between the actions Act1 in CIG_A and Act2 in CIG_B can be detected and physician can choose to manage it via the substitution of Act2 with a set of actions achieving the goal of Act2, but non-interacting with Act1. However, such a substitution must be performed only in case the execution of the two CIGs enforces the execution of both Act1 and Act2 (at times such that their effects may overlap in time). Indeed, if in CIG_A a path of actions not including Act1 has been selected for execution, there is no need to substitute Act2.

upper part of Fig. 2 shows simplified parts of the CIGs). Besides the CIGs, additional medical knowledge is available, including the triggers for patient exceptions. In our example, among them, we consider the exception for heart failure (notably, in this context, heart failure can be considered an exception: it is not statistically recurrent in PU and VT, thus its treatment is not contained into the original CIGs).

In our example, the CIGs for PU and VT are executed concurrently by two different physicians: Physician$_1$ manages PU, and Physician$_2$ manages VT. We consider a sample working section articulated as follows.

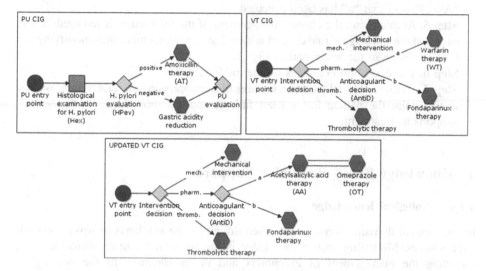

Fig. 2. Part of PU and VT original CIGs (above) and the updated version of VT after the managing of the interaction (below). Original figure in [23].

Step 1. We suppose that Physician$_1$, at a certain point of execution of PU and VT (e.g., at the beginning), decides to analyze the possible interactions between the two CIGs. To do so, Physician$_1$ exploits the Interaction Manager module (see Fig. 1) focusing on relevant parts of PU and of VT, and the Interaction Manager module detects an interaction between warfarin therapy (WT) in VT and amoxicillin therapy (AT) in PU.

Step 2. Physician$_1$ chooses to manage such an interaction replacing the action WT with an alternative plan, having the same goal. For instance, the new therapeutic plan may be the combination of acetylsalicylic acid (AA) therapy and omeprazole (OT) therapy. As we will see in the Sect. 5, the Interaction Manager module creates a trigger rule to implement such a management (if\when required).

Step 3. We suppose that Physician$_1$ goes on executions of PU and that the histological examination for H. pylori (Hex) fails, because the test must be executed through a biopsy and the patient does not accept it. Through the External Exception Manager, Physician$_1$ finds out a non-invasive examination, the Urea Breath Test (UBT), to substitute Hex. Thus, a trigger is created and executed, replacing Hex with UBT.

Step 4. Physician$_1$ and Physician$_2$ goes on with the independent executions of the CIGs. We suppose that in PU "UBT" and "HPev" are executed with exit "positive"; in the meanwhile, in VT "VT start", "intervention decision", with exit "pharm", and "AntiD" with exit "a" has been executed.

Step 5. At this point, the chosen management of the interaction is required, and is executed (i.e. the trigger rule created at step 2 above is executed, thus modifying the CIG as shown in the lower part of Fig. 2).

Step 6. The execution continues on the modified CIGs.

Step 7. To exemplify all the main features of our approach, we further suppose that at this point the patient has a heart failure, and we show how our framework supports its treatment.

4   Knowledge-Based Reasoning Supports

4.1   Ontological Knowledge

In the medical domain, decisions are often driven by the synthesis of several knowledge sources. Modelling such a knowledge is fundamental for many different tasks, including the management of *exceptions* and of *interactions*. In the ontological extension of GLARE [21], we decided to represent at least a part of such a medical knowledge through the development of an ontological model of clinical actions and, consequently, also of CIG actions. Our model is an extension of consensus medical ontologies (in our approach, we used SNOMED CT [37]).

In the ontological extension of META-GLARE, we characterize clinical actions (concept *Action* in Fig. 3). we distinguish among several types of actions. In this paper, we just mention some of them: pharmacological actions (concept *Pharmacological Action*; i.e., the administration of a drug), "common" actions (*Work Action*; e.g., surgery), and data requests (*Query Action*; e.g., a laboratory test, or a search of a data in the patient's clinical record). Notably, each category of action characterizes actions "in general". We have added the concept *CIGAction* (which is not mutually exclusive with the above categories) to denote the actions in a CIG. Each action, while occurring in a CIG, has an additional property: it has a specific intention (concept *Intention*) to achieve (relation *aimsTo*).

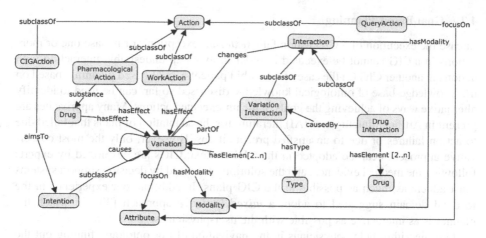

Fig. 3. Ontological Knowledge about actions, effects\intentions, and interactions.

Actions are characterized by several properties. In particular, *Work Action* and *Pharmacological Action* have one or more effects (*hasEffect* relation). We characterize such effects as variations (concept *Variation*), with certain modalities (concept *Modality*; e.g., increase, decrease) of patient state parameters (relation *focusOn*, concept *Attribute*). In our model, variations (and intentions) are hierarchically organized in an IS-A and PART-OF taxonomy. PART-OF relations allow to decompose "composite" intentions into their subcomponents.

Pharmacological actions are clinical actions (and, of course, may be also CIG actions) that are related with the drug (*substance* relation) they prescribe. Drugs are hierarchically organized following the ATC classification [38]. Also drugs are related to their effects (*hasEffect* relation) and, for integrity purpose, the action of administering a drug has the same effects (or super-concepts of them) of the drug it recommend. Data requests (concept *Query Action*) asks for (relation *focusOn*) values of specific attributes (*Attribute*).

In our model, interactions (concept *Interaction*) can be *Variation Interactions* or *Drug Interactions*. The first ones occur between (relation *hasElement*) effects or intentions of actions, i.e., between *variations*, and produce (relation *changes*) other *variations*. Interactions may have different types (*hasType* relation; *Type* concept). *Type* can be further refined into *Concordance*, *Discordance* and *Independence*. Drug Interactions occur between (*hasElement*) two drugs and can be caused by (*causedBy* relation) variation interactions. Following our model, two or more actions interact if two or more of their effects or intentions interact. Two or more pharmacological actions interact also if the drugs they prescribe have two or more interacting effects. It is worth stressing that, given such a model, interactions can be both imported from external repositories and inferred by performing some forms of reasoning on the model. In is worth stressing that the ontological model has been also extended with temporal information (e.g., with the temporal constraints between actions and their effects; see [22]). For the sake of brevity, here we do not discuss such an aspect.

4.2   Goal-Based Planning

In case the execution of a CIG action fails (*external* exception), or in case one or more actions in a CIG cannot be executed in order to avoid an undesirable interaction with actions in another CIG (in the case of comorbid patients), goal-based planning, based on the knowledge-base of ontological knowledge discussed so far, can be used to identify alternative ways of achieving the goals of the un-executed actions. Many approaches are present in Artificial Intelligence (AI) literature for the adaptation of plans that failed due to action failures or due to unsatisfied preconditions. However, only the most conservative approaches can be adopted in the CIG context: CIGs are developed by experts following the medical evidence, and the solutions proposed by decision support systems must adhere as much as possible to the CIG plans. In addition, our experience in the medical domain suggested to adopt a *mixed initiative* approach [39], in which the planner is as interactive as possible with the user-physicians.

Our algorithm helps physicians in the navigation of our ontology, finding out the relevant alternatives for the failed action, or the action(s) to be substituted.

First, let us focus on the basic case, in which the recovering involves only one (not decomposable) goal\intention.

In case the failed (or not executable) action is a *Work* or *Pharmacological* action, our algorithm retrieves in the ontological knowledge the actions that satisfy (*hasEffect* relation) the intention *int* of the failed\substituted action *a*. First, the intention *int* of the failed\substituted action is retrieved from the CIG model. Then, the set *actset* containing all the actions which have as effect (*hasEffect* relation, followed backward) *int* is retrieved from the ontological knowledge. Notice that the set *actset* also includes composite actions (i.e., actions whose components have been specified through the PART-OF taxonomy). Finally, *actset* is pruned by asking the user to discard uninteresting actions, in order to maintain only the relevant results. At the end of the algorithm, *actset* represents the set of possible alternatives to the failed action a, satisfying its intention and considered relevant by the physician.

In case *actset* is empty, there is no direct way to recover from the failure, or to "substitute" the action. However, a more flexible treatment of such an exception can be tried, in case the failed action *a* is part of a composite action *a'* in the CIG. In such a case, the basic algorithm can be applied considering *a'* as the failed action. Such a procedure can be recursively applied, until either one (or more) recovery action is found, or the highest level of abstraction in the CIG is reached.

The management of the case in which more than one goal\intention has to be considered requires some modifications in the basic algorithm, since two or more intentions must be satisfied by the proposed solution.

Finally, the case in which the failed (or not executable) action is a *Query* action is similar: the only difference with respect to the above procedure is that our algorithm retrieves alternative actions (*actset*) by navigating the *focusOn* relations instead of the *hasEffect* ones.

4.3   CIG Navigation Facilities

CIGs are large bodies of knowledge and, for achieving several different tasks, including the management of interactions, it is important to provide tools to navigate them. In GLARE, as well as in most CIG formalisms, CIGs are represented by hierarchical graphs, and alternative paths originate from decision actions. A crucial issue is the forward (for what if analysis) and backward (for the treatment of interactions) navigation on alternative paths. In particular, CIG navigation (henceforth indicated by "NAV") is important in order to support some forms of interaction management, in which physicians choose to avoid an interaction by choosing an alternative therapy (encoded as an alternative path stemming from a therapeutic decision in GLARE). The NAV facility is thus provided, to move back from an action in a CIG and to retrieve alternative CIG paths, stemming from previous therapeutic decisions. Standard graph searching algorithms (not discussed here for the sake of brevity) are used for NAV.

4.4   Temporal Reasoning

The goal of the temporal reasoner is to provide user-physicians with a general set of facilities in order to enable them to look for temporal interactions between CIGs. We provide the following facilities, to support physicians to:

1. (*Interaction?*) check whether two actions in two different CIGs may interact, certainly interact or certainly do not interact;
2. (*Interaction (what-if)?*) assume a hypothetical execution time for some future actions and check whether – given such an assumption – two actions in two different CIGs may interact, certainly interact or certainly do not interact;
3. (*Time of future actions to have (or to avoid) an interaction?*) determine the execution times of some future actions in order to have or to avoid some interactions;
4. (*Time of future actions to have (or to avoid) an interaction (what-if)?*), as (3), but assuming some temporal constraints concerning the execution of future actions.

Notice that the answers may be not crisp, in the sense that an interaction between two actions can be temporally necessary, temporally possible or temporally impossible.

Our treatment of temporal constraints is grounded on the STP framework [40]. In short, in STP a set of constraints is modelled as a conjunction of bounds on differences of the form $c \leq x - y \leq d$, which have an intuitive temporal interpretation, namely that the temporal *distance* between the *time points* x and y is between c (minimum distance) and d (maximum distance). Also strict inequalities are possible (i.e., <), and $-\infty$ and $+\infty$ can be used to denote infinite lower and upper bounds respectively.

Temporal reasoning on STP can be performed/computed by an "all-pairs shortest paths" algorithm such as the Floyd-Warshall's one. Such an algorithm provides as output the *minimal network* of the constraints, i.e., the minimum and maximum distance between each pair of points. In our approach, STP constraints are homogeneously adopted to represent (1) temporal constraints between actions in the CIGs; (2) exact dates of actions in the log, or temporal constraints between them; (3) temporal constraints in the ontology, and (4) temporal constraints on the hypothesized actions, if any.

In order to provide the temporal facilities in above, the first step is the *collection of* (relevant) *constraints* from the log (if present), from the CIGs and from the ontology. In the case of the log, each executed action is timestamped with its starting and ending time. The collection of constraints from the CIGs involves the navigation of the CIGs (expressed in GLARE) from the starting action A_s to the focused action A_f, and the collection of the constraints on the arc in the path connecting them. Finally, the knowledge base of ontological knowledge can be easily navigated in order to retrieve the temporal constraints between the focused actions and their focused effects.

After the collection of constraints (from log, CIGs and ontology) is performed, STP temporal reasoning can be performed on such constraints, to offer the above facilities to user-physicians.

To provide the different facilities mentioned above, we rely on Floyd Warshall's algorithm to propagate the temporal constraints and to evaluate the minimal network.

For example, in the following we show how the *Interaction (what-if)?* facility can be achieved, on the basis of temporal reasoning. The parameters *O, G1, G2, Var1, Var2, Log, Hyp* in the table represent the ontology, the two CIGs, the two interacting variations to be examined, the log and the hypothetical temporal constraints to be assumed, respectively.

```
Hypothetical Interaction?(O, G1, G2, Var1, Var2, Hyp)
   Extract temporal constraints
   Add the temporal constraints Hyp
   Propagate the constraints (Floyd-Warshall)
   Given minimal network:
   If there is necessarily an overlap between variation Var1
      and variation Var2 then return YES
   Else If variation Var1 necessarily does not temporally over-
      lap variation Var2 then return NO
      Else return MAYBE
```

5   Management of Interactions and Exceptions

5.1   Interaction Management Options

On the basis of the experience of physicians cooperating with GLARE, and considering the medical literature (see e.g., [41, 42]), we have identified a set of "*management options*" to manage interactions. Two aspects must be highlighted:

(i)   managements options are not mutually exclusive: in many cases, several options are possible, and the physicians have to choose between them.

(ii) when managing interactions, physicians' goal is to produce limited and controlled changes in the treatments that respect, as much as possible, the constraints suggested by the original CIGs. This is due to the fact that clinical guidelines (from which CIGs derive) are "best practice" care plans developed following medical *evidence*, and any change to them results in a non-evidence-based recommendation

The ontological knowledge in Sect. 4.1 can be exploited by physicians to discriminate between "desired" and "undesired" interactions.

In the medical literature, undesired interactions are usually *avoided* or are managed through *adjustments* of the CIGs. The avoidance of an interaction is required, e.g., when the interaction imperils the patient's life or when it compromises some of the intentions of an action, or when it causes undesired side effects. Two main options are used by physicians: the *safe alternative* option and the *temporal avoidance* option.

Safe Alternative: the *safe alternative* option consists in the choice of alternative CIG paths in which the considered interaction does not occur.

Temporal Avoidance: interactions can also be *temporally avoided*. To do so, interacting actions can be executed at times such that the interaction cannot actually occur (i.e., the two hypothetically interacting variations do not overlap in time – see also [22, 43]).

Not all the undesired interactions need to be avoided. In some cases, CIGs can be *adjusted* to manage the cases in which the interactions arise. We support three main management options to this purpose.

Dosage Adjustment: the *adjustment of the dosage* is particularly useful for those drug interactions that cause a deviation (increase/decrease) in the intention of one of the two interacting actions (see Sect. 4.1).

Effect Monitoring: in some cases, *monitoring the effects* of the interaction is enough (instead of, e.g., mitigating the effects through dosage adjustment). In particular, if an interaction causes a change of some parameters of the patient, they have to be monitored and evaluated by the physician during the span of time in which the interaction occurs. Obviously, if a serious risk is detected, other management options can be applied, e.g., the therapy can be suspended or the WAR dosage can be adjusted.

Interaction Mitigation: some interactions can cause undesired side effects. In such cases, a "shared" action that mitigates such effects can be added to the interacting CIGs.

On the other hand, *desired* interactions are those that, by *physician preference* or "by *CIG definition*", should happen. A physician may desire an interaction, for instance, because the effects of the interacting actions are enhanced by the interaction. On the other side, an interaction is desired "by CIG definition" when two (or more) actions in the different CIGs can be replaced by a "common" action achieving their intentions. We provide two types of alignment to manage such cases.

Interaction Alignment: to guarantee the occurrence of an interaction two requirements are needed: (i) the interacting actions must be executed and (ii) their execution times have to be such that their effects overlap in time.

Intention Alignment: in the case of intention alignment, the physician may want to "merge" two actions in a single one, executing it in a time that respects all the intentions of both the original actions. This alignment is useful, for instance, with duplicated actions and with actions that can be replaced by a third one, achieving both their intentions.

All the management options described above (except dosage adjustment) can be obtained on the basis of the above reasoning techniques shown in Sect. 4, as summarized in Table 1.

The **safe alternative** option can be achieved in two ways. (1) NAV is used to find the first (preceding) therapeutic decision action in each CIG originating an alternative path not causing the interaction. The decision actions are then annotated with the suggestion to follow alternative paths. (2) Goal-based planning (henceforth GBP) can be used to add non-interacting alternatives to CIG actions, searching plans that satisfy the intentions of one of the interacting actions.

Temporal avoidance can be obtained directly by applying the temporal reasoning facility (TR) facility.

In **effect monitoring**, a variation of GBP above (not described here for space constraint) is used in order to find out a monitoring action (*query* action in META-GLARE) for the patient status attribute changed by the given interaction. Such an action must be added (as a "shared action") to the two CIGs, together with the constraint stating that it must be executed during the interaction time. Such a time is determined by the temporal reasoner.

In **interaction mitigation**, GBP is used to determine a plan that satisfies an intention opposite (or discordant) with respect to the variation caused by the interaction. Then temporal reasoning is used to determine the temporal constraints such that the effects of the plan occur during the interaction.

In **interaction alignment**, NAV is used to retrieve all the paths that lead to the interaction and to suggest the physician to follow one of them, respecting the temporal constraints identified by the temporal reasoner.

In **intention alignment**, GBP is used to find out a plan that achieves all the intentions of the replaced actions. Then temporal reasoning is adopted to find out the temporal constraints (on the new plan) needed to enforce that the new plan achieves its intentions at the time required by the input CIGs.

Finally, the **dosage adjustment** is easier, since it does not require any of the previous reasoning techniques. In fact, the system suggests an adjustment of the drug dosage opposite with respect to the variation caused by the interaction (i.e., an increase of the dosage in case of decreased variation and vice versa).

Table 1 summarizes how the different techniques are composed to achieve the different modalities.

Table 1. Reasoning techniques adopted to support management options.

Safe alternative	Temporal avoidance	Dose adj.	Effect monitor.	Interact. mitigation	Interact. align.	Intention align.
NAV or GBP	TR	other	GBP and TR	GBP and TR	NAV and TR	GBP and TR

5.2   Mixed-Initiative Management of Interactions

The *Interaction Manager module* supports the detection and the definition of management for CIG interactions. It is composed by two modules (see Fig. 1): the *Interaction Analysis* and the *Management Definition*. The *Interaction Analysis* module (see [20]) operates in two steps. First, it provides physicians with a navigation tool (operating at the different abstraction levels supported by the given CIGs) supporting the choice of a specific part (called "focus") of the CIGs, the part currently of interest for the treatment of the current patient. Second, it provides a knowledge-based tool that automatically detects all the possible interactions between the actions in the "focus". Moreover, this module has been recently extended with a set of facilities to *temporally* analyze interactions [22], distinguishing among temporally certain, possible or impossible interactions and performing hypothetical reasoning. Once detected an interaction, the *Management Definition* module supports physicians in the selection of a management, choosing among the *management options* discussed so far. Notably, in our approach, managements are not applied immediately to CIGs, but through the creation of dynamic trigger rules (see the discussion in Sect. 3). The triggers have the form <Condition, Manag> where "Condition" indicates a Boolean condition on the execution of specific CIG action(s) or decision result(s), and "Manag" represents the actions to cope with such a situation. These actions can be described using a subset of primitives to operate on the global data structures. Such trigger rules are automatically generated by a specific component of the *Management Definition* module (the "Trigger Generator", not detailed in Fig. 3 for the sake of brevity and clarity). The "Trigger Generator" takes as input from the other modules the detected interacting actions, and the management options chosen to manage such an interaction, plus additional parameters. The Trigger Generator consists of a set of parametric procedures, one for each management option, to automatically generate a trigger, on the basis of the input parameters. Then, the trigger is sent as a message to the *Trigger Manager*.

For example, we show the trigger created by the Interaction Manager module to manage the interaction between WT and AT, with the *safe alternative* management option (see Sect. 5.1).

```
TR-WTAT:
    (1)<(Exec(AntiD)=a AND  (Exec(HPev)=positive OR NOT Ex-
        ec(HPev)),
    (2)(REMOVE_ACTION WT in VT;
    (3)ADD_ACTION AA to VT;
    (4)ADD_ACTION OT to VT;
    (5)ADD_ARC in VT from AntiD to AA;
    (6)ADD_ARC in VT from AA to OT;)>
```

The Condition part of TR-WTAT represents the conditions under which the interaction can occur. In particular, in our example, AT and WT interacts in case (line 1): (i) the decision AntiD has been taken, having as result to execute the path "a" which contains WT, and (ii) either the decision HPev has been taken with result "positive" (i.e. choosing the path containing AT), or HPev has not been already executed (in this last situation, the system preventively applies the management, avoiding the cases in which decision HPev is taken with "positive" result only after WT has been executed, impeding the application of the management). Notably, such a condition is automatically built by the Trigger Generator, through a navigation throughout the PU and VT CIGs. The Manag part of TR-WTAT is automatically built by the Trigger Generator on the basis of the management option chosen by Physician₁ and the new alternative plan. Specifically, the Manag part of TR-WTAT prescribes to (line 2) remove WT, and (lines 3-4) to add AA, OT and (lines 5-6) the corresponding arcs in the CIG VT(the result of the execution of TR-WTAT is shown in the lower part of Fig. 2).

5.3 Management of Exceptions

The treatment of exceptions is easier. As regards patient exceptions, they are managed through a set of <Condition, Manag> triggers, in which the Condition regards the state of the patient, and Manag is a plan (stored as a CIG) to be activated when a change in the status of the patient makes the Condition true. Such trigger rules are permanently stored within the Patient Exceptions knowledge base (see Fig. 1).

For example, among the others, the trigger TR-HF (i.e. the trigger for heart failure) may be stored in the Patient Exceptions knowledge base:

```
TR-HF:
    (1)  <(Heart Failure = TRUE),
    (2)  (ADD_NODE HF-PLAN TO GRAPH;
    (3)  ADD HF-PLAN TO YELLOW PAGES;
    (4)  ADD_ARC from HF-PLAN to VT;
    (5)  ADD_ARC from HF-PLAN to PU;)>
```

In TR-HF, the Condition (line 1) captures that the patient has a heart failure, the Manag (lines 2–5) describes the instructions that must be executed to manage it. In short, (2)–(5) encode the commands to activate a new CIG "HF-PLAN" suspending the execution of VT and PU.

On the other hand, the treatment of external exceptions involve the definition of <Condition, Manag> trigger rules directly associated with the actions in the CIGs. The Condition part specify a specific failure for the action (notably, a CIG action may fail in different ways), and the Manag part simply call GBP to determine a new action\plan achieving the same intention of the failed action. For instance, to create a trigger that manages the failure of action Hex, GBP retrieves from the ontological knowledge a set of query actions focusing on the attribute "H. pylori infection" (i.e., which verify whether the patient is infected by H. pylori or not). Then, GBP proposes to the user physician such a set. Hypothesizing that the physician choses the urea breath test (UBT), the resulting trigger is

```
TR-HEX:
 (1)<(Failed(Hex),
 (2)(REMOVE_ACTION Hex in PU;
 (3)ADD_ACTION UBT to PU;
 (4)ADD_ARC in PU from PUep to UBT;
 (5)ADD_ARC in PU from UBT to HPev;)>
```

6 Architecture for the Concurrent Execution of Multiple CIGs

6.1 The Architecture

In our overall approach, we aim at

(i) supporting a distributed execution of the patient treatments, since different CIGs can be managed by different physicians (i.e. each physician needs a client to manage her CIGs) and

(ii) supporting a global vision of patient treatments, and to "synchronize" them (such a vision will be stored and managed in the server).

To achieve such goals, we have chosen to base our approach on the client-server model. Notably, from an abstract point of view our approach can be described as an agent based system (i.e. each module can be seen as an agent).

For sake of clarity and brevity, in this paper we assume that all the CIGs are related to the same patient. The extension to cope with multiple patients is obvious. In our approach, the *server* (see Fig. 4) is composed by the following modules:

- a *"General Manager"* (in the middle of the "Server" in Fig. 4). The general manager maintains the global view of the patient and of her treatments (represented through global data structures). It interacts with the other modules to update such a view and to synchronize the treatments when necessary (the functionalities of such a module are described in more detail in Subsect. 6.2);
- the *"Executor Modules"* ("Exec CIG$_1$", "Exec CIG$_2$", and "Exec CIG$_3$", in the left part of the "Server" in Fig. 4; notably, there is one "Exec" module for each CIG under execution). Each Executor manages the execution of a CIG for a specific patient [6] (see Subsect. 6.3);
- the *"Interaction Manager"*. It supports the study of the interactions between CIGs and defines how they should be managed (see Subsect. 5.2 above);
- the *"External Exception Manager"*. It supports the definition of trigger rules to manage external exceptions.
- the *"Trigger Manager"*. It manages the triggers in the Trigger KB (see Subsect. 6.4).

Notably, the architecture of our framework is open, and can be extended by with the addition of new modules to provide new facilities, by specifying their communication API.

The **client** provides physicians with a GUI to support the execution of one or more CIGs (e.g. in Fig. 4 Client$_1$ allows to manage the execution of CIG$_1$ and CIG$_2$, while Client$_2$ supports the execution of CIG$_3$). Each *client* sends/receives messages to/from the *executor* module to manage the execution of the CIGs. Moreover, physicians can activate the *Interaction Manager* module to study and manage possible interactions between two or more CIGs (e.g. in Fig. 4, Client$_1$ activates it) or the *External Exception Manager* to manage external exceptions.

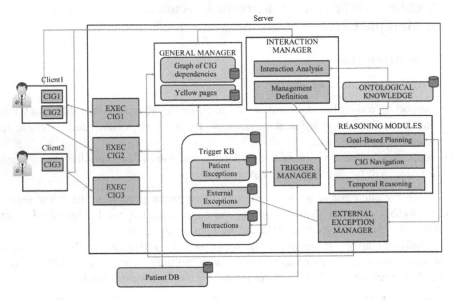

Fig. 4. General Architecture of our framework. The arrows show the flow of information between the different modules.

6.2   The General Manager Module

The *General Manager* is the core of the system. It supports the concurrent execution of CIGs on a given patient. To achieve such a goal, it manages the interplay between the other modules in the server by (i) sending\receiving messages, and (ii) maintaining a "global view" of the execution of the CIGs. Such a "global view" is provided by two data structures: (a) the **graph of CIG dependencies** and (b) the **yellow pages of CIGs**, that work as a *shared memory*. All the modules can *read* (a) and (b), while only the *General Manager* can *write* them.

The **graph of CIG dependencies** has two components: *nodes* and *arcs*. Each *node* represents a CIG under execution. *Arcs* represent the dependencies between such CIGs. An arc from a node A to a node B means that B is *suspended* by the execution of A. Thus, the *graph* represents the synchronization between CIGs: CIGs without entering arcs are *active*, while CIGs entered by an arc are temporarily suspended. We provide a set of primitives to update the *graph*:

- creation/deletion of a node,
- creation/deletion of an arc.

The *yellow pages of CIGs* store all the instances of CIGs currently in execution. The operations provided to update the *yellow pages* are:

- add a CIG,
- remove a CIG,
- update a pharmacological dosage,
- update a temporal constraint,
- add a node to a CIG,
- add an arc to a CIG.

The updates to the data structures are triggered by messages sent by the other modules in the server. A message represents a list of instructions expressed using the primitives described above. The **General Manager** manages messages units of work performed in an atomic way (i.e., as transactions). It performs all the updates required and then it notifies such updates to the modules to maintain the synchronization. The General Manager manages the message of updates using a FIFO policy.

6.3 The Executor Module

The *Executor* module manages the execution of a CIG instance for a specific patient. In our approach, there is an instance of Executor for each CIG under execution. The Executor of a CIG can be active or suspended depending on the current state (i.e. active/suspended) of the CIG represented in the *graph of dependencies*. Each instance of Executor takes in input (i) the instance of the CIG that it has to execute from the yellow pages, and (ii) the patient data from the *Patient DB*. The *Executor* interacts with a specific client to execute the current actions in the CIG. In case the CIG is terminated, the *Executor* sends a message to the *General Manager*, to remove the node (representing the CIG) from the graph, and remove the CIG from the *yellow pages*. Specifically, we use the executor of META-GLARE [5], but our methodology is mostly system-independent, and it can be adapted for use any CIG executor (such as, e.g., PROforma or Asbru [24, 25]).

6.4 The Trigger Manager

The *Trigger Manager* module manages the triggers. To achieve such a goal, it has

(i) to check whether the triggers stored in the Trigger *KB* fire and then to notify that the management had to be applied and
(ii) to maintain up-to-date the *Interactions* and the *External Exceptions* knowledge bases, since they are dynamic.

To achieves the goals at point (i), the *Trigger Manager* evaluates whether each rule <Condition, Manag> in the Trigger KB has to be executed. The *Trigger Manager* considers the patient status (from the Patient DB) and the execution status of the CIGs (in the yellow pages) and checks whether they satisfy the *Condition*. If so, the *Trigger Manager* sends a message to the *General Manager*. Such a message contains <Manag>

(i.e. the set of instructions to cope with the situation described in Condition, described in the second part of the <Condition, Manag> rule).

To achieve the goal (ii), the *Trigger Manager* adds a trigger to the *Interactions* knowledge base, when it receives a message from the *Interaction Manager* module. Each message contains a trigger that has to be added. The *Trigger Manager* manages the messages using a FIFO policy.

The triggers in the *Interactions* knowledge base are not permanent, since they are context and patient dependent. Thus, the *Interaction Manager* removes a trigger: (i) when it is used (in the case that it is not reusable, e.g. in the case it is applied to a repeatable part of the CIGs, it is removed when the repetitions of such a part is ended) or (ii) when one of the CIGs in its Condition ends.

The management of triggers in the External Exceptions knowledge base is similar.

7 Our System in Action: Managing the Case Study

We describe how our framework works on the case study described in Subsect. 3.3. The patient is affected by both Peptic Ulcer (PU) and deep Venous Thrombosis (VT) and two CIGs are executed to treat such diseases. Two physicians are involved: Physician$_1$, managing PU, and Physician$_2$, managing VT. In our framework, each physician interacts with the system via a client: (1) Physician$_1$ uses Client$_{PU}$ to execute the CIG PU via the executor instance Executor$_{PU}$, and (2) Physician$_1$ uses Client$_{VT}$, to execute the CIG VT via the executor instance Executor$_{VT}$. Suppose that both physicians are managing the first action in the CIG (but this is not restrictive at all). In such a context, *the graph of dependencies* contains two independent nodes (one for PU and one for VT), while the *yellow pages* contain the current instances of the CIGs. The *Interactions* and the *External Exceptions* knowledge bases are empty and Patient Exceptions knowledge base contains the triggers to manage the exceptions.

In our example, among the others, we suppose that the *External Exceptions* knowledge base contains the trigger TR-HF (i.e. the trigger for heart failure) presented in Sect. 5.3.

To analyze the possible interactions between the two CIGs, Physician$_1$ (through Client$_{PU}$) calls the *Interaction Manager module* and selects the relevant part of CIGs that the module has to analyse (i.e., the "focus"). The *Interaction Manager* identifies all the interaction between the actions in the "focus" via the *Interaction Analysis* module. In this specific example, the module finds an interaction between warfarin therapy (WT) and amoxicillin therapy (AT). Such an interaction increases the anticoagulant effect of warfarin and raises the risk of bleedings. As described in Sect. 5, we suppose that Physician$_1$ decides to apply the *safe alternative* management option, substituting WT with an alternative new plan. Such a new plan is automatically generated by the *Management Definition* module through the Goal-Based Planning. In our example, we suppose that, given the knowledge base of ontological knowledge, the planner outputs a new plan constituted by the combination of acetylsalicylic acid (AA) therapy and omeprazole (OT) therapy.

Then *the Trigger Generator* is invoked. It takes as input the PU and VT CIGs, the management option chosen *by* Physician$_1$ (i.e., the *safe alternative* option) and the new alternative plan, and automatically produces as output the trigger rule TR-WTAT described in Sect. 5.2 above.

Then, the *Interaction Manager* module sends a message containing the TR-WTAT rule to the *Trigger Manager*.

As a consequence, the *Trigger Manager* adds it to the *Interactions* knowledge base (see Fig. 4). Then, the two physicians can independently go on with the execution of the CIGs.

As an example of external exception, let us suppose that the execution of the action Histological examination for H. pylori (Hex in the PU CIG) by Physician₁ fails, because the test is executed through a biopsy and the patient does not accept it. The Executor$_{PU}$ notifies the failure of the action to the External Exception Manager, which invokes the Goal-Based Planning to manage the external exception. The Goal-Based Planning navigates the ontological knowledge to check what is the *Attribute* considered by the Hex action (*focusOn* relation). The "*H. pylori infection*" attribute is found out. At this point, the Goal-Based Planning navigates the ontological knowledge to identify other tests that *focusOn* "*H. pylori infection*". The urea breath test (UBT) is found out (notably, as shown in Subsect. 5.3, if more than one possibility is found, the user is asked to select one of them), so that the TR-HEX trigger rule (see Subsect. 5.3) as management is created and executed (replacing Hex with the alternative action UBT). The *Trigger Manager* sends a message to *General Manager* with the instructions in lines 2–5 of TR-HEX. The *General Manager* executes these instructions and replaces Hex with UBT in the instance of the PU CIG in the *yellow pages*. Finally, it notifies the Executor$_{PU}$ that the instance of PU in the *yellow pages* has been updated, and the Executor$_{PU}$ sends a message to Client$_{PU}$ to refresh the visualization of PU.

Then, let us suppose that physicians went on with the execution, in particular Physician₁ (through Client$_{PU}$) has executed the actions "PU start", "UBT" (to manage the previous exception), and "HPev", which results positive; in the meanwhile, Physician₂ (through client Client$_{VT}$) has executed "VT start", "intervention decision", with exit "pharm", and "AntiD" with exit "a". This situation triggers TR-WTAT (i.e. Condition in TR-WTAT is satisfied). Thus, the *Trigger Manager* sends a message to the *General Manager* containing the instruction to manage such an interaction (i.e. the Manag component in TR-WTAT, i.e. lines 2–6) and removes TR-WTAT from the *Interactions* knowledge base, since it is not reusable during the patient treatment.

Then, the *General Manager* executes as a unique transaction the instructions in the message, updating the global vision. In our example, the instance of VT in the *yellow pages* is updated by replacing WT with the alternative plan (see lines 2–6 in TR-WTAT), as shown in the lower part of Fig. 2. Thus, the *General Manager* notifies to Executor$_{VT}$ that the instance of VT in the *yellow pages* has been updated. As consequence, Executor$_{VT}$ sends a message to Client$_{VT}$ to refresh the visualization of VT, and let Physician₂ go on with the execution of the updated CIG.

Moreover, let us suppose that, during the execution of such CIGs, the patient has a heart failure. As a consequence, TR-HF is triggered by the *Trigger Manager*. Then the Trigger Manager sends a message to *General Manager* with the instructions to manage the heart failure (lines 2–5 in TR-HF). The *General Manager* executes these instructions. The first two instructions (lines 2–3 in TR-HF) generate (both in the graph of CIG dependencies and in the yellow pages of CIGs) the node corresponding to the CIG to treat heart failure. As a result of such a generation, our framework supports the search for a physician accepting the responsibility of executing the new CIG (following the approach in [44]), and generates a new instance of Executor module to manage the Heart Failure CIG. The selected physician can manage the execution of the CIG through a client. In case s/he is already executing a CIG for the specific patient, the Heart Failure CIG is added to its client, otherwise a new client is initialized for her/him. Moreover, the interpretation of lines 4–5 in TR-HF adds two (suspension) arcs in the graph of CIGs dependencies, then the *General Manager* notifies the suspension to Executor$_{VT}$ and to Executor$_{PU}$. Consequently, the two executors notify the suspension to the corresponding clients.

8 Conclusions

In the last 25 years, many different CIG execution engines have been developed, to support physician in the application of a specific CIG on a specific patient. However, such engines usually suppose an "ideal" situation, in which no exception arise, and the patient is not affected by any comorbidity. As a consequence, a single CIG must be executed, and no concurrency is needed, in addition the one directly involved by the CIG being executed. On the other hand, the treatment of "exceptions" and of comorbid patients demands for more extended supports. In this paper, we provide the first homogeneous framework for the management of "external exceptions", "patient exceptions" and CIG interactions (for comorbid patients). Indeed, our treatment exploit a knowledge-base of ontological knowledge, and three basic and task-independent reasoning modules: Goal-based Planning, CIG Navigation, and Temporal Reasoning. Additionally, a trigger manager is designed, to cope with both the trigger needed to cope with patient exceptions, and with the triggers dynamically built as the result of having chosen a specific management option to avoid an undesirable interaction. Our approach is modular, in that it adds a further layer building upon "traditional" execution engines for a single CIG. Though our framework is being built on top of META-GLARE, our methodology is general, and can be adapted for similar CIG systems (such as, e.g., PROforma [24] or Asbru [25]).

We are currently implementing our approach using Java. As soon as the implementation will be completed, we plan to develop an extensive experimentation of our framework, especially in the context of comorbidity treatment.

Acknowledgements. This research is original and has a financial support of the Università del Piemonte Orientale.

References

1. Field, M.J., Lohr, K.N. (eds.): Clinical practice guidelines: directions for a new program. National Academies Press (US), Washington (DC) (1990)
2. Peleg, M., et al.: Comparing computer-interpretable guideline models: a case-study approach. JAMIA. **10**, 52–68 (2003)

3. Bottrighi, A., et al.: Analysis of the GLARE and GPROVE approaches to clinical guidelines. In: Riaño, D., ten Teije, A., Miksch, S., Peleg, M. (eds.) KR4HC 2009. LNCS (LNAI), vol. 5943, pp. 76–87. Springer, Heidelberg (2010). https://doi.org/10.1007/978-3-642-11808-1_7

4. Peleg, M.: Computer-interpretable clinical guidelines: a methodological review. J. Biomed. Inform. **46**, 744–763 (2013)

5. Bottrighi, A., Terenziani, P.: META-GLARE: a meta-system for defining your own computer interpretable guideline system—architecture and acquisition. Artif. Intell. Med. **72**, 22–41 (2016)

6. Bottrighi, A., Rubrichi, S., Terenziani, P.: META-GLARE: a meta-engine for executing computer interpretable guidelines. In: Riaño, D., Lenz, R., Miksch, S., Peleg, M., Reichert, M., ten Teije, A. (eds.) KR4HC 2015. LNCS (LNAI), vol. 9485, pp. 37–50. Springer, Cham (2015). https://doi.org/10.1007/978-3-319-26585-8_3

7. Anselma, L., Terenziani, P., Montani, S., Bottrighi, A.: Towards a comprehensive treatment of repetitions, periodicity and temporal constraints in clinical guidelines. Artif. Intell. Med. **38**, 171–195 (2006)

8. Stantic, B., Terenziani, P., Governatori, G., Bottrighi, A., Sattar, A.: An implicit approach to deal with periodically repeated medical data. Artif. Intell. Med. **55**, 149–162 (2012)

9. Anselma, L., Bottrighi, A., Montani, S., Terenziani, P.: Managing proposals and evaluations of updates to medical knowledge: theory and applications. J. Biomed. Inform. **46**, 363–376 (2013)

10. Bottrighi, A., Giordano, L., Molino, G., Montani, S., Terenziani, P., Torchio, M.: Adopting model checking techniques for clinical guidelines verification. Artif. Intell. Med. **48**, 1–19 (2010)

11. Montani, S., Terenziani, P.: Exploiting decision theory concepts within clinical guideline systems: toward a general approach. Int. J. Intell. Syst. **21**, 585–599 (2006)

12. Anselma, L., Bottrighi, A., Molino, G., Montani, S., Terenziani, P., Torchio, M.: Supporting knowledge-based decision making in the medical context: the GLARE approach. IJKBO **1**, 42–60 (2011)

13. Terenziani, P., Montani, S., Bottrighi, A., Torchio, M., Molino, G., Correndo, G.: A context-adaptable approach to clinical guidelines. Stud. Health Technol. Inform. **107**, 169–173 (2004)

14. Michalowski, M., Wilk, S., Michalowski, W., Lin, D., Farion, K., Mohapatra, S.: Using constraint logic programming to implement iterative actions and numerical measures during mitigation of concurrently applied clinical practice guidelines. In: Peek, N., Marín Morales, R., Peleg, M. (eds.) AIME 2013. LNCS (LNAI), vol. 7885, pp. 17–22. Springer, Heidelberg (2013). https://doi.org/10.1007/978-3-642-38326-7_3

15. Fraccaro, P., Castelerio, M.A., Ainsworth, J., Buchan, I.: Adoption of clinical decision support in multimorbidity: a systematic review. JMIR Med. Inform. **3**, e4 (2015)

16. Riaño, D., Ortega, W.: Computer technologies to integrate medical treatments to manage multimorbidity. J. Biomed. Inform. **75**, 1–13 (2017)

17. Leonardi, G., Bottrighi, A., Galliani, G., Terenziani, P., Messina, A., Corte, F.D.: Exceptions handling within GLARE clinical guideline framework. In: AMIA (2012)

18. López-Vallverdú, J.A., Riaño, D., Collado, A.: Rule-based combination of comorbid treatments for chronic diseases applied to hypertension, diabetes mellitus and heart failure. In: Lenz, R., Miksch, S., Peleg, M., Reichert, M., Riaño, D., ten Teije, A. (eds.) KR4HC/ProHealth -2012. LNCS (LNAI), vol. 7738, pp. 30–41. Springer, Heidelberg (2013). https://doi.org/10.1007/978-3-642-36438-9_2

19. Sánchez-Garzón, I., Fdez-Olivares, J., Onaindía, E., Milla, G., Jordán, J., Castejón, P.: A multi-agent planning approach for the generation of personalized treatment plans of comorbid patients. In: Peek, N., Marín Morales, R., Peleg, M. (eds.) AIME 2013. LNCS

(LNAI), vol. 7885, pp. 23–27. Springer, Heidelberg (2013). https://doi.org/10.1007/978-3-642-38326-7_4

20. Piovesan, L., Molino, G., Terenziani, P.: Supporting multi-level user-driven detection of guideline interactions. In: Proceedings of the International Conference on Health Informatics (HEALTHINF-2015), pp. 413–422. Scitepress (2015)

21. Piovesan, L., Molino, G., Terenziani, P.: Supporting physicians in the detection of the interactions between treatments of co-morbid patients. In: Healthcare Informatics and Analytics: Emerging Issues and Trends, pp. 165–193. IGI Global (2014)

22. Anselma, L., Piovesan, L., Terenziani, P.: Temporal detection and analysis of guideline interactions. Artif. Intell. Med. **76**, 40–62 (2017)

23. Bottrighi, A., Piovesan, L., Terenziani, P.: A general framework for the distributed management of exceptions and comorbidities. In: Zwiggelaar, R., Gamboa, H., Fred, A.L.N., Badia, S.B.I (eds.) Proceedings of the 11th International Joint Conference on Biomedical Engineering Systems and Technologies (BIOSTEC 2018), vol. 5, HEALTHINF, Funchal, Madeira, Portugal, 19–21 January 2018, pp. 66–76. SciTePress (2018)

24. Fox, J., Johns, N., Rahmanzadeh, A.: Disseminating medical knowledge: the PROforma approach. Artif. Intell. Med. **14**, 157–182 (1998)

25. Shahar, Y., Miksch, S., Johnson, P.: The Asgaard project: a task-specific framework for the application and critiquing of time-oriented clinical guidelines. Artif. Intell. Med. **14**, 29–51 (1998)

26. Sutton, D.R., Fox, J.: The syntax and semantics of the PROforma guideline modeling language. J. Am. Med. Inform. Assoc. JAMIA **10**, 433–443 (2003)

27. Tu, S.W., Musen, M.A.: A flexible approach to guideline modeling. In: Proceedings of the AMIA Symposium, pp. 420–424 (1999)

28. Grando, A., Peleg, M., Glasspool, D.: A goal-oriented framework for specifying clinical guidelines and handling medical errors. J. Biomed. Inform. **43**, 287–299 (2010)

29. Quaglini, S., Stefanelli, M., Lanzola, G., Caporusso, V., Panzarasa, S.: Flexible guideline-based patient careflow systems. Artif. Intell. Med. **22**, 65–80 (2001)

30. Peleg, M., Somekh, J., Dori, D.: A methodology for eliciting and modeling exceptions. J. Biomed. Inform. **42**, 736–747 (2009)

31. Zamborlini, V., Hoekstra, R., da Silveira, M., Pruski, C., ten Teije, A., van Harmelen, F.: A conceptual model for detecting interactions among medical recommendations in clinical guidelines. In: Janowicz, K., Schlobach, S., Lambrix, P., Hyvönen, E. (eds.) EKAW 2014. LNCS (LNAI), vol. 8876, pp. 591–606. Springer, Cham (2014). https://doi.org/10.1007/978-3-319-13704-9_44

32. Wilk, S., Michalowski, M., Michalowski, W., Rosu, D., Carrier, M., Kezadri-Hamiaz, M.: Comprehensive mitigation framework for concurrent application of multiple clinical practice guidelines. J. Biomed. Inform. **66**, 52–71 (2017)

33. Riaño, D., Collado, A.: Model-based combination of treatments for the management of chronic comorbid patients. In: Peek, N., Marín Morales, R., Peleg, M. (eds.) AIME 2013. LNCS (LNAI), vol. 7885, pp. 11–16. Springer, Heidelberg (2013). https://doi.org/10.1007/978-3-642-38326-7_2

34. Jafarpour, B., Abidi, S.S.R.: Merging disease-specific clinical guidelines to handle comorbidities in a clinical decision support setting. In: Peek, N., Marín Morales, R., Peleg, M. (eds.) AIME 2013. LNCS (LNAI), vol. 7885, pp. 28–32. Springer, Heidelberg (2013). https://doi.org/10.1007/978-3-642-38326-7_5

35. Merhej, E., Schockaert, S., McKelvey, T.G., De Cock, M.: Generating conflict-free treatments for patients with comorbidity using ASP. In: KR4HC 2016. pp. 93–100 (2016)

36. Zhang, Y., Zhang, Z.: Preliminary result on finding treatments for patients with comorbidity. In: Miksch, S., Riaño, D., ten Teije, A. (eds.) KR4HC 2014. LNCS (LNAI), vol. 8903, pp. 14–28. Springer, Cham (2014). https://doi.org/10.1007/978-3-319-13281-5_2
37. International Health Terminology Standards Development Organisation: SNOMED Clinical Terms (2015). http://www.ihtsdo.org/snomed-ct
38. WHO Collaborating Centre for Drug Statistics Methodology: Anatomical Therapeutic Chemical classification system. http://www.whocc.no/atc/
39. Horvitz, E.: Uncertainty, action, and interaction: In: Pursuit of Mixed-Initiative Computing (1999)
40. Dechter, R., Meiri, I., Pearl, J.: Temporal constraint networks. Artif. Intell. **49**, 61–95 (1991)
41. Edwards, I.R., Aronson, J.K.: Adverse drug reactions: definitions, diagnosis, and management. Lancet **356**, 1255–1259 (2000)
42. Burger, D., et al.: Clinical management of drug-drug interactions in HCV therapy: challenges and solutions. J. Hepatol. **58**, 792–800 (2013)
43. Piovesan, L., Anselma, L., Terenziani, P.: Temporal detection of guideline interactions. In: HEALTHINF 2015, pp. 40–50. Scitepress (2015)
44. Bottrighi, A., Molino, G., Montani, S., Terenziani, P., Torchio, M.: Supporting a distributed execution of clinical guidelines. Comput. Methods Programs Biomed. **112**, 200–210 (2013)

A Multiagent-Based Model for Epidemic Disease Monitoring in DR Congo

Jean-Claude Tshilenge Mfumu[1](✉), Annabelle Mercier[2](✉),
Michel Occello[2](✉), and Christine Verdier[1](✉)

[1] Univ. Grenoble Alpes, CNRS, Grenoble INP, LIG, 38000 Grenoble, France
{jean-claude.tshilenge-mfumu,
christine.verdier}@univ-grenoble-alpes.fr
[2] Univ. Grenoble Alpes, Grenoble INP, LCIS, 26000 Valence, France
{annabelle.mercier,
michel.occello}@univ-grenoble-alpes.fr

Abstract. Any infectious diseases have been reported in sub-Saharan countries over the past decade due to the inefficiency of health structures to anticipate outbreaks. In a poorly-infrastructure country such as the Democratic Republic of Congo (DRC), with inadequate health staff and laboratories, it is difficult to respond rapidly to an epidemic, especially in rural areas. As the DRC's health system has three levels (peripheral, regional and national), from the production of health data at the peripheral level to the national level that makes the decision, meantime the disease can spread to many people. Lack of communication between health centres of the same health zone and Health zones of the same Health Provincial Division does not contribute to the regional response. This article, an extended version of [1], proposes a well elaborated solution track to deal with this problem by using an agent-centric approach to study by simulation how to improve the process. A new experiment is described by arranging twenty-eight health zones of Kinshasa to show how their collaboration can provide unique health data source for all stakeholders and help reducing disease propagation. It concerns also 47 health centres, 1 medical laboratory, 1 Provincial Health Division and 4 Rapid Riposte Teams. The simulation data, provided by Provincial Health Division of Kinshasa, concerned cholera outbreak from January to December 2017. The interaction between these agents demonstrated that Health Zone Agent can automatically alert his neighbours whenever he encountered a confirmed case of an outbreak. This action can reduce disease propagation as population will be provided with prevention measures. These interactions between agents have provided models to propose to the current system in order to find out the best that can help reducing decision time.

1 Introduction

Access to health care is a major concern in developing countries. The Democratic Republic of Congo ranks among the poorest countries according to its HDI[1] [2]. Despite its millions of hectares of arable land, this vast country of Central Africa is

---

[1] Human Development Index.

© Springer Nature Switzerland AG 2019
A. Cliquet jr. et al. (Eds.): BIOSTEC 2018, CCIS 1024, pp. 326–347, 2019.
https://doi.org/10.1007/978-3-030-29196-9_17

experiencing serious difficulties in improving the living conditions of its population, particularly in the field of basic health care. Life expectancy at birth is 50 and 53 respectively for men and women [3].

The country is currently divided into city-province of Kinshasa and 25 other provinces. The provinces are subdivided into territories which are divided into sectors. To facilitate the supervision of health structures, DRC health system is divided into three levels [4]: central, intermediate and peripheral. The nearest level to population is the peripheral area composed of 518 health zones (HZ) that coordinate the actions of health facilities. A Health Zone is divided into Health Area (HA) containing one or more Health Centers (HC) and a General Referral Hospital (GRH). The Central (national) level defines the policies, strategies and resources of the sector. It enforces strategies and policies at the peripheral level through the intermediate level called the Provincial Health Division (PHD), which coordinates primary health care and technical support activities for health zones in a province. Provincial Health Minister (PHM) is the political authority of the province.

Each Health Zone has a Health Information Bureau (HIB) which retrieves aggregated data from all its supervised Health Area to send to national level for decision measures. HIB has a Health Zone Executive Team (HZET) that organizes weekly meetings to discuss about suspicious cases to report to hierarchy if needed. Health Zone Executive Team manages health facilities (HF) that includes Health Center and GRH. Figure 1 represents three levels of DRC Health System in which each Health Zone Executive Team supervises many Health Center and one GRH at peripheral level. Provincial Health Division at intermediate level provides technical assistance to Health Zone Executive Team. Direction of Disease Control (DDC) at central level gives national policies to 26 Provincial Health Divisions. Provincial Health Minister plays also of political authority's role.

As WHO member country, DRC benefits from the technical and financial support of the partners to respond to epidemics under the conditions stipulated in the International Health Regulations (IHR) [5]. All cases of these four diseases must be automatically notified to WHO: smallpox, poliomyelitis due to wild-type poliovirus, severe acute respiratory syndrome (SARS) and cases of human influenza caused by a new subtype. On the ever-changing list of diseases provided by IHR, each country is free to add other diseases, with epidemic potential or not, which constitute a public health problem.

Access to basic care is difficult for a large part of population. People visit the health facilities in case of extreme emergency. This is more evident in rural areas where the diminishing resources of farmers do not allow them to consult medical services regularly. Most of time health care is provided during free medical workers' campaigns.

The most usual ways to collect data about cases that must be sent to the hierarchy for decision-making are described below [6]:

- Pharmacies must report when same medicines are increasingly purchased by population or when they detect some recurrent treatments;
- Schools reporting unusual rates of pupil absences due to strange signs and symptoms;

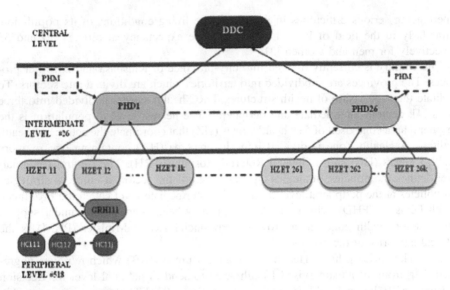

Fig. 1. Peripheral level contains health centre (HC) under the supervision of Health zone Executive Team (HZET). Provincial Health Division, the intermediate and Direction of Disease Control, the central or national level.

Figure 2 presents an exhaustive list of actors used in providing health data.

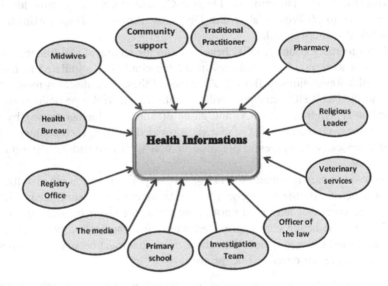

Fig. 2. Many structures are designated to produce Health data at each Health Zone [1].

Despite great efforts to improve disease surveillance and response, DRC faces big challenges in identifying, diagnosing and reporting infectious diseases properly due to the remoteness of communities, the inadequate transport and communication infrastructures, and the lack of qualified health staff and laboratory facilities to ensure accurate diagnosis.

The challenge, in this paper, is to find new solutions based on real population life and situation to improve health services organization and data sharing in order to detect infectious disease very quickly, organize the response and prevent the spread of disease.

2 Issues

In this paper, we present a part of this challenge. We propose a multi-agent system to simulate the interactions between actors working together to organize an optimal response to epidemic detection. When a new case of infectious disease is suspicious in Health Center, actors will collaborate to report it to Provincial Health Division through Health Zone Executive Team. The approach will be based on the current DRC heath system processes to extract relevant actors' tasks. The identification of these actors and their tasks will provide the opportunity to simulate a new system that distributes the entire competences of the old heath system to those actors in order to improve their collaboration and eventually shorten the making-decision time response. Work-sharing protocols will be proposed to simplify the complexity of the data sources.

This paper focuses precisely on improving the process of reporting health data from the peripheral level to the hierarchy for rapid decision-making and anticipate as much as possible the medical response using multi-agent systems (MAS). Hierarchical dependency between three levels forbids peripheral to directly transmit health data to National level for quick decision. As information must pass through intermediate level (Provincial Health Division), with defective means of communications, it drastically hampers the fight against a propagation of a disease. Since decision-making is pushed back to the central level, it can intervene belatedly at the risk of witnessing an alarming spread of an epidemic with high epidemic potential.

The next section shows the related work in healthcare and multiagent domains. Section 3 describes the healthcare system and problematic in DRC. The methodological approach and agent's models are explained in Sect. 4. The model is validated by a simulation presented in Sect. 5. Future research directions and conclusion are developed in Sect. 6.

3 Related Work

Information and Communication Technology is a powerful solution for health care in developing countries [7]. It made possible the improvement of remote patient follow-up [8], controlling the progression of malaria [9], improving the uptake of information from health systems [10]. Two main ways of research can be studied in this paper: the use of mobile phone as a relevant medium to rapidly transfer medical data and the multi-agent system that is powerful to simulate organizational skills to anticipate diseases spreading.

Mobile phone coverage in Africa grew from 10% in 1999, 65% in 2008 to more than 70% in 2012 [11]. This technology is used to cover numeric fraction. To improve drug adherence and suppression of plasma HIV-1 RNA load in Kenyan, mobile phone communication between health-care workers and patients starting antiretroviral therapy was set up [12] Text-message reminders sent to health workers' mobile phones improved and maintained their adherence to treatment guidelines for outpatient pediatric malaria [13].

Phone traces are powerful tools to estimate population migration while investigating an outbreak. These techniques were used to demonstrate the feasibility of rapid estimates and to identify areas at potentially increased risk of outbreaks in Haiti. They produced reports on SIM card movements from a cholera outbreak area at its immediate onset and within 12 h of receiving data. Results suggest that estimates of population movements during disasters and outbreaks can be delivered rapidly and with potentially high validity in areas with high mobile phone.

A trial of mobile phone text messaging for diabetes management in an eight-month period to transmit data such as blood glucose levels and body weight to a server that automatically answered with a monthly calculated glycosylated hemoglobin result. The trial results suggest that sms may provide a simple, fast and efficient adjunct to the management of diabetes.

In developed countries SMS messages have been widely used to remind patients of scheduled appointments Car and all, 2008). Similarly, more complex mobile phone applications have shown significant improvement in the follow-up of malaria patients in Thailand. The same approaches have been tested in Africa as part of the SMS reminder package to improve patients' adherence to antimalarial treatment schedules in .six sub Saharan countries [9].

Even if text-messaging is the simplest and the most widely easy to use technology function in reporting periodic data from the health system peripheral to control managers, it however needs to be experienced in interventions targeting individual patients, for whom a high facility workload or illiteracy may present a barrier.

A Multi-agent System is a set of agents situated in a common environment, which interact and try to reach a set of goals. Through these interactions, a global behavior, more intelligent than the sum of the local intelligence of multiagent system components, can emerge. By 'agent' we mean a software entity evolving in an environment that it can perceive and within which it reacts. There are several kinds of agents. A reactive agent reacts to the stimuli of the environment. Cognitive agents have a more developed intelligence: they manage knowledge and make decisions according to their internal states and according to their perception of the environment. It is provided with autonomous behaviors and some objectives. Autonomy is the main concept in the agent issue: it is the ability of agents to control their actions and their internal states. The agents' autonomy implies no centralized control [14]. When a MAS integrates agents on the fly dynamically during the execution, the system is qualified as an opened one. Otherwise, it is a closed one. One of the advantages of MAS is to model systems where a global description is not possible at any given moment. Multi-agent conception is well suitable to model actors described in Fig. 1.

Simulation based on MAS approach has wide potential applications in healthcare. First case, MAS approaches are suitable to applications where a complete control is unreachable, the high number of entities or the complexity of entities' behavior make hard to represent the overall system. The second case is related to the monitoring of the epidemics. In a general way, the model of each agents going into action in the system is designed in microscopic level. The environment, the agents' interactions and the social organizations are defined at the macroscopic level. In MAS domain, there are numerous methods to approach the analysis and the design of the software application. The methods come from various domains such as object oriented design, knowledge engineering or reproduction of behavior or natural phenomena. The first methods were AAII [15] which uses an external view (roles services, organization) and internal view (agent design bases on Belief Desire Intention architecture). Cassiopée [15] is a bottom-up approach based on natural behavior and DESIRE [16] is based on knowledge engineering. The method Vowels [17] allows obtaining modularity at the level of the multi-agents models by decomposing the problem into four elementary facets. Other method like Gaia [18] extends the concepts used in classical object engineering and provides a microscopic and a macroscopic view of the software system. There are also complete approaches for developing multi-agents systems from the analysis to the deployment by using MaSE [19] or Prometheus [20]. Moreover some models al-low the designer to develop the agent like AGR [19] based on Agent/Group/Role or BDI [21] based on Belief/Desir/Intention.

The main concept of all those approaches is the agent and the communication between agents to lead to the main objective of the software.

The general classification is clinical, operational, managerial and educational simulation. Managerial and operational simulations are closely interrelated. Both are the core components for healthcare process management. Some challenges and trends of simulation models in healthcare in the past two decades have been developed The design of a web-based clinical decision support system that guides patients with Low Back Pain in making suitable choices on self-referral has been experienced in Netherlands.

MAS is used to describe an approach to the analysis and development of telemedicine systems [22], to manage communications in wireless sensor networks [23], the epidemiological decision support system [24], the care of seniors at home [25], decision-making for monitoring and prevention of epidemics [26], evaluation of disaster response system [27], medical sensor modules in conjunction with wireless communication technology supporting a wide range of services including mobile telemedicine, patient monitoring, emergency management and information sharing between patients and doctors or among the healthcare workers [28].

MAS can be considered as a suitable technology for the realization of applications providing healthcare and social services where the use of data and remote collaborations among users are often the most requirements [29]. Cooperation in Agent Technology can provide better healthcare than the traditional medical system [30]. Real programs built on the multiagent paradigm are still evolving towards a complete maturity. The variety and complexity of the e-health scenario make it one of the most interesting application fields, able to check the advantages of their use to condition their evolution [31].

MAS was used to monitor a generic medical contact center for chronic disease environment, detect important cases, and inform the healthcare and administrative personnel via alert messages, recommendations, and reports, prompting them to action [32]. Developed MAS applications in healthcare can provide a reasonable way to mitigate the cost due to increased demand for services [33].

An Agent-Based Model (ABM) with Geospatial and Medical Details was used to evaluate the efficiency of disaster responders to rescue victims in a mass casualty incident situation in South Korea [27].

ABM can cooperate to share tasks between sensors observing a phenomena [34], to manage diabetes treatment between Caregivers and Patients. The usability evaluation of a collaborative information system for dementia assessment built using a user-centered design approach was experienced in Norway [35]. But from several research papers we have reviewed we didn't find a paper addressing ABM in sharing tasks from multisource health information to organize a rapid response to a high epidemic potential disease.

4 Health System in DRC

4.1 Administrative Structures

The patient health care and the reporting of suspicious cases are managed at the peripheral level by Health facilities (HF): health centers plus the general referral hospitals. Health data collected by the Health Facilities are transmitted to Health Zone Executive Team for consolidation, analyzes and decision-making. Aggregated data from entire Health Zone are also transmitted to Provincial Health Division. Each week this intermediate level structure convenes meetings to analyze data from each Health Zone, decide on actions to take. Provincial Health Division produces consolidated data for its province.

Provincial Health Division must transmit the health data from its province to the central level for a second analysis and national consolidation. If suspicious cases reported by Health Zone require deeper investigation, laboratory tests or kits intervention, Provincial Health Division will ask for technical and financial supports from central level.

Disease Control Direction (DCD) is a central respondent at central level. It also organizes weekly meetings to analyze health data from all provinces. It often provides advice and recommendations to Provincial Health Division to monitor suspicious cases in accordance with the national policy of the sector. Whenever Provincial Health Division asks for a help, DCD can approach government authorities, special programs, partners and even the international community, to fill up needs. Difficulties encountered by Health Facilities to better report information and structures dependency are well expressed at next section.

4.2 Structure Dependencies

The first challenge in managing epidemics begins with the multi-sources data processing at the Health Zone level. National policy has provided list of groups of individuals who can retrieve information from suspicious cases. This information transmitting by phone calls or narrative is not exhaustive. Hence, the interest in diversifying the mode of communication by adding text and voice sms, tweets and phone calls on green lines can enhance data completeness.

A second difficulty in an accurate identification of suspicious cases is the insufficient number of qualified health staff [36]. Despite training courses organized by Health Zone Executive Team for community relays and staff of health facilities, there are gaps in the implementation of the information brought to their attention. For example, the Provincial Health Division can conduct a thorough investigation with qualified staff as soon as the number of suspicious cases reaches the threshold for the pathology. Lack of information on the list of the nearest laboratories delays response time to confirm cases and ensure accuracy of diagnosis.

Hierarchical dependences do not favor communication between structures of the same level such as health areas of a same Health Zone or of contiguous health areas but belonging to different Provincial Health Division. This lack of dialogue can lead to the non-detection of an epidemic for the simple reason that the number of suspicious cases to organize investigation is not reached in an Health Zone. However, by combining number of suspicious case found in contiguous health areas, we could detect the pathology at the intersection of the provinces.

4.3   Collection and Response for Epidemic Surveillance

Structures authorized to report information relating to suspicious cases to Health Zone Executive Team are Health Facilities. But, community relays can also report their observations that need to be considered by Health Facilities. Reports concern pathologies described at International Sanitary Regulations (smallpox, poliomyelitis due to wild polio virus, human influenza and Severe Acute Respiratory Syndrome (SARS)) and local list of diseases with epidemic Eradication measures or Elimination and other chronic diseases provided by authorities.

4.4   Data Collection and Epidemics Response

As soon as it appears, suspicious cases must be transmitted to Health Zone Executive Team by all data providers indicated on Fig. 2. When number of suspicious cases in Health Zone equals to the threshold of observed pathology, a rapid riposte team (RRT) has to investigate some Health Center and the population of the concerned Health Area to make sure the allegation was correct. The investigation of Rapid Ripost Team could result to laboratory tests of some samples. In case of riposte many hierarchical structures such as Provincial Health Division or national level would intervene to provide technical and financial supports.

The process used to organize riposte simulation is heavily based upon computer science, mathematics, probability theory and statistics: yet the process of simulation modeling and experimentation remains very much an intuitive art. Simulation is a very general and somewhat ill-defined subject. For the purpose of this paper, we will define simulation as «the process of designing a computerized model of a system and conducting experiments for the purpose of understanding the behavior of the system and/or of evaluating various strategies for the operation of the system. Thus we will understand the process of simulation to include both the construction of the model and the analytical use of the model for studying a problem shortly described in Fig. 3. Health Zone Executive Team analyze the report of surveillance to determine if the number of suspicious case has reached the threshold to order an investigation. Rapid Ripost Team will research new cases at Health Area according to the clinical definition of case. It will find out new determinants of the outbreak to report to Provincial Health Division in other to realize the response.

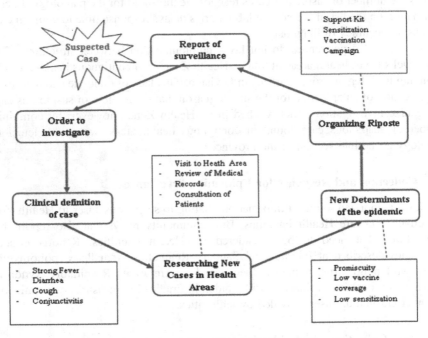

Fig. 3. Cycle of outbreak response [1].

A final evaluation of outbreak response presented as a report of the process can be shared with other Health Zone and Health Facilities.

This type of system is well suited to MAS using an AEIO representation. Real system is analyzed with four elements: **A**gent, **E**nvironment, **O**rganizations and **I**nteractions between agents. This model will be detailed in the next part.

5 Individual-Centered Models

The hierarchical organization of the healthcare system in DRC is a good candidate for a multiagent model because there are several kinds of agents with personal goals sharing the same global achievement. In the process described in Fig. 3, the agents use some knowledge and tasks to perform a main goal together: collecting data in order to respond with efficiency to epidemic.

At the stage of this research, the simulation's objective is to understand how the DRC's healthcare system reacts in Epidemic diseases. It is a preliminary work before (i) determining metrics to analyze process simulations and (ii) developing modules in embedded systems - phones or tablets- to assist the end-user in the data collection, coupled with the multiagent system. Multiagent-based-simulation (MABS) allows explicitly modeling the behavior of each individual and viewing the emergent system from the interactions between the individuals. Morvan in [37] proposes a survey on MABS and presents several multiagents platforms. In these existing platforms, we have not found solutions which can act as both a simulation system and a tool to end-users on embedded systems.

DIAMOND method and its associated simulator MASH – MultiAgent Software Hardware simulation - developed in LCIS Laboratory provided the capacity of testing a method in a tool of simulation [23, 34].

DIAMOND – Decentralized IterAtive Multiagent Open Network Design - is a method that guides the designer from the requirements to the implementation. It is based on A-E-I-O decomposition for Agent, Environment, Interactions and Organization of the system. The Agent dimension concerns the model of the reactive agent represented by a simple automaton, the cognitive agent manipulating information or a more complex agent based on a knowledge system. The Environment is the context in which the agent reacts, its geographic location. The Interaction dimension specifies the way the agents communicate; it mainly consists of protocols of interaction or the type of communication. The Organization dimension reflects the structural relations between the agents (group, hierarchy, market). These four key concepts are considered under a global angle (the society) and a local one (agent view).

The DIAMOND method proposes an analysis phase of the problem in four steps:

- *the situation phase* helps to find the society's circumference to be represented by defining the limits of the system, agents and environment;
- *the individual phase* concerns the internal functioning of the agents (behavior and the knowledge);
- *the social phase* defines the relations between agents, particularly by integrating into its knowledge communication protocols and information structures to understand the society organization and
- *The phase of socialization* consists of integrating *the individual agents* into the society by adding the social influences into its behavior (possible answers in the requests from the outside, the launch of interaction protocols and the choice to be made according to its position in the organization).

We decide to use this method because it allows explicitly designing the behavior of each individual. However, coupled with the MASH simulator platform, it is useful to view the emergent system from the interactions between the individuals. The process in Fig. 3 can be modelized by agents able to be simulated in the MASH simulator. The MASH simulation platform was used to simulate systems with embedded and software agents. It is suitable to our problem because we plan to provide a tool for collecting data with phones or tablets applications.

To have an individual-centered vision of the process is one of the advantages of this simulation. Afterwards, we will be able to contribute to the improvement of the process with an exterior view by proposing changes and ideas to reduce the response time for example.

This section shows the steps to break down multiagent system's elements.

5.1 Step 1: Agents' Tasks and Knowledge: The Internal Behavior

To start the analysis, each individual agent's behavior is studied. It is a way of seeing things at a micro level. The phenomenon at macro level does not change and the process remains the same even if observer's level changes.

The objective is to be able to adjust the behavior of each individual agent and probably to add some skills to certain nodes or node types.

The first step of this approach is to find out what to model as agents from information of the process. In our study context, agents are: health centers, General Referral Hospital, Health areas, Provincial Health Division, any national health entity related to the administrative structures, Health Zone Executive Team and Rapid Ripost Team for human team working group. Figure 4 shows for instance the internal behavior of one agent (Rapid Ripost Team).

For each agent, we have to list all its skills, what information will be required to store or to handle and how agent acquires this information. This information should be acquired directly by perception (e.g. the user grasps something) or on demand by asking other nodes (higher hierarchy or same level nodes).

In this step, we obtain for each agent a vision of the relevant knowledge to perform its individual tasks. That information is required by agents working in the same environment. The result is a set of tasks that an agent can perform. These tasks correspond to the skills of each node. Some skills are executed by one agent without the need of other agents. But to achieve a goal, an agent should have partial information and should ask to other agents to complete their goal. However, this will result to a cooperative behavior in place of an individual one which is entirely internal to agent. This kind of social behavior reflects an interaction between several agents: either to gain information or to share tasks.

5.2 Step 2: Agent's Sharing Data and Interactions

Social Behavior. In this second step, we will have to create interactions between nodes for example to back up information (Health Center to Health Zone Executive Team) or to receive orders (Health Zone Executive Team from Provincial Health Division). These interactions should intervene between different partner groups such as health areas. In the implementation, we define very simple interaction protocols for data exchange such as receiving information, answers/queries or order to perform a task. For some tasks, such as health alert surrounding areas, it is no longer just a request for information but cooperative behavior brings into play several kinds of agents. To communicate with others, agent uses interaction protocols. We will there-fore express how this behavior will be realized by defining a more sophisticated interaction protocol than query/response. Various protocols are available for negotiating, giving orders,

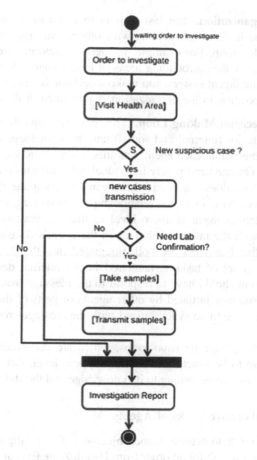

Fig. 4. Investigating an outbreak [1].

waiting for answers. The interaction patterns that will govern this cooperative behavior will be organized between the agents.

Interaction Protocols. The protocol is a part of the agents' knowledge. In our simulation, agents have a list of protocols they should initiate to answer others. For the moment, we use a simple protocol with two states as represented in Fig. 6: "inform" and "inform back". For example, Agent A1 launches an instance of protocol P1, with the state S1. The agent A2 receives a call from A1 with the performative "information" in the state S1. A2 knows the protocol and searches the next transition; it slips into state S2 and sends an acknowledgment to agent A1. A1 treats the message and the conversation finishes. The ACL FIPA compliant Performatives are used:

- *RDCMessage.ACL_QUERY_REF* for queries/answers,
- *RDCMessage.ACL_REQUEST* for an order to perform a task and,
- *RDCMessage.ACL_INFORM* for inform/acknowledgment.

Position in the Organization. The last step is to consider an agent's position in organization when he initiates interactions with others. An organization should be a hierarchy or a simple group. For example, to alert neighboring Health Zone, health center agents must know the surrounding areas of health zone, which is a group or an organization in the multiagent system, and make a decision based on its position in this group. The agent's position in the organization is integrated in the decision loop.

Agent's Internal Decision Making Loop. The previous steps showed agent's skills, agent's complex behavior (internal and social) and the knowledge of interaction protocols. On the hypothesis that each agent gets this information, we can now build the agent decision loop. On one hand purely individual behavior runs only with an agent's context information and does not need other agents to complete the agent goal. On other hand, social behavior involves relationships between agents. An individual-centered approach defines agent at micro level so that interactions with other agents have to be merged with the internal behavior in the agent's decision loop. The individual and cooperative behaviors are both integrated into the decision loop. In the individual behavior, a set of tasks is launched in the internal decision loop. In its decision loop, the agent should have to respond to the message from others, which are part of interaction protocols initiated by other agents or parts of the agent interaction patterns. These tasks have to be synchronized with the messages received from others agents.

As an external view, huge decision loops, which are decentralized in the several kinds of agents, seem to be synchronized at the system level. But in fact, each agent decides in what state to pass according to its knowledge and the state of its interactions.

5.3   Step 3: Collaborative Tasks of Agents

Agents would collaborate to achieve some objectives. To investigate on Health Area, Rapid Ripost Team must wait for an order from Health Zone Executive Team. The later receives health data every week from Health Center and checks if the threshold of the followed pathology has been reached. The same collaboration is needed between Rapid Ripost Team and Health Area, Rapid Ripost Team and Laboratory. The sequence diagram (Fig. 5) gives a snapshot of the kind of collaboration found in agents concerned with an outbreak investigation.

Message Format for Interaction. The messages exchanged between agents contain sender and receiver agents, protocol information and data to manage like *[sender; receiver; conversation; perform; protocol; inst_prot; state_prot; data]*. The data follow a format according to the performative.

To interact through a message sent by another agent, a simple protocol is established. For instance when Rapid Ripost Team asks a laboratory to perform exams, he has to first check its state to be convinced that it can answer his request. A simple protocol with acknowledgment is used.

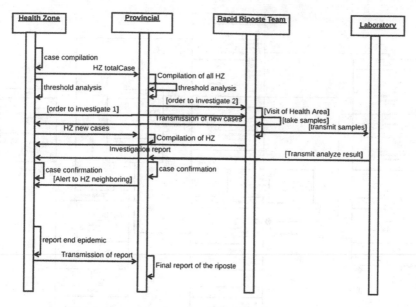

Fig. 5. Sequence diagrams of investigating an outbreak.

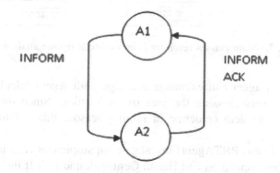

Fig. 6. Protocol for information with acknowledgment [1].

The agent changes state when he asks for information and when he receives answers to his request (Fig. 6). In a future simulation, a negotiation protocol with a call for proposal to several laboratories will be tested. However, the agent launching the conversation should negotiate among laboratories which one is available, near or powerful.

5.4 Overview of Agents in Process Analysis

The analyze of the cycle of outbreak response presented on 4.4 isolated some individuals playing different roles to achieve the objectives assigned to the riposte process. A simple class diagram (Fig. 7) gives a quick overview of main actors.

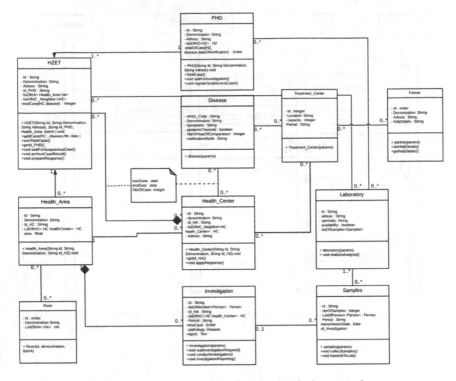

Fig. 7. Main classes resulting from outbreak riposte analyze.

Health Center as agent can exchange message with Agent 'Health Area' to get information about rivers crossing the area of its location. Since this knowledge is crucial to anticipate cholera epidemic in raining season, this collaboration is very important.

Rapid Riposte Team (RRTAgent) investigate on suspicious case in a Health Area which means visiting population and Health Centers found in it If the disease requires laboratory analyzes to confirm the case RRTAgent must take samples and transmit it to LaboratoryAgent available.

6 Simulation: Cholera Case Study

6.1 Cholera: A Plague Still Causing Major Epidemics

More than one million cases of cholera in Yemen have been reported to the World Health Organization since April 2017. The International Committee of the Red Cross does not hesitate to mention "the worst crisis humanitarian relief in the world "in this country. Despite the International Health Regulations, revised in 2005 to encourage countries to report events constituting a public health emergency, cases remain under-reported worldwide due to fear of economic consequences, often insufficient surveillance systems and a lack of standardized terminology to define a case of cholera.[2]

The disease results from the absorption by the mouth of water or food contaminated by the cholera vibrio. After a few hours to a few days of incubation, violent diarrhea and vomiting occur, without fever. In the absence of treatment, death occurs in 1 to 3 days, by cardiovascular collapse (fall in blood pressure) in 25 to 50% of cases. Mortality is higher among children, the elderly and vulnerable individuals.

The treatment consists essentially of compensating the digestive losses of water and electrolytes. Rehydration is given orally or intravenously, depending on the degree of dehydration. The improvement is noticeable after a few hours and healing, without sequelae, is obtained in a few days. Antibiotic therapy is recommended by WHO only for severe dehydration.

In 1973, since a first outbreak, V. cholerae serogroup O: 1 biotype El Tor was reintroduced several times in the Democratic Republic of Congo. 26 health zones in 6 provinces are identified as sanctuary areas. Kinshasa has recorded several outbreaks of the cholera epidemic. The 2017–2018's episode caused 56 deaths out of 1272 suspicious cases reported, as shown in Fig. 8.

6.2   Data Collection

DLM is a disease control direction located in Kinshasa which collects the national data for disease monitoring. It provided us with ten years data of cholera outbreak from 2008 to November 2017. We extracted the data for Kinshasa grouped on its 35 health zones to compare with Provincial Health Division's data.

Provincial Health Division's data contained more details about Health centers that reported the suspicious cases and theirs Health Area. We analyze the data from first January 2017 to December 30th 2017.

6.3   Methods

We reported cumulated data of each health zone to a map, as shown in Fig. 8, to find their neighboring and try to suggest the best way to establish collaboration between them in order to stop disease propagation.

We focus on two groups of health zones. In the first group we have Binza-Météo, Mont-Ngafula, Kokolo and Kintambo. The second contains Limete and Kingabwa.

Our hypothesis was: if actors from each heath zone could exchange disease information with their neighbors as soon as an outbreak happens, it would be possible to reduce the propagation. For example, epidemic began at Kintambo on January 2017. As the communication and sensitization weren't establish with its neighbors, some weeks after disease was reported from Kokolo and Binza-Météo.

---

[2] https://www.pasteur.fr/fr/journal-recherche/dossiers/cholera-fleau-encore-origine-epidemies-majeures.

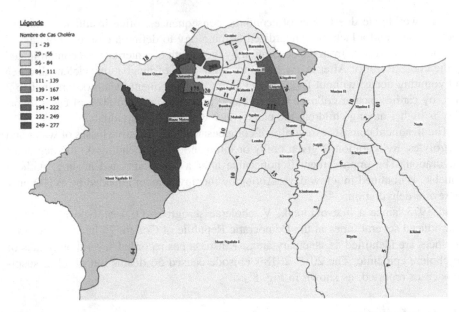

Fig. 8. From 01/01/2017 to 30/04/2018, Kinshasa's Health zones reported 1272 cases of Cholera outbreak with 56 dead.

6.4   Results

To test and evaluate our approach, we adapted MASH simulator developed by LCIS Lab for a wireless sensor multiagent system [34]. We focus our simulation to these health zones: Binza-Météo, Mont-Ngafula, Kokolo, Kintambo, Limete and Kingabwa.

The simulation concerns precisely Kintambo and Limete that register more suspicious case of cholera outbreak during 2017 and from them other neighboring health zones were affected. The main idea is to see how the future system would react if each actor of health system could perform its own task with autonomy. These experiences could result to many scenarios and the best of them will be proposed to DRC's Health System to reduce decision time as each actor can execute his talks according to the knowledge of the environment and the outbreak determinants he will be provided with.

We chose two Health-Zones of Kinshasa Provincial Health Division for the simulation. Kintambo and Limete are Health Zones that register respectively 57 and 64 suspicious cases with death in 2017. The epidemic began from them and the propagation of disease affected their neighbors with an important amount of suspicious cases. Kokolo counted 208 cases while Binza-météo registered 153 suspicious cases at the same period.

To respond to an outbreak noticed at a Health Center, health staff of the concerning Health Center must refer to Health Zone Executive Team. In their turn, Health Zone Executive Team must refer to Provincial Health Division and Provincial Health Division to central level. This chain of hierarchical contacts can enlarge time decision.

In our simulation, we worked with these hypotheses: (i) each Health Center actor must contact immediately its Health Executive Team as soon as it encountered a suspicious case; (ii) Health Zone Executive Team cumulate suspicious case and create an RRT when the disease's threshold is reached; (iii) RRT can contact the nearest LaboAgent able to answer to his request or to use his information to make decision. We considered twenty-eight Health Zone Executive Team in yellow or red, forty seven Health Center in green or blue, RRT in grey one Provincial Health Division and one medical test laboratories (LaboAgent). The first suspicious case was detected in Health Center #49 in green. Figure 9 illustrates those actors working as Agents. The below map represents Health zones in north of Kinshasa.

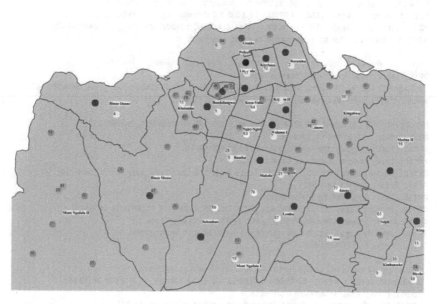

Fig. 9. Suspicious cases of cholera outbreak reported during 2017 by Kinshasa's Health Zones. (Color figure online)

The simulation trace file (Fig. 10) shows the communication between agents. As they are autonomous they perform their own tasks like "cumulate new cases", "conduct the investigation on Health Zone # 16" and manage messages like "realize analyzes from Health Center", "receive sample to_ analyze" or "report suspicious case detected". HZET Agents (#16 and #13) are waiting for a suspicious case message from any HC. Whenever Health Zone Executive Team Agent receives such a message he computes cases and compare with the threshold of disease monitoring to decide the necessity of building a RRT Agent able to investigate in Health Centers around suspicious case in Health Area. The visited health center will turn from green to blue color. RRT Agent could send samples to LaboAgent while searching for new cases in Health Areas. The organization of outbreak riposte could depend on the results from LaboAgent and investigation report from RRT Agent.

```
/*** Agent HC49: on loop 29000 29000 informed HZET a suspected case detected ***/
HC49: (Task): Suspicious case detected on 2017-01-30
(HCAgent: task) Agent HC50:  Next detection at: 85000, Case Number: 1
HC49: (sendMessage) : SEND : HZET16: [49;16;0;1;0;0;0;Suspiscious_case_detected 49 1]
         /** HZET cumulate all cases from other Health Center **/
HZET16: (Task): Wait for an Investigation request, cumulate: 2


/*** Agent HC49 : on loop 50000 50003 ***/
HC49: (Task): Suspicious case detected on 2017-02-20
HC49: (sendMessage) : SEND : HZET16: [49;16;0;1;0;0;0;Suspiscious_case_detected 49 1]
(HCAgent: task) Agent HC49:  Next detection at: 125000, Case Number: 2


/** as the threshold is reached, HZET16 sends an investigation team RRT80 **/
HZET16: (sendMessage) : SEND : RRT80 : [16;80;0;3;0;0;0;Investigation_request 16]
HZET16: (sendMessage) : SEND : PHD61 : [16;61;0;1;0;0;0;Suspiscious_case_detected  49 16]
HZET16: (Task): Wait for an Investigation request, cumulate: 5


/**starting the entity 80 – RRT must investigate Health Zone of Health Center**/
RRT80: (Task): Wait for an Investigation request!
(PHDAgent::receive) : PHD 61: RECEIVED message [16;61;0;1;0;0;0;Suspiscious_case_detected  49 16]
PHD61: (Task): Archives Case concerning HC 49 from HZET 16


(RRTAgent::receive) Agent : 80 RECEIVE : [16;80;0;3;0;0;0;Investigation_request 16]
RRT80: (Task): Go on the HC 16 zone!
RRT80: (Task): Conduct the Investigation on Health zone 16
RRT80: (Task): Reports Suspicious Case at HC 16!
RRT80: (sendMessage) : SEND : HZET16 : [80;16;0;1;0;0;0;Confirmed_suspiscious_case  16]
RRT80: (Task): Collect Samples!
RRT80: (Task): Transmit To a Laboratory!
RRT80: (sendMessage) : SEND : LABO62 : [80;62;0;2;0;0;0;Sample_to_analyze 16 80 16]
RRT80: (Task): Investigation Reporting by RRT 80about a case on zone 16!
RRT80: (sendMessage) : SEND : 16 : [80;16;0;1;0;0;0;Report_investigation 80]
RRT80: (Task): End Of Mission!


/**starting the entity 62. LABOAgent sends analyze results to HZET and PHD**/
(LABOAgent::receive) Agent : 62 RECEIVE : [80;62;0;2;0;0;0;Sample_to_analyze 16 80 16]
LABO62: (Task): Realizes Analysis from HC16
LABO62: (sendMessage) : SEND : 16: [62;16;0;1;0;0;0;Result_sample  16 80]
LABO62: (sendMessage) : SEND : PHD61: [62;61;0;1;0;0;0;Result_sample 16 16 80]


/** reception of results and alert to HCs **/
(PHDAgent::receive): PHD 61: RECEIVED message [62; 61; 0; 1;0;0;0;Result_sample 16 16 80]
HZET16: (sendMessage) : SEND : HC49 : [16;49;0;3;0;0;0;Apply_response]
HZET16: (sendMessage) : SEND : HC50 : [16;50;0;3;0;0;0;Apply_response]
HZET16: (sendMessage) : SEND : HC51 : [16;51;0;3;0;0;0;Apply_response]
HZET16: (sendMessage) : SEND : PHD61 : 16;61;0;3;0;0;0;Investigation_request 62


/** At the end of simulation every HZET can present its cumulate case **/
HZET16: (Task): Wait for an Investigation request, cumulate: 64
HZET20: (Task): Wait for an Investigation request, cumulate: 52
HZET20: (Task): Wait for an Investigation request, cumulate: 53
HZET1: (Task): Wait for an Investigation request, cumulate: 2
HZET3: (Task): Wait for an Investigation request, cumulate: 124
HZET3: (Task): Wait for an Investigation request, cumulate: 153
```

Fig. 10. Agents' collaboration to achieve the assigned objectives. Trace extracted from a simulation.

The agents operate independently: HCAgent transmits data to Health Zone Executive TeamAgent, RRTAgent completes a full investigation, LaboAgent conducts medical testing and transmits results to HZETAgent and PHDAgent which manages all information from Health Zone Executive Team under its supervision. Message synchronization between kinds of agent is done in the agent's decision loop. A protocol with two states is used and implements KQML-like performatives. The four numbers in the message are "1" for inform (give information), "2" for query information (ask for an information) and "3" for request (ask for a task to be done). The agents communicate and achieve their goal by reacting to messages from others or executing their inner task as response to a query.

With positive results from LaboAgent, Health Zone Executive Team sends warning and preventive measures to his all Health Centers. PHDAgent can also alert the surrounding Health Zone Executive Teams.

7 Conclusions

In this paper, we have showed how multi-agent system can improve the organizations' tasks in order to decrease the time to response when an epidemic disease is suspected or detected. A main research result can be highlighted: the use of a multi-agent method previously dedicated to wireless sensors and applied to human organizations.

We have proved that the method was generic enough and gave good results with real data and a hierarchical and complex health eco-system. MAS is often used in health domain and our paper's result complete the panel of applications with real data and under eco-system constraints.

Some limits must be underlined: (i) in order to adapt the method, we have defined hypothesis that strongly constraint the models; (ii) the stakeholders have been introduced in the method only with their job characteristics and adding their experience in the simulation can probably enhance the results. Nevertheless the multiagent method can cover only one part of the global problem. We discussed about an organizational method useful to enlarge all aspects of the problem laid down.

We propose in the future works to widen the approach to take into account different and complementary aspects: health data collection and transmission, health data quality, improvement of the complete riposte process, improvement of the health system organization. In order to, we propose a three-phases innovation method named Chicken useful to supervise and improve the epidemic disease riposte:

- Phase 1: define the life cycle of the epidemic disease to watch over.
- Phase 2: health data monitoring
- Phase 3: riposte and feed-back

Each phase of this innovation method is build with models, methods' fragments, tools coming from different sciences domains and proposes a road map to improve the riposte and the health data quality. Then the multiagent method becomes a method's fragment in the wider method Chicken.

References

1. Tshilenge Mfumu, J.-C., Mercier, A., Verdier, C., Occello, M.: Towards an agent-based model to monitor epidemics and chronic diseases in DR congo, pp. 83–93 (2018)
2. Programme des Nations Unies pour le Développement: Rapport sur le développement humain (2016). http://hdr.undp.org/sites/default/files/HDR2016_FR_Overview_Web.pdf. Accessed 05 Apr 2018
3. World health statistics 2014: Geneva: World Health Organization (2014)
4. Recueil des normes de la zone de santé: Ministère de la Santé (2006)
5. Weltgesundheitsorganisation (ed.): Règlement sanitaire international: 2005, 2nd edn. Organisation Mondiale de la Santé, Genève (2006)
6. Ministère de la Santé, RDC: Guide Technique pour la surveillance intégrée de la maladie et riposte (2011). http://www.luttecontrelamaladie.org/bvf/GUIDE%20SMIR.pdf. Accessed 26 Feb 2018
7. Greenberg, A.: ICTs for Poverty Alleviation: Basic Tool and Enabling Sector (2005)
8. Wouters, B., Barjis, J., Maponya, G., Martiz, J., Mashiri, M.: Supporting home based health care in South African rural communities using USSD technology. In: AMCIS 2009 Proceedings, p. 410 (2009)
9. Zurovac, D., Talisuna, A.O., Snow, R.W.: Mobile phone text messaging: tool for malaria control in Africa. PLoS Med. 9(2), e1001176 (2012)
10. Mutale, W., et al.: improving health information systems for decision making across five sub-Saharan African countries: implementation strategies from the African Health Initiative. BMC Health Serv. Res. 13(2), S9 (2013)
11. Aker, J.C., Mbiti, I.M.: Mobile phones and economic development in Africa. J. Econ. Perspect. 24(3), 207–232 (2010)
12. Lester, R.T., et al.: Effects of a mobile phone short message service on antiretroviral treatment adherence in Kenya (WelTel Kenya1): a randomised trial. Lancet Lond. Engl. 376 (9755), 1838–1845 (2010)
13. Zurovac, D., et al.: The effect of mobile phone text-message reminders on Kenyan health workers' adherence to malaria treatment guidelines: a cluster randomised trial. Lancet Lond. Engl. 378(9793), 795–803 (2011)
14. Wooldridge, M., Jennings, N.R., Kinny, D.: A methodology for agent-oriented analysis and design. In: Proceedings of the Third Annual Conference on Autonomous Agents, New York, NY, USA, pp. 69–76 (1999)
15. Kinny, D., Georgeff, M., Rao, A.: A methodology and modelling technique for systems of BDI agents. In: Van de Velde, W., Perram, J.W. (eds.) MAAMAW 1996. LNCS, vol. 1038, pp. 56–71. Springer, Heidelberg (1996). https://doi.org/10.1007/BFb0031846
16. Brazier, F.M.T., Dunin-Keplicz, B.M., Jennings, N.R., Treur, J.: Desire: modelling multi-agent systems in a compositional formal framework. Int. J. Coop. Inf. Syst. 06(01), 67–94 (1997)
17. Demazeau, Y.: "Voyelles," Mém. D'habilitation À Dir. Rech. INP Grenoble (2001)
18. Wooldridge, M.: The Gaia Methodology for Agent-Oriented Analysis and Design, p. 28
19. DeLoach, S.A.: Analysis and Design using MaSE and agentTool. Air Force Inst of Tech Wright-Patterson AFB, OH, School of Engineering and Management, April 2001
20. Padgham, L., Winikoff, M.: Prometheus: a methodology for developing intelligent agents. In: Giunchiglia, F., Odell, J., Weiß, G. (eds.) AOSE 2002. LNCS, vol. 2585, pp. 174–185. Springer, Heidelberg (2003). https://doi.org/10.1007/3-540-36540-0_14
21. Rao, A.S., Georgeff, M.P.: BDI Agents: From Theory to Practice, p. 8 (1995)

22. Mea, V.D.: Agents acting and moving in healthcare scenario - a paradigm for telemedical collaboration. IEEE Trans. Inf Technol. Biomed. **5**(1), 10–13 (2001)
23. Jamont, J.-P., Occello, M.: Designing embedded collective systems: The DIAMOND multiagent method. In: IEEE International Conference on Tools with Artificial Intelligence - ICTAI 2007, Patras, Greece, pp. 91–94 (2007)
24. Weber, A.: Modélisation et Gestion de Flux par Systèmes Multiagents: Application à un système d'aide à la décision en épidémiologie, Ecole Centrale de Lille (2007)
25. Mercier, A., Raievsky, C., Occello, M., Genthial, D.: Solutions multi-agents pour la prise en charge à domicile des séniors. Ingénierie Systèmes Inf. **18**(6), 83–112 (2013)
26. Younsi, F.-Z.: Mise en place d'un Système d'Information Décisionnel pour le suivi et la prévention des épidémies. Lyon (2016)
27. Bae, J.W., et al.: Evaluation of disaster response system using agent-based model with geospatial and medical details. IEEE Trans. Syst. Man Cybern. Syst. **48**, 1–16 (2017)
28. Han, B.-M., Song, S.-J., Lee, K.M., Jang, K.-S., Shin, D.-R.: Multi-agent system based efficient healthcare service. In: 2006 8th International Conference Advanced Communication Technology, vol. 1, pp. 5–51 (2006)
29. Bergenti, F., Poggi, A., Tomaiuolo, M.: Using multi-agent systems to support e-health services. In: Handbook of Research on ICTs for Human-Centered Healthcare and Social Care Services, pp. 549–567 (2013)
30. Jemal, H., Kechaou, Z., Ayed, M.B., Alimi, A.M.: A multi agent system for hospital organization. Int. J. Mach. Learn. Comput. **5**(1), 51–56 (2015)
31. Bergenti, F., Poggi, A., Tomaiuolo, M.: Multi-agent systems for e-health and telemedicine. In: Encyclopedia of e-Health and Telemedicine, pp. 688–699 (2016)
32. Koutkias, V.G., Chouvarda, I., Maglaveras, N.: A multiagent system enhancing home-care health services for chronic disease management. IEEE Trans. Inf Technol. Biomed. **9**(4), 528–537 (2005)
33. Shakshuki, E., Reid, M.: Multi-agent system applications in healthcare: current technology and future roadmap. Proc. Comput. Sci. **52**, 252–261 (2015)
34. Jamont, J.-P., Occello, M.: A multiagent tool to simulate hybrid real/virtual embedded agent societies. In: Proceedings of the 2009 IEEE/WIC/ACM International Joint Conference on Web Intelligence and Intelligent Agent Technology, Washington, DC, USA, vol. 02, pp. 501–504 (2009)
35. Smaradottir, B., Martinez, S., Holen-Rabbersvik, E., Vatnøy, T., Fensli, R.: Usability Evaluation of a Collaborative Health Information System - Lessons from a User-centred Design Process (2016)
36. Ministère du Plan de la RD Congo: Deuxième Enquête Démographique et de santé 2013–2014, September 2014. https://www.unicef.org/drcongo/french/00_-_00_-_DRC_DHS_2013-2014_FINAL_PDF_09-29-2014.pdf. Accessed 27 Feb 2018
37. Morvan, G.: Multi-level agent-based modeling - a literature survey. ArXiv12050561 Cs, May 2012

Predictive Modeling of Emerging Antibiotic Resistance Trends

M. L. Tlachac[1(✉)], Elke A. Rundensteiner[1], T. Scott Troppy[2], Kirthana Beaulac[3], Shira Doron[3], and Kerri Barton[2]

[1] Worcester Polytechnic Institute, Worcester, MA 01604, USA
{mltlachac,rundenst}@wpi.edu
[2] Massachusetts Department of Public Health,
Jamaica Plain, MA 02130, USA
{scott.troppy,kerri.barton}@state.ma.us
[3] Tufts Medical Center, Boston, MA 02111, USA
{kbeaulac,sdoron}@tuftsmedicalcenter.org

Abstract. Antibiotic resistance is constantly evolving, requiring frequent reevaluation of resistance patterns to guide treatment of bacterial infections. Antibiograms, aggregate antimicrobial susceptibility reports, are critical for evaluating the likelihood of antibiotic effectiveness. However, these antibiograms provide outdated resistance knowledge. Thus, this research employs predictive modeling of historic antibiograms to forecast the current year's resistance rates. Utilizing subsets of the expansive 15-year Massachusetts statewide antibiogram dataset, we demonstrate the effectiveness of using our model selector PYPER with regression-based models to forecast current antimicrobial susceptibility. A PYPER variant is effective since it leverages the fact that different antibiotic-bacteria-location combinations have different antimicrobial susceptibility trends over time. In addition, we discuss relative weighting of the regression-variant models, the impact of location granularity, and the ability to forecast multiple years into the future.

Keywords: Antimicrobial resistance · Antibiograms ·
Regression · Support vector regression ·
Autoregressive integrated moving average · Model selection

1 Introduction

1.1 Background on the Antibiotic Resistance Threat

Antibiotic resistance is becoming an increasing prevalent issue worldwide. Antibiotic resistance is a result of genetically mutated bacteria surviving exposure to antibiotics and propagating [13]. The reported levels of antimicrobial resistance are alarming according to the World Health Organization [19].

An estimated 700,000 people worldwide die from antibiotic resistance each year [13]. Conservative estimates from 2013 attribute 23 thousand deaths per

© Springer Nature Switzerland AG 2019
A. Cliquet jr. et al. (Eds.): BIOSTEC 2018, CCIS 1024, pp. 348–366, 2019.
https://doi.org/10.1007/978-3-030-29196-9_18

year within the United States to antibiotic resistance bacterial infections [4]. Patients with antibiotic resistant bacterial infections also experience more devastating health outcomes ranging from extended hospital stays to increased risk of death [19]. In addition, antibiotic resistant bacterial infections are more expensive to treat than other bacterial infections, costing the U.S. economy an estimated 20 billion dollars a year in direct healthcare costs as well as at least that much in loss of economic productivity [4].

The overuse of antibiotics is the main facilitator of antimicrobial resistance [4,18]. In particular, incorrectly prescribed antibiotics have been shown to be a major contributor of antimicrobial resistance [18]. Despite growing resistance, antibiotics remain one of the most prescribed human medicines [4]. Unfortunately, half of these prescriptions are either unnecessary or ineffective [4,18]. These inappropriate antibiotic prescriptions are unnecessarily hastening the increase in antibiotic resistance.

Antibiotics need to be prescribed more responsibly. Without action, it has been forecasted that by 2050, antibiotic resistant bacterial infections will cause 10 million deaths and cost 100 trillion per year worldwide [13]. One of the main steps to combat growing antimicrobial resistance is through more prudent antibiotic prescription practices. However, this can only be accomplished through up-to-date antibiotic susceptibility knowledge.

Antibiotic resistance is tracked using antibiograms, reports that provide the average percent susceptibility of select antibiotic tested against clinical isolates. Isolates are cultures of bacterial infections taken from hospital patients. Antibiograms are generated by microbiology laboratories most frequently for acute care hospitals. These antibiograms are then used to monitor epidemiological trends and for empirical antibiotic selection for patients who require treatment before patient specific laboratory data is available [7].

Despite the growing antimicrobial resistance crisis and the importance of antibiograms, there is a lack of both widespread data and analytics on longitudinal resistance patterns. There is no coordinated worldwide surveillance of antibiotic resistance bacterial infections and the surveillance that does exist tends to lack the prerequisite resources [13,19]. Although antimicrobial resistance data is monitored at the local level, the antibiograms used to inform antibiotic selection are often not be up-to-date.

For instance, the state of Massachusetts has collected a comprehensive set of antibiograms from acute care hospitals spanning 16 years. However, as antibiograms are collected annually and the collection process can span half a year, by the time these antibiograms are utilized for prescription purposes, the susceptibility information is at least one year old. While guided antibiotic treatment is greatly preferable over less informed decisions regarding antibiotic selection, antibiotics are unfortunately still being prescribed from outdated resistance knowledge.

Outdated resistance information facilitates the propagation of ineffective and inappropriate antibiotic use by suggesting antibiotics may be more or less effective than they are in reality. Inevitably, the responses to emerging resistance threats are delayed. The Centers for Disease Control and Prevention states that improving antibiotic prescribing by reducing the misuse and overuse of antibiotics is the most important of the four main actions to fight antimicrobial resistance [5]. Thus, predictive analytics needs to be applied to model existing susceptibility data and forecast current and future antibiotic susceptibility. This needs to be accomplished for as many antibiotic-bacteria pairs as possible as well as the most prevalent pairs. These forecasts can then be used to help guide prescription practices and prepare for future resistance threats. However, antimicrobial analytics is largely lacking in the literature, especially for short-term antibiotic resistance forecasts useful in treatment and for a variety of antibiotic-bacteria pairs.

1.2 Previous Antibiogram Analytics

The chi-square test is a popular statistical method to analyze antibiogram data as it determines if the change in susceptibility between two time periods is statistically different [6,8,14]. However, this test is limited in that it has no forecasting ability, rather it is a retrospective analysis.

Other antibiogram research incorporate machine learning methods, notably regression variants, to model the antibiotic resistance trends [1,2,6,10]. One of these studies uses multivariate logistic regression analysis to isolate the impact of time on antibiotic susceptibility for five bacterial infections with five years of data from Canadian hospitals [10]. There is also a study that uses logistic regression to determine for how many days the antibiogram was a reliable predictor of *Pseudomonas aeruginosa* susceptibility with eight years of data from Duke University Hospital [2]. Another study uses linear regression to forecast the future amount of antimicrobial infections based on five years of data from US nursing homes [6]. The Review on Antimicrobial Resistance estimated the number of deaths from three types of antimicrobial infections in 2050 with the assumption that resistance rates would become 100 percent in 15 years [13]. Lastly, a study uses Markov models to determine the likelihood that *E. coli* infection becomes resistant to six antibiotics over six months [14]. In addition to not utilizing the aforementioned methods for forecasting future percent susceptibility, these studies are all limited in either by the number of years of data or the number of antibiotic-bacteria pairs being studies.

There is only one prior project that has focused on forecasting future antibiotic susceptibility. This study used linear mixed models to predict *E. coli* and *K. pneumoniae* global susceptibility to carbapenems and third generation cephalosporins through 2030 [1]. While the method could be applied to more antibiotic-bacteria pairs given available data, this study fails to provide any validation of the methodology to suggest the accuracy of the forecast. In addition, this study made the assumption that these antimicrobial resistance trends are linear though no evidence was given to suggest antimicrobial resistance follows a linear trend.

1.3 Our Contribution

The objective of this work is to utilize, design, and evaluate predictive methods for their effectiveness to predict antimicrobial susceptibility. This work tackles predicting antimicrobial resistance on a much larger scale than previous works by both exploring a rich variety of predictive methods as well as applying these to a multitude of antibiotic-bacteria pairs. To achieve this, we leverage three datasets, all extracted from the Massachusetts statewide antibiogram (MA-SA) dataset. This expansive dataset, curated by the Massachusetts Department of Public Health (MDPH) since 1999, contains sufficient longitudinal data to predict the antimicrobial susceptibility multiple years into the future for more than 250 antibiotic-bacteria pairs.

Using the MA-SA dataset, we evaluate the ability of multiple regression-variants by comparing the predicted future antimicrobial susceptibility to the actual antimicrobial susceptibility. The effectiveness of the regression-based methods reveals the need for a strategy that automatically learns and utilizes the best prediction model for each antibiotic-bacteria pair. We address this using Previous Year Prediction Error Reduction with error distinction (PYPERed) model selector [16]. We designed this model selector to select the method that minimized the previous year's prediction error and it is thus more effective at predicting at predicting future percent susceptibility compared to existing methods. In addition, this paper specifically focuses on selecting models to be included in PYPER, weighting the regression-variant models by number of isolates, the impact of location granularity on prediction effectiveness, the importance of longitudinal data for forecasting, and the ability to forecast multiple years into the future.

2 Dataset and Methodologies

2.1 The Massachusetts Statewide Antibiogram Dataset

This research is conducted on 15 years of the Massachusetts statewide antibiogram (MA-SA) dataset. The antibiograms in this dataset were collected annually by the Massachusetts Department of Health (MDPH) from 2002 to 2015 from over 50 acute-care hospitals across Massachusetts [3]. Cultures of bacterial infections, called isolates, were collected by hospitals from both inpatients and outpatient populations. These isolates, tested in hospital microbiology laboratories, are considered susceptible or resistant to tested antibiotics based on the Clinical and Laboratory Standards Institute (CLSI) guidelines. The isolates collected from a hospital during a calendar year are aggregated to create a single antibiogram and reported to the MDPH annually.

Specifically, this expansive dataset contains 107, 968 reports consisting of an antibiotic, bacteria name, the year, the number of isolates, the percent susceptibility of the isolates, and the location. The 14 bacteria and 85 antibiotics in these reports combine to form 754 unique antibiotic-bacteria pairs, though the longitudinal amount of data for each pair differs. It is these reports we utilize in

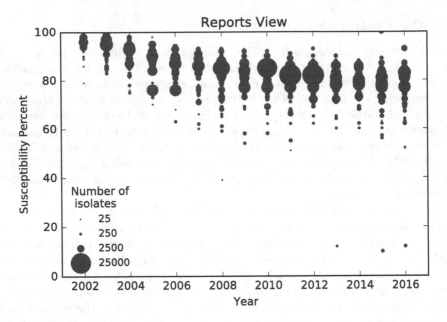

Fig. 1. Longitudinal state reports.

prediction methodology. The data can be analyzed at a state, county, or hospital granularity. Figure 1 shows the longitudinal reports at the state granularity for *E. coli* and levofloxacin.

The MA-SA dataset is used, among other things, to track antimicrobial susceptibility and prescribe antibiotics. These tasks are completed by considering the mean susceptibility for a given antibiotic-bacteria-location (A-B-L) combination over time. The actual mean susceptibility A, defined in Eq. 1, is calculated by taking the average percent susceptibility of each report weighted by the number of isolates in that report.

$$A = \frac{\sum_{i=1}^{n} s_i t_i}{\sum_{i=1}^{n} t_i} \tag{1}$$

where n is the number of reports, s_i is the percent susceptibility of the ith report, and t_{1i} is the number isolates of the ith report. The actual mean susceptibility A is a percent between 0 and 100.

The mean susceptibility is calculated to account for the disproportionate over or under representation of a hospital report based on the number of organisms cultured. The mean susceptibility over time with standard deviation at the state granularity is shown for *E. coli* and levofloxacin in Fig. 2.

While the MA-SA dataset is impressive in size and scope, data procurement occurring over 15 years and more than 50 hospitals varies in reliability. The most prevalent concern involves the microbiology laboratories' varied response times to implementing CLSI changes. However, policy changes have greatly

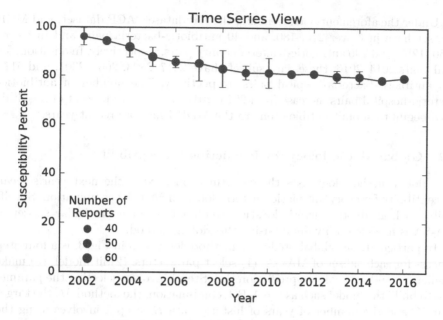

Fig. 2. Annual state mean susceptibility.

improved the quality and coverage of antibiograms submitted to the MDPH. For instance, due to these policies the number of duplicate isolates contained within the dataset have consistently decreased over time. Additionally the percent of hospitals submitting data has improved. Though due to original guidelines, some of these hospitals do not submit reports with fewer than 20 to 30 isolates to the MDPH.

As data quality has been consistently increasing over time, we have opted for minimal data cleaning. We only consider reports that have at least 20 isolates. In addition to matching the original antibiogram submission guidelines regarding the number of isolates per report, this requirement decreases the impact of an outlier bacterial infection. For modeling purposes, each antibiotic-bacteria pair must have at least 6 years of data. Specifically, each of these antibiotic-bacteria pairs must have at least one report per year in 2012–2014, 2013–2015, or 2014–2016 depending on the validation year.

We demonstrate our methods on three distinct subsets of the MA-SA dataset: all antibiotic-bacteria pairs (AP dataset), all clinically relevant antibiotic-bacteria pairs (ACP dataset), and the most clinically relevant antibiotic-bacteria pairs (MCP dataset). The MCP dataset contains *E. coli*, *Klebsiella pneumoniae*, and *Klebsiella oxytoca* susceptibility to antibiotics in the carbapenem, cephalosporin, fluroquinolone families. We also consider these subsets at different levels of location granularity resulting in unique antibiotic-bacteria, antibiotic-bacteria-county, and antibiotic-bacteria-hospital combinations.

Under the aforementioned cleaning, the AP dataset, ACP dataset, and MCP dataset have just over 270, 180, and 40 antibiotic-bacteria pairs and just over 1650, 1250, and 290 antibiotic-bacteria-county pairs, respectively. In addition, for final years 2014–2016, these data subsets have 2417–2823, 2000–2301, and 517–616 antibiotic-bacteria-hospital pairs, respectively. The number of antibiotic-bacteria-hospital pairs increase from 2014–2016 as a greater percent of hospitals have begun to submit antibiograms to the MDPH in more recent years.

2.2   Global Methodology for Predicting Susceptibility

The global methodology uses the same method predict the next year's mean susceptibility for every antibiotic-bacteria-location (A-B-L) combination. Specifically, each antibiotic-bacteria-location combination for a particular subset of MA-SA is modeled individually using the global method.

In particular, our global predictive methodology, seen in Fig. 3, is a four step process for each subset of MA-SA: (1) select parameters, (2) fit model, (3) make prediction, and (4) evaluate prediction [16]. Step 1 involves selecting the parameters to build the model such as the A-B-L combination, the method M, the target year Y, and the number of years of historic data H. Step 2 involves using the selected method M to establish a model D for the data using the historic years of data H. Step 3 involves using that model D to predict the mean susceptibility P for target year Y. Lastly, Step 4 involves utilizing evaluation metrics to measure the effectiveness of the model D in predicting current percent susceptibility for the A-B-L combination by comparing the predicted mean susceptibility P to the actual mean susceptibility A in target year Y. This methodology is repeated for each A-B-L combination in the dataset.

To ensure that the results of our methodology are not year specific, we implement a sliding window mechanism that enables us to repeat the methodology for multiple target years [16]. Specifically, we have chosen the three most recent years in the data as our target years: 2014, 2015, and 2016. The number of historic years of data H selected in methodology Step 1 is restricted by this sliding window mechanism. As 2014 is the earliest year in our target years and 2002 is the earliest year in MA-SA, the maximum number of years of historic data H is 12. Thus, the historic years of data H consist of twelve years $y_{-12}, ..., y_{-1}$ of susceptibility data. This historic susceptibility H is utilized to predict the subsequent percent susceptibility, otherwise known as the percent susceptibility for target year Y.

2.3   Regression-Based Models

We apply the above described global methodology with a variety of regression-based methods. Specifically, these include regression methods, support vector methods (SVR), and autoregressive integrated moving average models (ARIMA). As mentioned, the same method is applied uniformly to each A-B-L combination to create a set of predictive models. As these methods are modeling

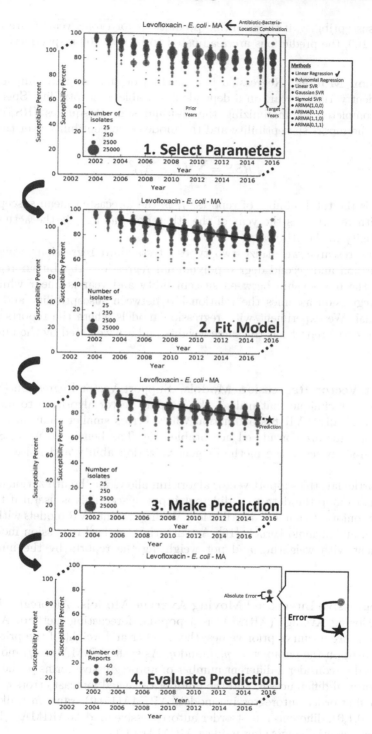

Fig. 3. Global methodology.

percent susceptibility, if the resulting predictions for target year Y are below 0 or above 100, the predictions are readjusted to be 0 or 100 respectively.

Regression Models. Regression is a method of analyzing the impact of an independent variable, year, on a dependent variable, susceptibility. Specifically, this is completed by minimizing the residual sum of squares (RSS), Eq. 2, between the report susceptibility and the modeled susceptibility over time [9].

$$RSS = \sum_{i=1}^{n} (f_i - A_j)^2 \tag{2}$$

where n is the total number of reports, f_i is the forecasted mean susceptibility for the ith report, j is the year of the ith report, and A_j is the actual mean susceptibility in the jth year.

In this research we utilize two types of standard regressions: simple linear regression and second degree polynomial regression [16]. Linear regression assumes the relationship between susceptibility and year is linear while polynomial regression assumes the relationship between susceptibility and year is polynomial. We experiment with regression models where the reports are not weighted- every report has the same weight- and are weighted by the number of isolates.

Support Vector Regression Models. Support Vector Regression (SVR) is a regression technique that utilizes the support vector algorithm to model the data. Specifically, SVR fits a function where errors smaller than an identified margin of error are considered acceptable [15]. The benefit to using SVR for predictive analytics is the method's generalization ability and noise tolerance [20].

In particular, the support vector algorithm allows for the utilization of kernel functions to map the data to a different input space. This is useful if the data does not conform to a linear distribution. We implement SVR models with linear, Gaussian, and sigmoid kernels [16]. As with the standard regression models, we experiment with weighting and not weighting the reports by the number of isolates.

Autoregressive Integrated Moving Average Models. Autoregressive Integrated Moving Average (ARIMA) is a popular forecasting method. ARIMA's predictions are a sum of prior values; the number and weight of the prior values is dependent on the parameters p, d, and q. As such, ARIMA(p,d,q) models can be tailored to consider a different number of autoregressive terms p, the number of nonseasonal differences d, and the number of lagged forecast errors q [12]. We consider first-order autoregressive models ARIMA(1,0,0), random walk models ARIMA(0,1,0), differenced first-order autoregressive models ARIMA(1,1,0), and simple exponential smoothing models ARIMA(0,1,1).

2.4 Customized Methodology for Predicting Susceptibility

The global methodology assumed that every A-B-L combination should be modeled using the same method. However, model selectors offer the flexibility for different A-B-L combinations to be modeled using different methods. Thus, in addition to the global methodology, we propose a customized methodology which leverages model selectors to select among a set of predictive methods for each A-B-L combination.

The customized methodology is composed of seven steps for each subset of MA-SA: (1) choose model selector parameters, (2) select model parameters, (3) building models, (4) choose best method, (7) update model, (6) make prediction, (7) evaluate prediction. Step 1 involves choosing the set of methods $\{M_1, ..., M_k\}$ that the model selector can select amongst and the strategy for selecting a model S. Step 2 involves selecting the parameters to build the models such as the A-B-L combination, the target year Y, and the number of years of historic data H. Step 3 involves using each of the methods in the method step $\{M_1, ..., M_k\}$ to establish a model set $\{D_1, ..., D_k\}$ for the data using the historic years of data H. Step 4 involves using the strategy S to select a model $D_d \in \{D_1, ..., D_k\}$. Step 5, which is optional depending on the model selection strategy S, involves using the method $M_d \in \{M_1, ..., M_k\}$ that built D_d to establish an updated model D. Step 6 involves using the updated model D to predict the mean susceptibility P for the target year Y. Lastly, Step 7 involves utilizing evaluation metrics to measure the effectiveness of the model D in predicting current percent susceptibility for the A-B-L combination by comparing the predicted mean susceptibility P to the actual mean susceptibility A in target year Y. This methodology is repeated for each A-B-L combination in the dataset.

As with the global methodology, we implement a sliding window to avoid overfitting. Specifically, we use 12 years of historic data to make predictions for 2014, 2015, and 2016.

2.5 Model Selectors

Tailoring the method with a model selector involves two unique challenges: deciding the methods to be included within the model selector and determining the best manner to select the model. In our previous work, we determined that choosing the model that minimized the mean squared error was not effective [16]. For this reason, we will focus on the model selector we designed called Previous Year Prediction Error Reduction (PYPER) and the variant with error distinction (PYPERed) [16].

PYPER. PYPER aims to select the method that builds a model that will produce the smallest error in the subsequent year. This is accomplished by selecting the method that built the model that minimizes the absolute error in the prior year to make predictions for the target year Y [16].

Specifically, in step 3 of the customized methodology, PYPER utilizes susceptibility data in years $y_{-12}, ..., y_{-2}$ to build the model set $D_1, ..., D_k$. The strategy PYPER implements in step 4 to select the model is to determine which model produces the lowest absolute error when predicting the susceptibility in year y_{-1}; if there is a tie, the global method the lowest error when applied to all antibiotic-bacteria-location combinations is selected. As such, step 5 of the customized methodology is necessary to build an updated model with susceptibility data in years $y_{-12}, ..., y_{-1}$.

PYPERed. PYPERed, a variant of PYPER model with error distinction, capitalizes on the fact that for some A-B-L combinations the susceptibility changes minimally over time. As such, PYPERed employs the customized methodology when the actual mean susceptibility in year y_{-1} is different from the actual mean susceptibility in year y_{-2} by a predetermined threshold T. Otherwise, in this research, PYPERed assumes that the susceptibility in year Y will be similar to the susceptibility in year y_{-1}.

The threshold T we use for this research is the standard deviation (SD) of the reports in year y_{-1}, shown in Eq. 3 [9]. PYPER is only employed if the change in susceptibility between year y_{-1} and y_{-2} is greater than the standard deviation in year y_{-1}. Otherwise, the average susceptibility in year y_{-1} is used as the small standard deviation indicates a stable resistance trend.

$$SD(y_{-1}) = \sqrt{\frac{1}{n_{y_{-1}}} \sum_{k=1}^{n_{y_{-1}}} (s_i - \bar{s})^2} \tag{3}$$

where $n_{y_{-1}}$ is the number of reports in year y_{-1} for the given A-B-L combination, s_i is the percent susceptibility of the kth report in year y_{-1}, and $\bar{s}$ is the

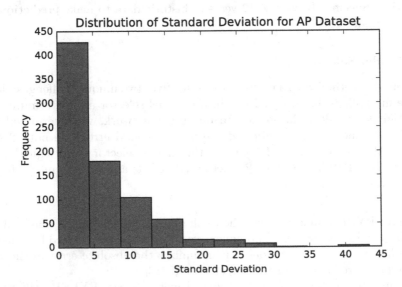

Fig. 4. Distribution of the susceptibility standard deviation for AP state dataset.

average susceptibility of all reports in year y_{-1}. This average susceptibility is different than the actual mean susceptibility as it is not weighted by the number of isolates. The standard deviation for report susceptibility of the AP dataset at the state granularity ranges from 0 to 43.3, the distribution of which is shown in Fig. 4.

2.6   Evaluation Metrics

We evaluate the prediction ability of the models by comparing the actual mean susceptibility A to our forecasted mean susceptibility f for target year Y for each antibiotic-bacteria-location combination in the dataset. We accomplish this using a common evaluation metric for assessing the quality of numeric predictions: mean absolute error (MAE) [11].

MAE, defined in Eq. 4, will both be used to compare methods and interpret the usefulness of the forecast. It is useful for health professionals to know the average error when determining whether to use the prediction method.

$$MAE = \frac{1}{n} \sum_{i=1}^{n} |f_i - A_j| \tag{4}$$

where n is the total number of reports, f_i is the forecasted mean susceptibility for the ith report, j is the year of the ith report, and A_j is the actual mean susceptibility in the jth year.

2.7   Software Tools and Availability

The code for this work was implemented with Python 3.5.2. The libraries used were Pandas (v.0.18.1), Numpy (v.1.11.1), scikit-learn (v.0.17.1), Statsmodels (v.0.9.0), and Matplotlib (v1.5.1). We have released the code along with additional plots at https://github.com/mltlachac/CCIS2018.

3   Results

For each antibiotic-bacteria pair in the all antibiotic-bacteria pairs (AP) dataset, we use the global regression-based methods constructed with between 6 and 12 years of data to make predictions for the subsequent year. We evaluate the 813 predictions for 2014, 2015, and 2016 with MAE, as seen in Table 1.

All four of the ARIMA methods perform better than any of the other regression and SVR methods. Except for polynomial regression, the weighted version of these regression-based methods performed better than the unweighted version of the regression-based methods. Specifically, linear regression, linear SVR, and Gaussian SVR have the lowest MAE of these weighted regression-based methods; the 2016 absolute errors of these methods for antibiotic-bacteria pairs containing *E. coli* in the MCP dataset are compared in Fig. 5.

From Fig. 5, we can see that different methods perform better for different antibiotic-bacteria pairs, motivating the use of model selectors. As such,

Table 1. Global methods for AP state dataset.

Method	MAE
Unweighted Linear Regression	2.699
Unweighted Poly. Regression	2.679
Unweighted Linear SVR	2.747
Unweighted Gaussian SVR	3.028
Unweighted Sigmoid SVR	3.275
Weighted Linear Regression	2.524
Weighted Poly. Regression	3.505
Weighted Linear SVR	2.622
Weighted Gaussian SVR	2.585
Weighted Sigmoid SVR	3.131
ARIMA(1,0,0)	2.502
ARIMA(0,1,0)	2.143
ARIMA(1,1,0)	2.280
ARIMA(0,1,1)	2.494

Table 2. Customized methods for AP state dataset.

Method	MAE
PYPER (L-Reg,L-SVR,G-SVR)	2.099
PYPERed (L-Reg,L-SVR,G-SVR)	1.882
PYPER (ARIMA)	2.100
PYPERed (ARIMA)	2.043

we apply PYPER and PYPERed on weighted regression-based methods and ARIMA variations, the results of which are in Table 2. The model selectors with weighted regression-based methods only include linear regression (L-Reg), linear SVR (L-SVR), and Gaussian SVR (G-SVR); including polynomial regression and Sigmoid regression cause PYPER to perform worse.

PYPERed with weighted linear regression, weighted linear SVR, and weighted Gaussian SVR has the lowest MAE. We compared the absolute errors of PYPERed and the weighted regression-based models using a t-test with a significance level of 0.05. PYPERed has a statistically significantly lower absolute errors than weighted linear regression, weighted linear SVR, and weighted Gaussian SVR. PYPERed 2016 absolute errors for antibiotic-bacteria pairs containing *E. coli* in the MCP dataset are shown in Fig. 6.

Even though at the global level the ARIMA models had lower errors than the other regression models, PYPERed with ARIMA performs worse than PYPERed with the other regression models. As such, PYPER and PYPERed will further refer to the use of these model selectors with the methods linear regression,

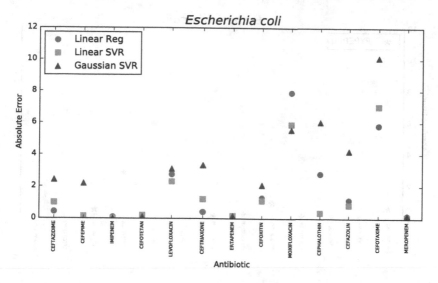

Fig. 5. Comparison of 2016 absolute errors for different weighted regression-based methods.

Table 3. Model comparison for state level datasets.

Method	ACP	MCP
Linear Regression	1.844	1.384
Linear SVR	2.073	1.675
Gaussian SVR	2.102	2.135
PYPERed	1.453	1.293

linear SVR, and Gaussian SVR. Using PYPERed, we are able to forecast the susceptibility in the target year Y on average within 1.882 percent susceptibility for the AP dataset at the state level.

3.1 Clinically Relevant Data Subsets

PYPERed remains an effective method at reducing susceptibility forecasting error at the state level regardless of the data subset selected. Table 3 compares PYPERed's error to linear regression, weighted linear SVR, and weighted Gaussian SVR for the all clinically revelent antibiotic-bacteria pairs (ACP) and most clinically relevant antibiotic-bacteria pairs (MCP) datasets. The state ACP dataset contains 543 predictions and the state MCP dataset contains 124 predictions for target years 2014, 2015, and 2016.

Regardless of the clinical significance of the antibiotic-bacteria pairs in the three datasets, implementing PYPERed proves to produce better forecasts than any of the individual regression-based methods. PYPERed has a MAE of 1.822 (Table 2), 1.453 (Table 3), and 1.293 (Table 3) for the AP, ACP, and MCP state level datasets respectively. In other words, as the clinical significance of the

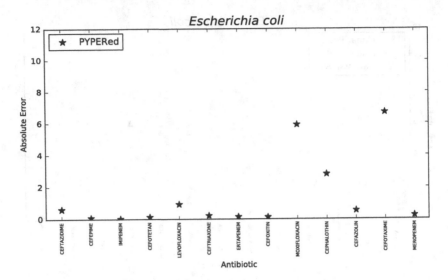

Fig. 6. 2016 absolute errors for PYPERed.

Table 4. PYPERed comparison at different location granularities.

Granularity	AP	ACP	MCP
State	1.822	1.453	1.293
County	2.490	2.479	1.657
Hospital	2.934	2.911	2.396

antibiotic-bacteria pairs increases, the MAE of the subsequent year forecasts decreases.

3.2 Location Granularity

We can analyze the data at the state, county, and hospital levels for the AP, ACP, and MP data subsets. The PYPERed MAE of these data subsets at the different location granularities are displayed in Table 4. In addition, Table 5 contains the number of predictions for the antibiotic-bacteria-location (A-B-L) combinations for target years 2014, 2015, and 2016.

For every combination of dataset and location granularity, PYPERed MAE is lower than any globally applied regression-based methods. Consistent with the conclusions of Sect. 3.1, as the clinical significance of the A-B-L combination increases, the MAE decreases for every location granularity. Additionally, for every dataset, as the location becomes more granular, the error increases. This makes sense given that the number of predictions for the A-B-L combinations increases greatly as the location becomes more granular. For instance, we can forecast within 1.822 percent susceptibility for 813 antibiotic-bacteria pairs and within 2.934 susceptibility percent for 7779 antibiotic-bacteria-hospital combinations.

Table 5. Number of A-B-L predictions at different location granularities.

Granularity	AP	ACP	MCP
State	813	543	124
County	4981	3772	875
Hospital	7779	6392	1677

Table 6. State level forecasting MAE for different length time series with PYPERed.

Prior years	AP	ACP	MCP
6–12	1.822	1.453	1.293
3–12	1.940	1.462	1.294
3–9	1.965	1.469	1.124
6–9	1.920	1.473	1.110

3.3 Longitudinal Data Importance

We use the state datasets to explore the importance of longitudinal data in forecasting future antibiotic susceptibility. In particular the MCP dataset is ideal for this task as, since the antibiotic-bacteria pairs are most relevant, the number of years of data has little impact to the number of antibiotic-bacteria pairs. We explore the impact of using between 6–12, 3–12, 3–9, and 6–9 years of historic data, seen in Table 6.

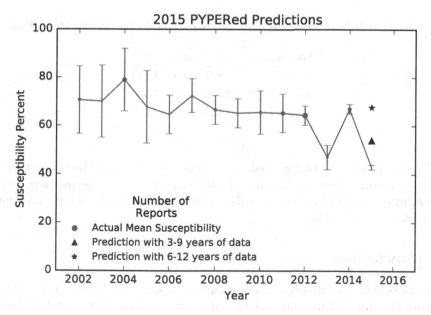

Fig. 7. Cephalothin and *Klebsiella oxytoca* susceptibility.

For both the AP and ACP datasets, using between 6–12 years, as was done in prior portions of the paper, has the lowest mean absolute error MAE of all of longitudinal restrictions. This is not true for the MCP dataset; not permitting more than 9 years of data reduces the error. However, the MCP dataset only contains a maximum of 45 antibiotic-bacteria pairs per year so this may be the influence of a single antibiotic-bacteria pair: Cephalothin and *Klebsiella oxytoca*. As seen in Fig. 7, with 6–12 years of data and 3–9 years of data, PYPERed predicted the 2015 with an absolute error of 24.667 and 11.008, respectively.

We can attribute the results for the MCP data subset in Table 6 in part to the outlying mean susceptibilities in the resistance trend for Cephalothin and *Klebsiella oxytoca*. Thus, we conclude that it is advisable to use as much data as possible when making predictions for future antibiotic susceptibility.

3.4 Forecasting Multiple Years into the Future

When forecasting multiple years into the future, we use between 6 and 12 years of historic data to forecast the three subsequent years at the state level for each data subset. Specifically, we use prior years of data y_{-12} to y_{-1} to forecast target years Y_0, Y_{+1}, and Y_{+2}. The sliding window works such that forecasts Y_0, Y_{+1}, and Y_{+2} are still for years 2014, 2015, and 2016. Given that the MA-SA dataset only contains 15 years of data, this means that there may not be up to 12 years of data available with which to make these forecasts. As seen in Sect. 3.3, this would likely reduce the forecasting ability for AP and ACP datasets even without forecasting further into the future. These forecasts multiple years into the future are seen in Table 7.

Table 7. State level forecasting multiple years into the future with PYPERed.

Forecast year	AP	ACP	MCP
$Year_0$	1.822	1.453	1.293
$Year_1$	2.506	1.939	1.500
$Year_2$	3.134	2.459	2.047

For all three datasets, forecasting an additional year into the future consistently increases the error by around a quarter to a third of the previous error. These future forecasts indicate trends and would allow for health professionals to prepare for outbreaks.

4   Conclusions

Using three different subsets of the Massachusetts statewide antibiogram dataset varying by clinical significance of the antibiotic-bacteria pairs, we determined that our model selector <u>P</u>revious <u>Y</u>ear <u>P</u>rediction <u>E</u>rror <u>R</u>eduction with <u>e</u>rror distinction(PYPERed) was effective at forecasting the antibiotic susceptibility for the subsequent years. In particular, we discovered that weighted linear regression, linear SVR, and Gaussian SVR were the best methods to include within PYPERed. We were able to predict the current susceptibility of over 270 antibiotic-bacteria pairs on average within 1.882 percent susceptibility of the actual mean susceptibility using PYPERed.

In addition, PYPERed performed better than the globally applied regression-based models regardless of the data subset or the location granularity. Specifically, we discovered that the mean absolute error (MAE) decreased as the subset contained antibiotic-bacteria pairs that were more clinically relevant and increased as the location granularity became smaller.

PYPERed can be implemented to predict the antimicrobial susceptibility in the current year. These predictions can be used to guide antibiotic prescription practices. Thus, antibiotics will be prescribed based on updated resistance knowledge which is an important piece of reducing the misuse and overuse of antibiotics. As stated, this is a key action in fighting antimicrobial resistance [5].

Our next step is, instead of predicting the future percent susceptibility, predicting if the change in antimicrobial susceptibility between years will be clinically and statistically significant [17]. Other future antibiogram work would involve forecasting with data is that collected either more or less frequently. As seen in Sect. 3.3, outlier mean susceptibilities greatly impact predictive ability; detecting, removing, and predicting outlying mean susceptibilities is a future step in this area of research. Additionally, PYPERed should be applied to forecasting problems on other datasets. In other domains a different subset of methods or a different error threshold may prove to be more effective.

Acknowledgements. This work is supported by WPI and the US Department of Education P200A150306: GAANN Fellowships to Support Data-Driven Computing Research. We thank Jian Zou, PhD and Tom Hartvigsen at WPI, Matthew Tlachac at University of Minnesota, and Alfred DeMaria, MD and Monina Klevens, DMD at MDPH for their input on this work. We thank the DSRG community at WPI for providing a stimulating research environment.

References

1. Alvarez-Uria, G., Gandra, S., Mandal, S., Laxminarayan, R.: Global forecast of antimicrobial resistance in invasive isolates of Escherichia coli and Klebsiella pneumoniae. Int. J. Infect. Dis. **68**, 50–53 (2018)
2. Anderson, D., Miller, B., Marfatia, R., Drew, R.: Ability of an antibiogram to predict pseudomonas aeruginosa susceptibility to targeted antimicrobials based on hospital day of isolation. Infect. Control Hosp. Epidemiol. **33**(6), 589–593 (2012)
3. Bureau of Infectious Disease and Laboratory Sciences: 2015 statewide antibiogram report. Massachusetts State Public Health Laboratory (2016). Accessed 24 Jan 2017
4. Centers for Disease Control and Prevention: Antibiotic resistance threats in the United States, 2013. U.S. Department of Health and Human Services (2015). https://www.cdc.gov/drugresistance/pdf/ar-threats-2013-508.pdf

5. Centers For Disease Control and Prevention: About Antimicrobial Resistance. Antibiotic/Antimicrobial Resistance (2018). https://www.cdc.gov/drugresistance/about.html. Accessed May 2018
6. Crnich, C., Safdar, N., Robinson, J., Zimmerman, D.: Longitudinal trends in antibiotic resistance in US nursing homes, 2000–2004. Infect. Control Hosp. Epidemiol. **28**(8), 1006–1008 (2017)
7. Food and Drug Administration: Stewardship guidelines. The National Antimicrobial Resistance Monitoring System (2016)
8. Hastey, C., et al.: Changes in the antibiotic susceptibility of anaerobic bacteria from 2007–2009 to 2010–2012 based on CLSI methodology. Anaerobe **42**, 27–30 (2016)
9. James, G., Witten, D., Hastie, T., Tibshirani, R.: An Introduction to Statistical Learning with Applications in R, 1st edn. Springer, New York (2013)
10. Lagace-Wiens, P., et al.: Trends in antibiotic resistance over time among pathogens from Canadian hospitals: results of the CANWARD study 2007–11. J. Antimicrob. Chemother. **6**, i23–i29 (2013)
11. Moore, D.: The Basic Practice of Statistics, 4th edn. WH Freeman, New York (2007)
12. Nau, R.: Statistical forecasting: notes on regression and time series analysis. Fuqua School of Buisness, Duke University, (2018). https://people.duke.edu/~rnau/411home.htm. Accessed May 2018
13. O'Neill, J.: Tackling Drug-Resistant Infections Globally: Final Report and Reccomendations. The Review on Antimicrobial Resistance (2016). https://amr-review.org/sites/default/files/160525_Final%20paper_with%20cover.pdf
14. Seidman, S., et al.: Longitudinal comparison of antibiotic resistance in diarrheagenic and non-pathogenic Escherichia coli from young Tanzanian children. Front. Microbiol. **7**, 1420 (2016)
15. Smola, A., Scholkopf, B.: A tutorial on support vector regression. Stat. Comput. **14**(3), 199–222 (2014)
16. Tlachac, M., Rundensteiner, E., Barton, K., Troppy, S., Beaulac, K., Doron, S.: Predicting future antibiotic susceptibility using regression-based methods on longitudinal Massachusetts antibiogram data. In: Proceedings of the 11th International Conference on Health Informatics (2018)
17. Tlachac, M., et al.: CASSIA: an assistant for identifying clinically and statistically significant decreases in antimicrobial susceptibility. In: 2018 IEEE EMBS International Conference on Biomedical & Health Informatics (BHI) (2018)
18. Ventola, L.: The antibiotic resistance crisis. Pharm. Ther. **40**(4), 277–283 (2015)
19. World Health Organization: Antimicrobial resistance global report on surveillance 2014. World Health Organization (2014). http://apps.who.int/iris/bitstream/handle/10665/112642/9789241564748_eng.pdf
20. Yang, H., King, L.: Localized support vector regression for time series prediction. Nuerocomputing **72**(10–12), 2659–2669 (2009)

Exploring the Value of Electronic Health Records from Multiple Datasets

Olga Fajarda[1] (ID), Alina Trifan[1] (ID), Michel Van Speybroeck[2],
Peter R. Rijnbeek[3] (ID), and José Luís Oliveira[1(✉)] (ID)

[1] DETI/IEETA, University of Aveiro, Aveiro, Portugal
jlo@ua.pt
[2] Janssen Pharmaceutica NV, Beerse, Belgium
[3] Erasmus MC, Rotterdam, The Netherlands

Abstract. During the last decades, most European countries dedicated huge efforts in collecting and maintaining Electronic Health Records (EHR). With the continuous grow of these datasets, it became obvious that its secondary use for research may lead to new insights about diseases and treatments outcomes.

EHR databases can be used to speed up and reduce the cost of health research studies, which are essential for the advance and improvement of health services. However, many times, a single observational data source is not enough for a clinical study, thus data interoperability has a major impact on the exploration of value of EHRs. Despite the recognized benefit of data sharing, database owners remain reluctant in conceding access to the contents of their databases, mainly due to ownership, privacy and security issues.

In this paper, we exploit two major international initiatives, the European Medical Information Framework (EMIF) and the Observational Health Data Sciences and Informatics (OHDSI), to provide a methodology through which multiple longitudinal clinical repositories can be queried, without the data leaving its original repository.

Keywords: Electronic Health Records · Observational studies ·
Data interoperability · Clinical research · Secondary use

1 Introduction

Health research studies are determinant for the advance of health science and the improvement of health services. Pharmaceutical and public health surveillance, the development of new treatments, the expansion of knowledge about diseases and the monitoring of health crises are essentially done using health research studies [17]. The secondary use of clinical data opens the door to translational research, which can be considered a two-way path. The first is from "Bench to Bedside", that is, translate research discoveries into clinical practice; the second is from "Bedside to Bench", i.e., the other direction, using clinical practice to

A. Cliquet jr. et al. (Eds.): BIOSTEC 2018, CCIS 1024, pp. 367–383, 2019.
https://doi.org/10.1007/978-3-030-29196-9_19

assist research. The reuse of clinical digital data is advantageous in both ways, as it allows time saving and cost reduction, and prevents redundant data collection.

Over the past two decades the use of electronic health record systems has significantly increased in many countries around the world. This increase translates into a proliferation of electronic health databases containing a wide collection of diversified clinical digital data. Beyond the undeniable value that EHRs have for the direct health care of patients, i.e. beyond primary clinical care, the secondary use of these data brings great benefit to scientific, clinical and translational research. The use of these databases for health research studies has, beside turning the research more efficient by saving time and money, the advantage to increase the quality of the research, especially when combining data from several databases [20]. Furthermore, the use of existing databases prevents the collection of duplicate data and gives the researcher access to a larger, more diversified population, as well as to certain groups of people, which may not participate in clinical trials, such as children and older people [24].

EHRs can also be reused to conduct observational studies, such as retrospective cohort studies and case-control studies. A cohort study is a form of longitudinal study used to investigate the incidence, causes, and prognosis of a given clinical condition. In a retrospective cohort study, one or more groups of patients are followed up backwards to examine medical events or outcomes [12]. Drug safety surveillance, are, essentially, done using EHRs, given that some adverse drug events are only observed after the release of the drug to a larger, diversified population [28]. In the development of new therapies, the secondary use of clinical digital data can improve the clinical trial design and accelerate the complex process of identifying clinical trial participants [18, 19].

Despite the recognized value of the secondary use of EHR, it is still nearly impossible to obtain access to digital clinical data. Lopes et al. [11] reviewed initiatives and projects focusing on the exploration of patient-level data and pointed out that even data obtained through public research funding projects are not shared with the research community. There are several socio-technological reasons behind this hardship. One impediment is the existence of database silos. Over the years, as clinical digital data were collected in different countries and institutions, many isolated silos were created due to the lack of regulation and primitive technological implementation [15].

Apart from this, clinical digital data are also widely distributed and fragmented. A patient's clinical history may be fragmented and distributed among multiple electronic systems, such as the patient's pharmacy, insurance companies, care providers and others [22]. These distributed, decentralized and autonomous EHR systems lead to the existence of multiple highly heterogeneous databases. Every system collects and stores the data in an application-specific or vendor-specific format without considering information sharing. The heterogeneity of the databases can be found at several levels, namely, in the technologies and data models employed, in the query languages supported and the terminologies recognized.

Another major impediment relates to privacy issues due to legal, ethical and regulatory requirements [2]. Data privacy protection is a very important and sensitive matter because a minimal break in privacy can have dramatic consequences for individuals' lives, healthcare providers and subgroups within society. Moreover, legislation differs from one country to another and it may be difficult to develop a protocol that conforms to all of them [14]. The recently EU General Data Protection Regulation (GDPR)[1] tries to address this caveat.

Having identified the importance and the challenges of EHR data interoperability and reuse, we intend to contribute to this research area by providing a methodology through which interoperable yet geographically dispersed EHR datasets can be queried, without data leaving their original repositories. Although an increasing number of providers and developers have worked towards providing solutions for leveraging the secondary use of EHR datasets, longstanding challenges have become better understood and new challenges have been identified.

Our ambition evolved around the realization that clinical and research studies and trials conducted in a traditional fashion can take up to several years to be completed. The common pipeline of a research study involves several time consuming and expensive tasks, namely, the identification and recruitment of consenting subjects, and the gathering of the data, which in some cases means following the recruited subjects over a long period of time. However, health research studies can be speed up and much cheaper, if they are done using data collected for other purposes, like data from health-related registry systems or data collected from previous studies [1]. A feasibility trial normally starts by asking data custodians or physicians if they have patients who meet research eligibility criteria. For a clinical trial to be scientifically and statistically valid, the number of participants must be sufficiently large [10], and so this process can be very slow and expensive.

The use of EHR data can reduce the time and cost of this process. Besides, a pre-trial feasibility analysis using EHR data also allows a redefinition of criteria in order to increase the number of participants [4]. Some adverse drug events are only observed after its release to a large and diverse population because a clinical trial has only a reduced number of participants. Moreover, every clinical trial puts the research subjects through some risk and, therefore, the substitution, when possible, of clinical trial by the secondary use of clinical digital data, prevents unnecessary risk [5].

For the success of clinical translational research, it is imperative to develop solutions that enable the querying of distributed and heterogeneous EHR databases without losing data and patients' privacy. In this paper, which is an extended version of a previous work [6], we present a methodology to semi-automatically query several distributed, heterogeneous databases. When followed, this methodology has to potential to drastically improve the necessary time and resources involved in a study. It reinforces data interoperability and reuse, by bringing together two initiatives concerned with ensuring overall better

---

[1] http://www.eugdpr.org/.

healthcare throughout Europe. In our approach the EMIF Platform[2] sides with open source tools designed by OHDSI[3] for querying EHR databases converted to the Observational Medical Outcomes Partnership Common Data Model (OMOP CDM)[4]. Both of these initiatives are discussed in detailed in Sect. 2, along with an overview of other current efforts in making electronic health data reusable. We expose our methodology in Sect. 3 and discuss results in Sect. 4. Section 5 outlines our final remarks.

2   EHR Interoperability and Reuse

As awareness of the value of secondary use of EHR increased, several projects emerged to develop solutions for secure sharing of information across different databases. Given the wide adoption of electronic health records, there is a great need for improving the interoperability of EHR databases to better integrate clinical research and patient care [25].

Mini-Sentinel [21] is a project developed by the U.S. Food and Drug Administration (FDA) to perform active safety surveillance of FDA-regulated medical products using routinely collected electronic health record data from multiple sources. The developed system uses data from public and private organizations, centralized in a secure container. A common data model was designed so that each data partner is able to transform local source data into this model. Several complementary software tools have been developed to support specific research questions, related to identification and evaluation of the exposure of medical products and possible associated health issues. However, the setup of these technologies requires some technical expertise and field knowledge.

The Informatics for Integrating Biology and the Bedside (i2b2) [16] is a U.S. project launched with the aim to develop tools that can help clinical researchers integrate medical records and clinical research data in the genomics age. The i2b2 team developed a web application which allows cohort estimation and feasibility determination by querying de-identified and aggregate EHR data. The i2b2 team also developed the Shared Health Research Information Network (SHRINE) [13,29], a distributed query system that allows researchers to query synchronously several databases containing everyday clinical data. SHRINE provides obfuscated, aggregated counts of patients, which facilitates population-based research and assessment of potential clinical trial cohorts. The software developed by the i2b2 is open source, freely available and can be adapted to query other groups of databases.

The Electronic Health Records for Clinical Research (EHR4CR), was a European public-private project that developed a platform to assist researchers in clinical trials' feasibility assessment and patient recruitment [3]. Through a distributed real-time querying system, multiple clinical data warehouses across Europe containing de-identified EHR data, can be synchronously queried to

---

[2] www.emif-catalogue.eu.
[3] www.ohdsi.org.
[4] https://github.com/OHDSI/CommonDataModel/wiki.

obtain aggregated results. The platform may enable a trial sponsor to predict the number of eligible patients for a candidate clinical trial protocol, to assess its feasibility and to locate the most relevant hospital sites.

Due to historical reasons and genuine differences in citizen attitudes and preferences across the country, state privacy laws vary, often widely, in ways that inhibit both within-state as well as cross-state information sharing. With time, however, we expect that technologies and processes will mature to the point that they both ease the flow of clinical information and give providers and patients greater control over how such information is used [7].

2.1 The European Medical Information Framework

Most of the solutions presented combine data from healthcare centers which adopt the same data model and allow the integration or distributed query of databases. However, data sharing cannot be taken for granted, and it might even be impossible for many centers. Data custodians' desire to share clinical data for research is usually hindered by legal and governance issues, and they do not engage in solutions that, for instance, use centralized data warehouses or real-time query systems. Therefore, clinical research is still hindered by the limited and fragmented access to health data repositories. The methodology we present allows clinical researchers to query several heterogeneous databases while keeping patient health data private in each healthcare institution.

The European Medical Information Framework (EMIF)[5] is one of the most recent European projects, aiming to facilitate the reuse and exploitation of patient-level data from different EHR systems and cohorts, for research purposes. The EMIF Platform intends to be an integrated system to allow researchers to browse information at three different conceptual levels. The first level refers to browsing a catalog containing database fingerprints, i.e. a general characterization of the databases, the second level will allow the extraction of aggregated data from several databases and the third level will allow drilling down to the individual patient level in those databases [27]. Currently, the EMIF Catalogue includes information from 8 research communities, with more than 400 datasets, from population-based data sources (e.g. electronic health records, regional databases) up to disease-specific ones (e.g. Alzheimer). The methodology that we propose was developed within the EMIF initiative in order to leverage clinical studies conducted within the aim of the project.

2.2 Observational Health Data Sciences and Informatics

The second driving force that made possible the development of the methodology that we propose, is the Observational Health Data Sciences and Informatics initiative (OHDSI). OHDSI's overall approach is to create an open network of observational data holders, and require that they translate their data to the

---

[5] http://www.emif.eu.

OMOP CDM. In return, this approach creates a unique opportunity of implementing a number of existing data exploration and evidence generation tools and participating in world-wide studies because any given query can be executed at any site without modification [8].

Single observational data source provides a comprehensive view of the clinical data a patient accumulates while receiving healthcare, and therefore none can be sufficient to meet all expected outcome analysis needs. Interoperability refers to more than just information exchange. For two EHR systems to be truly interoperable, they must be able to exchange and then use the data. For this to occur, the message transmitted must contain standardized coded data so that the receiving system can interpret it. However, lack of standardized certainly limits the ability to share data electronically for patient care [23]. This explains the need for assessing and analyzing multiple data sources concurrently using a common data standard. This standard is provided by the OMOP CDM, a data model through which healthcare data coming from diverse sources can be represented in a consistent and standardized way.

In this data model, medical terms were categorized into seven types including four entities (Condition, Observation, Drug, Procedure) and three attributes (Qualifier, Measurements, Temporal constraints). Each attribute has a close relationship with a corresponding entity. For instance, a relation of has value shows a quantitative measurement value of one entity. The four entities consist of medical terms with similar characteristics, while the three attributes differ from each other [25]. CDM supports implementation of standardized analytics across organizations with different database structures. Besides the common data model, the OHDSI community has been developing several analytic tools, such as Achilles, Achilles Web, HERMES, CIRCE and ATLAS.

The EMIF initiative invested consistent effort in converting several European EHR databases to OMOP CDM. This efforts empower the methodology that we present in this paper since they led to a harmonized view over biomedical datasets otherwise geographically scattered across Europe. Moreover, by having the databases converted to OMOP CDM, all OHDSI open source tools can be used on these data.

3   Methodology

The methodology we present enables semi-automatically querying of several distributed, heterogeneous EHR databases at once, which streamlines the entire request process. This approach is semi-automatic so that every data custodian can maintain control of their database and only share the data they consider to fulfill the legal, ethical and regulatory requirements. Moreover, it uses partially existing solutions and open-source software, which significantly reduces the cost involved in the process.

Data are retained at the participant's site, simplifying patient and business privacy issues. Instead, the analyses are carried out locally and the results are transmitted to the coordinating center, where they can be studied on a population level and aggregated as appropriate [8].

3.1   The EMIF Platform

The EMIF Platform was designed as a portal for all EMIF provided function-alities and incorporates a web interface that links to other relevant components such as a federated query module (ATLAS) and a workflow manager (TASKA), among others (Fig. 1). Its main purpose is to facilitate biomedical data exposure and sharing, on one hand, and data discovery and reuse, on the other [26]. This translated into a one-stop platform, which we denominate as a biomedical mar-ketplace, where data custodians can share their data and researchers can easily discover these data to support their clinical studies. The data custodian controls right upfront in how much detail s/he wants to expose a data source. Several levels of information can be exposed, from summarized views to raw data, acces-sible in a controlled and possibly remote environment. Moreover, a role-based access control (RBAC) assures that an access policy can be tailored to combine the access constraints with the needs of biomedical researchers.

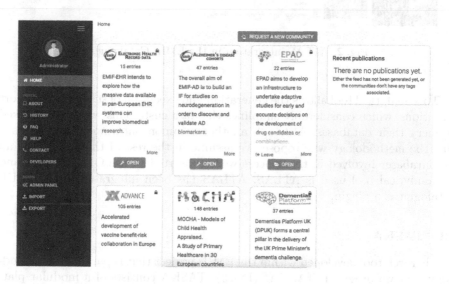

Fig. 1. Landing page of the EMIF Catalogue.

3.2   ATLAS

Recent emergence of Common Data Models (CDMs) facilitated creation of tools that provide syntactic integration (shared information model) and in some cases also semantic integration (shared set of target terminologies used by structured data) [9]. One such tool is ATLAS[6] (Fig. 2), a web-based platform which inte-grates features from various previously developed OHDSI applications. This

---

[6] http://www.ohdsi.org/web/atlas.

platform allows database exploration, standardized vocabulary browsing, cohort definition, and population-level analysis of observational data converted to the OMOP CDM.

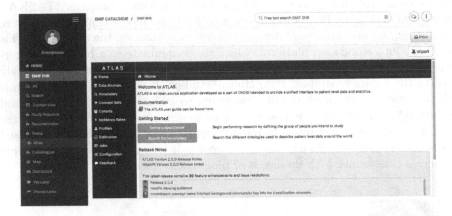

Fig. 2. ATLAS integration in the EMIF Catalogue.

This analytical tool allows the generation and execution of scripts with cohort definitions, which considerably simplifies the data custodians' work when asked to query their databases. Although another common data model can be used with the methodology we propose, we assume in the rest of the paper that all the databases involved in the process were converted to the OMOP CDM and the analytical tool used is ATLAS. ATLAS has been integrated in the EMIF Catalogue as a plugin.

3.3   TASKA

Another web tool developed within the EMIF project that is part of the methodology that we present is TASKA[7] (Fig. 3). TASKA consists of a modular platform that allows collaboration between different users through a user-friendly web-based interface, while keeping a strong focus on the relation between the tasks that users perform. Within the methodology that we propose, TASKA is a key player for managing all people, tasks and interactions involved in a research study. Just like ATLAS, TASKA is integrated and directly accessible from the EMIF Catalogue. This means that users of this methodology do not have to worry about installing different software tools, the pipeline that we propose is achievable by only making use of the EMIF Platform and the tools that it integrates.

---

[7] https://emif-catalogue.eu/taska/.

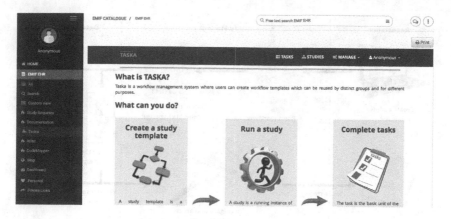

Fig. 3. TASKA integration in the EMIF Catalogue.

3.4 Methodology Break-Down

Our approach assumes that the EMIF Catalogue is the main entry and management solution, where researchers can search for data sources, submit a study request, choose the databases to engage with, and follow the progress of the study, while more advanced users are handling the data extraction job. So all communication between all users is through this application. In addition, TASKA is used to perform and monitor all the tasks involved in the process. Our methodology has three main actors:

- the *Researcher*, the person who wants to query one or several patient-level databases;
- the *Data Custodian* (DC), the person responsible for managing a database;
- the *Study Manager* (SM), the person who leads and manages the research study and moderates the tasks between the researcher and the Data Custodian.

Other actors can be involved in the process, e.g. the SM can delegate some of their tasks and responsibilities to others.

Figure 4 presents the main workflow of this methodology. The researcher starts by formulating a study request, which can be done by simply specifying a question. This request is made using the EMIF platform where the researcher also has access to a catalogue of databases that can be chosen.

The SM manages the entire query process. They receive all the study requests, evaluate their suitability and also the DCs' willingness to participate, create an ATLAS script that defines the cohort, share it with the DCs, and after receiving the DCs' response, reply to the study request. The SM is a community expert that knows the characteristics of the different databases that are part of the group, and is familiar with the technologies and software needed to query these databases, namely the EMIF Platform and ATLAS.

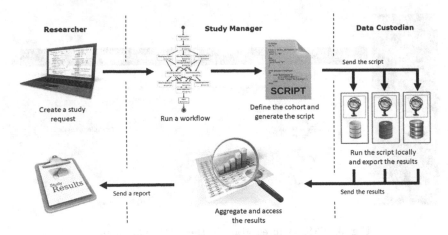

Fig. 4. Workflow of the querying process.

The DC is responsible for the local running of the script sent by the SM and determines if the results of a query can be shared. Since this methodology does not require all the data to be centralized, nor does it need to previously de-identify the data, the DC keeps autonomy and control of its database and the executing and sharing of query results.

Afterwards, the SM analyses the study request and decides if they can fulfill the request or if they need more detailed information about the request in order to accurately define the cohort, in which case they contact the researcher using the platform. The SM can also make suggestions on how to formulate the study request in order to be accepted. After accepting the request, the SM uses a workflow management tool to create a workflow with the tasks necessary to perform the query process and designate the participants in the process, namely the data custodians. During this phase, a governance board approval and other administrative issues can also be included in the protocol. The next step is to use ATLAS to create a script that defines the cohort and send it to the data custodians through the workflow execution.

After receiving the script, the DC runs it locally, using a local installation of ATLAS, and generates the results. Subsequently, the DC evaluates the results and decides if these can be shared or not. The workflow management tool can be used to inform the SM of the rejection and the respective reason. Otherwise, the DC sends the results to the SM using the same workflow management tool.

Once all data custodians have completed the local queries and returned aggregate results, the SM uses ATLAS to visualize the results and compiles them in a document that is sent to the researcher, completing the query process.

4   Results and Discussion

The worldwide proliferation of EHR systems leads to the existence of an increasing number of digital clinical data repositories. Despite the recognized value of these repositories for secondary use, and their undeniable importance for clinical research, it is still very difficult to access these data. There are several reasons that make sharing these data so difficult: the existence of database silos, the difficulty in locating EHR databases, the distribution and fragmentation of the data, and privacy issues due to legal, ethical and regulatory requirements.

Technical solutions for health data integration typically use a centralized data warehouse, with replicas of original EHRs, or a real-time distributed query system, which relies on complex governance agreements and institutions' trust. These solutions are time consuming or imply governance models that might not be allowed by most data custodians. Moreover, in both cases, data custodians lose control of their data. Other approaches are designed for a specific type of database and are difficult to adapt to other types. More recently, solutions that operate based on OHDSI open source tools, such as the ARACHNE Research Network[8] started to address the complexity of running a research study and proposed a leveraging solution. However, the solution proposed comes as a software package. This adds to the difficulties generated by the technical complexity of such solutions that organizations experience, due to the lack of technical skills or knowledge on how to use them.

Nonetheless, existent solutions that have individual benefits, can lead to global advances when advanced. The EMIF Catalogue, for example, enables researchers to find multiple distinct databases. The OHDSI tools can transform data from different databases into a CDM, thereby allowing queries across a set of databases. Joining these initiatives and adding TASKA, a workflow management system, provides a universal methodology for performing a research study over multiple datasets in a short amount of time compared to traditional approaches.

To overcome the difficulties that we have identified in the secondary use of EHRs, we developed a methodology to perform semi-automatic distributed EHR database queries. Our methodology does not use centralized data warehouses, but rather it is semi-automatic so that every data custodian can maintain control of their database and only share the data they consider to fulfill the legal, ethical and regulatory requirements. Moreover, our methodology relies on existing solutions and open-source software, which significantly reduces the cost involved in the process.

Next, we present a simple example of a feasibility study involving the various actors (R, SM, and DCs), i.e. a study to identify how many patients of one or more databases fulfill some criteria. Here, we ignore governance and contractual aspects, although they can be incorporated at any stage of this workflow.

- Step 1 (R): Research Question
  - After logging into the EMIF Catalogue, the user (researcher) fills out a form describing the research question and the objective of the study (Fig. 5).
  - As an example, we may take a research question such as "How many patients, with prostate cancer, had prostate cancer screening" involving

---

[8] https://github.com/OHDSI/ArachneUI.

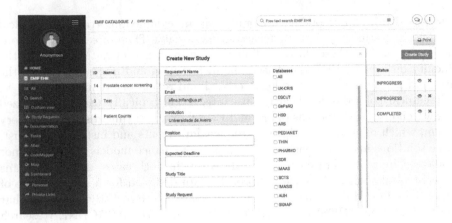

Fig. 5. Study Request form in the EMIF Catalogue. In this form, the user can choose one or multiple databases of interest, ask a research question with regard to these databases and indicate a tentative deadline for the answer s/he expects.

three databases. Other information, such as the expected delivery deadline, the user's e-mail, institution and position, among others, also need to be provided.
- The three databases of interest can be a-priori identified using the search and compare features available in the EMIF Catalogue.

– Step 2 (SM): Feasibility Assessment
- The study manager(s) receives a notification about the existence of a new study request. In the EMIF Catalogue each of the 8 available communities can name one or more study managers.
- They log into the EMIF Catalogue and evaluate the feasibility of this request.
- Through an internal messaging system, the SM has the option to ask the researcher for more information or details, in order to better understand the scope of the study. The study manager can also make suggestions on how to improve the request. Ideally, the SM has a general knowledge over the databases in a community and is able to either reach a conclusion on his own, or mount a network of experts in a controlled amount of time that can support him in providing a conclusion about the feasibility of the request.
- After this step is concluded, the study can start internally. The management of the study is the responsibility of the SM.

– Step 3 (SM): Define the Cohort Template
- The study manager enters the ATLAS installation available in the EMIF Catalogue.
- They start by creating the Concept Sets needed for the Cohort definition, namely, "Prostate cancer screening" and "Prostate cancer".
- The Concept Sets created are used to specify the inclusion criteria when the study manager defines the cohort. Figure 6 presents a possible cohort definition for this study.

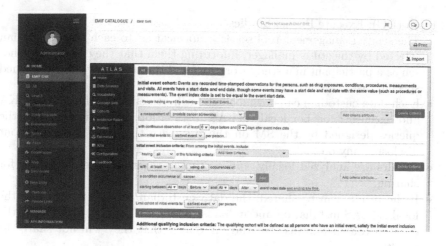

Fig. 6. Example of a cohort definition using ATLAS.

- The cohort definition is then exported by the SM in a JSON format and will be share with DCs of the three databases of interests in the next steps.

– Step 4 (SM): Create and Initiate the Study Workflow
- Using TASKA, the study manager creates a new study (Fig. 7).
- They select the participants, namely, the data custodians of the selected databases, assigning them the tasks.
- After initiating the workflow, the study manager shares through TASKA the cohort definition that he created using the ATLAS installation in the EMIF Catalogue.

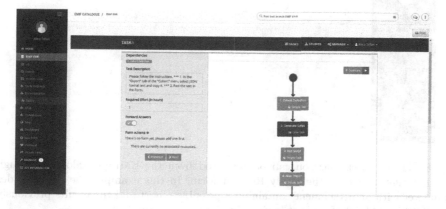

Fig. 7. Example of a TASKA template used for conducting a research study. The image focuses on the second task of the template, which is the export of a JSON file in ATLAS, followed by its upload in TASKA. The details of a specific task are listed on the left side of the page.

– Step 5 (DC): Execute Partial Studies
  • The study management tool sends a notification to each data custodian selected by the study manager, informing them that they have been chosen as a participant in a study workflow and that they have been assigned specific tasks.
  • Each data custodian can download the cohort definition through TASKA and execute it on her local ATLAS installation. Like this, he runs the queries designed by the SM on the database that s/he owns, without disclosing any data.
  • Results are analyzed locally, and evaluated regarding the possibility for sharing.
  • If the results can be shared, the data custodian exports them using the local ATLAS installation and uploads them into TASKA. Otherwise, the data custodian informs the study manager that they will not share the results.
– Step 6 (SM): Result integration and reporting
  • After all data custodians complete their tasks, the workflow management tool notifies the study manager.
  • If individual results have been shared, the study manager uploads them into the ATLAS installation of the EMIF Catalogue.
  • The study manager visualizes the results of the study, using the ATLAS installation of the EMIF Catalogue, and elaborates a report based on these results.
  • Through an internal messaging system, the study manager sends the report back to the researcher (Fig. 8).

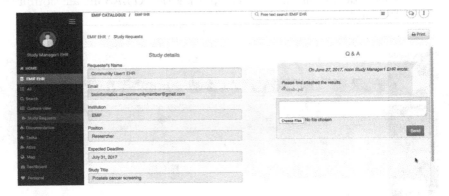

Fig. 8. The research question can be answered from the EMIF Catalogue, through the chat that is part of the Study Request form. In this example, the SM provides an answer with an attachment containing a possible report and the results previously visualized in ATLAS, if consent is given by data custodians.

- Step 7 (R): Results evaluation
  - The researcher receives a notification informing that the results are available.
  - They access the results and analyze them.
  - If needed, the researcher can ask for clarification or additional information, through the internal messaging system.

The presented methodology allows managing and simplifying the execution of research studies over multiple EHRs databases, addressing one of the core concerns for the sharing of clinical data for research, i.e. by preserving local governance.

5 Conclusion

In this paper we presented a methodology to perform semi-automatic distributed EHR database queries that uses preexisting partial solutions and open-source software. The query process presented enables the researcher to formulate a feasibility question and obtain statistical and aggregated information about data from different databases without accessing these data directly or contacting the various data custodians.

The proposed methodology can be fully followed using the EMIF Catalogue and two of the tools already integrated in this platform: (a) ATLAS, an open source OHDSI tool used for defining biomedical queries over CDM converted databases; and (b) TASKA, a workflow management system that helps researchers orchestrate the complexity of a research study. The described use case is integrated as a pipeline in the EMIF Catalogue, which is publicly available.

Acknowledgements. This work has received support from the EU/EFPIA Innovative Medicines Initiative Joint Undertaking (EMIF grant n. 115372), and from the Integrated Programme of SR&TD 'SOCA' (CENTRO-01-0145-FEDER-000010), co-funded by Centro 2020 program, Portugal 2020, European Union, through the European Regional Development Fund.

References

1. Cheng, H.G., Phillips, M.R.: Secondary analysis of existing data: opportunities and implementation. Shanghai Arch. Psychiatry **26**(6), 371 (2014)
2. Cushman, R., Froomkin, A.M., Cava, A., Abril, P., Goodman, K.W.: Ethical, legal and social issues for personal health records and applications. J. Biomed. Inform. **43**(5), S51–S55 (2010)
3. Daniel, C., et al.: Cross border semantic interoperability for clinical research: the EHR4CR semantic resources and services. AMIA Summits Transl. Sci. Proc. **2016**, 51 (2016)
4. Doods, J., Botteri, F., Dugas, M., Fritz, F.: A European inventory of common electronic health record data elements for clinical trial feasibility. Trials **15**(1), 18 (2014)

5. Doolan, D.M., Winters, J., Nouredini, S.: Answering research questions using an existing data set. Med. Res. Arch. **5**(9), 1–14 (2017)
6. Fajarda, O., Silva, L.B., Rijnbeek, P., Van Speybroeck, M., Oliveira, J.L.: A methodology to perform semi-automatic distributed EHR database queries. In: 11th International Joint Conference on Biomedical Engineering Systems and Technologies (BIOSTEC 2018), vol. 5, pp. 127–134 (2018)
7. Gini, R., et al.: Data extraction and management in networks of observational health care databases for scientific research: a comparison of EU-ADR, OMOP, Mini-Sentinel and MATRICE strategies. Egems **4**(1), 1189 (2016)
8. Hripcsak, G., et al.: Observational health data sciences and informatics (OHDSI): opportunities for observational researchers. Stud. Health Technol. Inform. **216**, 574 (2015)
9. Huser, V., Kahn, M.G., Brown, J.S., Gouripeddi, R.: Methods for examining data quality in healthcare integrated data repositories. In: Pacific Symposium on Biocomputing (PSB), pp. 628–633 (2017)
10. Köpcke, F., Prokosch, H.U.: Employing computers for the recruitment into clinical trials: a comprehensive systematic review. J. Med. Internet Res. **16**(7), e161 (2014)
11. Lopes, P., Silva, L.B., Oliveira, J.L.: Challenges and opportunities for exploring patient-level data. BioMed Res. Int. **2015**, 11 (2015)
12. Mann, C.: Observational research methods II: cohort, cross sectional, and case-control studies. Research design. Emerg. Med. J. **20**(1), 54–60 (2003)
13. McMurry, A.J., et al.: SHRINE: enabling nationally scalable multi-site disease studies. PLoS One **8**(3), e55811 (2013)
14. Meystre, S., Lovis, C., Bürkle, T., Tognola, G., Budrionis, A., Lehmann, C., et al.: Clinical data reuse or secondary use: current status and potential future progress. IMIA Yearb. **26**, 38–52 (2017)
15. Miller, A.R., Tucker, C.: Health information exchange, system size and information silos. J. Health Econ. **33**, 28–42 (2014)
16. Murphy, S.N., et al.: Serving the enterprise and beyond with informatics for integrating biology and the bedside (i2b2). J. Am. Med. Inform. Assoc. **17**(2), 124–130 (2010)
17. Nass, S.J., Levit, L.A., Gostin, L.O., et al.: The value, importance, and oversight of health research. In: Beyond the HIPAA Privacy Rule: Enhancing Privacy Improving Health Through Research (2009)
18. Ohmann, C., Kuchinke, W.: Meeting the challenges of patient recruitment. Int. J. Pharm. Med. **21**(4), 263–270 (2007)
19. Pakhomov, S., Weston, S.A., Jacobsen, S.J., Chute, C.G., Meverden, R., Roger, V.L., et al.: Electronic medical records for clinical research: application to the identification of heart failure. Am. J. Manag. Care **13**(6 Part 1), 281–288 (2007)
20. Piwowar, H.A., Chapman, W.W.: Public sharing of research datasets: a pilot study of associations. J. Informetr. **4**(2), 148–156 (2010)
21. Platt, R., Carnahan, R.: The us food and drug administration's mini-sentinel program. Pharmacoepidemiol. Drug Saf. **21**(S1), 1–303 (2012)
22. Pringle, S., Lippitt, A.: Interoperability of electronic health records and personal health records: key interoperability issues associated with information exchange. J. Healthc. Inf. Manag.: JHIM **23**(3), 31–37 (2009)
23. Reisman, M.: EHRs: the challenge of making electronic data usable and interoperable. Pharm. Ther. **42**(9), 572 (2017)
24. Schneeweiss, S., Avorn, J.: A review of uses of health care utilization databases for epidemiologic research on therapeutics. J. Clin. Epidemiol. **58**(4), 323–337 (2005)

25. Si, Y., Weng, C.: An OMOP CDM-based relational database of clinical research eligibility criteria. Stud. Health Technol. Inform. **245**, 950 (2017)
26. Silva, L.B., Trifan, A., Oliveira, J.L.: MONTRA: an agile architecture for data publishing and discovery. Comput. Methods Programs Biomed. **160**, 33–42 (2018)
27. Trifan, A., Díaz, C., Oliveira, J., et al.: A methodology for fine-grained access control in exposing biomedical data. Stud. Health Technol. Inform. **247**, 561–565 (2018)
28. Trifirò, G., et al.: Combining multiple healthcare databases for postmarketing drug and vaccine safety surveillance: why and how? J. Intern. Med. **275**(6), 551–561 (2014)
29. Weber, G.M., et al.: The shared health research information network (SHRINE): a prototype federated query tool for clinical data repositories. J. Am. Med. Inform. Assoc. **16**(5), 624–630 (2009)

Application of a Rule-Based Classifier to Data Regarding Radiation Toxicity in Prostate Cancer Treatment

Juan L. Domínguez-Olmedo[1], Jacinto Mata[1(✉)], Victoria Pachón[1],
and Jose L. Lopez Guerra[2]

[1] Department of Information Technologies, University of Huelva, Huelva, Spain
{juan.dominguez,mata,vpachon}@dti.uhu.es
[2] University Hospital Virgen del Rocío, Seville, Spain
chanodetriana@yahoo.es

Abstract. In this work we describe a rule-based classifier (DEQAR-CC), which employs a combination of selected rules after a two-phase training process, and without the need of a previous discretization for the numerical variables. It was compared in the application to a real imbalanced dataset regarding the toxicity during and after radiation therapy for prostate cancer. In this comparison with other predictive methods (rule-based, artificial neural networks, trees, Bayesian and logistic regression), DEQAR-CC showed a better global prediction performance than the rest of classifiers, in an evaluation regarding several performance measures and by using cross-validation. Finally, it was employed to obtain a predictive model for genitourinary toxicity, obtaining an interpretable classification scheme which simply combines two rules with two variables.

Keywords: Rules discovery · Imbalanced data classification · Prostate cancer

1 Introduction

Machine learning is an area of artificial intelligence that uses a variety of algorithmic techniques that allow computers to learn from past observations and detect patterns in datasets. One of the methods we can employ to extract knowledge from data is the use of *association rules*, whose purpose is to extract strong and interesting relationships between patterns in a set of data. An association rule takes the form $A \rightarrow C$, where A (the antecedent) and C (the consequent) express a condition (or a conjunction of conditions) on variables of the dataset [1, 2]. The measures *support* and *confidence* are used to assess the quality and importance of the association rules. The support evaluates the number of cases in which both the antecedent and the consequent of the rule hold. The confidence is the ratio between the support of the rule and the number of cases in which the antecedent holds.

Subgroup discovery is a type of descriptive induction whose objective is to generate models based on rules using a predictive perspective. It emerged as the task of discovering properties of a population by obtaining simple (but significant) rules, using only one variable in the consequent: the class or target variable [3, 4].

© Springer Nature Switzerland AG 2019
A. Cliquet jr. et al. (Eds.): BIOSTEC 2018, CCIS 1024, pp. 384–398, 2019.
https://doi.org/10.1007/978-3-030-29196-9_20

Another task in machine learning is *classification*, which deals with assigning observations into discrete categories. In the simplest case, there are two possible categories, and this case is known as binary classification. Numerous techniques have been proposed for classification problems. Some examples of predictive methods are artificial neural networks, decision trees, logistic regression and Bayesian networks, among others [5, 6]. In classification tasks with imbalanced data, most algorithms are not usually capable of obtaining good results for the minority class and, therefore, the overall classification performance does not usually reach adequate values [7, 8].

Prostate cancer (PC) is the most common cancer in men, and the third leading cause of death in men in Europe [9]. Although there is an improvement in tumor control rates using radiation dose escalation, PC radiotherapy is limited by the proximity of surrounding normal tissues and because of the observed dose-effect association with toxicity. It is essential to understand the true complications associated with doses delivered to normal anatomy, to ensure the delivery of a sufficient dose with minimal complications.

In this work we describe a rule-based classifier (DEQAR-CC), and its application to a real imbalanced dataset regarding the toxicity during and after radiation therapy for PC. The rest of the paper is organized as follows. Section 2 gives a description of the methods employed in this work. The experimental setup is presented in Sect. 3. Section 4 describes the experimental results and discussion. And the last section presents the conclusions.

2 Methods Employed

2.1 Description of DEQAR-CC

The classifier DEQAR-CC is a rule-based method that works by using a list of selected rules and a default class, both of them obtained during the training process of the classifier. Figure 1 illustrates this training process, which is composed of two phases.

In the first phase, "rule generation", DEQAR-CC generates rules from the training dataset. This generation of rules is based on a method developed to extract knowledge in the form of association rules [10, 11], later adapted for subgroup discovery tasks in the method DEQAR-SD [12, 13]. As in DEQAR-SD, DEQAR-CC uses the parameters *minsens* (minimum sensitivity), *maxAttr* (maximum number of variables) and *delta*, in order to manage the exhaustivity of the process, controlling the search for rules and conditions for the numerical variables.

It employs a deterministic approach to generate rules without a previous discretization of the numerical variables. Instead of discretizing, what may result in suboptimal results [4], the process uses a dynamic generation of conditions. DEQAR-CC obtains an ordered list of rules (called *ranking*) for each possible value of the class variable, storing separately the best rules in each class according to their values of confidence and support. The parameter *rankingSize* defines the maximum number of rules to be stored in each of these rankings.

In the second phase, "rule selection", the algorithm selects the rules that will be part of the classifier. A description of such process is shown in Algorithm 1. In order to select rules for different classes, we have used a value of "cumulative confidence" (*cumConf*) for each class, to try not to choose all the rules from the same class.

The process iteratively checks one rule from each ranking, starting with the first of each of them, provided that they cover at least one additional case to those already covered by the previously chosen rules (lines 4–7). The product between the confidence of the rule and the cumulative confidence of its class is calculated, and the rule with the highest value for this product is chosen (lines 8–12). In each iteration, the value of the cumulative confidence for the class corresponding to the last selected rule is updated, and the value of the cumulative confidence for the rest of the classes is set to 1 (lines 25–26). The process ends when all the rules of all the rankings have been processed (lines 19–21). Finally, the default class is established as the class with the highest number of cases not covered by any of the selected rules. In case that all the cases had been covered, the majority class in the training data would be chosen (lines 30–34).

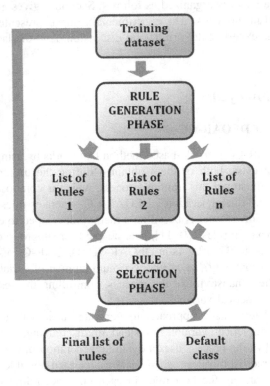

Fig. 1. Training process in DEQAR-CC [8].

Algorithm 1. Rules selection in DEQAR-CC.

Input: Training data (T), rankings of rules
Output: Final list of rules, default class

1: initialize the vector *cumConf* to 1 and *stop* to FALSE
2: **while** NOT *stop* **do**
3:      $maxCumConf \leftarrow 0$
4:      **for each** class c **do**
5:          **if** ranking c has more rules to process **then**
6:              $R \leftarrow$ next rule in ranking c
7:              **if** rule R covers at least one case in T **then**
8:                  **if** confidence(R) $\cdot$ *cumConf*[c] > *maxCumConf* **then**
9:                      $maxR \leftarrow R$
10:                     $maxC \leftarrow c$
11:                     $maxCumConf \leftarrow$ confidence(R) $\cdot$ *cumConf*[c]
12:                 **end if**
13:             **else**
14:                 move to next rule in ranking c
15:             **end if**
16:         **end if**
17:     **end for**
18:     **if** $maxCumConf = 0$ **then**
19:         **if** all the rules were processed **then**
20:             *stop* $\leftarrow$ TRUE
21:         **end if**
22:     **else**
23:         add the rule *maxR* to the final list of rules
24:         $T \leftarrow T$ - cases covered by the rule *maxR*
25:         *cumConf*[*maxC*] $\leftarrow$ *maxCumConf*
26:         set *cumConf* to 1 except in the class *maxC*
27:         move to next rule in ranking *maxC*
28:     **end if**
29: **end while**
30: **if** $T \Leftrightarrow \emptyset$ **then**
31:     *defaultClass* $\leftarrow$ majority class in T
32: **else**
33:     *defaultClass* $\leftarrow$ majority class in training data
34: **end if**
35: **return** the final list of rules and *defaultClass*

In Fig. 2 an example of such rule selection is illustrated. As can be seen in the final list of rules, the first rule of the second ranking has been inserted before the second of the first, even though it has lower confidence, because its value (0.5) is higher than the corresponding product for the first ranking ($0.6 \cdot 0.7$).

Ranking #1 (+)

1: $A_1 = 20$ AND $A_3 \geq 15$ → class = '+'
   (confidence = 0.7)

2: $A_2 = $ 'HIGH' → class = '+'
   (confidence = 0.6)

Ranking #2 (-)

1: $A_4 \leq 5$ AND $A_3 \leq 10$ → class = '-'
   (confidence = 0.5)

2: $A_2 = $ 'LOW' → class = '-'
   (confidence = 0.4)

Final list of rules

1: $A_1 = 20$ AND $A_3 \geq 15$ → class = '+'

2: $A_4 \leq 5$ AND $A_3 \leq 10$ → class = '-'

3: $A_2 = $ 'HIGH' → class = '+'

4: $A_2 = $ 'LOW' → class = '-'

Fig. 2. Example of rule selection in DEQAR-CC.

The classification process for a given case is described in Algorithm 2. The final list of rules is inspected, looking for the first rule in which the case matches its antecedent, and the class of that rule is selected (lines 2–8). In case that no rule applies to the case, the default class is selected (lines 9–11).

Algorithm 2. Classification process in DEQAR-CC.

Input: A case
Output: Predicted class

1:   *matched* ← FALSE
2:   **while** (NOT *matched* AND NOT all the rules were processed) **do**
3:      *R* ← next rule in the list
4:      **if** (the case matches the antecedent of rule *R*) **then**
5:         *predictedClass* ← class of the rule *R*
6:         *matched* ← TRUE
7:      **end if**
8:   **end while**
9:   **if** (NOT *matched*) **then**
10:      *predictedClass* ← default class
11:   **end if**
12:   **return** *predictedClass*

2.2   Classifiers Used in the Comparison

We have used several predictive methods in a comparison with DEQAR-CC. Methods based on rules (*ZeroR*, *PART*), artificial neural networks (*MultilayerPerceptron*), trees (*J48*, *RandomForest*), Bayes (*BayesNet*, *NaiveBayes*) or logistic regression (*Logistic*) have been used. Some of their characteristics are shown below:

- *ZeroR*. It is a classification method that only relies on the target variable (class), simply predicting the majority class. It can be useful to determine a baseline performance.
- *PART*. It generates a decision list by using a separate-and-conquer strategy [14].
- *MultilayerPerceptron*. A classifier that uses an artificial neural network with backpropagation. The nodes in this network are all sigmoid [15].
- *J48*. It uses a pruned or unpruned C4.5 decision tree [16]. A decision tree builds a classification model in the form of a tree structure.
- *RandomForest*. It constructs a forest of random trees, an ensemble learning method for classification, regression and other tasks [17].
- *BayesNet*. It employs a Bayes network, a probabilistic graphical model that represents a set of random variables and their conditional dependencies [18].
- *NaiveBayes*. It is based on Bayes theorem with independence assumptions between predictors. Despite its simplicity, it often outperforms more sophisticated classification methods [19].
- *Logistic*. It builds a multinomial logistic regression model with a ridge estimator [20].

3   Experimental Setup

3.1   Dataset Description

In this work, we have applied DEQAR-CC to a dataset about the toxicity effects during and after treatment of PC [21]. This dataset includes the clinical (i.e. age), pathological (i.e. Gleason score, T score), and therapeutic (i.e. radiation dose, fractionation, whole pelvic lymph node irradiation, radiation technique) information as well as the out-come (acute genitourinary [GU] toxicity) of 162 PC patients treated with arc radiation therapy from June 2006 through May 2012 at two institutions from different nationalities (Europe and Latin-America).

The names of the 17 variables in the dataset are shown in Table 1. There are 10 numerical variables and the class variable is binary ('+' for a toxicity grade ≥ 2, '−' for a toxicity grade <2), with a distribution for class '+' of 23.5% of the cases. Therefore, it is an imbalanced dataset with a 3:1 ratio of negative/positive cases.

For ethical considerations, all identifiable information about the patients was adequately removed from the data to preserve anonymity.

Table 1. Variables and units of the dataset [8].

Variable	Units/values
Age	Years
Indication treatment	Post-prostatectomy, primary prostate cancer, recurrence
Radiation technique	Tomotherapy, rapid arc
T stage	T1, T1b, T1c, T2, T2a, T2b, T2c, T3, T3a, T3b, T4
Diagnosis PSA	ng/mL
Risk	Low, intermediate, high
ADT	No ADT, short term, long term
Radiation time	Days
Planning tumor volume	Cc
Prostate radiation dose	Gy
Fractionation	Gy
Pelvic treatment	Yes, no
Bladder volume	cc
Bladder mean dose	Gy
Bladder median dose	Gy
GU acute toxicity	+, −

3.2   Evaluation Criteria

For a binary classification problem, such as the one we are dealing with, we can denote with TP (True Positive) the number of positive cases correctly classified, with TN (True Negative) the number of negative cases correctly classified, with FN (False Negative) the number of positive cases incorrectly classified, and with FP (False Positive) the number of negative cases incorrectly classified.

The following evaluation measures were employed in the comparison: accuracy, kappa index, Matthews correlation coefficient, the average value of sensitivity and specificity, precision, recall and F-measure. A description of these measures is presented below:

- Accuracy. The proportion of true results (both true positives and true negatives) among the total number of cases examined [8].

$$accuracy = \frac{TP + TN}{TP + TN + FN + FP} \tag{1}$$

- Kappa. Cohen's kappa is a widely used index for assessing agreement between raters [22].

$$kappa = \frac{accuracy - randomAccuracy}{1 - randomAccuracy} \tag{2}$$

$$randomAccuracy = \frac{(TN + FP) * (TN + FN) + (FN + TP) * (FP + TP)}{(TP + TN + FN + FP) * (TP + TN + FN + FP)} \tag{3}$$

- MCC. Matthews correlation coefficient, which can be used as measure of the quality of binary classifications [8, 23].

$$MCC = \frac{TP * TN - FP * FN}{\sqrt{(TP + FP) * (TP + FN) * (TN + FP) * (TN + FN)}} \tag{4}$$

- Average value of sensitivity and specificity. Sensitivity (Se) is the proportion of positives cases that are correctly identified as such, and specificity (Sp) is the proportion of negatives cases that are correctly identified as such [8].

$$avg(Se, Sp) = \left(\frac{TP}{TP + FN} + \frac{TN}{TN + FP} \right) * 0.5 \tag{5}$$

- Precision. Analogous to positive predictive value (PPV) [8].

$$precision = \frac{TP}{TP + FP} \tag{6}$$

- Recall. Analogous to sensitivity [8].

$$recall = \frac{TP}{TP + FN} \tag{7}$$

- F-measure. The harmonic mean of precision and recall [8].

$$F - measure = \frac{precision * recall}{precision + recall} * 2 \tag{8}$$

4 Experimental Results

4.1 Comparative Results

We have evaluated the classifiers previously described in the task of predicting the toxicity effects in the radiotherapy treatment of PC. The evaluation measures were calculated by using stratified 10-fold cross-validation. Cross-validation reduces the variance of the estimates and improves the estimation of the generalization performance. In k-fold cross-validation, the original data is partitioned into k equal size subsets. Then, a single subset is retained as the validation data and the remaining k-1 subsets are used as training data. The process is repeated k times, with each of the k subsets used exactly once as the validation data [24]. At the end, the final validation result is calculated from all the partial results.

We employed the machine learning software *Weka* [25] to run the classifiers ZeroR, PART, MultilayerPerceptron, J48, RandomForest, BayesNet, NaiveBayes and Logistic. For a fair comparison, the values of the parameters used in each classifier were the ones that yielded the best results after testing several combinations of values (grid search).

The results for accuracy, kappa, MCC and average value of sensitivity and specificity are displayed in Table 2 and Fig. 3. As can be seen, DEQAR-CC obtained excellent results, which seems to support the proposed selection of high confidence-support rules for each class, not only to obtain high values of general accuracy but also to get a satisfactory prediction for both classes. The imbalance in the dataset (38 positive cases and 124 negative ones) adds more difficulty to the classification task. The results of DEQAR-CC were the best regarding these evaluation measures. Although RandomForest has the same accuracy, the difference in the other measures reveals a better classification performance for both classes. The classifiers NaiveBayes and MultilayerPerceptron also obtained good results, but the difference for kappa and MCC, in comparison with DEQAR-CC, is important. Matthews correlation coefficient is generally regarded as being one of the best measures to describe the confusion matrix of true and false positives and negatives by a single number, especially suitable to the case of imbalanced data learning [26].

Table 2. Results for accuracy, kappa index, Matthews correlation coefficient and average value of sensitivity and specificity.

Classifier	Accuracy	Kappa	MCC	Avg(Se, Sp)
ZeroR	0.765	0.000	0.000	0.500
PART	0.710	0.185	0.185	0.592
MultilayerPerceptron	0.710	0.199	0.199	0.601
J48	0.698	0.117	0.118	0.556
RandomForest	**0.772**	0.135	0.184	0.550
BayesNet	0.710	0.185	0.185	0.592
NaiveBayes	0.698	0.208	0.210	0.611
Logistic	0.716	0.130	0.132	0.559
DEQAR-CC	**0.772**	**0.358**	**0.358**	**0.677**

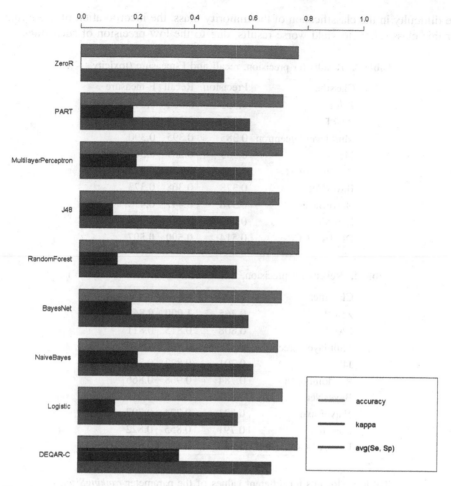

Fig. 3. Results for accuracy, kappa index and average value of sensitivity and specificity.

The results for the measures associated with each particular class (precision, recall and F-measure) are shown in Tables 3 and 4. DEQAR-CC did not obtain the best F-measure result for negative toxicity (the majority class); but its result was close to the best, and obtained the best precision. Regarding the positive toxicity, DEQAR-CC obtained the best recall and F-measure; the classifier RandomForest was the one with the best precision, but with a low recall. As can be seen, the F-measure for this minority class was not very high in all the classifiers, and only DEQAR-CC surpassed the value 0.5.

The values employed for the parameters in DEQAR-CC were the following ones: *minsens* = 0.7, *delta* = 0.05, *maxAttr* = 2 and *rankingSize* = 1. If *rankingSize* is 1, the list of rules for each class simply keeps the best rule found for that class, so the final classifier will have a list of rules with two rules (in the case of binary classes). To check how the parameter *rankingSize* affects to the results, we have registered the classifier's performance for several values of it, and they are displayed in Table 5. It can be seen how the results improve when the value of this parameter is lower. In this dataset, given the difficulty in the classification of the minority class, the incorporation of more rules for this class seems to yield worse results, due to the low precision of such rules.

Table 3. Results for precision, recall and F-measure (toxicity '+').

Classifier	Precision	Recall	F-measure
ZeroR	0.000	0.000	0.000
PART	0.378	0.368	0.373
MultilayerPerceptron	0.385	0.395	0.390
J48	0.333	0.289	0.310
RandomForest	**0.556**	0.132	0.213
BayesNet	0.378	0.368	0.373
NaiveBayes	0.378	0.447	0.410
Logistic	0.357	0.263	0.303
DEQAR-CC	0.514	**0.500**	**0.507**

Table 4. Results for precision, recall and F-measure (toxicity '−').

Classifier	Precision	Recall	F-measure
ZeroR	0.765	**1.000**	**0.867**
PART	0.808	0.815	0.811
MultilayerPerceptron	0.813	0.806	0.810
J48	0.791	0.823	0.806
RandomForest	0.784	0.968	0.866
BayesNet	0.808	0.815	0.811
NaiveBayes	0.821	0.774	0.797
Logistic	0.791	0.855	0.822
DEQAR-CC	**0.848**	0.855	0.851

Table 5. Results for different values of the parameter *rankingSize*.

RankingSize	Accuracy	Kappa	MCC	Avg(Se, Sp)
10	0.722	0.247	0.247	0.627
5	0.728	0.295	0.298	0.658
3	0.741	0.315	0.317	0.666
2	0.747	0.326	0.327	0.670
1	0.772	0.358	0.358	0.677

4.2   Prediction Model

After the comparison of these classifiers was carried out, we also used the whole dataset to obtain a prediction model for the GU toxicity. DEQAR-CC was executed with the same parameters that achieved the best results in cross-validation. After this execution, two rules were selected (see Table 6) and the default class was set to '−'.

It can be observed the low confidence value of the second rule (0.33), associated to the prediction of the minority class (high toxicity). In spite of this, the prevalence of high toxicity in the data is 23.5%, so the *lift* value of the rule is 1.4. Since this rule is only considered when the antecedent of the first one is not matched (in that case the class '−' would be predicted), its antecedent would really be "*NOT (Radiation technique = Tomotherapy AND Planning tumor volume* ≤ *218.62) AND Prostate radiation dose* ≥ *70.02 AND Bladder volume* ≥ *63.67*". Calculating the confidence of this rule, it turns out to be 0.512, similar to the precision obtained in cross-validation for high toxicity cases.

Apart from the good results obtained by DEQAR-CC in the measures evaluated, it should be noted the simplicity of the generated model. It employs only two rules with two variables in the antecedent, plus the default class. If it is compared with other classifiers, its simplicity is evident. For example, the RandomForest classifier obtained the best results by using 2000 trees. Figure 4 shows one of the simplest of those trees, and as can be seen, it is not so easy to analyze which variables and conditions may have the greatest influence on the classification.

Table 6. Rules in the final predictive model.

Rule	Confidence	Support
Radiation technique = *Tomotherapy* AND Planning tumor volume ≤ 218.62 → Toxicity = '−'	0.882	0.556
Prostate radiation dose ≥ 70.02 AND Bladder volume ≥ 63.67 → Toxicity = '+'	0.329	0.167

```
RandomTree
==========

Radiation technique = ArcTherapy
|   Planning tumor volume < 44.5 : - (13/0)
|   Planning tumor volume >= 44.5
|   |   Radiation time < 63.5
|   |   |   Age < 69.5 : + (15/0)
|   |   |   Age >= 69.5
|   |   |   |   Radiation time < 61
|   |   |   |   |   Age < 77 : + (4/0)
|   |   |   |   |   Age >= 77 : - (1/0)
|   |   |   |   Radiation time >= 61 : - (7/0)
|   |   Radiation time >= 63.5
|   |   |   Indication treatment = Post-prostatectomy : + (1/0)
|   |   |   Indication treatment = PrimaryProstateCancer
|   |   |   |   Age < 76.5 : - (9/0)
|   |   |   |   Age >= 76.5
|   |   |   |   |   Gleason score < 7.5 : - (2/0)
|   |   |   |   |   Gleason score >= 7.5 : + (1/0)
|   |   |   Indication treatment = Recurrence : + (0/0)
Radiation technique = Tomotherapy
|   Age < 62.5
|   |   Radiation time < 41.5
|   |   |   Diagnosis PSA < 4.75 : - (2/0)
|   |   |   Diagnosis PSA >= 4.75 : + (4/0)
|   |   Radiation time >= 41.5 : - (15/0)
|   Age >= 62.5
|   |   Radiation time < 54.5 : - (57/0)
|   |   Radiation time >= 54.5
|   |   |   Radiation time < 57.5
|   |   |   |   Gleason score < 6.5 : + (4/0)
|   |   |   |   Gleason score >= 6.5 : - (6/0)
|   |   |   Radiation time >= 57.5 : - (12/0)
```

Fig. 4. One of the trees obtained by the classifier *RandomForest*.

From the sixteen independent variables in the dataset, only four of them are employed in the model: *Radiation technique, Planning tumor volume, Prostate radiation dose*, and *Bladder volume*. They can be considered of great relevance in this model for GU toxicity, because the predictions only depend on the values for these variables. These variables and their associated values could be seen as risk factors for GU toxicity. These risk factors are mostly confirmed by the literature [27, 28], which may corroborate the value of the method employed.

5   Conclusions

In this paper, we have described a rule-based classifier (DEQAR-CC), which works without the need of a previous discretization of the numerical variables, and employs the best rules found for each class to arrange a list of rules and a default class.

In an experimental setup, this method was applied to a dataset regarding the toxicity of radiation therapy for prostate cancer, and compared to other classifiers by using several evaluation measures. In this classification task, DEQAR-CC presented a better global prediction performance than the rest of classifiers. Considering the imbalance in the cases of the two classes, which adds more difficulty to the classification process, the proposed method obtained the best F-measure value for the minority class (high toxicity).

It was also employed to obtain a predictive model using the whole dataset. The simplicity of the resulting model (two rules with two variables) also makes it more interpretable, which may be useful for applying it into the clinical practice. Prostate cancer patients with low-risk toxicity (e.g., men treated with Tomotherapy and having a lower prostate volume) might be able to receive a more intense treatment. Additionally, we could better define the individual patient subgroups that benefit from specific components of radiation therapy.

Acknowledgments. The research presented in this paper was partially funded by the Regional Government of Andalusia (Junta de Andalucía) under grant number TIC-7629 and Spanish Ministry of Education and Science (Grant Number: TIN2009-14057-C03-03).

References

1. Agrawal, R., Imielinski, T., Swami, A.: Mining association rules between sets of items in large databases. In: Proceedings of ACM SIGMOD ICMD, pp. 207–216 (1993)
2. Zhang, M., He, C.: Survey on association rules mining algorithms. In: Luo, Q. (ed.) Advancing Computing, Communication, Control and Management. Lecture Notes in Electrical Engineering, vol. 56, pp. 111–118. Springer, Berlin (2010). https://doi.org/10.1007/978-3-642-05173-9_15
3. Wrobel, S.: An algorithm for multi-relational discovery of subgroups. In: Komorowski, J., Zytkow, J. (eds.) PKDD 1997. LNCS, vol. 1263, pp. 78–87. Springer, Heidelberg (1997). https://doi.org/10.1007/3-540-63223-9_108
4. Grosskreutz, H., Rüping, S.: On subgroup discovery in numerical domains. Data Min. Knowl. Disc. **19**(2), 210–226 (2009)

5. Hastie, T., Tibshirani, R., Friedman, J.: The Elements of Statistical Learning: Data Mining, Inference, and Prediction. Springer, New York (2009)
6. Liu, B., Hsu, W., Ma, Y.: Integrating classification and association rule mining. In: Proceedings of Fourth International Conference on Knowledge Discovery and Data Mining, pp. 80–86 (1998)
7. Sun, Y., Wong, A.K.C., Kamel, M.S.: Classification of imbalanced data: a review. Int. J. Pattern Recognit. Artif. Intell. 23(4), 687–719 (2009)
8. Domínguez-Olmedo, J.L., Mata, J., Pachón, V., Lopez Guerra, J.L.: A rule-based method applied to the imbalanced classification of radiation toxicity. In: Proceedings of the 11th International Joint Conference on Biomedical Engineering Systems and Technologies, vol. 5, HEALTHINF, pp. 147–155 (2018)
9. Ferlay, J., et al.: Cancer incidence and mortality patterns in Europe: estimates for 40 countries in 2012. Eur. J. Cancer 49(6), 1374–1403 (2013)
10. Domínguez-Olmedo, J.L., Mata Vázquez, J.: Comparison of standard discretization with a new method for quantitative association rules. IEEE Lat. Am. Trans. 14(4), 1879–1885 (2016)
11. Domínguez-Olmedo, J.L., Mata, J., Pachón, V., Maña, M.J.: A deterministic approach to association rule mining without attribute discretization. In: Snasel, V., Platos, J., El-Qawasmeh, E. (eds.) ICDIPC 2011. CCIS, vol. 188, pp. 140–150. Springer, Heidelberg (2011). https://doi.org/10.1007/978-3-642-22389-1_13
12. Domínguez-Olmedo, J.L., Mata Vázquez, J.: Obtaining significant and interpretable rules for subgroup discovery tasks. IEEE Lat. Am. Trans. 15(10), 2012–2016 (2017)
13. Domínguez-Olmedo, J.L., Vázquez, J.M., Pachón, V.: Deterministic extraction of compact sets of rules for subgroup discovery. In: Jackowski, K., Burduk, R., Walkowiak, K., Woźniak, M., Yin, H. (eds.) IDEAL 2015. LNCS, vol. 9375, pp. 138–145. Springer, Cham (2015). https://doi.org/10.1007/978-3-319-24834-9_17
14. Frank, E., Witten, I.H.: Generating accurate rule sets without global optimization. In: Proceedings of the Fifteenth International Conference on Machine Learning, pp. 144–151 (1998)
15. Rumelhart, D.E., Hinton, G.E., Williams, R.J.: Parallel Distributed Processing: Explorations in the Microstructure of Cognition, pp. 318–362. MIT Press, Cambridge (1986)
16. Quinlan, R.: C4.5: Programs for Machine Learning. Morgan Kaufmann Publishers, San Mateo (1993)
17. Breiman, L.: Random forests. Mach. Learn. 45(1), 5–32 (2001)
18. Pearl, J.: Bayesian networks: a model of self-activated memory for evidential reasoning. UCLA Computer Science Department (1985)
19. John, G.H., Langley, P.: Estimating continuous distributions in Bayesian classifiers. In: Proceedings of the Eleventh Conference on Uncertainty in Artificial Intelligence, San Mateo, pp. 338–345 (1995)
20. Le-Cessie, S., van Houwelingen, J.C.: Ridge estimators in logistic regression. Appl. Stat. 41(1), 191–201 (1992)
21. Lopez Guerra, J.L., et al.: Ethnic difference in risk of toxicity in prostate cancer patients treated with dynamic arc radiation therapy. Tumori 101(4), 461–468 (2015)
22. Cohen, J.: A coefficient of agreement for nominal scales. Educ. Psychol. Meas. 20(1), 37–46 (1960)
23. Matthews, B.W.: Comparison of the predicted and observed secondary structure of T4 phage lysozyme. Biochimica et Biophysica Acta (BBA)-Protein Structure 405(2), 442–451 (1975)
24. Arlot, S., Celisse, A.: A survey of cross-validation procedures for model selection. Stat. Surv. 4, 40–79 (2010)

25. Frank, E., Hall, M.A., Witten, I.H.: Data Mining: Practical Machine Learning Tools and Techniques. Morgan Kaufmann, Burlington (2016)
26. Powers, D.M.W.: Evaluation: from precision, recall and F-measure to ROC, informedness, markedness and correlation. Int. J. Mach. Learn. Technol. **2**(1), 37–63 (2011)
27. Acevedo-Henao, C.M., Lopez, J.L., Matute, R., Azinovic, I.: Image-guided radiation therapy based on helical tomotherapy in prostate cancer: minimizing toxicity. Oncol. Res. Treat. **37** (6), 324–330 (2014)
28. Ahmed, A.A., et al.: A novel method for predicting late genitourinary toxicity after prostate radiation therapy and the need for age-based risk-adapted dose constraints. Int. J. Radiat. Oncol. Biol. Phys. **86**(4), 709–715 (2013)

Detecting MRSA Infections by Fusing Structured and Unstructured Electronic Health Record Data

Thomas Hartvigsen[✉], Cansu Sen, and Elke A. Rundensteiner

Worcester Polytechnic Institute, Worcester, MA 01609, USA
{twhartvigsen,csen,rundenst}@wpi.edu

Abstract. Methicillin-resistant Staphylococcus aureus (MRSA), an antibiotic resistant bacteria, is a common cause of one of the more devastating hospital-acquired infections (HAI) in the United States. In this work, we study the practicality of leveraging machine learning methods for early detection of MRSA infections based on a rich variety of patient information commonly available in modern Electronic Health Records (EHR). We explore heterogeneous types of data in EHRs including on-admission demographics, throughout-stay time series and free-form clinical notes. On-admission data capture non-clinical information (e.g., age, marital status) while Throughout-stay data include vital signs, medications, laboratory studies, and other clinical assessments. Clinical notes, free-from text documents created by medical professionals, contain expert observations about patients. Our proposed system generates dense patient-level representations for each data type, extracting features from each of our data types. It then generates scores for each patient, indicating their risk of acquiring MRSA. We evaluate prediction performance achieved by core Machine Learning methods, namely Logistic Regression, Support Vector Machine, and Random Forest, when mining these different types of EHR data retrospectively to detect patterns predictive of MRSA infection. We evaluate classification performance using MIMIC III – a critical care data set comprised of 12 years of patient records from the Beth Israel Deaconess Medical Center Intensive Care Unit in Boston, MA. Our experiments show that while all types of data contain predictive signals, the fusion of all sources of data leads to the most effective prediction accuracy.

Keywords: MRSA · Machine learning ·
Early prediction · Feature fusion

1 Introduction

1.1 Antibiotic Resistance and Methicillin-Resistant Staphylococcus Aureus

Addressing the threat posed by antibiotic resistance is an essential task for the 21st century. Antibiotics treat bacterial infections and have transformed

© Springer Nature Switzerland AG 2019
A. Cliquet jr. et al. (Eds.): BIOSTEC 2018, CCIS 1024, pp. 399–419, 2019.
https://doi.org/10.1007/978-3-030-29196-9_21

medicine, saving millions of lives in total [28]. Over time, however, the use of antibiotics has resulted in the selection and spread of antibiotic-resistant organisms which are becoming more difficult to treat. They may also require the use of more expensive and potentially toxic alternative therapies, if any are available [22].

Staphylococcus aureus is a common cause of Hospital-Acquired Infections (HAIs). It accounted for a roughly 12% of HAIs between 2011–2014 and caused over 80,000 infections in the United States in 2011 alone [8,30]. Methicillin-resistant Staphylococcus aureus (MRSA) is one antibiotic-resistant strain of this bacteria. MRSA infections may result in serious complications such as sepsis or death. Unfortunately, hospitals are known to be high-risk zones for the spread of MRSA because contamination may lay dormant within a carrier, going undetected for quite some time. Worse yet, many hospitalized patients are at an increased risk of infection [19] due to their weakened immune systems.

1.2   Leveraging EHR Collections for Early Detection of MRSA

The construction of intelligent infection prediction systems using machine learning presents one important opportunity for confronting the challenges of antibiotic resistance and the spread of infections such as MRSA in healthcare environments [27]. Such systems have been shown to successfully identify early signals for other infections, such as *Clostridium difficile* [25]. Before caregivers recognize and then request a test for MRSA for a patient, machine learning algorithms have the potential to function as an inexpensive means of identifying likely MRSA cases in advance based on patterns learned from the medical information of previous cases. Such early detection would facilitate (1) early isolation of a potentially infected patient to reduce spread of resistant strains within the healthcare facility; (2) more precisely targeted antibiotic usage; and (3) earlier initiation of optimal treatments to improve a patient's outcome. Using insights created through intelligent prediction systems, healthcare professionals could decide to initiate precautionary measures or alter treatment plans. For example, at the point of admission, high-risk patients could benefit from *contact precautions*, such as gloving, gowning, and environment alterations or from *patient placement precautions*, such as patient assignment decisions based on risk factors [26]. Machine learning-guided patient assessment thus offers an enhanced range of intervention points to contain or possibly prevent the spread of MRSA.

Electronic Health Records (EHR) systems have been universally adopted by medical facilities across the United States as a result of the Health Information Technology for Economic and Clinical Health (HITECH) Act [6] and the Centers for Medicare and Medicaid EHR Incentive Programs [5]. These EHR collections are the perfect source of data for effectively deploying machine learning systems. One of the main challenges presented by these EHR databases is that they are heterogeneous data sources containing distinct types of data. The majority of EHR records consist of highly structured data (e.g., age, recorded once, or heart rate, recorded many times repeatedly). This is the most straightforward type of EHR data from which meaningful information can be extracted. However, unstructured data in the form of free-hand notes recorded by clinicians often makes up a large portion of EHR databases. Such text data, being a popular form of data entry for medical staff, often includes the intuition behind actions of experts, shown in general to be potentially rich with information. Effectively extracting information from complex unstructured notes and combining it with the already-structured information present in EHR data has the potential to vastly improve the predictive power of infection-prediction systems.

To date, however, data accumulated within these systems has been largely underutilized for predictive analytics [3]. The widespread digitalization of health records presents a unique opportunity for healthcare innovation [14,24]. It is evident that there are signals embedded in these complex patient data that could indicate the likelihood of an evolving infection or other medically important conditions [14,24]. Thus, in this work we focus on one critical application, namely the prediction of hospital-acquired MRSA infections using machine learning methods.

1.3 State-of-the-Art Methods for MRSA Prediction

Previous research efforts have begun to explore the study of computational methods that use EHR data for HAI prediction. In one such investigation, EHR data was analyzed to generate predictions for HAI occurrence without specific determination of infection type [4]. This method used 16 patient characteristics recorded at the beginning of the hospital stay and classified patients using Logistic Regression and Artificial Neural Networks. Even using this limited set of patient variables, the authors reported high predictive accuracy. In another study [23], only admission information was used to identify multi-drug resistant bacterial infections using Logistic Regression methods.

For MRSA infection prediction, [10] used statistical methods such as Bayes' Theorem and a Maximum Probability Rule to predict MRSA cases from medical-sensor data with high accuracy. However, these authors did not focus on early detection. Instead, they used data available right up to the microbiological confirmation of MRSA. Last-minute detection has limited clinical value since it does not give clinicians adequate time to alter their actions and prevent the spread of infection. Another study by [26] used EHR data collected at the time of admission to diagnose community-acquired MRSA using Logistic Regression and simple Artificial Neural Networks, however this approach did not incorporate information obtained from patients after entering the hospital. Unlike previous works [4,10,26] and our own previous study [13], we now make use of state-of-the-art text modeling methods to incorporate rich unstructured sources of useful information when predicting MRSA infections. Such text modeling approaches promise to allow for more extensive use of EHR data across many tasks.

1.4 Scope of This Work

In this study, we use Logistic Regression, consistent with earlier diagnostic prediction studies [4,26], along with additional machine learning methods such as

Support Vector Machines [7] and Random Forests [2] due to their previous use in detecting other infections [17, 18, 31, 32]. Each of these was also tested in our previous work on MRSA as well [13]. These algorithms are also known to be interpretable, a standard requirement for many clinical prediction tasks. In contrast to earlier work, however, we focus on developing clinically translatable models along with integrating three valuable data types: structured on-admission, structured throughout-stay time series, and unstructured throughout-stay text. Previous studies have either used data taken immediately before diagnosis, achieving high predictive accuracy, or have used only data collected upon admission, preventing the identification of conditions that evolve throughout hospitalization.

In contrast to our previous work in this area [13], we perform experiments on a cohort involving patients who have associated clinical notes, using their information as input to our prediction strategy. By including clinical notes, we expect to better emulate decisions made in hospitals by clinicians in that these are their sources of information when assessing the state of a patient. To include textual information, we make use of a state-of-the-art neural network-based architecture for learning dense representations of clinical words, referred to as *word embeddings* [20]. Such word embeddings encode abstract concepts into concise low-dimensional vector representations. These methods, shown to be highly promising for Natual Language Processing (NLP) have not been extensively used for infection prediction tasks. Our objective in this investigation is to combine three distinct data types (on-admission, throughout-stay, and clinical notes), teaching classification algorithms to detect MRSA infections far in advance.

We evaluate our techniques on the MIMIC III database, a publicly-available critical-care data set collected over 12 years from the Beth Israel Deaconess Medical Center Intensive Care Unit in Boston, MA [15]. We find that core machine learning methods are indeed effective at identify high-risk MRSA patients. We generate accurate predictions at least one days prior to microbiological confirmation of MRSA and on average over four days in advance. We report AUC scores of over 0.76 using a dataset fusing on-admission, throughout-stay, and clinical note information. We also see *Accuracy* values over 70%. We conclude that Random Forests outperforms Logistic Regression and Support Vector Machines with a linear kernel function. These findings underscore the potential for machine learning techniques to detect MRSA infections soon after patients are admitted into an Intensive Care Unit.

2   Patient Level Feature Representations

2.1   The Dataset

The Medical Information Mart for Intensive Care III (MIMIC III) is a publicly available critical care database collected from the Beth Israel Deaconess Medical Center Intensive Care Unit (ICU) between 2001 and 2012 [15]. It contains 58,000 admissions comprised of the following information:

– Billing: Coded data recorded for billing and administrative purposes (CPT, DRG, ICD codes).

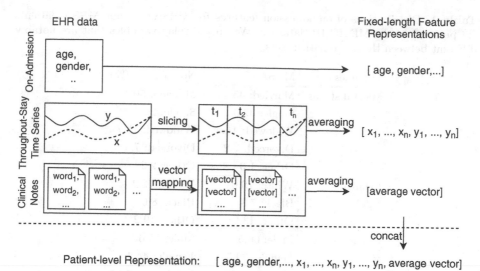

Fig. 1. Feature fusion strategy.

- Descriptive Data: Demographic detail, admission and discharge times and information, and dates of death.
- Physiologic Data: Nurse-verified vital signs such as heart rate and blood pressure.
- Intervention: Procedures such as dialysis and placement of lines.
- Laboratory: Blood chemistry, hematology, urine analysis, and microbiology test results.
- Medications: Administration records of intravenous medications and medication orders.
- Notes: Free-form text notes such as provider progress notes and hospital discharge summaries.

Information in MIMIC dataset contains many known risk factors for MRSA infections. We display known risk factors for MRSA and their availability in MIMIC in Table 2 [1].

2.2 Feature Extraction from Structured EHR Data

The EHR collection for a patient mostly consists of structured data. Two main groups of data types exist in the structured part of EHR records: Tabular numerical on-admission data, and multivariate time series throughout-stay data.

On-Admission Features. Certain patient information is known at the time of admission and does not change during a patient's hospital stay. We refer to this as *on-admission* or *static* data. The only known on-admission risk factor accessible in the MIMIC III database is *age*. Instead of making predictions based only on this known factor, we extract seven extra features, grouped in the following way:

Table 1. Distributions of on-admission features for MRSA and non-MRSA patients (in percent) in the MIMIC III database. We only display variables that are notably different between these two patient sets.

Variables	MRSA (%)	Non-MRSA (%)
Marital status	Married: 45.1	Married: 50.1
	Single: 32.0	Single: 26.6
	Widowed: 14.4	Widowed: 13.7
	Divorced: 7.2	Divorced: 7.4
	Other: 1.3	Other: 2.2
Ethnicity	White: 79.0	White: 72.2
	Black: 7.8	Black: 8.6
	Other: 13.2	Other: 19.2
Gender	Male: 60.5	Male: 55.6
	Female: 39.5	Female: 44.4
Insurance	Medicare: 67.2	Medicare: 55.5
	Private: 22.7	Private: 32.4
	Medicaid: 9.2	Medicaid: 10.3
	Other: 0.9	Other: 1.8
Admiss. type	Emergency: 92.0	Emergency: 74.8
	Elective: 6.7	Elective: 14.7
	Newborn: 0	Newborn: 8.2
	Urgent: 1.3	Urgent: 2.3
Age (av ± std)	68.5 ± 15.9	59.6 ± 23.9

– **Demographic features** are immutable patient features. These include *age*, *gender*, *ethnicity*, *marital status*, and *religion*.
– **Stay-specific features** describe a patient's admission such as admission location, allowing inference on the patient's condition. Stay-specific data could be different for the same patient upon readmission. We extracted 3 such features: *admission type* (e.g., Emergency), *admission location* (e.g., Transfer from another hospital), and *insurance* (e.g., Medicaid).

We extracted a total of eight on-admission features and display the six that best contrast the MRSA-positive and MRSA-negative patients in Table 1. As machine learning methods require numerical inputs and these variables are categorical, follow the standard method for converting categorical features to numerical: creating binary flag variables for each possible value of each of the seven categorical variables. For example, as *gender* has two potential values in this database: *Male* or *Female*, we create one binary feature *Gender:Male* which contains the value 1 if the patient is Male and 0 otherwise. This leads to a total of 30 on-admission features containing the information of eight features, one of which is numerical (age), the others being categorical.

Table 2. Known risk factors for MRSA [11]. The **Available** column indicates if we can extract this information, and the **Source** column indicates the relational table in the MIMIC database.

Risk factors	Available	Table
Old age	Yes	Admission
Nursing home residence	Unknown	Unknown
Receipt of transfusion	Yes	Services
Placing of central line	Yes	Chart
Respiratory failure	Yes	Chart
Open wounds	Unknown	Unknown
Severe bacteremia	Yes	Lab Tests
Organ impairment	Yes	Services
Previous hospital stay	Yes	Admission
Treatment with antibiotics	Yes	Medications

Table 3. Throughout-stay feature descriptions.

Feature	Explanation	Example
Lab tests	Daily average results of 20 lab tests	White Blood Cell ct.
Vital signs	Daily average results of 49 vital signs	Heart Rate
Micro. tests	Daily average results of 14 microbiology tests	Enterococcus Sp.

Throughout-Stay Features. Throughout the hospital stay of a patient, observations such as laboratory results and vital signs are recorded frequently. These data, referred to as *throughout-stay* data, create multivariate time series. We use 83 throughout-stay variables as summarized in Table 3.

One challenge with such data is that the variables (e.g., heart rate) are *irregularly spaced*. The frequency at which measurements are taken varies between patients (e.g., once a day vs. multiple times a day). This variation is a function of **(1)** the variable itself (lab tests may be taken only once a day while vital signs may be measured multiple times a day); **(2)** patient's condition (more severely ill patients must be monitored more closely); and **(3)** the time of the day (nurses are less likely to wake up patients in the middle of the night unless there is a reason or concern to do so).

To make these data comparable across patients and processable by computational ML methods, cleaning and aggregation are required. To address these challenges, we roll up all observations into evenly sampled averages, resulting in one value per hour. If there are no measurements for an hour, they are considered missing values. To handle these empty spaces, we reassign that value to be 0. All values are then scaled to 0–1 interval. We use data from the first 24 h of hospitalization as this will ensure early detection of the infection. Our previous work [13] indicated that even one-day worth of data can be predictive for MRSA detection. Having 83 variables and 24 time stamps for each of them, we generate $83 * 24 = 1992$ throughout-stay features in total per patient.

2.3   Feature Extraction from Unstructured EHR Data

Unstructured components of EHRs consist of different types of clinical notes, such as nursing reports and radiology reports. For each patient, a series of free-form text documents are created by doctors and nurses during hospital stay of the patients. We describe how we generate patient level representations from a series of clinical notes below.

Vector Representations of Words. To input words into machine learning algorithms, numerical representations of words or phrases are necessary. One-hot-encoding, commonly used in text mining domain, is a way of forming a vocabulary-size vector for each word in the vocabulary where one specific bit of the vector is 1 and other bits are 0. This is a very sparse representation in the order of the number of possible words in the alphabet. As a consequence, this creates non-scalable input vectors. In addition, since the set-bit location is random, we lose the contextual information contained across words. Furthermore, when using one-hot encoding, two very similar words can be represented with very different vectors whereas two unrelated words can correspond to two very similar vectors. Word embeddings are dense numerical representations of words, mapping them into a continuous vector space such that similar words are mapped to similar vectors. Word2vec [20] is the most commonly used algorithm to learn word embeddings from raw text.

Learning Word Embeddings from Clinical Notes. We learn word embeddings with the skip-gram model of the "word2vec" algorithm [20] using the clinical notes of our MRSA cohort. The skip-gram model is trained using a binary classification objective (logistic regression) to discriminate the real target words w_t from k imaginary (noise) words $\tilde{w}$, in the same context:

$$J = \log Q_D(D = 1|h, w_t) + k \underset{\tilde{w} \ P_{noise}}{\mathbb{E}} [\log Q_D(D = 0|\tilde{w}, w_t)] \tag{1}$$

where $\log Q_D(D = 1|w, h)$ is the binary logistic regression probability under the model of seeing the word w in the context h in the dataset D, calculated in terms of the learned embedding vectors θ. Then, using the embedding vector θ, words are mapped into vectors in the following way: $x_{ij} = \theta w_{ij}$.

Using all clinical notes recorded for our cohort before the diagnosis of MRSA, we train a skip-gram model and learn dense vectors for words. We choose to map each word into a 32-dimensional space. Figure 2 visualizes reduced-dimension vectors for a randomly-selected 500 words. We see many meaningful word clusters in this figure. For example, all numbers are clustered together and within this specific cluster, numbers are seemingly sorted in order. Furthermore, we notice that different typings for the same numbers have similar vectors, as seen in "00" - "0" and "01" - "1". Another cluster consists of different forms of auxiliary verbs (e.g., have, has, had) and other verbs (e.g., were) representing past time in a sentence. These are especially important in clinical notes where it is essential to know if a condition exists now or if it is a part of the medical history.

We hypothesize that learning word embeddings using a medical dataset achieves better results compared to using general purpose word embeddings (e.g., those learned on Wikipedia). We can see the usefulness of this from the fact that similar medical concepts are grouped together. For example, "catheter", "central line", and "picc" are the same concept described in different ways. We see that these phrases are represented with very similar vectors. These example clusters can be seen in Fig. 3.

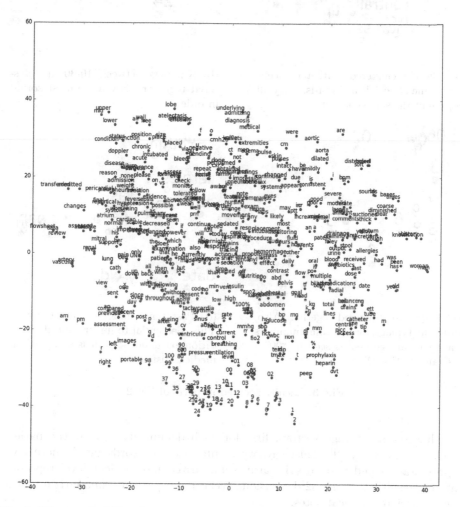

Fig. 2. Word embeddings learned using the MRSA Cohort from the MIMIC dataset. Zoomed-in version of important parts can be seen in Fig. 3.

Patient-Embeddings. After learning word embeddings, we generate a feature vector per patient in the following way. The clinical notes for each patient create a set of documents. Using the word embeddings we learn, we first replace each word in a note with its vector representation. We then compute the

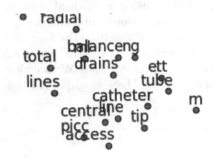

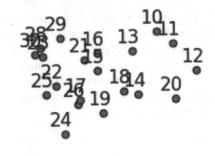

(a) Closely clustered 'catheter', 'central', 'line', 'picc', 'tube' words. They all represent the same concept.

(b) Numbers between 10-30 are clustered together, they are almost sorted in order.

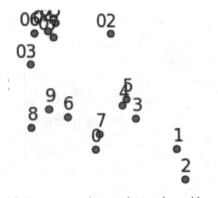

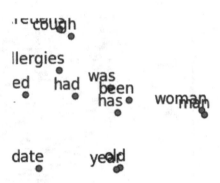

(c) Digits are clustered together. Also, different typings for the same numbers have similar vectors, as seen in "00" - "0" and "02" - "2".

(d) Past tense indicators are grouped. This is essential to understand if a condition exists now or if it is a part of the medical history.

Fig. 3. Locally zoomed-in parts of Fig. 2.

coordinate-wise average vectors, first for each document, then at the patient level, motivated by [9]. This way, we summarize the words into a note level representation and then are similarly summarized into patient level representations, resulting in one 32-dimensional vector per patient, summarizing all of their associated clinical notes.

2.4   Fusion of Features

Once we have feature vectors for all three types of data, each of which summarizes the patient's health with regards to that data type, the task is to combine these vectors to create one merged representation of each patient's overall health. As there are different numbers of features for each data type (30 for on-admission data, 1992 for throughout-stay data, and 32 for clinical notes), we cannot take the average. Thus, here we tackle this by concatenating the vectors together. In our experiments, we try different data type combinations (e.g., on-admission + throughout-stay = 2022 features). Our process of extracting features from each data type and then fusing them together is illustrated in Fig. 1.

3 Classification Methodology

3.1 Ground Truth

In supervised machine learning, each data instance must have an associated label, indicating the outcome. In this work, the outcome is a binary flag indicating the diagnosis of MRSA (1 for MRSA, 0 for non-MRSA), stored in a vector with one value per patient. Positive MRSA microbiology test is used to constitute ground truth labels.

3.2 Classification

In classification tasks, the goal is to divide data points into predefined classes. As we have two classes, *MRSA-positive*, labeled as 1, and *MRSA-negative*, labeled as 0, this creates a binary classification task, where we attempt to learn the relationship between each patient's historical EHR and their associated label. Predicted labels were generated using three different machine learning methods: Logistic Regression, Support Vector Machines, and Random Forests. Generated predictions lie between 0 and 1, requiring transformation into an integer, either 0 or 1 to be directly comparable to the binary label vector for evaluation metrics *Accuracy, Precision, Recall, F1-Score*, and *Area Under the Receiver Operating Characteristic Curve (AUC)*. In this work, if a prediction is ≥ 0.5, then it is converted to 1. Otherwise it is converted to 0.

L2-Regularized Logistic Regression. Logistic Regression is a classic machine learning method based on the odds ratio of how the change in individual features affects the outcome. This algorithm is commonly used for diagnosis prediction [4,26,29,32]. In our setting, each input is a vector, x, containing a patient's historical information which will in turn be weighted by θ, a vector of coefficients, as shown in Eq. 2, where n is the number of patients and p is the number of variables. We also use *L2-Regularization*, controlled by parameter λ, to normalize the values of θ, ensuring direct comparisons between the variable weights. The data is then mapped from input to prediction per formula $f(x)$, shown in Eq. 2.

$$f(\mathbf{x}) = \frac{1}{1 + e^{-\theta^\top \mathbf{x}}} + \lambda \sum_{i=1}^{p} \theta_i^2 \tag{2}$$

Finally, the difference between the predictions made and the true label vector y is minimized. The task is to learn the proper coefficients that project positively labeled data close to 1, and negatively labeled data close to 0. In this setting, the value predicted for a patient can be considered their probability of MRSA infection.

Soft-Margin Support Vector Machine Classification. Support Vector Machine Classification is another popular solution to binary classification problems, also commonly used for diagnosis [31,32]. In contrast to Logistic Regression, this algorithm makes classifications based on distances between data instances. In this case, we compute the coefficients for a hyperplane that divides the dataset based on the labels and the distance from the hyperplane to a few select data instances, termed *support vectors*. To accomplish this task, we again tune the elements of a vector θ, which will subsequently be multiplied by the patient vector, $\mathbf{x}$, to divide the data by label. This is accomplished by minimizing Eq. 3, where n is the number of support vectors, $\mathbf{x}_i$ is each support vector in turn, y_i is the corresponding label for each support vector, λ is a regularizing parameter, and b is a bias variable. The linear kernel was used for all SVM experiments in this work, the minimization task for which is shown in Eq. 3, where y_i is the true label, θ is a vector of tunable parameters, x_i is the input data for example i, b is a bias vector, λ is a regularization term for constraining the size of parameters θ.

$$\min \left[\frac{1}{n} \sum_{i=1}^{n} \max \left[0,\ 1 - y_i \left(\theta^\top \mathbf{x}_i - b \right) \right] \right] + \lambda \|\theta\|_2^2 \qquad (3)$$

Random Forests. Random Forests are the *bootstrap aggregating* implementation of decision trees, a well known and interpretable classification algorithm [2]. They have been shown to be effective in a variety of classification tasks across many domains including prediction of infections [17,18] while allowing easy access to relative variable importances. To generate classifications, random subsets of both data instances and variables are iteratively used to generate decision trees and make predictions on a training set. Then, once a set of decision trees has been generated, testing instances are input into each decision tree and the predictions from each tree are recorded. Finally, the predictions made by each decision tree are combined into one prediction, typically via majority voting. This ensemble learning technique emphasizes high levels of randomness, aiding the generalizability of our models.

3.3   Evaluation Criteria

To evaluate the performance of our classifiers, we use a multitude of standard metrics, namely *Accuracy, Area under the ROC Curve (AUC), Precision, Recall,* and *F-1 Score*. We define and explain each of them below, where TP is the number of True Positive predictions, FP is the number of False Positive predictions, TN is the number of True Negative predictions, and FN is the number of False Negative predictions.

$$\text{Accuracy} = \frac{TP + FP}{TP + FP + TN + FN} \tag{4}$$

$$\text{Precision} = \frac{TP}{TP + FP} \tag{5}$$

$$\text{Recall} = \frac{TP}{TP + FN} \tag{6}$$

$$\text{F1} = \frac{2 * TP}{2 * TP + FP + FN} \tag{7}$$

Accuracy is between 0 and 1, with 0.5 indicating random predictions. Any consistent score higher than 0.5 indicates that the model is not guessing and has learned some pattern. In our setting, it shows what percentage of the patients are correctly predicted (as MRSA or non-MRSA). While *Accuracy* is a common metric in the machine learning domain, more specific metrics may be more informative for clinical application. For example, *Precision* shows among the patients who are predicted as MRSA, what percentage actually has MRSA. *Recall* shows among the actual MRSA patients, what percentage is correctly classified as MRSA. *F1 Score* is the harmonic mean of Precision and Recall, thus capturing success in them both.

The *Receiver Operating Characteristic (ROC) Curve* quantifies the performance of a binary classifier using the *True Positive Rate* (Eq. 8) and *False Positive Rate* (Eq. 9). An ROC curve is used to examine how TPR and FPR change as the decision criterion varies from 0 to 1. The sum of the Area Under the Curve (AUC) quantifies the ability of a classifier to distinguish between two classes. An AUC score of 0.5 indicates a randomly-guessing classifier, and an AUC score of 1 indicates perfect classification.

$$\text{True Positive Rate (TPR)} = \frac{TP}{TP + FN} \tag{8}$$

$$\text{False Positive Rate (FPR)} = \frac{FP}{TN + FP} \tag{9}$$

When a binary classifier makes a probabilistic prediction between 0 and 1, a decision criterion (a.k.a. probability cutoff) decides which probabilities to assign to which class. For example, setting cutoff = 0.5 means that *class* = 1 if probability > 0.5 while for smaller probability values, *class* = 0. Based on the decision criterion, a binary prediction can be made and TPR (sensitivity) and FPR (1-specificity) can be calculated. When evaluating the performance of a clinical test, sensitivity quantifies the ability of a test to correctly identify cases. Specificity reflects the ability of a test to correctly rule out the condition of interest.

AUC is widely used in clinical diagnosis prediction and risk stratification tasks due to several advantages it brings [12,31]. First, it quantifies the success of a classifier independent of a decision criterion. Second, sensitivity and specificity can be easily considered together by examining the curve. Finally, for risk prediction tasks, the optimal cut-off value can be determined using the ROC curve analysis to determine at-risk patients.

3.4 Software and Availability

All preprocessing and machine learning are implemented in Python 3.5. Specifically, Pandas 0.18 and Numpy 1.13 are used for preprocessing, Scikit-Learn 0.18 is used to train machine learning algorithms and Matplotlib 1.5 is used for visualizations. Tensorflow is used to learn word embeddings. PostgreSQL 9.5 is used for data storage and extraction. The scripts used in this work are available at https://github.com/wpi-dsrg/MRSA-prediction-ccis.

4 Experimental Results

4.1 Cohort Construction

To identify MRSA patients, we extract the microbiology test associated with the organism **80293** (MRSA) found in the *Microbiology Events* table. We use the microbiology test, as opposed to the ICD9 code, to extract the time of diagnosis. The presence of this test in a patient's record indicates a positive result. Of 1,304 patients with a positive MRSA test, 643 have this test on the first day of their hospitalization. We exclude these patients and use the ones who are diagnosed with MRSA on day 2 or later of their hospital stay. Of these remaining patients, half are detected on day 2 and the remaining half range up to day 80. Thus, correctly-predicted instances will be at least 1 day early and many will be much earlier. From the remaining patients, 476 of them have data for all three data types we explore: on-admission, throughout-stay and clinical notes. These 476 patient form our MRSA-positive population. As the vast majority of MIMIC consists of patients who do not contract MRSA, the entire negative dataset would be highly imbalanced. To overcome this, we randomly subsample 476 patients who have no record of a test for organism 80293, obtaining a balanced dataset. For consistency, we also only use one-day worth of data for negative patients.

After obtaining a cohort of 952 patients, we split these into training (%80) and testing (%20). We use 5-fold cross validation over the training patients to tune hyper-parameters (Fig. 5). Finally, we report prediction accuracies on the previously-unseen testing patients. This split is maintained across all experiments and all reported performance is obtained on the same test set (Fig. 4, Table 4).

4.2 On-Admission Stratification

To evaluate how successfully we can predict likely MRSA-positive patients directly upon a patient's admission, we train a set of models based only on admission-time data. This essentially captures maximally-early predictions. Non-random predictions would indicate a demographic divide between MRSA-positive and MRSA-negative patients in the context of the classification task.

Current clinical practice emphasizes assessment of MRSA risk factors and observation of signs of infection. We capture these risk factors (e.g., age), but also include other non-risk factors (e.g., marital status) which may help the classifiers find patterns and potentially list new previously-unknown risk factors for some cohorts.

We show results in Table 4 that using only the on-admission data leads to results roughly 10% better than random. Interestingly, using Logistic Regression leads to very high *Recall* of 1.0, and using the Linear SVM results in very low Recall and the highest *Precision* of any model, 0.8. These results show that, we can assign a MRSA risk score to patients during their admission to an ICU.

4.3 Throughout-Stay Stratification

Throughout each patient's stay, data are recorded that quantify a patient's condition. These data may relate to the evolving risk of MRSA acquisition. We train each machine learning algorithm using only throughout-stay features.

We see in Table 4 that across all evaluation metrics, predicting MRSA based on the 24-h worth of 83 variables taken over the course of the first day of a patient's stay in the ICU does not lead to strong predictions. Almost all results are nearly-random, indicating that this is not an excellent source of predictive power.

4.4 Clinical Note Stratification

To evaluate how successful we can predict MRSA infections based only on clinical notes, we train a set of models using only patient-level vectors generated from clinical notes. Based on the results presented in Fig. 4, using only clinical notes achieves an accuracy 4% higher than on-admission time and 16% higher than throughout-stay time series data. This is a promising result indicating that clinical notes carry expert insights about patients that cannot be found elsewhere in EHR collections.

4.5 Fusing Feature Sets for Maximally-Informed Models

We consider combinations of these feature sets, extracted from different types of data, to understand which sources of data are leading to better predictions, and whether or not combining the features leads to improvement. We experiment with four combinations of feature sets: on-admission + throughout-stay, on-admission + clinical Notes, throughout-stay + clinical notes, and all three together, on-admission + throughout-stay + clinical notes. We hypothesize that the model trained using features from all three data types will lead to the best predictions since the classifiers are maximally informed in this setting.

First, in Fig. 4 we show the final *Accuracy* computed on the testing set. This indicates the model performance on previously-unseen data. Test results show that any combination of features including on-admission features slightly surpass any of our three single feature sets on average. When combining all three feature sets, we see the highest *Accuracy* (.71), the highest AUC (.76), and the highest

Table 4. Classification results on the testing dataset from combining data types.

Feature set		Classification method		
		Random Forest	Log. Regression	Lin. SVM
On-admission	Accuracy	.60	.55	.47
	AUC	.66	.67	.67
	F1	.63	.71	.07
	Precision	.63	.55	**.8**
	Recall	.63	**1.0**	.04
Throughout-stay	Accuracy	.48	.53	.51
	AUC	.52	.55	.44
	F1	.48	.55	.37
	Precision	.53	.57	.61
	Recall	.43	.54	.27
Clinical Notes	Accuracy	.64	.63	.47
	AUC	.69	.64	.64
	F1	.66	.72	.09
	Precision	.68	.62	.71
	Recall	.64	.87	.05
On-admission + Throughout-stay	Accuracy	.66	.65	.56
	AUC	.76	.70	.68
	F1	.69	.74	.43
	Precision	.69	.63	.72
	Recall	.69	.89	.31
On-admission + Clinical Notes	Accuracy	.64	.61	.46
	AUC	.71	.67	.67
	F1	.67	.73	0
	Precision	.68	.59	0
	Recall	.65	.98	0
Throughout-stay + Clinical Notes	Accuracy	.54	.52	.52
	AUC	.58	.54	.54
	F1	.51	.55	.40
	Precision	.61	.57	.30
	Recall	.43	.53	.30
On-Admission + Throughout-stay + Clinical Notes	Accuracy	**.71**	.65	.57
	AUC	**.76**	.70	.69
	F1	**.74**	**.74**	.45
	Precision	.72	.33	.75
	Recall	.76	.89	.32

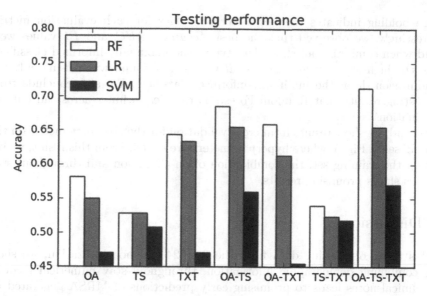

Fig. 4. Comparing accuracy across feature fusion options. OA indicates on-admission, TS indicates throughout-stay, and TXT indicates clinical notes.

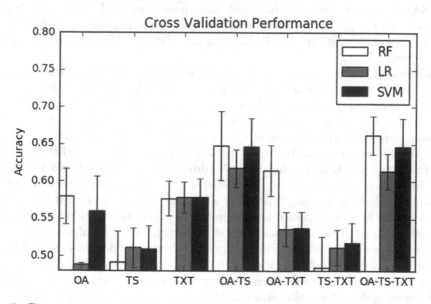

Fig. 5. Comparing accuracy across feature fusion options from cross validation over the training data. OA indicates on-admission, TS indicates throughout-stay, and TXT indicates clinical notes.

F1 score (.74, a tie between Random Forest and Logistic Regression). We also note that the full combination is consistently superior to all other feature sets. A more comprehensive summary of the experimental findings is shown in Table 4, where bolding indicates the best-observed values for each evaluation metric. Interestingly, we observed that the best *Accuracy*, *AUC*, and *F1* values were found when combining all three data types, the maximally-informed classifiers, while the highest *Precision* and *Recall* values were found when using only the on-admission data, the minimally-informed classifiers. We also conclude from our testing results that Random Forests is the clear winner across all dataset combinations.

Second, we show results from cross-validation for the *Accuracy* metric on the training set in Fig. 5, where hyperparameters are tuned. From this result, we see that on the training set, the combination of on-admission and throughout-stay features shows promising results.

5   Discussion

In this work, only using data from the first 24 h of hospitalization, we show that combining demographic information, throughout-stay numerical records, and clinical notes leads to promising early predictions of MRSA generated by core machine learning algorithms. Building a MRSA risk prediction system fusing three key data types has potential to provide effective risk assessments of MRSA infections while providing a risk score indicating to clinicians whether or not patients are likely to develop a MRSA infection using only their first day's records. We show that even this limited amount of information can provide useful predictions.

Clinical decision-making can be significantly aided by intelligent infection prediction systems (such as one that predicts MRSA infections) that process EHRs and support clinicians. EHR systems such as Epic are becoming increasingly popular world-wide, resulting in massive data lakes containing too many patient records for clinicians to efficiently analyze and detect long-term trends [16]. With a machine learning based system like ours, MRSA predictions could be integrated into EHR platforms. Such additions to EHR platforms save costs and improve the quality of care for patients [21]. For instance, such a system could easily include warning reports for a patient that are generated when their risk score for MRSA surpasses some user-set threshold, thus making efficient use of staff resources. This information would in turn enhance the information at the hands of clinicians, providing a means for the reduction of needless antibiotic use or for increased levels of sanitation on a patient-by-patient basis. This strategy offers promise for the development of integrated systems that retrieve, analyze, and report useful information contained within records of thousands of patients. Combining these health record systems with infection prediction could permit medical diagnoses and assist in the identification of hospital-specific risk factors for different infections.

Methods for combining vastly different data types contained in EHRs, such as highly structured demographic information and unstructured clinical notes, are essential to the success of advanced EHR systems. As each data type requires different methods of analysis, focusing on how to best combine these feature types, particularly in the context of infection prediction, promises to better-emulate intuition by clinicians, as these are the types of data they actually use in practice to assess the status of a patient. By increasing the scale at which patient records are analyzed via machine learning (i.e., from one-by-one by a human to thousands by a computer) doors open to understand long-term trends in hospital databases.

A limitation of the current study is that our data come from intensive care units in one hospital in the United States. As such, these patients do not necessarily represent the conditions of general hospitalized populations or the demographics of other regions. The stay-specific data (See Table 1) indicate that while there are diverse groups within the data set, the majority of patients are ethnically white and their gender is predominantly male. In the future, we intend to evaluate the performance of our MRSA risk prediction system using multiple EHR datasets and to ensure generalizability through transfer learning techniques. We also plan to expand these models to predict multiple HAIs concurrently to better serve current hospital needs. An all-encompassing prediction system is the ultimate future goal of this research.

6   Conclusion

Early-warning systems can be used in real time for risk stratification as well as early HAI detection. In this study, we show a prediction system that generates MRSA risk scores from large amounts of EHR data. Mixing clinical time series data, demographic information collected upon admission, and state-of-the-art clinical text modeling method leads to strong predictions for MRSA infections many days before the infections are confirmed. Three binary classification algorithms were trained using EHR data, leading to highly accurate predictions (Mean $AUC = 0.72$, Mean $Accuracy = 0.64$, Mean $F1\text{-}Score = .64$, Mean $Precision = .6$, Mean $Recall = .66$) using only information from the first day of each patient's stay. These results outweigh average results using any of the single-feature-set groups. We successfully trained machine learning algorithms to detect MRSA nearly as far in advance of MRSA diagnosis dates as possible by using on-admission data mixed with the first day of throughout-stay data and of clinical notes collected on that day. Our results indicate that an early warning system could be implemented for hospital patients, to be updated with stay progression, generating reliable risk scores one day into patient stays to aid clinical decision-making and facilitate clinicians in preventing MRSA infections.

Acknowledgements. Thomas Hartvigsen thanks the US Department of Education for supporting his PhD studies via the grant P200A150306 on "GAANN Fellowships to Support Data-Driven Computing Research", while Cansu Sen thanks WPI for granting her the Arvid Anderson Fellowship (2015–2016) to pursue her PhD studies. We also thank the DSRG and Data Science Community at WPI for their continued support and feedback.

References

1. Aureden, K., Arias, K., Burns, L., et al.: Guide to the Elimination of Methicillin-Resistant Staphylococcus Aureus (MRSA): Transmission in Hospital Settings. APIC, Washington, D.C. (2010)
2. Breiman, L.: Random forests. Mach. Learn. **45**(1), 5–32 (2001)
3. Celi, L.A., Mark, R.G., Stone, D.J., Montgomery, R.A.: "Big Data" in the intensive care unit. Closing the data loop. Am. J. Respir. Crit. Care Med. **187**(11), 1157–1160 (2013)
4. Chang, Y., et al.: Predicting hospital-acquired infections by scoring system with simple parameters. PLoS ONE **6**(8), e23137 (2011)
5. CMS: Electronic health records (EHR) incentive programs (2011). https://www.cms.gov/Regulations-and-Guidance/Legislation/EHRIncentivePrograms/index.html
6. Congress of the United States: American Recovery and Reinvestment Act (2009). www.healthit.gov/policy-researchers-implementers/health-it-legislation
7. Cortes, C., Vapnik, V.: Support-vector networks. Mach. Learn. **20**(3), 273–297 (1995)
8. Dantes, R., et al.: National burden of invasive Methicillin-resistant Staphylococcus aureus infections, United States, 2011. JAMA Intern. Med. **173**(21), 1970–1978 (2013)
9. Dubois, S., Kale, D.C., Shah, N., Jung, K.: Learning effective representations from clinical notes. arXiv preprint arXiv:1705.07025 (2017)
10. Dutta, R., Dutta, R.: Maximum probability rule based classification of MRSA infections in hospital environment: using electronic nose. Sens. Actuators B: Chem. **120**(1), 156–165 (2006)
11. Fukuta, Y., Cunningham, C.A., Harris, P.L., Wagener, M.M., Muder, R.R.: Identifying the risk factors for hospital-acquired methicillin-resistant Staphylococcus aureus (MRSA) infection among patients colonized with MRSA on admission. Infect. Control Hosp. Epidemiol. **33**(12), 1219–1225 (2012)
12. Hajian-Tilaki, K.: Receiver operating characteristic (ROC) curve analysis for medical diagnostic test evaluation. Caspian J. Intern. Med. **4**(2), 627 (2013)
13. Hartvigsen, T., Sen, C., Brownell, S., Teeple, E., Kong, X., Rundensteiner, E.: Early Prediction of MRSA Infections using Electronic Health Records. HealthInf, Valletta (2018)
14. Jensen, P.B., Jensen, L.J., Brunak, S.: Mining electronic health records: towards better research applications and clinical care. Nat. Rev. Genet. **13**(6), 395 (2012)
15. Johnson, A.E., et al.: MIMIC-III, a freely accessible critical care database. Sci. Data **3**, 160035 (2016)
16. Jones, D.A., Shipman, J.P., Plaut, D.A., Selden, C.R.: Characteristics of personal health records: findings of the Medical Library Association/National Library of Medicine joint electronic personal health record task force. JMLA: J. Med. Libr. Assoc. **98**(3), 243 (2010)
17. Khalilia, M., Chakraborty, S., Popescu, M.: Predicting disease risks from highly imbalanced data using random forest. BMC Med. Inform. Decis. Mak. **11**(1), 51 (2011)
18. Lebedev, A., et al.: Random forest ensembles for detection and prediction of Alzheimer's disease with a good between-cohort robustness. NeuroImage: Clin. **6**, 115–125 (2014)

19. Maree, C., Daum, R., Boyle-Vavra, S., Matayoshi, K., Miller, L.: Community-associated methicillin-resistant Staphylococcus aureus isolates and healthcare-associated infections. Emerg. Infect. Dis. **13**(2), 236 (2007). https://doi.org/10.3201/eid1302.060781

20. Mikolov, T., Sutskever, I., Chen, K., Corrado, G.S., Dean, J.: Distributed representations of words and phrases and their compositionality. In: Advances in Neural Information Processing Systems, pp. 3111–3119 (2013)

21. Murdoch, T., Detsky, A.: The inevitable application of big data to health care. JAMA **309**(13), 1351–1352 (2013)

22. Neu, H.C.: The crisis in antibiotic resistance. Science **257**(5073), 1064–1074 (1992)

23. Nseir, S., Grailles, G., Soury-Lavergne, A., Minacori, F., Alves, I., Durocher, A.: Accuracy of American Thoracic Society/Infectious Diseases Society of America criteria in predicting infection or colonization with multidrug-resistant bacteria at intensive-care unit admission. Clin. Microbiol. Infect. **16**(7), 902–908 (2010)

24. Raghupathi, W., Raghupathi, V.: Big data analytics in healthcare: promise and potential. Health Inf. Sci. Syst. **2**(1), 3 (2014)

25. Sen, C., Hartvigsen, T., Rundensteiner, E., Claypool, K.: CREST - risk prediction for clostridium difficile infection using multimodal data mining. In: Altun, Y., et al. (eds.) ECML PKDD 2017. LNCS (LNAI), vol. 10536, pp. 52–63. Springer, Cham (2017). https://doi.org/10.1007/978-3-319-71273-4_5

26. Shang, J.S., Lin, Y.E., Goetz, A.M.: Diagnosis of MRSA with neural networks and logistic regression approach. Health Care Manag. Sci. **3**(4), 287 (2000)

27. Sintchenko, V., Coiera, E., Gilbert, G.L.: Decision support systems for antibiotic prescribing. Curr. Opin. Infect. Dis. **21**(6), 573–579 (2008)

28. Ventola, C.L.: The antibiotic resistance crisis: Part 1: causes and threats. Pharm. Ther. **40**(4), 277 (2015)

29. Visser, H., le Cessie, S., Vos, K., Breedveld, F.C., Hazes, J.M.: How to diagnose rheumatoid arthritis early: a prediction model for persistent (erosive) arthritis. Arthritis Rheumatol. **46**(2), 357–365 (2002)

30. Weiner, L., et al.: Antimicrobial-resistant pathogens associated with healthcare-associated infections: summary of data reported to the National Healthcare Safety Network at the centers for disease control and prevention, 2011–2014. Infect. Control Hosp. Epidemiol. **37**(11), 1288–1301 (2016)

31. Wiens, J., Guttag, J., Horvitz, E.: Learning evolving patient risk processes for c. diff. colonization. In: ICML Workshop on Machine Learning from Clinical Data (2012)

32. Wu, J., Roy, J., Stewart, W.F.: Prediction modeling using EHR data: challenges, strategies, and a comparison of machine learning approaches. Med. Care **48**(6), S106–S113 (2010)

Multi-layered Learning for Information Extraction from Adverse Drug Event Narratives

Susmitha Wunnava[1](✉), Xiao Qin[1](✉), Tabassum Kakar[1](✉), M. L. Tlachac[1],
Xiangnan Kong[1](✉), Elke A. Rundensteiner[1](✉), Sanjay K. Sahoo[2](✉),
and Suranjan De[2](✉)

[1] Worcester Polytechnic Institute, Worcester, MA, USA
{swunnava,xqin,tkakar,mltlachac,xkong,rundenst}@wpi.edu
[2] Center for Drug Evaluation and Research, U.S. Food and Drug Administration,
Silver Spring, MD, USA
{sanjay.sahoo,suranjan.de}@fda.hhs.gov

Abstract. Recognizing named entities in Adverse Drug Reactions narratives is a crucial step towards extracting valuable patient information from unstructured text and transforming the information into an easily processable structured format. This motivates using advanced data analytics to support data-driven pharmacovigilance. Yet existing biomedical named entity recognition (NER) tools are limited in their ability to identify certain entity types from these domain-specific narratives, resulting in poor accuracy. To address this shortcoming, we propose our novel methodology called Tiered Ensemble Learning System with Diversity (TELS-D), an ensemble approach that integrates a rich variety of named entity recognizers to procure the final result. There are two specific challenges faced by biomedical NER: the classes are imbalanced and the lack of a single best performing method. The first challenge is addressed through a balanced, under-sampled bagging strategy that depends on the imbalance level to overcome this highly skewed data problem. To address the second challenge, we design an ensemble of heterogeneous entity recognizers that leverages a novel ensemble combiner. Our experimental results demonstrate that for biomedical text datasets: (i) a balanced learning environment combined with an ensemble of heterogeneous classifiers consistently improves the performance over individual base learners and (ii) stacking-based ensemble combiner methods outperform simple majority voting based solutions by 0.3 in F1-score.

Keywords: Pharmacovigilance · Adverse Drug Reaction ·
Class imbalance · Ensemble learning

We are grateful for funding to in part support this research, including by the Seeds of STEM at WPI via the Institute of Education Sciences, U.S. Department of Education grant R305A150571, Oak Ridge Associated Universities (ORAU) for two ORISE Fellowships to conduct research with the U.S. Food and Drug Administration, and the Department of Education GAANN fellowship grant P200A150306.

A. Cliquet jr. et al. (Eds.): BIOSTEC 2018, CCIS 1024, pp. 420–446, 2019.
https://doi.org/10.1007/978-3-030-29196-9_22

1 Introduction

1.1 Motivation and Background

Adverse Drug Reactions (ADRs) refer to unwanted, and often immensely dangerous, effects caused by the administration of drugs. In fact, ADRs not revealed during clinical trials are one of the leading causes of death worldwide [23]. ADRs can be the result of a single administered drug or a combination of administered drugs.

The FDA Adverse Event Reporting System (FAERS) is responsible for overseeing the safety and effectiveness of drugs in the post marketing phase. As such, the FDA leverages the FAERS system to monitor the ADR incidences submitted by consumers, healthcare professionals and drug manufacturers. The FAERS reports are manually reviewed by FDA staff to identify potential drug safety concerns and, when necessary, to recommend appropriate actions to improve product safety.

FAERS features the MedWatch[1] report form, illustrated in Fig. 2, for reporting an adverse drug event [39]. The MedWatch form contains both structured fields as well as unstructured narratives. These narratives tend to contain information that either is left blank in the structured fields and/or simply goes beyond the information meant for the structured meta fields. Even more important, these narratives contain a wealth of detailed information regarding the adverse events, as seen in Fig. 1 [39].

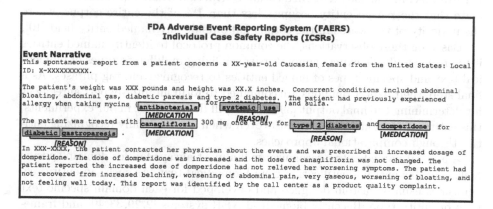

Fig. 1. A sample FAERS report highlighting detailed information on the ADR incident within the narrative [39].

FAERS received over 1.7 million ADR incident reports in 2015, a number that is increasing annually [11]. This growing volume of reports and the vital information stored within the unstructured narratives makes the manual review process

---

[1] https://www.fda.gov/safety/medwatch/.

ever more challenging. Thus, to ensure that drug safety signals are effectively identified in a timely manner from the exploding quantity of reports with limited human resources, the future review processes must be enhanced by advanced data mining and visualization technologies [12,28,37].

Most existing technologies rely on information organized in a structured format. As such, it is vital that the unstructured text in the ADR report narratives are first processed and converted into a structured format. This extraction is mandatory for the aforementioned advanced analytics and crucial for timely detection, assessment, and prevention of future incidents of ADRs. In this study, we focus on the problem of Named Entity Recognition (NER) – a fundamental task in this process to identifying the appropriate information in the narratives and then filling it into the information categories [39].

A major obstacle of processing biomedical narratives within medical reports is that the unstructured text is comprised of different formats and styles depending on the report source. Two specific challenges rise in this context that we address in this research project. First, a named entity phrase may be expressed as a combination of entity-specific medical terms in addition to non-medical descriptive text. For example, in the named entity phrase "*coronary artery disease related event prophylaxis*", the words "related" and "event" are descriptive text while the remaining words are medical terms. These named entity phrases can cause ambiguity even during the manual annotation process. Second, the narratives are predominately composed of large segments of text with only a rather small number of phrases specific to the named entities [39] interleaved. For example, in the 2009 i2b2 Medication Extraction Challenge dataset, we estimate that the *reason* entity occupies less than 1% of the entire corpus, where the majority of the words in the corpus fall outside any named entity field [10].

Based on these observations, the common protocol to identify named entities is to engage multiple expert annotators specializing in different types of biomedical text and specific types of named entities to recognize and tag phrases. As a final step, their expert opinions are combined to form an inter-expert agreement for determining the final output [39]. As we will demonstrate in our experiments, this entity extraction problem persists even when automatically recognizing entities through computational approaches.

A general named entity recognizer will almost always fail for domain specific tasks, such as entity identification from biomedical text. As such, an entity recognizer is usually custom designed and developed for each domain specific text type or entity type. Recently biomedical NER systems [2,29,33,40] and frameworks [13] have been customized for the biomedical domain and specific entity types. To the best of our knowledge, there is no comprehensive study to date on how to automatically adapt and integrate the strength of a relevant and yet diverse set of named entity recognizers to tackle a new domain-specific NER task [39].

1.2   Related Work

Existing approaches to biomedical NER can be categorized into three different methods: (1) rule-based, (2) machine learning based, and (3) hybrid.

The rule-based methods leverage user-defined pattern matching rules supported with semantic knowledge resources [39]. MedLEE [14] and MedEx [40] are rule-based systems that use a medical knowledge base and a linguistic approach to extract relevant medical information from clinical text. The benefits of rule-based systems are that they perform well when identifying known patterns. However, these systems are limited in their ability to generalize so they fail to identify previously unknown words and patterns. Given the rapid development of scientific discoveries, the list of applicable semantic categories is continually changing and growing – a hurdle for rule-based systems that depend on the semantic knowledge resources [31].

Machine learning based methods for entity recognition leverage features extracted from words. As such, these methods have a better generalization ability than the rule-based methods. A study [35] demonstrated that machine learning approaches can outperform rule-based systems for assertion classification in clinical text. Unfortunately, the machine learning methods require large annotated corpora for training [39].

Despite this challenge, some studies have implemented machine learning methods for biomedical entity recognition. Ramesh et al. developed a biomedical named entity tagger using Support Vector Machines (SVM) to extract medication and ADR information from FAERS narratives [27]. Ghiasvand et al. leveraged Conditional Random Fields (CRF) to label diseases and disorders in clinical sentences [16]. Halgrim et al. used a Maximum Entropy model to extract relevant medical information [17]. Most recently, Jagannatha and Yu implemented Recurrent Neural Networks to extract medical events from Electronic Health Records (EHR) and showed they significantly outperformed CRF models [19].

Hybrid approaches that utilize both rule-based and machine learning methods have also began to be explored [39]. For instance, Doan and Xu developed an SVM based method that utilizes the semantic tags of the words obtained from MedEx as features to recognize medication-related entities from discharge summaries.

We introduced our novel methodology called Tiered Ensemble Learning System with Diversity (TELS-D) to address the challenges associated with NER [39], namely, class imbalance and lack of a best performing method as further described in Sect. 1.3. This paper delves deeper into our previous work described in a conference paper [39] by offering enhanced explanations and additional analysis.

1.3   Challenges of Automating Biomedical Entity Recognition

The focus of our research is on implementing supervised machine learning methods for effective biomedical NER and classification. In particular, we focus on a two-class, binary classification task to recognize and classify named entities [39].

Biomedical NER and classification is challenging due to the specific characteristics of the task [39]. In this research we tackle two of the most critical challenges: (1) the lack of positive class instances & class imbalance and (2) the lack of a single best performing classification method.

Lack of Positive Class Instances and Class Imbalance. A challenge in classifying named entities in any biomedical text, but especially in clinical text, is that the data has class imbalance. The training dataset is predominately composed of non-medical text containing only a small percentage of entity-specific medical text. This results in highly skewed and imbalanced class distributions.

Typically in the biomedical domain, the positive class – the class of interest that represents the medical named entity – is minimally represented in the text and is a stark minority compared to the negative class [39]. For example, consider the "reason" vs non-reason instances in the narratives, such as in Fig. 1, where the vast majority of the words in the text do not belong to the reasons category.

Research [20, 24] has found that learning on imbalanced training datasets can cause a significant deterioration in the performance of the supervised machine learning methods, particularly when classifying instances belonging to the underrepresented class [39]. As such, this imbalance must be addressed to build effective NERs.

Lack of a Single Best Performing Classification Method. Selecting the appropriate learning algorithm to train to classify named entities in text is challenging because every method has different advantages and drawbacks. Conventional approaches to biomedical NER tend to use a single machine learning method such as SVM, CRF, Maximum Entropy (ME) [5] for entity classification. However, these methods differ significantly in their performances based on the context. An i2b2 challenge demonstrated that teams using different supervised machine learning methods obtained significantly different results from each other [33].

In addition, the performance of a single system has been shown to differ across diverse named entities. For instance, Uzuner et al. [33] concluded from the aforementioned i2b2 challenge that while the state-of-the-art natural language processing systems perform well extracting certain named entities (such as medication and dosages), the extraction of other medical entities (such as duration and reason for administration) has been shown to be more challenging. As machine learning methods perform significantly different from each other and performance is reliant on the particular named entity being targeted, there is no single classification method that is best for every named entity in the biomedical domain.

1.4   The Scope of This Work

The general problems of class imbalance and ensemble learning systems for classification have been addressed in the literature [15]. However, in the context of

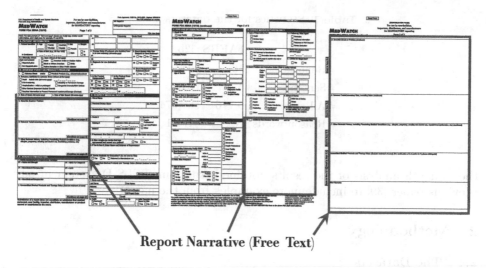

Report Narrative (Free Text)

Fig. 2. FAERS report – Medwatch 3500A [39].

biomedical NER, an integrative approach that deals with both the class imbalance problem and the limitations of any one individual classification method has not previously been studied [39].

In this paper, we thus explore a novel methodology called Tiered Ensemble Learning System with Diversity, or in short TELS-D, that we designed to address the above challenges in NER, with the methodology briefly introduced in our previous paper [39]. TELS-D involves four core steps:

1. Create a balanced training environment: to address the class imbalance inherent in medical data used for machine learning training, we create a balanced training environment by applying undersampling techniques.
2. Generate an ensemble of classifiers: by training a set of heterogeneous learning algorithms in this balanced training environment, we generate an ensemble of diverse classifiers.
3. Create a meta-training feature set: we combine the intermediate results generated by each of the classifiers in the ensemble to create a meta-training feature set.
4. Train a meta-algorithm: we train a *"learner-over-learners"* meta-algorithm over the meta-level features to correctly learn and classify the named entities in the narratives.

To evaluate our proposed methodology TELS-D, we perform comprehensive experiments on datasets of biomedical reports. Our experiments demonstrate that TELS-D outperforms each of the individual learners that contribute to the ensemble. TELS-D achieves a higher accuracy of 0.52 in F1-score compared to any of the individual classifiers with F1-score ranging from 0.22-0.33, in recognizing the relevant information categories from the narratives. We have extended

Table 1. Statistics for the datasets [39].

	FAERS	i2b2
#Reports	16	242
#Sentences	678	8,050
#All words	6,116	67,074
#Reason words	NA	1,881

the in-depth analysis of the results obtained from our TELS-D system in our previous paper [39] to include more examples from the narratives.

2   Methodology

2.1   The Datasets

The FAERS Adverse Event Report Narratives. The FAERS database contains reports with information about adverse events and medication errors. These reports are submitted to the FDA from various sources such as patients, medical professionals, and drug manufacturers.

A report contains sections to enter both structured content as well as free-form text. The areas available for this unstructured text in an example Med-Watch report form, supported by FAERS, can be seen in Fig. 2. Many studies have indicated [18] that the text narratives serve to provide either (1) supplementary information or (2) primary information. To elaborate, when the structured fields have been completed, the narrative becomes supplementary material to that structured content. However, in many cases the individual making the report provides a detailed narrative in the form of unstructured text without manually entering information into all of the structured fields.

It is important to collect all of the relevant medical knowledge available in a structured format so it can easily be processed. Therefore, there is a need for identifying information related to the adverse event case from the free text in these FAERS report narratives.

While we have access to 925 FAERS reports, they are not annotated and not redacted. As such, these reports are not available to the general public due to privacy concerns. In addition to these reports, we also work with 16 redacted reports provided by the FDA, briefly described in Table 1.

The i2b2 Annotated Patient Discharge Summaries. In addition, to assure reproducibility, we leverage the publicly available data set used during the 2009 Medication Extraction Challenge from the Third i2b2 Workshop on Natural Language Processing Challenges for Clinical Records [33,34]. This i2b2 data set is composed of patient discharge summaries provided by Partners Healthcare.

A total of 696 reports were released for training purposes as part of the Medication Extraction Challenge. Of these reports, 17 were annotated by the i2b2 organizers. An additional 251 reports, annotated by the participating teams, were released as the testing data set.

The annotated entities include *medication name, dosage, mode, frequency, duration,* and *reason for administration.* Our research involves 242 of these annotated reports (9 from the training set and 233 from the testing set) which are briefly described in Table 1. Since the goal of this study is to develop an information extraction strategy from the text, we focus on the annotated narrative section of each report.

2.2 *Reason* Entity

In this study, we specifically focus on identifying a single vital entity: the *"reason"*. This entity is the *reason* thought to be the cause of the administration of the medication as per the FAERS report narrative. In the i2b2 discharge summaries, this entity corresponds to the *reason* for the administration of a drug.

The *reason* entity has been routinely hailed as one of the most important fields to extract from text narratives. However, as mentioned in Sect. 1.3, it has also proved among the most challenging of entities to identify. The particular difficulties in extracting the *reason* entity stem from the diversity and often not well scoped vocabulary [17,33].

The i2b2 discharge summaries feature a heavy class imbalance in regards to the *reason* entity. In other words, words tagged as belonging to the *reason* class represent only about 1% of all words in these narratives. The challenges associated with lack of positive class instances is mentioned in Sect. 1.3.

2.3 Data Pre-processing

Data pre-processing is a vital first step for transforming the raw textual narratives into format suitable for natural language processing. We perform the following pre-processing steps on each report in the corpus:

1. *Sentence Segmentation*: Each narrative is separated into sentences to decompose the structure.
2. *Word Tokenization*: Each sentence is separated into tokens (words) as tokens are our unit of processing.
3. *Punctuation Removal*: All tokens that represent punctuations are removed.
4. *Token Offsets*: For each token, its starting and ending character positions within the report are recorded. Additionally, we generate the word offsets which include both the global (report level) and local (sentence level) positions of each token.

2.4 Feature Extraction

A rich set of features are required for machine learning methods to learn the meaning of the tokens. For each token obtained from the preprocessing module (Fig. 3), we generate the following feature sets:

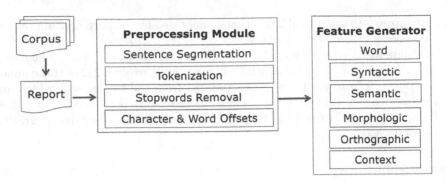

Fig. 3. Preprocessing and feature extraction.

1. *Word Features*: The token is converted into a bag-of-words representation based on the vocabulary of the entire corpus. We form a vocabulary for the entire corpus by converting all of the words in the corpus to lowercase and then stemming them using the NLTK Porter Stemmer [4].
2. *Syntactic Features*: A constituency parse tree is created using Charniak-Johnson parser [8]. The token is then tagged with its respective parts-of-speech (POS) and lexical categories. Figure 4 illustrates an example of a constituency parse tree. For example, the syntactic features of the word "domperidone" are: 1. POS is "NN" indicating it is a noun and 2. phrasal class "NP" indicating it is a noun phrase.
3. *Semantic Features*: Semantic categories of the token are then obtained through lexicon lookup from medication lexicons. These include side effect lexicons such as SIDER [22] as well as UMLS Metamap [2].
4. *Context Features*: In the narrative, adjacent words to the token provide valuable information regarding the context in which the token is actually used. As words have multiple definitions, the same word may be labeled differently at different points within the narrative. This feature is helpful to differentiate when a word has multiple labels. A context window of size five words – two words before and two words after the token – are coded using bag-of-words representation. A boolean value is used as a binary flag to indicate whether the token occurs before or after certain so called "trigger words". As such, we identify trigger words that may indicate the presence of the named entity *reason* [39].
5. *Morphological Features*: We consider a maximum of 3 characters of the suffix and prefix of the token. The prefix and suffix of a token can provide useful information about the token. For example, in the case of words with prefix of "dys" indicate something is abnormal, such as dyspnea. Similarity, words with a suffix of "ing" may indicate a condition or symptom, such as bloating.
6. *Orthographic Features*: Boolean values are used to indicate if this token contains capital letters, digits, special characters, etc.

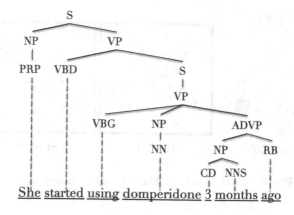

Fig. 4. An example of constituency parse tree.

2.5   Base Machine Learning Models

After each token has been characterized by descriptive features as described in Sect. 2.4 the tokens form feature vectors. These feature vectors and their corresponding label indicating class type (*reason* or *non-reason*) are then used to train the models.

These machine learned models are then leveraged to classify the new feature vectors representing the tokens in the input narrative into *reason* or *non-reason* type. Given a new input feature vector representing a token in the new narrative, these machine learned models are then leveraged to classify tokens characterized by the same set of features.

Different machine learning models have different sets of assumptions and ways of modeling the data, resulting in different degrees of effectiveness for different classification tasks. In our study, we assume that different models are able to capture different aspects of the data [39]. Thus having them compliment each other in an assembly fashion will achieve better accuracy than any of them working individually. We build our base classifiers using multiple popular machine learning models, namely, Decision Tree (DT), Logistic Regression (LR) and SVM [1], illustrated in Fig. 5 [39].

Decision Tree. A decision tree is a tree structure classification model using a branching method to classify the feature vector. Figure 5(a) shows a decision tree that classifies a token to *reason* or *non-reason*. The input token comes in the form of feature vector. The model is to traverse the decision tree from the root node to a leaf node. Each non-leaf node D_i conditions the traverse direction by evaluating some feature values of the input token. The leaf node to which the token goes represents the final classification decision made by the model on this particular token. The decision tree model is intuitive in that the tree consists of decision rules which are human interpretable. Moreover, it is designed to handle categorical feature types and non-linear features. However, this model is highly biased. And it does not provide a ranking score for the input w.r.t different classes.

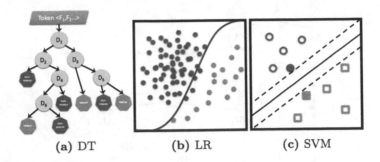

(a) DT   (b) LR   (c) SVM

Fig. 5. Illustration of machine learning models [39].

Logistic Regression. A logistic regression model is a regression model that estimates the probability of a binary response (*reason* or *non-reason*) based on the input feature vector (token). Figure 5(b) shows an example of a logistic regression classifier (curved line) that classifies the tokens (points) into two classes. The logistic regression model provides convenient probability scores for each token indicating the degree of it being in a particular class. Such score provides richer information than only a binary decision. It thus can be used to rank the tokens. The LR model can be trained efficiently compared to other machine learning models. However, it does not perform well if the number of features for each input is too large. And it does not handle categorical feature types well.

Support Vector Machine. A support vector machine is a discriminative classifier formally defined by a separating hyperplane. Figure 5(c) shows a maximum-margin hyperplane and margins for an SVM trained with feature vectors (tokens) from two classes (*reason* and *non-reason*). Feature vectors on the margin (solid shapes) are called the support vectors. The SVM model is able to handle input with large number of features and is designed to process non-linear feature. As illustrated in Fig. 5(c), the learned model does not reply on the entire dataset since it is constructed based on a few support vectors. However, SVM is not efficient with a large number of input feature vectors. Moreover, tuning its parameter, e.g., kernel selections, to achieve high accuracy is not trivial.

2.6   Ensemble of Classifiers

Ensemble of classifiers is a collection of diverse classifiers whose classification recommendations are aggregated to achieve more accurate classification [1,26]. The goal of an ensemble system to achieve more accurate classification is accomplished by combining the results of many diverse classifiers into a single consensus result.

The ensemble of classifiers outperforms each of the individual classifiers by reducing the generalization error of individual classifiers and thus the misclassification rate. The success of an ensemble of classifiers assumes that the base learners perform better than random guessing, in other words, these learners have an accuracy greater than 50% [32].

Model Diversity. The generalization error of the ensemble system tends to be lower than that of the individual classifiers when there is sufficient diversity in the ensemble. To elaborate, this diversity exists when the base learners have different prediction accuracy on different data instances. There are two distinct approaches to generate a diverse set of classifiers for an ensemble of classifiers:

1. Heterogeneous Learning Methods: The first approach to generating a diverse set of classifiers is to train different learning methods on the same training set. Provided the performance of each of these methods varies significantly, the results obtained are diverse in nature. We simultaneously overcome the limitations and take advantage of the respective strengths of each learning algorithm by combining the classifiers into an ensemble of classifiers.
2. Heterogeneous Training Datasets: Another common approach to generating a diverse set of classifiers is to create different subsets of the original training dataset and then to train a single learning method on each of those subsets of training data. Bagging [7] and Boosting [30] are examples of algorithms that tackle the need for a diverse set of classifiers by sub-setting the original dataset.

Given our data set suffers from a heavy class imbalance problem and the amount of *reason* tokens are limited, restrict our options for generating a diverse set of classifiers. For instance, boosting and bagging are not suitable design options for our task as they further reduce the data to smaller subsets of data.

Thus, in this study we follow the methodology for heterogeneous learning methods. Specifically, we form an ensemble of models obtained with the models described in Sect. 2.5: SVM, LR, and DT learning models. Our experiments in Sect. 3.8 confirm that an ensemble of these base classifiers outperforms any of these individual classifiers.

Model Assembly. There are multiple combination techniques that can be used to aggregate the results of the diverse learning methods in the ensemble of classifiers to obtain a single aggregated consensus. We explore two such techniques:

1. Majority Voting: Majority Voting (MV) is the most commonly used combination technique. The selected class is the class that receives the most votes from all of the individual learning methods by simple counting. MV can involve either simple voting where each base learner is given the same weight or weighted voting where the base learners are given different weights. In both cases, the average is taken.

2. <u>Stacked Generalization</u>: Another combination technique is Stacked Generalization [38], also known as Stacking. This technique is a *learning over learners* method to procure the final result. Specifically, stacking is a meta-learning algorithm that leverages the prediction patterns of the base learners. The class predictions from the base learners are passed as input data to the meta-algorithm to learn the correct output.

In our study, we experiment with both Majority Voting and Stacking techniques as model combiners. Ultimately, we demonstrate that the Stacking method outperforms Majority Voting method. Therefore, Stacking is a promising strategy to adopt for combining the models into an ensemble.

2.7   Strategies for Addressing the Class Imbalance Problem

In biomedical named entity recognition tasks, frequently the training datasets are very skewed [25]. In other words, these datasets suffer from a heavy class imbalance. This occurs when the positive class, typically the class of interest, is in stark minority to the negative class. When machine learning methods are trained over datasets with class imbalance, their performance tends to be greatly affected by the class imbalance. In particular, the result tends to be the minority class not being well learned and hence mostly misclassified. As such, class imbalance tends to influence the performance of the machine learning method by favoring the majority negative class. Approaches to deal with class-imbalanced datasets include balancing with class weights, class instances, and classier ensembles.

Balancing with Class Weights. One common method to dealing with class imbalance is to balance the class weights within the classifier, thereby giving more importance (or weight) to the errors of the minority class. The higher class-weights emphasize the importance of the minority class. That is, the weights penalize the model more for making classification mistakes on instances of the minority class than the majority class during training. Thus, these penalties function to bias the model to pay more attention to the minority class.

Usually, when the dataset is balanced, both classes are given an equal weight of one. However, for imbalanced datasets, the class weights can be balanced by performing a grid search with different class weight combinations to find the optimal class weights. These weights are then used to bias the decision making process of the learning method.

Balancing with Class Instances. Another approach to minimize the effect of class imbalance is to re-sample the original training dataset to create a new modified training dataset with balanced class distribution. Random over-sampling and random under-sampling are examples of common re-sampling techniques [9]. In both cases, the objective is to reduce the impact of the highly skewed class distribution by creating a balance between the number of majority and

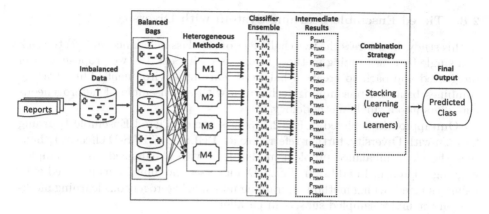

Fig. 6. TELS-D tiered ensemble learning system with diversity [39].

minority class instances. This enables the classifier to give equal importance (or weight) to both of the classes during the training phase.

However, the random under-sampling and random over-sampling techniques have limitations. Under-sampling poses the risk of potentially disregarding important data instances of the majority class. Over-sampling increases the size of the training dataset, randomly repeating instances in the minority class until there are the same number of instances in both classes.

As *reason* instances compose only around 1% of the tokens in the i2b2 discharge summaries, as discussed in Sect. 2.2, over-sampling would almost double the already numerous number of tokens. In addition, each of the *reason* tokens would be repeated many times. As such, we have opted to re-sample the dataset with the random under-sampling technique.

Balancing with Classifier Ensembles. The final approach to handle class imbalance that we discuss is to leverage ensemble methods to generate a classifier ensemble with the ability to create a balanced learning environment for the learning algorithm. [6]. Under-Bagging [3] and Over-Bagging [36] are examples of such ensemble techniques. Both approaches deal with class imbalance in the learning phase through a combination of data re-sampling and bagging approaches, known as "balanced bagging".

To the best of our knowledge, the diversity of the ensemble with regards to the aforementioned existing methods is typically generated through training a single homogeneous learning algorithm on all balanced subsets of the training data. The Majority Voting combination method is then used to aggregate the results from the ensemble of classifiers. In this study, while we will employ the basic idea of "balanced bagging", we will also extend this approach to simultaneously train a diverse set of heterogeneous learning algorithms.

2.8   Tiered Ensemble Learning System with Diversity

In this study, we address the two challenges of (1) class imbalance and (2) the lack of a single best performing method, as discussed in Sect. 1.3, we propose a novel integrated approach to create a balanced learning environment. This strategy combines balanced re-sampling techniques with an ensemble of heterogeneous classifiers into a single methodology.

Our approach, depicted in Fig. 2.8 [39], is named **T**iered **E**nsemble **L**earning **S**ystem with **D**iversity, further referred to as **TELS-D**. TELS-D effectively handles the class imbalance problem in the data with a balanced under-sampled bagging approach. In addition, TELS-D addresses the limitations involved with using a single learning method by training multiple heterogeneous learning methods on the under-sampled subsets in parallel.

TELS-D Implementation. We define the class imbalance level (IM) for the dataset in (Eq. 1). This IM is the ratio of the number of majority negative class instances to the number of minority positive class instances. It indicates how many times more majority class instances than there are minority class instances.

$$Imbalance\ Level\ (IM) = \frac{\#\ Negative\ class\ tokens}{\#\ Positive\ class\ tokens} \tag{1}$$

The imbalance level of our dataset informs our under-sampling to create multiple smaller subsets of the original dataset that each individually exhibit a balanced class distribution. To elaborate, these balanced subsets include *all* of the available positive class instances as well as an equal number of randomly sampled negative class instances. This re-sampling enables us to learn the features inherent in the minority positive class of interest without getting overwhelmed by the typical characteristics of the majority negative class instances.

The number of subsets formed is determined by the IM of our dataset. For example, in Fig. 6 [39], the negative class contains five times as many instances as the positive class. Hence, the original unbalanced training dataset (DB) is split into five smaller balanced subsets, further referred to as "balanced bags" (BB). During this splitting process we ensure that we do not discard any instances from either of the classes. In other words, $\cap_{i=1}^{5} BB \neq \emptyset$ and $\cup_{i=1}^{5} BB = DB$. For example, if the imbalance level in the dataset is N, then we create N (N > 1) balanced training sets, BB. If we have M (M > 1) base learning methods, we train T = N × M base learners in the first layer of the ensemble [39]. Thus, instead of creating an ensemble of just N diverse models or just M diverse models as discussed in Sect. 2.6), our proposed TELS-D strategy creates a collection of T diverse models.

TELS-D Advantage. The advantage of TELS-D approach is that we generate more diversity in the ensemble while balancing the class distribution [39]. Given the diversity of the base learners, the importance of which is explained in Sect. 2.6, we anticipate each of the T base classifiers makes different errors on different data instances. We then combine the results from these T diverse base learners to form an input for the second layer stacking meta-algorithm [39]. As such, the meta-learner has the opportunity to learn the patterns required to predict the correct class, thereby reducing the total error.

2.9   Evaluation Metrics

We adapt the evaluation criteria commonly used for evaluating classification methods to apply to the token-granularity level: Precision (Eq. 2) and Recall (Eq. 3). Since we desire to achieve both high precision and high recall, we additionally consider the *F1-score* (Eq. 4).

$$Precision\ (P) = \frac{\#\ Correctly\ predicted\ positive\ tokens}{\#Total\ predicted\ positive\ tokens} \tag{2}$$

$$Recall\ (R) = \frac{\#\ Correctly\ predicted\ positive\ tokens}{\#\ Total\ real\ positive\ tokens} \tag{3}$$

$$F-measure\ (F1) = \frac{2(P\ x\ R)}{(P\ +\ R)} \tag{4}$$

3   Results

3.1   Experimental Setup

Data Sets. In this study, we have leveraged the annotated patient discharge summaries from i2b2 as discussed in Sect. 2.1 to build and evaluate our classification approaches. This dataset has been augmented with ground truth labels which are mandatory for supervised machine learning strategies.

We implement a holdout test set approach with a 90/10 split. The 242 reports we use from the i2b2 corpus, as described in Table 1, are split accordingly. 90% (217) of the reports are randomly selected for training and building our proposed model. The remaining 10% (25) reports are used as the holdout for the subsequent testing so that we can evaluate the effectiveness of our methods. In this section, we discuss our empirical results of our methodology on this holdout test set from the i2b2 corpus.

In addition to these i2b2 discharge summaries, we have access to 16 redacted FAERS reports, also described in Table 1. We use these FAERS reports as a second test set. However, these reports are not annotated so we lack the ground truth labels present in the i2b2 corpus. As such, we manually evaluate of the results of our methodology on the FAERS reports and present a case study as part of the discussion of the results.

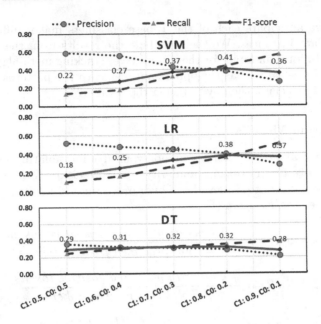

Fig. 7. Grid search results for balancing *Reason* class weight in *i2b2* dataset [39].

Parameter Tuning. Base learners, such as SVM and LR, must first have their parameters tuned. For SVM, we selected a linear kernel function. In LR, the *c-value* parameter controls the trade off between model complexity and misclassified instances. We obtained a *c-value* of 1.0 after performing 10-fold cross-validation with *c-values* ∈ {0.001, 0.01, 0.1, 1, 10} [21]. The decision tree parameters we use include *best* split at each node strategy with *gini* impurity measure to determine the quality of the split [32].

In order to select the optimal class_weight setting, we use 10-fold cross-validation to perform a systematic grid search with a set of class weights for each class. The effect of balancing different *class_weight* values on the individual learning methods – SVM, LR, and DT from Sect. 2.5 – is depicted in Fig. 7 [39]. C1 denotes the weight for the *reason* class and C0 denotes the weight for the *non-reason* class. We observe that for all of the base learners, the precision and recall correspond with a higher F1-score at the *class weight* setting of {C1 : 0.8, C0 : 0.2}. Thus, we set the weight for the class *reason* to 0.8 and the weight for the class *non-reason* to 0.2 for all further experiments where we balance the class within the learning methods.

Experiments. In Sects. 3.2–3.6, we conduct experiments to explore the effectiveness of different strategies in tackling the class imbalance problem. These experiments involve: (1) Unbalanced class distributions, (2) Balancing with class weights, (3) Balancing with class instances, (4) Balancing with classifier ensembles, and (5) Balancing with TELS-D. We compare these approaches in Sect. 3.7

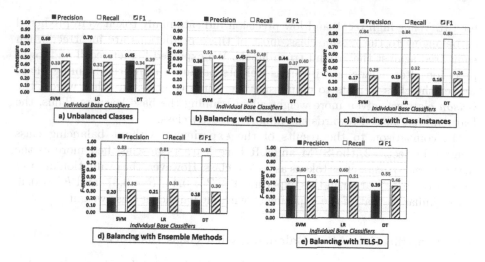

Fig. 8. The precision, recall, and F1-score of different classification strategies [39].

before proceeding to implement TELS-D on the i2b2 discharge summaries and the FAERS narratives.

3.2 Classification with Unbalanced Class Distribution

We conduct this experiment to obtain a baseline to compare the different approaches explained in Sect. 2.7. The individual base learners are trained on the original training set (DB) without balancing the class weights or instances. In Fig. 8(a) shows the effect of a skewed class distribution [39].

The precision P is much higher than the recall R for all base learners in the results of this experiment. This is especially true for SVM (P:0.68/R:0.33) and LR ($P = 0.70/R = 0.31$). High precision and low recall implies that while very few tokens were predicted as belonging to *reason* class, most of these predictions are correct when compared against ground truth labels. This result is expected due to the class imbalance in the training data as the large majority of the tokens were in the *non-reason* class. Thus, when the class imbalance problem is not rectified, the base classifiers are biased towards the *non-reason* class and tend to misclassify many of tokens in the minority *reason* class.

3.3 Classification After Balancing with Class Weights

The purpose of this experiment is to evaluate the effectiveness of balancing class weights as a strategy for addressing the data imbalance problem. The *class weight* parameter is set to $\{C1 : 0.8, C0 : 0.2\}$ for the individual base learners, as discussed in Sect. 3.1. We train the base learners on the original training set (DB). The results are seen in Fig. 8(b)[39].

In this experiment, the recall R is now higher than the precision P for two of the base learners. Specifically, (P:0.38/R:0.51) for SVM and (P:0.45/R:0.53) for LR. While high recall and low precision indicate many token were predicted as belonging to the *reason* class, most of these predictions are incorrect when compared against the ground truth labels. We expected higher recall and lower precision after balancing with class weights because during the training phase we set the class weights to emphasize the minority class. In other words, the *reason* class was given more weight when training the base learners. Thus, the learners were biased towards the minority *reason* class.

In comparison to the results of the experiment without balancing class weights in Sect. 3.2, the SVM and LR base learners misclassified more of the majority *non-reason* class tokens as *reason* class. However, the evaluation metrics for the DT base learner in this experiment – $P = 0.44$, $R = 0.37$, and $F1 = 0.40$ – are similar to that of the experiment without balancing class weights.

3.4   Classification After Balancing with Class Instances

In this experiment, we evaluate the effect of balancing class instances rather than class weights to handle the class imbalance problem. We achieve balanced classes by performing random under-sampling on the original training dataset (DB). This creates a single balanced subset of the training data with an equal number of positive *reason* and negative *non-reason* class instances.

Figure 8(c) shows the results of using this balanced subset to train the base learners. The recall R is much higher than precision P for all base learners: (P:0.17/R:0.84) for SVM, (P:0.19/R:0.84) for LR, and (P:0.16/R:0.83) for DT. In fact, the precision is much lower and the recall much higher than in the previous two experiments.

The low precision in this experiment indicates that most of the tokens were predicted as belonging to the *reason* class, although the majority of these tokens actually belong to the *non-reason* class. This also explains the very high recall. During under-sampling only a random subset of negative *non-reason* tokens were included in the balanced subset. As such, our training subset does not include many potentially informative instances important for learning the classes. In this scenario, the base learners would be unable learn the predominant characteristics of the negative class well explaining why these instances are often misclassified.

3.5   Classification After Balancing with Classifier Ensembles

This next experiment evaluates the effect of balancing with ensemble of homogeneous classifiers to address the class imbalance problem. We balance with Ensemble of Homogeneous Classifiers by performing Under-Bagging strategy on the original training dataset (DB). This creates multiple under-sampled subsets of the training data as mentioned in Sect. 2.7. Then we train each base learner on all of these subsets and combine their predictions with Majority Voting.

Similar to the experiment where we balanced the class instances (Sect. 3.4), the recall R is much higher than the precision P for all base learners. As seen in Fig. 8(d) [39], the results for SVM are (P:0.20/R:0.83), LR are (P:0.21/R:0.81)

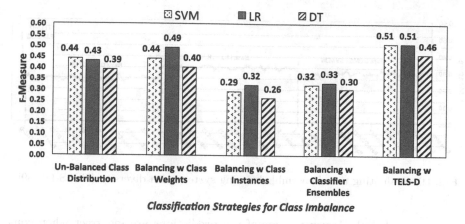

Fig. 9. Comparison of classification strategies for class imbalance [39].

and DT are (P:0.18/R:0.81) in this experiment. As ensemble of classifiers approach uses multiple balanced subsets, it does not eliminate potentially important negative class instances which was the limitation encountered when balancing the class instances in Sect. 3.4.

Unfortunately, the effectiveness of balancing with ensemble of classifiers relies on well performing base classifiers. As we see in Fig. 8(c), the precision of the base learners on a single balanced subset is very low. The Under-Bagging approach in this experiment uses majority voting to aggregate the results obtained from training the base classifiers on multiple subsets. Thus, while we rely on the majority vote of N classifiers, the ensemble of classifiers strategy is unable to overcome the erroneous predictions of the individuals classifiers.

3.6 Classification After Balancing with TELS-D

Our proposed approach TELS-D is a multi-layer framework, discussed in Sect. 2.8. The first layer in TELS-D creates a balanced learning environment to handle class imbalance in the training dataset [39].

As such, this experiment evaluates effectiveness of the first layer in TELS-D in comparison to the other balancing strategies. Balancing in TELS-D is achieved by creating multiple balanced subsets (BB) of the original training data (DB). The number of subsets is based on the imbalanced level (IM) in the training set. We train each base learner on the balanced subsets (BB). We combine these trained learners with Stacking using another meta-algorithm, namely, logistic regression. In contrast to Under-Bagging which uses simple majority voting, TELS-D employs stacking method to combine the results from the base learners and make the final predictions (Fig. 8(e)) [39].

In the TELS-D balancing experiment, the recall R is only a little higher than precision P for all base learners. Specifically, the results – SVM (P:0.45/R:0.60), LR (P:0.44/R:0.60), and DT (P:0.39/R:0.55) – indicate many of the tokens were

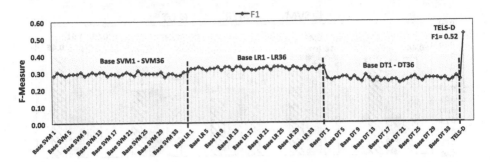

Fig. 10. Evaluating tiered ensemble learning system with diversity (TELS-D) [39].

correctly predicted. However, some of the predictions are incorrect when compared against the ground truth labels due to the small learning bias towards the minority *reason* class. This bias is expected because since we give priority to learning the minority *reason* class during the training phase by training on multiple subsets that have the same minority instances.

3.7   Comparing Classification Strategies for Class Imbalance

In Sects. 3.2–3.6 we conduct experiments to learn the effectiveness of different approaches for dealing with class imbalance. We compare the experimental results of these approaches on the base learners using the F1-score evaluation metric. F1-score, Eq. 4, gives a weighted average of the precision and recall scores. The F1-score can range from 0 to 1 where 1 indicates perfect precision and recall. As such, an increase in the F1-score indicates an equilibrium point where the base learners correctly classify more instances and thereby reduce the number of incorrectly classify instances.

Figure 9 [39] shows the F1-score of the experimental results on each of the base learners. The F1-scores for classifying after balancing with class instancing and after balancing with classifier ensembles are much lower than F1-scores of the other experiments due to the extreme differences in the values of precision and recall. We can see in Fig. 9 [39] that our proposed **TELS-D** approach is the most effective solution for the class imbalance problem. The TELS-D F1-scores for all three base learners – 0.51 for SVM, 0.51 for LR, and 0.46 for DT – are higher than the F1-score for the other approaches.

3.8   Analysis of TELS-D Results on i2b2 Discharge Summaries

The second layer in TELS-D is designed to create and combine an ensemble of heterogeneous classifiers with the goal to improve the accuracy over the individual base learners as discussed in Sect. 2.8. The second layer of TELS-D is built on the output from the first layer, the base learners trained over all balanced subsets. The predictions of these trained base learners are combined with Stacking using a meta-algorithm, in this case, Logistic Regression.

Table 2. Examples of Reason class labels predicted by TELS-D.

Example	Sentence from the Narrative	True Positive (TP)	False Positive (FP)	False Negative (FN)
1)	The patient was treated with canagliflozin for type 2 diabetes and domperidone for diabetic gastroparesis	type, diabetes, diabetic, gastroparesis		2
2)	The patient had previously experienced allergy when taking mycins (antibacterials for systemic use)	systemic		use
3)	Concurrent conditions [abdominal] [pain], [diabetic] paresis.		abdominal, pain, diabetic	
4)	The patient was restarted on Coumadin for known paroxysmal atrial fibrillation.	known, paroxysmal, atrial, fibrillation		
5)	She was continued on Celexa for depression.	depression		
6)	She was continued on her Cymbalta , which was for her history of depression	depression		
7)	Given her history of atrial fibrillation as well as depressed ejection fraction , she was restarted on Coumadin.	atrial, fibrillation		depressed, ejection, fraction
8)	This pain was well controlled with the combination of Dilaudid and oxycodone.	pain		
9)	Lactulose and Colace to prevent constipation while taking narcotics.	constipation		
10)	He received aspirin and Zocor for coronary artery disease related event prophylaxis.	coronary, artery, prophylaxis		disease, related, event
11)	Blood pressure was controlled with isosorbide dinitrate, Norvasc, lisinopril, and Lopressor.	pressure		Blood
12)	[Prophylaxis]: He was initially treated with Lovenox 40 mg sub-Q. q. day for a prophylaxis against DVTs.	prophylaxis, against, DVTs	Prophylaxis	
13)	Hypercholesterolemia: He was continued on his Zocor throughout the hospitalization.			Hypercholesterolemia
14)	The patient's [pain] in her left hand existed and she was treated with tramadol and Tylenol for this pain.	pain	pain	
15)	The [hyperkalemia] resolved		hyperkalemia	

Figure 10 shows F1-score of: (1) Individual base classifiers generated by training the three base learners on all balanced subsets, (2) Ensemble combined with majority voting (for comparison only) and, (3) Ensemble combined with Stacking [39]. The F1-scores of individual base classifiers range from 0.28–0.33 and the F1-scores for Ensemble with Majority voting is 0.22. This is in stark contrast to the F1-score of the ensemble with stacking, which is 0.52. TELS-D performed much better than any of the other classifiers.

This application demonstrates the impressive ability of an ensemble learning system that leverages a learning-over-learners combiner called meta-algorithm in the final step. The meta-algorithm learns from the errors generated by the base classifiers to output the correct result [39]. Majority voting, in contrast, performs poorly since simply counting votes only combines the errors of the base classifiers and thus makes the final result more erroneous. As such, TELS-D is preferred for this biomedical Named Entity Recognition task.

We compared our results from TELS-D with an existing study [10] conducted on the same i2b2 test dataset. The study demonstrated with MedEx only and SVM-based NER including MedEx [10]. The results showed that for recognizing the *reason* entity from the narratives, the rule-based MedEx system achieved a F1-score of 0.43 while the SVM combined with MedEx achieved 0.48. Our results from TELS-D approach show an improvement over both MedEx and SVM including MedEx with the F1-score of 0.52 [39]. Examples 4–15 in Table 2 demonstrate the ability of TELS-D on sample sentences from the i2b2 corpus.

3.9   Analysis of TELS-D Results on FAERS Narratives

Due to lack of ground truth labels for the FAERS reports, we manually evaluated the TELS-D predictions on some of the redacted FAERS reports. We analyze errors on these FAERS narratives below with references to examples in Table 2.

- **True Positives:** True Positives (TP) are token correctly predicted as belonging to the *reason* class. For instance, in the first two examples in Table 2, all tokens predicted to be a *reason* did indeed belong to the reason class. Notice that the many of the ground truth labeled words in these sentences are purely medical text with a certain sentence structure.
- **False Positives:** False positives (FP) – tokens incorrectly predicted as belonging to the *reason* class – mostly occurred when the token was not associated with a medication and therefore by definition not a *reason*. For instance, in example 3 the medical text was not associated with a medication name, leading to the incorrectly predicted tokens. Such cases remain challenging to classify, indicating a need for additional feature engineering.
- **False Negatives:** Our evaluation showed that false negatives (FN), the tokens incorrectly predicted as the *non-reason* class, occurred primarily due to mixtures of medical and non-medical words. These FN tokens tend to be embedded or part of TP tokens. Note, in examples 1 and 2, the words "2" and "use" are commonly present in regular text.

4   Discussion

4.1   Lack of Annotated FAERS Narratives

To be published, FAERS narratives must be redacted due to privacy concerns. Report redaction requires massive amount of cautious effort to ensure no private information remains the text. Since the redaction process demands perfect *recall* and utmost *precision*, any automation of this task still involves significant manual intervention. As such, it is challenging to create a large corpus of redacted FAERS narratives.

In addition, annotating FAERS narratives requires reviewers with deep domain knowledge and annotating experience. Machine learning models deployed for FAERS NER must be trained on a large dataset of annotated FAERS narratives. This annotating must be completed by the FDA's safety reviewers whose annotating strategy reflects specific annotation guidelines. Due to limited resources, this annotating would be a monumental task requiring significant time and effort.

Given the aforementioned challenges, at this time there exists no publishable FAERS reports annotated by FDA staff to be used for training and testing purposes. Thus, to prove the concept and ensure the reproducibility of this study, we trained our model and evaluated our methodology using a public benchmark dataset, namely, the i2b2 2009 discharge summaries. We also tested the trained model on a small sample of redacted FAERS narratives. Since discharge summaries do not necessarily share the same vocabulary as the FAERS narratives, we expect this change of datasets to be reflected in the results.

4.2   Practical Application of This Research for the FDA

The FDA recognizes automatic identification of high value information from biomedical text as a key step for the future of its regulatory and supervisory tasks. As such, the FDA has been partnering with research instustite and technology companies to develop text mining and natural language processing tools customized for the various types of biomedical text collected by the FDA. These texts include the vaccine ADR reports (VAERS) as well as the FAERS narratives.

Due to the distinct nature of these texts, the tools and methodologies must be highly customized to handle particular text types. Additionally, in comparison to the other biomedical texts, the FAERS narratives have a relatively complex structure in terms of size, vocabulary, and writing style. Thus, to cope with the complexity of the FAERS narratives, we propose a machine learning framework that combines a selection of internally available tools to extract entities in an ensemble fashion. These extracted results can then be utilized by advanced data mining or visualization techniques to enhance the drug review process [39].

Availability of reliable drug safety information from accredited sources such as FAERS will certainly aid health-care practitioners and consumers in making informed therapeutic decisions while prescribing or using drugs and thus lead to a cutback in the recurrence of AEs. Most of the time, FAERS report narratives provide a 360° view of the AE with patient personal experiences. Case examples may serve as useful teaching tools for improving the safe use of medicines. Information that includes patients' subjective experiences of adverse reactions would be most useful to patients and to prescribers of medicines. FAERS reports are reviewed for similar adverse events occurring with a particular drug, adverse reaction, indication or a specific age group. Often medications listed within the FAERS narratives are associated with indications (reasons) for its use and/or its side effects or ADRs. For example, the reviewers might want to find out "What indications for use are frequently reported on?" or "reports where a specific indication for use (such as hypertension) was mentioned?".

In this work we discussed the importance of using machine learning especially an ensemble learning approach to automatically recognize and extract information on indications (*reasons*) from the medical narratives. If such information can be easily detected, thereby cutting down the time-consuming and in-efficient manual review process, has the potential to aid in effective post marketing drug surveillance.

5   Conclusions

In this paper, we describe $\underline{T}$iered $\underline{E}$nsemble $\underline{L}$earning $\underline{S}$ystem with $\underline{D}$iversity (TELS-D), a novel approach for biomedical named entity recognition (NER) from Adverse Event Reports. To solve this crucial NER task, TELS-D leverages an ensemble of diverse heterogeneous classification models to recognize named entities in text. Simultaneously, our proposed approach handles the critical problem of skewed class distribution of the named entities in the training datasets compared to normal words.

When applied to biomedical reports to extract the *reason* entity, TELS-D outperformed simple majority voting based solutions by 0.3 in F1-score. These promising results indicate that an ensemble approach would be a better choice for NER in the context of binary classification. In particular, our results support that an ensemble approach is especially useful for NER tasks involving datasets with a class imbalance.

References

1. Alpaydin, E.: Introduction to Machine Learning. MIT Press, Cambridge (2014)
2. Aronson, A.R.: Effective mapping of biomedical text to the UMLS Metathesaurus: the MetaMap program. In: Proceedings of the AMIA Symposium, p. 17. AMIA (2001)
3. Barandela, R., Valdovinos, R.M., Sánchez, J.S.: New applications of ensembles of classifiers. Pattern Anal. Appl. **6**(3), 245–256 (2003)
4. Bird, S., et al.: Natural Language Processing with Python: Analyzing Text with the Natural Language Toolkit. O'Reilly Media Inc., Sebastopol (2009)
5. Bishop, C.M.: Pattern Recognition and Machine Learning. Springer, Heidelberg (2006)
6. Błaszczyński, J., Stefanowski, J., Idkowiak, Ł.: Extending bagging for imbalanced data. In: Burduk, R., Jackowski, K., Kurzynski, M., Wozniak, M., Zolnierek, A. (eds.) Proceedings of the 8th International Conference on Computer Recognition Systems CORES 2013. Advances in Intelligent Systems and Computing, vol. 226, pp. 269–278. Springer, Heidelberg (2013). https://doi.org/10.1007/978-3-319-00969-8_26

7. Breiman, L.: Bagging predictors. Mach. Learn. **24**(2), 123–140 (1996)
8. Charniak, E., Johnson, M.: Coarse-to-fine n-best parsing and MaxEnt discriminative reranking. In: Proceedings of the 43rd Annual Meeting on ACL, pp. 173–180. ACL (2005)
9. Chawla, N.V.: Data mining for imbalanced datasets: An overview. In: Maimon, O., Rokach, L. (eds.) Data Mining and Knowledge Discovery Handbook, pp. 875–886. Springer, Boston (2009). https://doi.org/10.1007/978-0-387-09823-4_45
10. Doan, S., Xu, H.: Recognizing medication related entities in hospital discharge summaries using support vector machine. In: Proceedings of the 23rd International Conference on Computational Linguistics: Posters, pp. 259–266. ACL (2010)
11. FDA: FAERS (FDA adverse event reporting system) (2016)
12. Feng, X., et al.: Assessing pancreatic cancer risk associated with dipeptidyl peptidase 4 inhibitors: data mining of FDA adverse event reporting system (FAERS). J. Pharmacovigilance **1**, 1–7 (2013)
13. Ferrucci, D., Lally, A.: UIMA: an architectural approach to unstructured information processing in the corporate research environment. Nat. Lang. Eng. **10**(3–4), 327–348 (2004)
14. Friedman, C., Alderson, P.O., Austin, J.H., Cimino, J.J., Johnson, S.B.: A general natural-language text processor for clinical radiology. JAMIA **1**(2), 161–174 (1994)
15. Galar, M., Fernandez, A., Barrenechea, E., Bustince, H., Herrera, F.: A review on ensembles for the class imbalance problem: bagging-, boosting-, and hybrid-based approaches. IEEE Trans. Syst. Man Cybern. Part C (Appl. Rev.) **42**(4), 463–484 (2012)
16. Ghiasvand, O.: Disease name extraction from clinical text using conditional random fields. Ph.D. thesis, The University of Wisconsin-Milwaukee (2014)
17. Halgrim, S.R., Xia, F., Solti, I., Cadag, E., Uzuner, Ö.: A cascade of classifiers for extracting medication information from discharge summaries. J. Biomed. Semant. **2**(3), S2 (2011)
18. Harpaz, R., et al.: Text mining for adverse drug events: the promise, challenges, and state of the art. Drug Saf. **37**(10), 777–790 (2014)
19. Jagannatha, A.N., Yu, H.: Bidirectional RNN for medical event detection in electronic health records. In: Proceedings of the conference. ACL. North American Chapter. Meeting, vol. 2016, p. 473. NIH Public Access (2016)
20. Japkowicz, N., Stephen, S.: The class imbalance problem: a systematic study. Intell. Data Anal. **6**(5), 429–449 (2002)
21. Kohavi, R., et al.: A study of cross-validation and bootstrap for accuracy estimation and model selection. In: Ijcai, Stanford, CA, vol. 14, pp. 1137–1145 (1995)
22. Kuhn, M., Letunic, I., Jensen, L.J., Bork, P.: The sider database of drugs and side effects. Nucleic Acids Res. **44**(D1), D1075–D1079 (2015)
23. Lazarou, J., Pomeranz, B.H., Corey, P.N.: Incidence of adverse drug reactions in hospitalized patients: a meta-analysis of prospective studies. JAMA **279**(15), 1200–1205 (1998)
24. Longadge, R., Dongre, S.: Class imbalance problem in data mining review. arXiv preprint arXiv:1305.1707 (2013)
25. Nguyen, H., Patrick, J.: Text mining in clinical domain: dealing with noise. In: KDD, pp. 549–558 (2016)
26. Polikar, R.: Ensemble learning. Scholarpedia **4**(1), 2776 (2009). https://doi.org/10.4249/scholarpedia.2776. revision #91224

27. Ramesh, B.P., Belknap, S.M., Li, Z., Frid, N., West, D.P., Yu, H.: Automatically recognizing medication and adverse event information from food and drug administration's adverse event reporting system narratives. JMIR Med. Inform. **2**(1), e10 (2014)

28. Sakaeda, T., Tamon, A., Kadoyama, K., Okuno, Y.: Data mining of the public version of the FDA adverse event reporting system. Int. J. Med. Sci. **10**(7), 796 (2013)

29. Savova, G.K., et al.: Mayo clinical Text Analysis and Knowledge Extraction System (cTAKES): architecture, component evaluation and applications. JAMIA **17**(5), 507–513 (2010)

30. Schapire, R.E.: The strength of weak learnability. Mach. Learn. **5**(2), 197–227 (1990)

31. Simpson, M.S., Demner-Fushman, D.: Biomedical text mining: a survey of recent progress. In: Aggarwal, C., Zhai, C. (eds.) Mining Text Data, pp. 465–517. Springer, Boston (2012). https://doi.org/10.1007/978-1-4614-3223-4_14

32. Tan, P.N., et al.: Introduction to Data Mining. Pearson Education India, New Delhi (2006)

33. Uzuner, Ö., Solti, I., Cadag, E.: Extracting medication information from clinical text. JAMIA **17**(5), 514–518 (2010)

34. Uzuner, Ö., Solti, I., Xia, F., Cadag, E.: Community annotation experiment for ground truth generation for the i2b2 medication challenge. JAMIA **17**(5), 519–523 (2010)

35. Uzuner, Ö., Zhang, X., Sibanda, T.: Machine learning and rule-based approaches to assertion classification. JAMIA **16**(1), 109–115 (2009)

36. Wang, S., Yao, X.: Diversity analysis on imbalanced data sets by using ensemble models. In: Proceedings of the IEEE Symposium on Computational Intelligence and Data Mining, CIDM, pp. 324–331 (2009)

37. Wilson, A.M., Thabane, L., Holbrook, A.: Application of data mining techniques in pharmacovigilance. BJCP **57**(2), 127–134 (2004)

38. Wolpert, D.H.: Stacked generalization. Neural Netw. **5**(2), 241–259 (1992)

39. Wunnava, S., et al.: One size does not fit all: an ensemble approach towards information extraction from adverse drug event narratives. In: Proceedings of the 11th International Joint Conference on Biomedical Engineering Systems and Technologies - Volume 5: HEALTHINF, pp. 176–188. INSTICC, SciTePress (2018). https://doi.org/10.5220/0006600201760188

40. Xu, H., Stenner, S.P., Doan, S., Johnson, K.B., Waitman, L.R., Denny, J.C.: MedEx: a medication information extraction system for clinical narratives. JAMIA **17**(1), 19–24 (2010)

Application of Sample Entropy of Pulse Waves in Identifying Characteristic Physiological Patterns of Parkinson's Disease Sufferers

Mayumi Oyama-Higa[1], Tokihiko Niwa[2], Fumitake Ou[3(✉)],
and Yoshifumi Kawanabe[4]

[1] Chaos Technology Research Laboratory,
5-26-5 Seta, Otsu, Shiga 520-2134, Japan
oyama00@gmail.com, mhiga@chaotech.org
[2] Kwansei Gakuin Senior High School, 1-155 Uegahara Ichibancho,
Nishinomiya, Hyogo 662-0891, Japan
niwa@kwansei.ac.jp
[3] PricewaterhouseCoopers Aarata LLC, 1-1-1 Otemachi,
Chiyoda-ku, Tokyo 100-0004, Japan
wangwb10@yahoo.co.jp
[4] Shizuoka General Hospital, 4-27-1 Kita Ando,
Aoi-ku, Shizuoka 420-8527, Japan
bwh5255725@yahoo.co.jp

Abstract. While there are plenty of studies on clinical diagnosis of Parkinson's disease, little literature is available on the possibility of simple tests that can help distinguish Parkinson's disease sufferers from healthy individuals. In our study, by making use of pulse wave data, we identify physiological patterns characteristic of Parkinson's disease patients. We observe that the sample entropy values of pulse waves, with certain parameters fixed, is statistically different between Parkinson's disease sufferers and healthy individuals. We also find significant difference between the two groups in values of the largest Lyapunov exponent computed from the same pulse wave data. In addition, we introduce an Android tablet that in which the real-time measurement and analysis functions are incorporated. With this device, it takes only 5 s to produce a test result.

Keywords: Parkinson's disease · Sample entropy ·
Border of Parkinson Entropy (BPE) · Largest Lyapunov Exponent (LLE) ·
Android tablet for real-time health check

1 Introduction

1.1 Background and Clinical Diagnosis of Parkinson's Disease

Japan has a rapidly aging population: as of October 1, 2015, the population aged 65 and over has reached about 34 million, accounting for nearly 1/3 of the total population, and this percentage has kept rising since 1950 and is expected to increase in the future [1]. As a result, incidence of various aging-related diseases is becoming increasingly frequent. Parkinson's disease is one of them [24].

© Springer Nature Switzerland AG 2019
A. Cliquet jr. et al. (Eds.): BIOSTEC 2018, CCIS 1024, pp. 447–463, 2019.
https://doi.org/10.1007/978-3-030-29196-9_23

Parkinson's disease is caused by the disruption of dopaminergic neurotransmission in the basal ganglia [9]. Concerning the clinical diagnosis, assessment is generally based on the patient's motor features - Tremor at rest, Rigidity, Akinesia (or bradykinesia) and Postural instability, under the well-known acronym "TRAP" as four primary symptoms [5].

In Japan, following a medical interview and a neurological examination, the potential patient will often receive an image inspection, and it is common to use a SPECT (single-photon emission computed tomography) gamma scanner to directly observe the amount of dopaminergic neurons in the subject's brain. As the following figure shows, a Parkinson's disease patient has significantly less amount of dopaminergic neurons than a healthy individual (Nishi-Niigata Chuo National Hospital [8]) (Fig. 1).

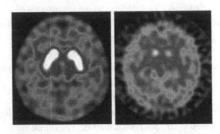

Fig. 1. SPECT images of dopaminergic neurons of a healthy individual (left) and a Parkinson's patient (right).

1.2   Possibility of a Simple Test Using Pulse Waves

The SPECT imaging is widely applied in Japan's hospitals in diagnosing Parkinson's disease, but for the patients, the SPECT scan procedure seems not a comfortable experience. Injection of gamma-emitting radioisotope (RI) is required. After the injection, the patient normally has to wait 3 to 6 h in order for the RI to take effect in the brain. Then, the SPECT scan itself needs approximately 30 min to complete (Nihon Medi-Physics Co., Ltd. [7]). In addition, such inspection is relatively expensive: an insured patient under 70 years old (the applicable coinsurance rate is 30%) has to pay about 25,000 JPY (about 200 EUR under the exchange rate 1 EUR = 125.44 JPY).

It would be beneficial for the potential patients if a simple – less time-consuming and expensive – test can help distinguish Parkinson's disease sufferers from healthy individuals. However, little literature, if any, is available on this subject.

Studies have shown that non-motor symptoms are also common in Parkinson's disease. Two categories of these symptoms are autonomic dysfunction [25] and cognitive and neurobehavioural abnormalities. The latter includes depression [6] and dementia [2].

Meanwhile, in our recent studies, we have discovered indicators – the largest Lyapunov exponent (LLE) and the autonomic nerve balance (ANB), both computed from pulse wave data – for identifying mental status changes [13, 23] and mental disorders, including dementia [11, 13, 17] and depression [4, 13, 18]. A comprehensive explanation is available in Oyama's 2012 book [10] and a review article [15].

Inspired by the relevance of Parkinson's disease to mental disorders and the effectiveness of the pulse wave analysis in detecting mental disorders, we have made an attempt to observe if any characteristic patterns of Parkinson's disease sufferers exist in their pulse waves.

This study has succeeded in discovering such characteristic patterns, by comparing the sample entropy computed from the pulse wave data. More precisely, what we applied is the sample entropy with two parameters – the length of subsequences of the data sequence and the tolerance – set to certain fixed values. We define this indicator as "border of Parkinson Entropy (BPE)". Besides, in addition to BPE, statistically significant difference is also in the LLE values from the same pulse wave data.

Furthermore, we have incorporated the function of BPE computation and result display into "Alys", an application installed on an Android tablet that we developed for real-time mental health check-up [16]. With "Alys", not only status of mental health, but also risk of Parkinson's disease can be checked in a convenient and economical way. In particular, it takes only 5 s to show the test result on the screen.

2 Computational Methods

In this study, we mainly propose two indicators – the border of Parkinson entropy (BPE) and the largest Lyapunov exponent (LLE). We begin with the introduction of sample entropy.

2.1 Sample Entropy

As a conventional method for studying the complexity in biological time series, the sample entropy is defined as the opposite of the natural logarithm of the conditional probability that two sequences that are similar for certain points within a given tolerance still remain similar when one consecutive point is included [19].

To begin with, given a time-series sequence

$$\{x(1), \ldots, x(N)\}, \tag{1}$$

its subsequence with a length of m can form a vector

$$X_m(i) = (x(i), x(i+1), \ldots, x(i+m-1)) \tag{2}$$

and, in the same fashion, an (m + 1) subsequence can be denoted as

$$X_{m+1}(i) = (x(i), x(i+1), \ldots, x(i+m)). \tag{3}$$

Here, the range of i is from 1 to $N - m$ so that both (2) and (3) are well-defined. Next, the distance between two m-long subsequences $X_m(i)$ and $X_m(j)$ is defined as

$$|X_m(i) - X_m(j)| = \max_{0 \leq k \leq m-1} |x(i+k) - x(j+k)| \tag{4}$$

For a given $X_m(i)$, its r-neighbourhood is

$$\{X_m(j) : |X_m(i) - X_m(j)| < r\} \tag{5}$$

Let $B_i^m(r)$ denote the probability that another subsequence is in its r-neighbourhood. Thus,

$$B_i^m(r) = \frac{\#\{X_m(j) : |X_m(i) - X_m(j)| < r, 1 \leq j \leq N - m, j \neq i\}}{N - m - 1} \qquad (6)$$

Note that when counting the number of such subsequences in the numerator of (6), since $X_m(i)$ itself should be excluded, there are a total of $N - m - 1$ candidates. Hence the denominator $N - m - 1$. Regarding $X_{m+1}(i)$, we use a different notation $A_i^m(r)$ to denote the probability that another $(m + 1)$-long subsequence is in its r-neighbourhood:

$$A_i^m(r) = \frac{\#\{X_{m+1}(j) : |X_{m+1}(i) - X_{m+1}(j)| < r, 1 \leq j \leq N - m, j \neq i\}}{N - m - 1} \qquad (7)$$

For the whole time-series sequence (1), the probability corresponding to (6) or (7) can be given as an average taken over all subsequences, from $i = 1$ to $i = N - m$, as follows.

$$B^m(r) = \frac{1}{N - m} \sum_{i=1}^{N-m} B_i^m(r) \qquad (8)$$

$$A^m(r) = \frac{1}{N - m} \sum_{i=1}^{N-m} A_i^m(r) \qquad (9)$$

with tolerance r for m-long subsequences of an N-point time-series sequence is therefore computed by the following formula.

$$SampEn(m, r, N) = -\ln \frac{A^m(r)}{B^m(r)} \qquad (10)$$

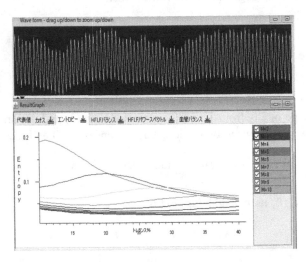

Fig. 2. Display of sample entropy with "Lyspect".

In our recent studies on the indication of mental health from pulse waves, the device "Lyspect" (developed by Chaos Technology Research Laboratory) has been frequently applied [12]. We have upgraded the device to make the computation of sample entropy possible. The following shows the value of sample entropy (vertical axis) as a function of the tolerance r (horizontal axis), with the length of subsequence m fixed. A total of 9 graphs are displayed, for $m = 2$ to 10 (Fig. 2).

2.2 Border of Parkinson Entropy

We define the border of Parkinson entropy (BPE) as the sample entropy with $m = 2$ and $r = 10\%$, namely,

$$BPE = SampEn(2, 10\%) \tag{11}$$

(The length of the time series sequence, N, is dropped for convenience.) These two parameters were decided this way after trials and errors in search for an ideal indicator that shows statistically significant difference between Parkinson's disease sufferers and healthy individuals. This will be explained in Sect. 4.1.

As mentioned at the end of Sect. 1, we have imbedded the function of BPE computation in our device "Alys". A normalized result display, in a range of 0–10, is applied with a semi-circular graph, in consistency with the display of largest Lyapunov exponent and autonomic nerve balance. We will introduce this new performance in Sect. 5.

2.3 Largest Lyapunov Exponent

The mathematical definition and computation of the largest Lyapunov exponent (LLE) is elaborated in almost each of our papers on the indication of mental health from pulse waves (for the most updated work, refer to [16] and [15]). In this article, although we mainly study the BPE, we still examine whether a relevant result holds from the viewpoint of the LLE behaviour. The following is a brief explanation on the definition and computational method of the LLE.

Consider the same time-series sequence (1). If we let τ denote a constant delay and d be the embedding dimension, then the phase space can be reconstructed with vectors represented as

$$\begin{aligned} X(i) &= (x(i), x(i - \tau), \ldots, x(i - (d - 1)\tau)) \\ &= \{x_k(i)\}_{k=1,\ldots,d} \end{aligned} \tag{12}$$

where

$$x_k(i) = x(i - (k - 1)\tau), k = 1, \ldots, d. \tag{13}$$

Regarding the fingertip pulse waves, the optimal choices for the constant delay and the embedding dimension are determined from the autocorrelation coefficient of the wave [21, 22]:

$$\tau = 50\,\mathrm{ms} \tag{14}$$

and

$$d = 4. \tag{15}$$

Then the LLE is defined by the following formula.

$$LLE = \lim_{t \to \infty} \lim_{\epsilon \to 0} \frac{1}{t} \log \frac{|\delta X_\epsilon(t)|}{|\epsilon|} \tag{16}$$

where

$$\delta X_\epsilon(t) = X(t) - X_\epsilon(t) \tag{17}$$

represents the divergence of the trajectories, with initial condition of

$$\epsilon = X(0) - X_\epsilon(0) \tag{18}$$

In our studies, the method proposed by [20] is applied for estimating the LLE.

In our devices "Lyspect" [12] and "Alys" [16], the value of LLE is normalized to a range of 0–10 in the result display.

Our previous studies have shown important results concerning the LLE as a mental health indicator. The values of LLE of a mentally healthy individual fluctuate from 2 to 7, centred at 5. When LLE is abnormally high, the mental immunity of the individual is so strong that he or she is likely to go to extremes: such individual can be easily irritated and take unexpected actions. On the other hand, when it is abnormally low, the mental immunity is so weak that the individual is prone to mental illnesses. In other words, a high LLE indicates a mental status of adapting to the external environment (we simply called it "external adaptation" in some of our previous articles), while a low LLE indicates a status of "internal focusing".

2.4   Autonomic Nerve Balance

The autonomic nerve balance (ANB) is another important indicator in our recent studies [16] and [15].

We consider the high frequency (HF, 0.15–0.40 Hz) component and the low frequency (LF, 0.04–0.15 Hz) component, which represents parasympathetic nerve activity and sympathetic nerve activity, respectively. Then, we define the autonomic nerve balance (ANB) as a normalized index ranging from 0 to 10 as follows.

$$ANB = 10\,B/3.5, \tag{19}$$

where

$$B = \ln(LF) / \ln(HF). \tag{20}$$

From the ranges of LF and HF, we can clearly observe that B ranges from 1, when both LF and HF take the value 0.15, to approximately 3.5, when LF reaches its minimum while HF is at its maximum. Therefore, ANB goes from approximately 2.86 to 10.

In our devices, like LLE, we apply a 0–10 valued graph to display the result of ANB. $ANB < 5$ indicates predominance of parasympathetic nerve while $ANB > 5$ indicates sympathetic predominance.

The computation method has also been embedded in the devices "Lyspect" and "Alys", and it has been registered as a U.S. patent [3].

3   Experiment

3.1   Devices

We apply an infrared sensor (UBIX Corporation) to take in pulse waves from the subjects, and computer software "Lyspect" (Chaos Technology Research Laboratory) to analyse the data.

The pulse waves are taken in as 200 Hz analogue data, saved as text file, and then input to "Lyspect" for analysis. To reduce noise from the external environment (such as the power supply), the fast Fourier transform is applied in order that only data with frequency less than 30 Hz (It has been shown by additional trials that 8 Hz will suffice to produce the same analytical results) is to be analysed.

3.2   Subjects

Two groups of subjects, the Parkinson's disease patients and healthy individuals, are studied.

The former group consists of 45 patients diagnosed as Parkinson's disease, aged from 40 to 65. The latter group consists of 113 healthy university students, aged from 19 to 20.

3.3   Process of Measurement

Informed consent was obtained from all subjects in the measurement.

For each subject, a 2-min measurement was performed for 2 to 3 times in a relaxed condition at room temperature (25 °C) and the average result of measurement was used for analyse. Specifically, for the healthy students, it was sufficient to take 2 times because their results were stable, while for each of the Parkinson's disease sufferers, measurement was performed 3 times at intervals.

For a part of the Parkinson's disease sufferers, in order to reduce measurement errors due to tremor, a common symptom of the disease, the sensor was attached to the subject's earlobe instead of fingertip.

4 Analysis and Result

4.1 Comparison of Sample Entropy

As introduced at the end of Sect. 2.1, "Lyspect" can display the sample entropy values *SampEn* (m, r) as a function of r, for different m's. We observed that as m increases, the range of *SampEn* (m, r) tends to concentrate and less sensitive to r, so we decided to apply $m = 2$. In the following, *SampEn* $(2, r)$ is compared between the two groups.

The following graph shows *SampEn* $(2, r)$ for the group of 113 healthy individuals. We observe that when the tolerance r changes from a small value over 0 to a little more than 40%, the sample entropy value with $m = 2$ monotonically decreases and the range of *SampEn* $(2, r)$ is bounded in $(0, 0.4)$ for each subject of this group.

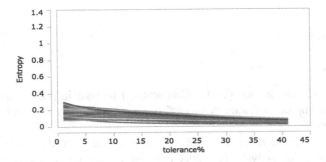

Fig. 3. Graph of *SampEn* $(2, r)$ for healthy individuals.

Similarly, *SampEn* $(2, r)$ for the group of Parkinson's disease suffers is shown in the following graph. The tolerance changes in the same way as the above. *SampEn* $(2, r)$ is monotonically decreasing, but the range of *SampEn* $(2, r)$ is remarkably wider than the healthy individuals' group.

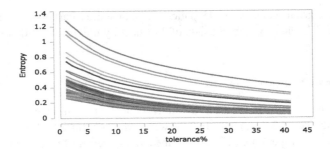

Fig. 4. Graph of *SampEn* $(2, r)$ for Parkinson's sufferers.

In hopes of finding an ideal indicator to distinguish Parkinson's disease sufferers from healthy individuals, based on the data from our measurement, we have performed analysis of variance (ANOVA) for various r's. Consequently, through trial and error, we found that when $r = 10\%$, the result of ANOVA shows highly statistically significant difference in *SampEn* (2, 10%) between Parkinson's disease sufferers and healthy individuals. The basic information of *SampEn* (2, 10%) values for the analysis are given in the following Table 1.

Table 1. SampEn (2, 10%) data information.

Group	Number of Data Points	Mean			Standard Deviation
		Total	w/o the largest 5%	w/o the smallest 5%	
Healthy	113	0.17267	0.14588	0.19945	0.01356
Parkinson's	45	0.44105	0.39861	0.48350	0.02149

The ANOVA for the difference in *SampEn* (2, 10%) between the two groups produces the following result (Table 2).

Table 2. ANOVA for the difference in *SampEn* (2, 10%).

Source	Degree of Freedom	Sum of Squares	Mean Sum of Squares	F statistic	p value
Regression	1	2.3181505	2.31815	111.5685	<.0001*
Residual	156	3.2413411	0.02078		
Total	157	5.5594916			

Since the p value is less than 0.0001, the *SampEn* (2, 10%) values between the two groups are statistically different at 0.01% significance level, or at 99.99% confidence level. This is why we call *SampEn* (2, 10%) border of Parkinson's entropy, or BPE. The distribution of BPE values for the two groups can also be compared in the following figure. One can clearly observe that the Parkinson's disease sufferers exhibit a significantly higher BPE than the healthy students.

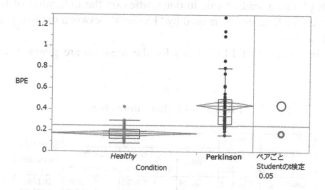

Fig. 5. Comparison of distribution of BPE values.

4.2   Sample Entropy and Progression of Parkinson's Disease

Another observation made is that the sample entropy value tends to increase as the Parkinson's disease sufferer deteriorates.

The following shows the status of *SampEn* (2, *r*) for a same Parkinson's disease sufferer on two different dates of measurement. On July 31, 2016, there was no particular problem reported, but after 3 months, on November 1, 2016, the patient reported difficulty to move and occurrence of drooling, which interfered the patient's daily life. We clearly observe that for each tolerance *r*, *SampEn* (2, *r*) (and thus BPE in particular) on the latter date is higher than that on the former date.

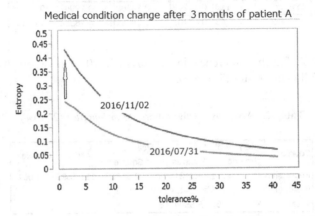

Fig. 6. Graph of *SampEn* (2, *r*) for a Parkinson's sufferer in different condition of disease progression.

Therefore, for a same patient, BPE may be a potential indicator for checking the progression of Parkinson's disease. Doctors may refer to the BPE value when they conduct medical examination by interview.

4.3   Comparison of LLE and ANB

Since LLE has played a leading role in our studies on the indication of mental health from pulse waves, LLE values computed by "Lyspect" between the two groups are also compared and analysed.

The basic information of LLE values for the analysis are given in the following Table 3.

Table 3. LLE data information.

Group	Number of Data Points	Mean			Standard Deviation
		Total	w/o the largest 5%	w/o the smallest 5%	
Healthy	113	4.52024	4.27080	4.76970	0.12627
Parkinson's	45	2.91475	2.51950	3.31000	0.20009

Recall from Sect. 2.3 that the LLE value is normalized to range from 0 to 10. Next, the result of ANOVA for the difference in LLE between the two groups is stated in the following Table 4.

Table 4. ANOVA for the difference in LLE.

Source	Degree of Freedom	Sum of Squares	Mean Sum of Squares	F statistic	p value
Regression	1	82.95642	82.9564	46.0469	<.0001*
Residual	156	281.04406	1.8016		
Total	157	364.00048			

Since the p value is less than 0.0001, the LLE values between the two groups are statistically different at 0.01% significance level, or at 99.99% confidence level. The following figure compares the distribution of LLE values between the two groups. Obviously, the LLE of the group of Parkinson's disease patients is significantly lower than that of the healthy individuals' group.

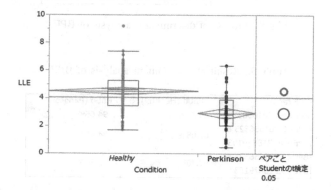

Fig. 7. Comparison of distribution of LLE values.

The above result is consistent with the fact that depression is a common symptom of Parkinson's disease [6] and the result we have obtained in our recent studies that a low LLE indicates weakness in mental immunity which leads to depression [10].

In addition, we have also looked over ANB computed from the same data. Like in BPE and LLE, we have obtained statistically significant difference in the ANB values between the two groups. However, since medicine that the patients are taking can affect the nervous system and thus influence the result of ANB, we withhold further analysis.

4.4 Discriminant Analysis of BPE

As presented in Sect. 4.1, the BPE can provide as an indicator for identifying Parkinson's disease sufferers. Next, discriminant analysis is carried out, with the help of statistical software, in order to determine critical values of BPE to distinguish

Parkinson's disease sufferers from healthy individuals. The process and result of the discriminant analysis are shown below (Table 5).

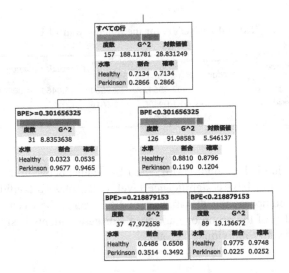

Fig. 8. Process of discriminant analysis of BPE.

Table 5. Result of discriminant analysis of BPE.

BPE range	Ratio (Healthy)	Ratio (Parkison's)
BPE>=0.301656325	5.35%	94.65%
BPE<0.301656325 & BPE>=0.218879153	65.08%	34.92%
BPE<0.301656325 & BPE<0.218879153	97.48%	2.52%

From the result, we conclude that our pulse wave data infer that if BPE $\geq$ 0.3017, the probability of suffering Parkinson's disease is 94.65%, and if BPE < 0.2189, the probability of not suffering Parkinson's disease is 97.48%.

5 Checking BPE with "Alys"

In this section, we introduce our upgraded version of "Alys", with which the analysis and result display of BPE have become possible. We explain the procedure of visualizing BPE with "Alys".

1. Start "Alys"

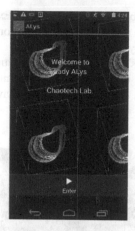

Fig. 9. The welcoming window of "Alys".

2. Connect the sensor to the tablet through a USB connector

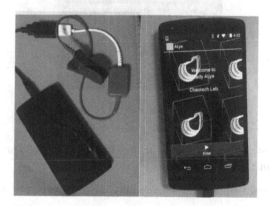

Fig. 10. Connection of the sensor and the tablet.

3. Click the tool mark on the upper right, select "Set Properties" and then select "Compute BPE" from the "Execution of Analysis Mode"

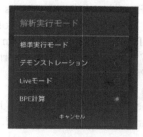

Fig. 11. Option list of "Execution of Analysis Mode".

The 4 options, from top to bottom, are "Standard Execution Mode", "Demonstration Mode", "Live Mode" and "BPE Computation". The "BPE Computation" comes at last as it is a newly added function.

4. Back to the "Set Properties" menu, set the measurement time (in second) and determine the critical value of BPE that is to be normalised to 5.0 in the result display. When this setting is done once, it will be saved so users need not set each time

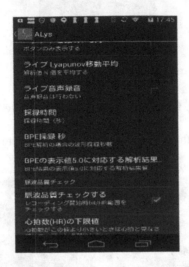

Fig. 12. Option list of "Set Properties".

In the above figure, the items shown in "Set Properties" Menu are interpreted, from top to bottom, in the following.

- Moving average of real-time Lyapunov (Here Lyapunov simply means the LLE.)
- Real-time sound recording
- Measurement time (in second)
- Critical value of BPE that is to be normalized to 5.0 in the result display
- Quality check for pulse waves.

Regarding the "Measurement time (in second)", we have improved the system so that analytical result of BPE can be obtained with as short as 5 s of measurement. Concerning "Critical value of BPE that is to be normalized to 5.0 in the result display", from the result of discriminant analysis in Sect. 4.4, we may use 0.31 (slightly higher than 0.3017) as the critical value corresponding to 5.0, the central value of the normalized BPE.

5. Start to take the pulse from a fingertip
   When the measurement time set in the previous step has elapsed, the measurement will end and a semi-circular graph will be displayed.

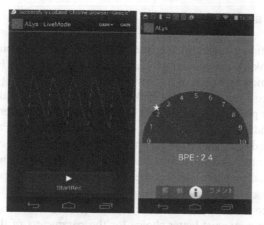

Fig. 13. (Left) Display of waveform during a measurement; (Right) graph for normalized BPE.

The BPE is normalized to range from 0 to 10, centred at 5.0, which corresponds to the critical BPE value set at the previous step. From the above figure we observe that the subject's normalized BPE is 2.4, which is less than 5.0, so this subject may not be a Parkinson's disease sufferer.

6. Other options

Users may view their records of BPE values taken in the past in both "List Mode" and "Graph Mode". The former makes a list of all recent records, while the latter displays all results on the same semi-circular graph.

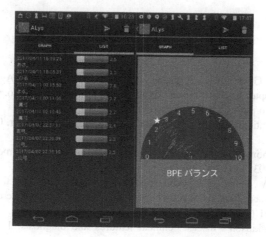

Fig. 14. Display of past records in "List Mode" (left) and "Graph Mode" (right).

Moreover, the data saved in the tablet can be attached to email or sent to Cloud.

6 Conclusion and Remark

In this study, we firstly reviewed the background of the occurrence of Parkinson's disease in Japan, taking the demographic state into consideration. Following that, we presented the common approach of its clinical diagnosis. Observing the role of mental disorders as a bridge – the relevance of Parkinson's disease to mental disorders, and the effectiveness of the pulse wave analysis in detecting mental disorders – we proposed a new indicator for identifying Parkinson's disease, the border of Parkinson's entropy (BPE). We collected a considerable number of pulse wave data, computed the BPE values with our device, and performed statistical analysis to obtain persuasive result. The analysis reached a conclusion that the BPE can provide as a potentially effective indicator of Parkinson's disease.

However, since this indicator is newly proposed, there is much room for improvement: there may exist better choice for the parameters of the sample entropy, and statistical analysis needs to be performed based on larger samples in order to obtain more convincing result. We will strive to collect and analyse more data in the future.

In regard to the upgraded "Alys", since 5 s will suffice to produce analytical result, we believe it can enable users to conduct self-check in a convenient and economical way, without time and space limitation. Test results of BPE may provide a reference for doctors conducting a medical examination for a potential patient. Moreover, the result of LLE, together with BPE, may also be a worthwhile reference.

Declaration

This article is a revised and extended version of a previous paper [14]. Figures 3, 4, 5, 6, 7, 8, 9, 10, 11, 12, 13 and 14, Formulae 1 to 11 and all Tables are borrowed from the original paper.

References

1. Cabinet Office, Government of Japan: Annual Report on the Aging Society: 2016 (Summary) (Chapter 1: Situation on Aging) (2017). http://www8.cao.go.jp/kourei/english/annualreport/2016/pdf/c1-1.pdf. Accessed 1 May 2018
2. Emre, M.: Dementia in Parkinson's disease: cause and treatment. Curr. Opin. Neurol. **17**(4), 399–404 (2004)
3. Higa, M.: Autonomic nervous balance computation apparatus and method therefor, U.S. Patent US 2011/0313303 A1 (2011)
4. Hu, Y., Wang, W., Suzuki, T., Oyama-Higa, M.: Characteristic extraction of mental disease patients by nonlinear analysis of plethysmograms. In: AIP Conference on Proceedings, vol. 1371, pp. 92–101 (2011)
5. Jankovic, J.: Parkinson's disease: clinical features and diagnosis. J. Neurol. Neurosurg. Psychiatry **79**(4), 368–376 (2008)
6. Lemke, M.R., Fuchs, G., Gemende, I., Herting, B., Oehlwein, C., Reichmann, H., Rieke, J., Volkmann, J.: Depression and Parkinson's disease. J. Neurol. **251**(6 Suppl.), vi24–vi27 (2004)
7. Nihon Medi-Physics Co., Ltd. For the diagnosis and treatment of Parkinson's disease. http://www.nmp.co.jp/public/pk/02.html. Accessed 1 May 2018

8. Nishi-Niigata Chuo National Hospital. Inspection of Parkinson's disease. http://www.masa. go.jp/contents/shinryouka/parkinsoncenter/test.html. Accessed 1 May 2018
9. Nutt, J.G., Wooten, G.F.: Diagnosis and initial management of Parkinson's disease. N. Engl. J. Med. **353**, 1021–1027 (2005)
10. Oyama, M.: Psychology of Mental Flexibility, (English edition, Kindle) edn. Amazon Services International Inc., Seattle (2012)
11. Oyama-Higa, M., Miao, T.: Discovery and application of new index for cognitive psychology. In: 2006 IEEE Conference on Systems, Man, and Cybernetics Proceedings, vol. 4, pp. 2040–2044 (2006)
12. Oyama-Higa, M., Miao, T., Kaizu, S., Kojima, J.: Mental health self-check system using "Lyspect". In: Proceedings of the Sixth International Symposium on e-Health Services and Technologies, (EHST 2012), Geneva, pp. 9–18 (2012)
13. Oyama-Higa, M., Miao, T., Tsujino, J., Imanishi, A.: Possibility of mental health self-checks using divergence of pulse waves. In: Proceedings of the First International Conference on Biomedical Electronics and Devices, BIOSIGNALS 2008, Funchal, pp. 361–370 (2008)
14. Oyama-Higa, M., Niwa, T., Wang, W., Kawanabe, Y.: Identifying characteristic physiological patterns of Parkinson's disease sufferers using sample entropy of pulse waves. In: Proceedings of the 11th International Joint Conference on Biomedical Engineering Systems and Technologies, vol. 5, pp. 189–196. (HEALTHINF) (2018)
15. Oyama-Higa, M., Ou, F.: Indication of mental health from fingertip pulse waves and its application. J. Healthc. Eng. **2018**, 17 (2018). https://doi.org/10.1155/2018/7696458. Article ID 7696458
16. Oyama-Higa, M., Wang, W., Kaizu, S., Futaba, T., Suzuki, T.: Smartphone-based device for checking mental status in real time. In: Proceedings of the 9th International Joint Conference on Biomedical Engineering Systems and Technologies, (BIOSIGNALS), vol. 4, pp. 207–214 (2016)
17. Pham, T.D., Oyama-Higa, M., Truong, C.T., Okamoto, K., Futaba, T., Kanemoto, S., Sugiyama, M., Lampe, L.: Computerized assessment of communication for cognitive stimulation for people with cognitive decline using spectral-distortion measures and phylogenetic inference. PLoS ONE **10**(3), e0118739 (2015)
18. Pham, T.D., Thang, T.C., Oyama-Higa, M., Nguyen, H.X., Saji, H., Sugiyama, M.: Chaos and nonlinear time-series analysis of finger pulse waves for depression detection. In: Proceedings of the International Conference on Bio-Inspired Systems and Signal Processing, BIOSIGNALS 2013, Barcelona, pp. 298–301 (2013)
19. Richman, J.S., Moorman, J.R.: Physiological time-series analysis using approximate entropy and sample entropy. Am. J. Physiol. - Heart Circ. Physiol. **278**(6), H2039–H2049 (2000)
20. Rosenstein, M.T., Collinsa, J.J., De Luca, C.J.: A practical method for calculating largest Lyapunov exponents from small data sets. Physica D **65**, 117–134 (1993)
21. Sano, M., Sawada, Y.: Measurement of the Lyapunov spectrum from a chaotic time series. Phys. Rev. Lett. **55**, 1082 (1985)
22. Sumida, T., Arimitu, Y., Tahara, T., Iwanaga, H.: Mental conditions reflected by the chaos of pulsation in capillary vessels. Int. J. Bifurcat. Chaos **10**, 2245–2255 (2000)
23. Wang, W., Hu, Y., Oyama-Higa, M., Suzuki, T., Miao, T., Kojima, J.: Analysis of electroencephalogram and pulse waves during music listening. In: Proceedings of the Sixth International Symposium on e-Health Services and Technologies, (EHST 2012), Geneva, pp. 31–35 (2012)
24. Yamawaki, M., Kusumi, M., Kowa, H., Nakashima, K.: Changes in prevalence and incidence of Parkinson's disease in Japan during a quarter of a century. Neuroepidemiology **32**(4), 263–269 (2009)
25. Zesiewicz, T.A., Baker, M.J., Wahba, M., Hauser, R.A.: Autonomic nervous system dysfunction in Parkinson's disease. Curr. Treat. Options Neurol. **5**(2), 149–160 (2003)

META-GLARE's Supports to Agent Coordination

Luca Anselma[1], Alessio Bottrighi[2], Luca Piovesan[2(✉)],
and Paolo Terenziani[2]

[1] Dipartimento di Informatica, Università di Torino,
corso Svizzera 185, Torino, Italy
anselma@di.unito.it
[2] DISIT, Università del Piemonte Orientale, Viale Teresa Michel 11,
Alessandria, Italy
{alessio.bottrighi, luca.piovesan,
paolo.terenziani}@uniupo.it

Abstract. Clinical Guidelines (GLs) provide evidence-based recommendations
to suggest to physicians the "best" medical treatments, and are widely used to
enhance the quality of patient care, and to optimize it. In many cases, the
treatment of patients cannot be provided by a unique healthcare agent, operating
in a unique context. For instance, the treatment of chronic patients is usually
performed not only in the hospital, but also at home and\or in the general
practitioner's ambulatory, and many healthcare agents (e.g., different specialist,
nurses, family doctor) may be involved. To grant the quality of the treatments,
all such agents must cooperate and interact. A computer-based support to GL
execution is important to provide facilities for coordinating such different
agents, and for granting that, at any time, the actions to be executed have a
"proper" person in charge and executor, and are executed in the correct context.
Additionally, also facilities to support the delegation of responsibility should
also be considered. In this paper we extend META-GLARE, a computerized GL
management system, to support such needs providing facilities for (1) treatment
continuity (2) action contextualization, (3) responsibility assignment and delegation (4) check of agent "appropriateness". Specific attention is also devoted to
the temporal dimension, to grant that each action is executed according to the
temporal constraints possibly present in the GL. We illustrate our approach by
means of a practical case study.

Keywords: Computer-Interpretable guidelines · Agent coordination ·
Temporal reasoning

1 Introduction

The rationalization of the healthcare system is a task of fundamental importance in
order to grant both the quality and the standardization of healthcare services, and the
minimization of costs. *Evidence-based* medicine and clinical guidelines (GLs) have
gained a major role in this context. Clinical guidelines (GLs) are *"systematically
developed statements to assist practitioner and patient decisions about appropriate*

© Springer Nature Switzerland AG 2019
A. Cliquet jr. et al. (Eds.): BIOSTEC 2018, CCIS 1024, pp. 464–496, 2019.
https://doi.org/10.1007/978-3-030-29196-9_24

healthcare under specific clinical circumstances" [1]. In short, GLs provide evidence-based recommendations to suggest to physician the set of diagnostic/therapeutic actions to be executed to cope with a specific disease, supporting their decision-making activity. Thousands of GLs have been devised in the last years. For instance, the Guideline International Network (http://www.g-i-n.net) groups 103 organizations representing 47 countries from all continents, and provides a library of more than 6400 CPGs. Despite such a huge effort, CPGs have not provided all the expected advantages to clinical practice yet. Recent research has shown that Computer Science can help to drastically improve the impact of GLs in the clinical practice. The adoption of *computer-interpretable clinical guidelines* (**CIGs** henceforth) and computerized approaches to acquire, represent, execute and reason with CIGs can further increase the advantages of CPGs, providing crucial advantages to:

(1) patients, enabling them to receive the best quality medical treatments;
(2) physicians, providing them with a standard reference which they may consult, as well as advanced support for their decision-making and\or coordination activities;
(3) hospitals, and healthcare centers, providing them with tools to enable the quality and the standardization of their services.

Many different systems and projects have been developed to this purpose (see e.g. [2–4]). Such systems usually provide facilities to acquire, represent and/or execute CIGs, and are mainly developed to support physicians in patient care.

Different forms of support may be provided. In particular, a lot of attention has been devoted to decision support facilities (such as "what if" analysis [5] or cost-benefit analysis [6]). However, CIG systems have quite neglected the problem of properly supporting the coordination of different healthcare agents in the execution of CIGs (see, however, the discussion in Sect. 7). In most cases, CIG systems assume that the CIG is executed in a unique location (usually, in a hospital) under the responsibility of a unique agent (usually, a physician). However, such a simplified assumption does not hold for many different GLs. For example, GLs dealing with chronic disorders require that the patient treatment is continued in time, and is carried on in *different contexts* (e.g. at home, or in the general practitioner's ambulatory), under the responsibility of *different agents* (not only physicians, but also nurses, family doctors, family members). In such cases, it is crucial that the different healthcare agents communicate and coordinate themselves in an effective way, so that, at any moment, there is a "proper" person in charge (henceforth, "responsible person" or "responsible" for short) for the GL actions to be executed, operating in the right context, and having the appropriate role and qualification. Additionally, the responsible might have the possibility of transferring the responsibility to other agents, or to delegate the responsibility or the execution of actions. None of the available computerized GL systems fully addresses such needs. Notably, there are several multi-agent approaches for healthcare in the literature (see e.g. the survey in [7]), but they consider agents as autonomous software entities. In our approach, we consider agents as a representation of real persons and use a *multi-agents view* to describe and support a distributed GL execution.

In this paper, we describe how we have extended META-GLARE, [8], a recent evolution of GLARE (Guideline Acquisition, Representation and Execution), a domain-independent CIG system for GL acquisition and execution [9], to provide such support to healthcare agents. However, although we have implemented our approach in META-GLARE, it is worth stressing that the methodology we propose is general and application-independent.

First, we identify the extensions to the CIG formalism needed to represent the different pieces of information required to manage the above phenomena. In particular, our representation formalism supports the specification, for each action, of the *context* in which it must be executed, and of the *qualification* and *competences* required to its *responsible*, to its *delegate* (if any) and to its *executor*.

Then, we describe the facilities we have provided to support the coordination of the different agents involved in the execution of a CIG on a patient. The main goal of such facilities is to grant that a proper treatment is assured to the patient. While "standard" CIG systems support physicians by suggesting the proper action to be executed at a given time on the patient, our approach further enhances such a support to grant that the actions are executed in the proper context, under the responsibility of a proper (i.e., having the correct qualification and competences) agent, and are executed by a proper agent. To achieve such a goal, our facilities support:

(1) *treatment continuity,*
(2) *action contextualization,*
(3) *responsibility assignment and delegation,*
(4) *check of agent and executor "appropriateness".*

Last, but not least, our approach is the first one in the literature that explicitly manages the **temporal dimension** within the coordination process. Indeed, actions are delegated and executed at specific times, so that, to implement a realistic and useful coordination process, systems have to explicitly manage the "window" of time in which actions have to be executed (given the temporal constraints in the CIG, and given the execution times of the previous actions in the CIG). For instance, before accepting a delegation\execution, it is important (and realistic) that the agents have also the information about when they will have to manage such an action. Without such an information, their acceptance is just a "generic" one (and not a strong commitment to manage the action) since they cannot grant to be available at the time when the action will have to be executed. Therefore, our approach also proposes temporal facilities to

(5) *associate with each action (during the coordination process) the window of time when it has to be executed, and*
(6) *check that the actions are executed at "proper" times (i.e., at times consistent with the temporal constraints in the CIG).*

Notably, the facilities (5) and (6) constitute a major advance with respect to the other approaches in the literature, since they require not only the representation of the temporal constraints in the CIG, but also the development of temporal reasoning algorithms, and their integration into the delegation\execution process. In particular, temporal reasoning is necessary in order to associate with each GL action a "window" of time in which it has to be executed. Notably, such a "window" cannot be evaluated once-and-for-all, since the execution of other actions may further "restrict" the window of execution of a given one. In our approach, we suggest that such a temporal window has to be evaluated (i) whenever an agent is looking for a responsible\delegate\executor of an action, to check whether the new agent accepts the task in the specified window of time, and (ii) whenever an action has to be effectively executed, to grant that it is executed in a time consistent with the temporal constraints in the CIG and with the times of execution of the previously executed actions in the CIG.

As a running example, in this paper we show the application of our approach to the "management of harmful drinking and alcohol dependence in primary care" GL developed by the Scottish Intercollegiate Guidelines Network (SIGN) [10], which we have adapted to the Italian context.

The paper is structured as follows: in Sect. 2 we describe the main features of GLARE and META-GLARE. In Sect. 3 we describe our extensions to the META-GLARE representation formalism. In Sect. 4, we specifically discuss the temporal reasoning support. In Sect. 5 we describe the different facilities we provide to support the distributed execution of a CIG, and the coordination of the involved agents, with specific emphasis on the temporal issues. In Sect. 6 we exemplify a practical application of our approach considering the treatment of alcohol-related disorders. Finally, in Sect. 7 we address related work and concluding remarks.

2 GLARE and META-GLARE

META-GLARE is an evolution of GLARE, a domain-independent system for acquisition and execution of GLs [9], which we have been developing since 1997, in collaboration with the physicians of Azienda Ospedaliera San Giovanni Battista in Torino, Italy.

The main goals of the GLARE systems are:

(i)   to be domain-independent. In particular, GLARE has been already applied to deal with a wide range of CIGs ranging from asthma to ischemic stroke;

(ii) to be user-friendly. GLARE is intended to be a tool to support physicians (in particular, regarding decision making), and not to replace them. Such a goal has several implications, including the facts that (i) CIGs representation language must be as close as possible to the physicians' way of looking at it, and (ii) the "technological" complexity of the system must be hidden to the user-physicians, through a user-friendly and easy-to-use interface;

(iii) to be easily extendable. Indeed, physicians should be provided with plenty of facilities concerning CIGs. Thus, the system architecture must be modular and easily extendable.

2.1 GLARE's Kernel

The core of GLARE (see the box on the left of Fig. 1) is based on a modular architecture. CG_KRM (Clinical Guidelines Knowledge Representation Manager) is the main module of the system: it manages the internal representation of CIG, and operates as a domain-independent and task-independent knowledge server for the other modules; moreover, it permanently stores the acquired CIG in a dedicated Clinical Guidelines Database (CG-DB).

The Clinical Guidelines Acquisition Manager (CG_AM) provides expert-physicians with a user-friendly graphical interface to introduce the CIGs into the CG_KRM and to describe them. It may interact with four databases: the Pharmacological DB, storing a structured list of drugs and their costs; the Resources DB, listing the resources that are available in a given hospital; the ICD DB, containing an international coding system of diseases; the Clinical DB, providing a "standard" terminology to be used when building a new CIG, and storing the descriptions and the set of possible values of clinical findings.

GLARE's acquisition module provides expert-physicians with a user-friendly and easy-to-use tool for acquiring a CIG. In order to achieve these goals, GLARE provides: (i) a graphical interface, which supports primitives for drawing the control information within the CIGs, and ad-hoc windows to acquire the internal properties of the objects; (ii) facilities for browsing the CIGs; (iii) an "intelligent" help and consistency-checking facilities including name and range checking, logical design criteria checks.

The execution module (CG-EM) executes a CIG for a specific patient, considering the patient's data (retrieved from the Patient DB). It adopts the "agenda technique" (see [11]). Basically, through the "agenda technique", GLARE is able to identify all the next actions to be executed in the current CIG, and the window of time when they have to be executed.

Notably, the schema of the Patient DB mirrors the schema of the Clinical DB. Therefore, the interaction with the Clinical DB during the acquisition phase makes it possible to automatically retrieve data from the Patient DB at execution time. CG-EM stores the execution status in another DB (CG Instances) and interacts with the user-physician via a graphical interface (CG-IM).

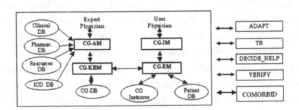

Fig. 1. Architecture of GLARE. Rectangles represent computation modules, and ovals data/knowledge bases (original figure in [12]).

2.2   GLARE's Extended Architecture

GLARE's architecture is open: new modules and functionalities can be easily added if \when necessary. In the last years, several new modules and\or methodologies have been added to cope with different phenomena.

The **ADAPT** module [13] copes with automatic resource-based contextualization. Indeed, contextualization is an essential step to be taken before a guideline manager is actually adopted in clinical practice. One of the most relevant obstacles to the exploitation and dissemination of GLs is the gap between the generality of the GLs themselves (as defined, e.g., by physicians' committees) and the peculiarities of the specific contexts of application. ADAPT supports the adaptation of general guidelines to the local setting, by (automatically) taking into account local resources (e.g. diagnostic instrumentation) unavailability, and locally applied procedures, which may require to discard some alternatives.

The temporal reasoning module **TR** [11] deals with the temporal constraints in the CIGs. As already discussed in the introductory section, the temporal dimension is essential in the management of CIGs. A detailed description of this module, and how it is exploited in the coordination process, is presented in Sects. 4 and 5 of this paper.

The decision making support module **DECIDE_HELP** [14] provides further support to physicians for their decision-making activities, focusing on therapy selection. In many cases, when executing a CIG on a given patient, a physician can be faced with a choice among different therapeutic alternatives, and identifying the most suitable one is often not straightforward. In several situations no alternative is actually "better" than the others from a strictly clinical viewpoint, and CIGs are only meant to present all the range of choices, leaving to the user the responsibility of selecting the "right" one.

In clinical practice, various selection parameters (such as the costs and effectiveness of the different procedures) are sometimes available when executing a CIG, but the task of comparing and balancing them is typically left to the physician.

Decision theory seems a natural candidate as a methodology for affording this analysis; to this end, we have realized a mapping between the CIG representation primitives and decision-theory concepts (in particular we represent CIGs as Markov Decision Processes), and we have developed a decision-theory tool for supporting therapy selection in GLARE. In particular, the GLARE decision-theory facility enables the user to: (1) identify the optimal policy, and (2) calculate the expected utility along a path, by exploiting classical dynamic programming algorithms.

The module **VERIFY** [15] supports *model-based verification* of CIGs. Indeed, CIGs are very large and complex bodies of knowledge, so that, after they have been acquired, it is important to be able to check automatically whether they satisfy different types of properties (e.g., their eligibility to treat specific classes of patients). The general methodology we propose is to exploit the capabilities of a model checker (specifically, we adopt SPIN [16]) by loosely integrating with it a CIG system. Such a loose integration is achieved by defining a module for the automatic translation of any GLARE CIG into the corresponding CIG represented in the model-checker format. The translation of a CIG can be performed a priori and once and for all. After that, the model-checker can be used in a standard way in order to verify any property (that can be expressed in the model-checker property language) on any of the translated CIGs. It is important to stress that the properties need not to be defined a-priori: the user can directly express a new property and ask the model-checker to verify it.

Finally, the **COMORBID** module [17, 18] is devoted to the treatment of comorbid patients, i.e., of patients having more than one disease.

Computer Interpretable Guidelines (CIGs) are consolidated tools to support physicians with evidence-based recommendations in the treatment of patients affected by a specific disease. However, the application of two or more CIGs on comorbid patients is critical, since dangerous interactions between (the effects of) actions from different CIGs may arise. **COMORBID** is the *first* tool supporting, in an integrated way, (i) the knowledge-based detection of interactions, (ii) the management of the interactions, and (iii) the final "merge" of (part of) the CIGs operating on the patient. **COMORBID** is characterized by being very supportive to physicians, providing them support for focusing, interaction detection, and for an "hypothesize and test" approach to manage the detected interactions. To achieve such goals, it provides advanced Artificial Intelligence techniques.

Testing. GLARE has been already tested considering different domains, including bladder cancer, reflux esophagitis, heart failure, and ischemic stroke. The acquisition of a GL using GLARE is reasonably fast (e.g., the acquisition of the GL on heart failure required 3 days).

2.3   GLARE Representation Formalism

In the GLARE project, a GL is represented through the set of actions composing it. GLARE distinguishes between *atomic* and *composite* actions. Atomic actions can be regarded as elementary steps in a CIG, in the sense that they do not need a further decomposition into sub-actions to be executed. Composite actions are composed by other actions (atomic or composite). Four different types of atomic actions can be distinguished in GLARE: *work* actions, *query* actions, *decisions* and *conclusions*. Work actions are basic atomic actions which must be executed on the patient, and can be described in terms of a set of attributes, such as name, (textual) description, cost, time, resources, goals. Query actions are requests of information, which can be obtained from the outside world (physicians, databases, knowledge bases). Decision actions are specific types of actions embodying the criteria which can be used to select alternative paths in a CIG. In particular, diagnostic decisions are represented as an open set of triples <diagnosis, parameter, score> (where, in turn, a parameter is a triple <data, attribute, value>), plus a threshold to be compared with the different diagnoses' scores. On the other hand, therapeutic decisions are based on a pre-defined set of parameters: *effectiveness*, *cost*, *side-effects*, *compliance*, *duration*. Finally, conclusions represent the output of a decision process. Composite actions are defined in terms of their components, via the "has-part" relation. Control relations establish which actions might be executed next and in what order. We distinguish among four different control relations: *sequence*, *constrained*, *alternative* and *repetition*. The description of sequences usually involves the definition of the minimum and maximum delay between actions. Complex temporal constraints between actions (e.g., *overlaps*, *during*) can be specified using constrained control relations. In particular, action *parallelism* is also supported through this feature.

2.4   META-GLARE

In the last years, a new CIG system, META-GLARE, has been designed, on top of GLARE. Basically, METAGLARE takes in input a CIG formalism (based on the Task-Network Model approach), and provides as output a CIG system for acquiring and executing CIGs expressed through the input language. The core idea of our meta-approach is:

(i)   To define an open library of elementary components (e.g., textual attribute, Boolean condition, Score-based decision), each of which is equipped with methods for acquiring, consulting and executing them,

(ii) To provide system-designers with an easy way of aggregating such components to define node and arc types (constituting the representation formalism of a new system),

(iii) To devise general and basic tools for the acquisition, consultation and execution of CIGs, represented by hierarchical directed graphs which are parametric over the node and arc types (in the sense that the definitions of node and arc types are an input for such tools).

In such a way, META-GLARE provides users with several advantages:

- Using META-GLARE, users can easily define their own systems, basically by defining the nodes and arcs types as an aggregation of components (called *attributes*) from the library. No other effort (e.g., building acquisition or execution modules) is needed.

- The extension of a system can be easily achieved by adding new node/arc types, or adding components to already existing types (with no programming effort at all).

- User programming is needed only in case a new component (*attribute type*) has to be added to the component library. However, this addition is modular and minimal: the programmer has just to focus on the component to be added, and to provide the code for acquiring, consulting, and (if needed) executing it (while the "general" acquisition, consultation and execution engines have not to be modified).

In short, META-GLARE is a "meta" system, in that it takes in input a CIG representation formalism, and automatically generates a CIG system to acquire and execute CIGs expressed in the input formalism. To test it, an extended formalism has been used (see [8]). In the following, we refer to such an extended formalism as "META-GLARE formalism". In particular, the META-GLARE formalism extends GLARE's one with the possibility of specifying not only 1:1 arcs (i.e., arcs with just one input action and one output action), but also 1:n, n:1 and n:n arcs. Such an additional feature is very useful to easily model the parallelism between actions.

GLARE and META-GLARE have been developed in Java, to take advantage of its portability. As a consequence, GLARE can run similarly on any hardware/operating-system platform.

3   CIG Annotations

Our approach aims at supporting the coordination of multiple healthcare agents in the execution of a CIG on a given patient, granting at the same time that each action is managed by "proper" agents. To achieve such a goal, each action has to specify a set of properties (that we call annotations), to specify what are the characteristics of a "proper" execution in terms of (i) what are the "proper" (in terms of qualification and competences) agents that can manage the action (either the responsible, or the executor), (ii) what are the "proper" execution contexts, and (iii) when applicable, also additional constraints to cope with the continuity of treatments (in terms of the agents managing them). In META-GLARE, such properties are managed as additional attributes to be added to the description of actions.

In the following, we describe such additional attributes in detail.

First of all, META-GLARE actions can be annotated with the possible *contexts* in which they can be executed.

- **Context** annotation: it specifies where the action can be executed (e.g. in-patient care, community medicine). Notably, a context is not necessarily a physical place, but it might also indicate an operative environment. For example, community medicine can refer to the patient's home or to the general practitioner's ambulatory. In META-GLARE, each action can be annotated with a set of contexts. In such a case, we intend that the action can be executed in any one of the contexts in the set;

Regarding the agents that have to take care of a given action (or set of actions) in a CIG, META-GLARE supports the distinction among three different *roles*: *responsible*, *delegate*, and *executor*.

The *responsible* of an action (or of a whole part of a CIG; for instance, the head physician of a hospital department) is, indeed, the agent that retains the whole responsibility of the management of the action, and who also has the responsibility of determining the responsible of the next actions. Of course, a responsible can delegate an action (or a set of actions) to a delegate agent. A delegate has the "local" responsibility of the action, but, after managing it, s\he has to return the responsibility to the responsible of the action. Both responsibles and delegates are not necessarily the physical executors of actions. Indeed, in many cases, the responsibility (and, possibly, the delegation) is given to physicians, but the physical execution is demanded to nurses or lab technicians.

To be a "proper" responsible, delegate or executor of an action, an agent must have a given *qualification*, and, possibly, some specific *competences*. To cope with such issues, we extended the META-GLARE formalism with six additional annotations:

- **responsible_qualification** (e.g. neurologist, gastroenterologist, ...), **delegate_qualification** (e.g. neurologist, gastroenterologist, ...), **executor_qualification** (e.g., nurse): such annotations specify what the qualification of the responsible, delegate, and executor of the action must be. A list of qualifications can be specified, meaning that the agent must have (at least) one of the qualifications in the list;
- **responsible_competence, delegate_competence, executor_competence:** they specify that the agent must have specific abilities (e.g. expert in the alcohol-related disorders management). Such an attribute is optional. A list of competences can be specified, meaning that the agent must have *all* the competences in the list.

When a CIG is being acquired, we impose that each action in it is annotated with a specification of a list of possible contexts and of a list of possible qualifications of responsibles and executors. This is mandatory, and the acquisition module is extended to support the acquisition of such annotations (see Sect. 4). On the contrary, competence annotations are optional. In case the competence list is empty, no specific restriction needs to be applied; otherwise, only the agents having the required competences are allowed to be responsible for or to execute the action at hand.

Example 1. The action "Brief intervention for hazardous and harmful drinking" (see action 11 in Fig. 4) in the alcohol-related disorders treatment GL [10] is described as follows:

- responsible_qualification: physician
- responsible_competence: \
- delegate_qualification: physician
- delegate_competence: \
- executor_ qualification: physician, nurse
- executor_competence: \
- context: community medicine, SERT medicine (SERT is the acronym for "SERvizio per le Tossicodipendenze", an Italian service similar to the Mental Health Service in U.S.A.), in-patient care, hospital ambulatory care.

In many practical cases, behind coordination of agents, it is also important to support the continuity of treatments. Indeed, it is preferable to assign "homogeneous" sets of actions in a CIG to the same responsible (or, in some cases, executor). For instance, it might be preferable that the same neurologist is responsible of all the neurological activities performed on a given patient, and that the different EMG examinations of a patient are executed by the same specialist. Notably, continuity constraints are interpreted as "preferential" constraints by our system (see Sect. 4), and admit violations (e.g., after a period, a physician may, for any reason, be unable to continue to treat a given patient). In META-GLARE, we support such a need through an independent data structure, which annotates CIGs with *"continuity constraints"*, which specifies sets of actions that should have (preferably) the same responsible, delegate and\or executor.

In the next sections, we will present how *annotations* are formalized in our approach, and how they are treated by META-GLARE.

3.1   Ontology of Annotations

GL *annotations* can be modeled on the basis of three taxonomies, and of the relations between them. Part of the taxonomies and relations are graphically shown in Fig. 2. The ontology of *contexts* is a "part-of" taxonomy, in which each context can be further specified by its components. For instance, in Fig. 2, FAMILY, HOSPITAL and COMMUNITY MEDICINE are three possible contexts, and NEUROLOGY, GASTROENTOROLOGY and INTERNAL MEDICINE are some of the departments that are part of a hospital. *Qualifications* can be modeled through a standard "isa" taxonomy, in which each qualification can be further refined (*isa* relation) by its specializations. For instance, in Fig. 2, NURSE and PHYSICIAN are two possible qualifications. In turn, NEUROLOGIST, GASTROENTEROLOGIST and INTERNIST are specializations of PHYSICIAN. Analogously, also *competences* are modeled by an "is-a" taxonomy. For instance, in Fig. 2, (the competence in) PERIPHERAL NEUROPATHY is a specialization of (competence in) NEUROLOGY, which is a specialization of MEDICAL COMPETENCE.

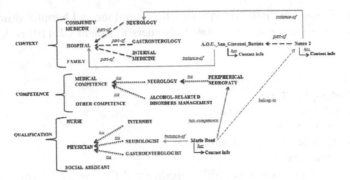

Fig. 2. Ontology of contexts, qualifications and competences and their instances (original figure in [12]).

Besides concepts, which denote classes of entities, the ontology also includes instances, denoting specific entities. Each instance is connected to its class through an "instance-of" relation. For example, in Fig. 2, Neuro2 is an instance of NEUROLOGY in Azienda Ospedaliera San Giovanni Battista (which is an instance of Hospital); Mario Rossi is an instance of NEUROLOGIST (thus, given the transitivity of the *isa* relation, Mario Rossi is also an instance of PHYSICIAN). It is worth noticing that, while the entities in the context and qualification taxonomies have instances, competences do not have them (they are individual concepts). Besides *part-of*, *isa* and *instance-of* relations, other relations are useful to represent the domain. *Agents* (which are instances of Qualifications) are related to the contexts they belong to by the *belong-to* relation. Additionally, agents may have competences, and this fact is represented by the *has-competence* relation. For instance, in Fig. 2, Mario Rossi belongs to Neuro2, and has specific competence about Peripheral Neuropathy. Contexts and persons have *contacts* (usually phone numbers).

Continuity constraints model the fact that, preferably, "homogeneous" sets of actions in a GL should be performed by the same agent. Such constraints are typically GL-dependent, and can be easily formalized in an independent data structure, to store three different partitions of the GL actions into subsets, to model:

  (i)   the sets of actions which should (preferably) have the same responsible;
  (ii) the sets of actions which should (preferably) have the same delegate;
  (iii) the sets of actions which should (preferably) have the same executor.

The definition of continuity constraints is a refinement process. First, the users can define the continuity constraints concerning the responsibles. Then, within each responsible-level continuity group, they can further specify continuity groups for possible delegates. Finally, continuity execution groups can be defined, within the delegate-level continuity groups.

Temporal constraints play a fundamental role in clinical guidelines. For example, temporal indeterminacy, constraints about duration, delays between actions, and periodic repetitions of actions are essential in order to cope with clinical therapies. As a matter of fact, in most therapies, actions have to be performed according to a set of temporal constraints concerning their relative order, their duration, and the delays between them. Additionally, in many cases, actions must be repeated at regular (i.e., periodic) times. For instance, consider Example 1. In Example 1, the instances of the melphalan treatment must respect the temporal pattern "twice a day, for 5 days", but such a pattern must be repeated for six cycles, each one followed by a delay of 23 days, since the melphalan treatment is part of the general therapy for multiple myeloma.

Example 2. The therapy for multiple myeloma is made by six cycles of 5-day treatments, each one followed by a delay of 23 days (for a total time of 24 weeks). Within each cycle of 5 days, two inner cycles can be distinguished: the melphalan treatment, to be provided twice a day, for each of the 5 days, and the prednisone treatment, to be provided once a day, for each of the 5 days. These two treatments must be performed in parallel.

Coping with such temporal constraints involves two main challenges:

(1) Developing a representation formalism to capture them,
(2) Developing temporal reasoning algorithms to reason with them (e.g., to check their consistency, and to make explicit the implied constraints).

Notably, only in case the temporal reasoning algorithms are proved to be correct and complete (with respect to the representation formalism) one can assure that:

(i) the constraints are consistent (notably, if they are not, there is no execution of the CIG containing them that can satisfy all of the constraints)
(ii) the window of time associated with CIG actions is correct with respect to the constraints (i.e., it does not contain any time that is not "legal", given the temporal constraints in the CIG)
     (see the discussion in [11] for more details).

As a consequence, a fundamental step in the development of a manager for temporal constraints is the analysis of the trade-off between the expressiveness of the representation formalism and the tractability of correct and complete temporal reasoning algorithms [19].

4 Temporal Reasoning

4.1 Representing CIG Temporal Constraints

As regarding the representation formalism, the main challenge is how to represent the constraints about repetitions, and how to integrate such a representation with the representation of the "standard" temporal constraints (i.e., the temporal constraints between non-repeated actions).

"Standard" Temporal Constraints. We have chosen to model the temporal constraints concerning "standard" (i.e., non-repeated) actions in the CIGs, using a well-known and widely-used AI framework, namely STP [20].

In STP, a set of constraints is modeled as a conjunction of bounds on differences of the form $c \leq x - y \leq d$, which have an intuitive temporal interpretation, namely that the temporal distance between the time points x and y is between c (minimum distance) and d (maximum distance). In STP the correct and complete propagation of the constraints (e.g., for consistency checking) can be performed in a time cubic in the number of time points, and the *minimal network* of the constraints is provided as output (i.e., the minimum and maximum distance between each pair of points) [20]. The minimal network can be computed by an "all-to-all shortest paths" algorithm such as the Floyd-Warshall's one. The STP framework can be used to model precise or imprecise temporal locations (dates), durations, delays between points, and different forms of qualitative temporal constraints between time points and/or time intervals (see [21, 22]). Unfortunately, constraints about repeated actions cannot be easily captured by the STP framework.

Temporal Constraints about Repetitions. In our approach, the constraints on repetitions and periodicities are temporal constraints of the form

   <nRepetitions, I-Time, repConstraints, conditions>.

nRepetitions represents the number of times that the action must be repeated; **I-Time** represents the time span in which the repetitions must be included; **repConstraints** may impose a pattern that the repetitions must follow; **conditions** allows to express conditions that must hold so that the repetition can take place. Informally, we can roughly describe the semantics of the quadruple as the natural language sentence *"repeat the action **nRepetitions** times in exactly **I-Time** according to **repConstraints**, if conditions hold"*.

repConstraints$_i$ is a (possibly empty) set of pattern constraints, representing possibly imprecise repetition patterns. Pattern constraints may be of type:

- **fromStart(min, max)**, representing a (possibly imprecise) delay between the start of the I-Time and the beginning of the first repetition;
- **toEnd(min, max)**, representing a (possibly imprecise) delay between the end of the last repetition and the end of the I-Time;
- **inBetweenAll(min, max)** representing the (possibly imprecise) delay between the end of each repetition and the start of the subsequent one;
- **inBetween((min$_1$, max$_1$), ..., (min$_{nRepetitionsi-1}$, max$_{nRepetitionsi-1}$))**, representing the (possibly imprecise) delays between each repetition and the subsequent one.

For example, the temporal constraint modeling the repetition of the chemotherapy (as a whole) in Example 1 is

   <6, 6wk, {inBetweenAll(23d, 23d), toEnd(23d, 23d)}, $\emptyset$>.

Notably, our formalism to represent repetitions is recursive, in the sense that one can specify repetitions of repetitions, as a list of specifications **<<nRepetitions$_1$, I-Time$_1$, repConstraints$_1$, conditions$_1$>, ...,<nRepetitions$_k$, I-Time$_k$, repConstraints$_k$, conditions$_k$>>** as above.

For example, the temporal constraint modeling the melphalan cycle is the following:

   <<5, 5d, $\emptyset$, $\emptyset$>, <2, 1d, $\emptyset$, $\emptyset$>>.

Integrated Representation of Temporal Constraints. The formalism we propose to consider both "standard" constraints and constraints about repetitions is the STP-tree [11]. In an STP-tree, we model the constraints regarding repeated actions into separate

STPs, one for each repeated action. The root of the tree (node N1 in the example in Fig. 3) is the STP which homogeneously represents the constraints (including the ones derived from the control-flow of actions in the guideline) between all the actions in the guideline (e.g., in N1, the fact that the duration of the chemotherapy is 168 days), except repeated actions. Each node in the tree is an STP, and has as many children as the number of repeated actions it contains. Each edge in the tree connects a pair of endpoints in an STP (the starting and ending point of a repeated action) to the STP containing the constraints between its subactions, and it is labeled with the list of properties describing the temporal constraints on the repetitions. For example, in Fig. 3, we show the STP-tree representing the temporal constraints involved by Example 2 above.

Additionally, an independent STP must be used in order to represent the temporal constraints about the specific instances of the actions of the guidelines, as emerging from the executions of the guidelines on specific patients.

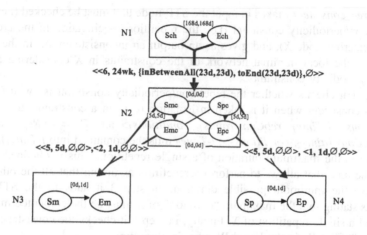

Fig. 3. STP-tree for the multiple myeloma chemotherapy guideline in Example 2. Edges inside STPs represent STP constraints; edges between STPs represent repetitions. *Sch, Ech, Smc, Emc, Spc, Epc, Sm, Em, Sp* and *Ep* stand for the starting (*S*) and ending (*E*) points of chemotherapy, melphalan cycle, prednisone cycle, melphalan treatment and prednisone treatment, respectively.

4.2 Temporal Reasoning

In order to propagate the temporal constraints in the STP-tree, and to check their consistency, it is not sufficient to check the consistency of each node separately. In such a case, in fact, we would neglect the repetition/periodicity information. Temporal consistency checking, thus, proceeds in a top-down fashion, starting from the root of the STP-tree. Basically, the root contains a "standard" STP, so that the Floyd-Warshall's algorithm can be applied to check its consistency. Thereafter, we proceed top-down towards the leaves of the tree. For each node X in the STP-tree (except the root), we progress as shown in the algorithm *STPs_tree_consistency* in Algorithm 1.

```
function STP_tree_consistency(X: STPNode, RepSpec = (R₁ =
<nRepetitions₁, I-Time₁, repConstraints₁, conditions₁>, …,
Rₙ = <nRepetitionsₙ, I-Timeₙ, repConstraintsₙ, condi-
tionsₙ>)) : STP
    1. check that the repetition/periodicity constraint is
       well-formed (i.e., that repetitions nest properly)
    2. compute Max, i.e. the maximum duration of a single
       repetition of X according to RepSpec
    3. impose in X that the maximum distance between each
       pair of points is less or equals Max
    4. X ← FloydWarshall(X)
    5. if X = INCONSISTENT then return INCONSISTENT else
       return X
```

Algorithm 1. Algorithm for checking the consistency of a guideline (represented as an STP-tree).

STP_tree_consistency takes in input the STP-node that must be checked (i.e. *X*) and the repetition/periodicity constraint (i.e., the repetition specification in the arc of the STP-tree entering node *X*), and gives as an output an inconsistency or, in the case of consistency, the local minimal network of the constraints in *X* considering also the repetition/periodicity constraints.

In step 1 it checks whether the repetition/periodicity constraint is "well-formed", i.e. if it is consistent when it is taken in isolation (e.g., in a constraint such as $R_1 =$ <*nRepetitions₁, I-Time₁, repConstraints₁, conditions₁*> and $R_2 =$ <*nRepetitions₂, I-Time₂, repConstraints₂, conditions₂*>, *I-Time₂* must be contained into *I-Time₁*). In step 2 it computes the maximum duration of a single repetition. This is obtained by considering the time that allows to perform a repetition assuming that all the other repetitions have the minimum possible duration. In step 3 it adds to the STP *X* the constraints stating that the maximum "duration" of *X* must be the computed maximum duration of a single repetition of *X*. Finally, in step 5 it checks the consistency of the "augmented" STP *X* via the Floyd-Warshall's algorithm.

Complexity. Considering that the number of nesting levels, in the worst case, is less than the number of classes, the algorithm is dominated by step 4, that is $O(C^3)$, where *C* is the number of actions in the guideline.

Property 1. The top-down visit of the STP-tree is complete as regards consistency checking of the constraints in the STP-tree.

Proof (sketch). The all-to-all-shortest-paths algorithm is complete for STP frameworks. The only constraints relating actions (or, better, time points) in different STPs in the tree are located on the arcs of the tree, and, by definition, the STP-tree does not allow loops between STPs. Since, in our approach, I-Times (if any) must be provided in a precise (exact) way, they cannot be further "restricted" by constraint propagation.

Thus, there is no need to propagate forward and backward the constraints along the tree, and a top-down visit of the tree is sufficient[1].

5 Agent Coordination Facilities

In the previous section, we have discussed the extensions to (i) the META-GLARE language and to (ii) the META-GLARE basic ontology to cope with the "annotations" required to support agent coordination. Indeed, such extensions to the knowledge representation languages must be paired with software modules to acquire and navigate them, and to use them to support agents in the coordinated execution of CIGs. In the following, we detail such modules. In Sect. 5.1, we discuss the tools we provide to navigate the ontological knowledge. Such tools are exploited by the acquisition module (discussed in Sect. 5.2) to acquire proper and "standardized" annotations for the actions of the CIGs. In Sect. 5.3, we discuss how we have extended the META-GLARE execution engine in order to support agent coordination. Last, but not least, in Sect. 5.4 we discuss the facilities we provide to the healthcare agents.

5.1 Navigation Module

The ontology pointed out in Sect. 3.1 is important for two main tasks:

(i) during the acquisition of CIGs, to support "standardized" annotations of CIGs with qualifications, contexts and competences taken from the ontology, and

(ii) during the execution of a CIG action, to support the search of agents having the properties required for the management (as a responsible, delegate, or executor) of such an action (as specified by the action's annotations).

To manage such needs, we have developed two different facilities to navigate the ontology:

(1) schema browsing,
(2) instance browsing.

The *schema browsing* facility is used at acquisition time, and allows experts to navigate the ontology (using the *part-of* and *is-a* relations) and to find qualifications/contexts/competences needed to annotate the CIG actions.

The *instance browsing* facility is used at execution time to support agent coordination in the selection of "proper" agents. It allows users to find a specific agent on the basis of the relations *part-of, is-a, instance-of, has-competence, belong-to*. For example, it supports the search of an agent on the basis of a qualification (e.g. Physician), a context (e.g. Neurology) and, possibly, a competence (e.g. Peripheral Neuropathy). This facility can give in output (i) one or more agents (and their contact information)

---

[1] Notice, however, that the above reasoning mechanism does not provide the minimal network between all the actions in the STP-tree.

satisfying the requirements, or (ii) one or more specific contexts, in which agents having the required qualification and competences operate.

5.2   Acquisition

We have extended META-GLARE with an ***annotation support***, supporting the acquisition of CIG annotations. We have developed a user-friendly Graphical User Interface (GUI). Such a GUI takes advantage of the schema browsing facility discussed in Sect. 5.1 to find in the ontology the proper qualifications, contexts and competences needed to annotate actions.

Moreover, we have developed an ad-hoc module to support the definition and the acquisition of ***continuity constraints***. The user can use this module to browse the CIG and to specify the set of actions in the CIG which belong to a continuity constraint by selecting such actions in the graphical representation of the CIG.

5.3   Execution Engine

The execution engine of META-GLARE has been deeply extended in order to support coordination in the execution of CIGs. Specifically, we provide facilities to support the identification of the responsible(s), of the delegate(s) and of the executor(s) for the next action(s) according to the CIG annotations, and to consider the window of time when the actions have to be executed, according to the temporal constraints in the CIG and to the times when the previous CIG actions have been executed.

The main data structure supporting CIG execution is an ***agenda*** [13], containing a set of pairs $\{(A_1, T_{A1}), \ldots, (A_k, T_{Ak})\}$ representing the actions to be executed next $(A_1, \ldots, A_k)$, and the window of time within which the actions have to be executed $(T_{A1}, \ldots, T_{Ak})$. Notably, (i) more than one pair may appear in the set, to support concurrent execution, and (ii) the time window of the action is evaluated by a temporal reasoner, as described in Sect. 4 above.

To support the management of responsibilities\delegations\executions, the agenda has to be integrated with additional data structures. First of all, to grant the continuity of treatments (as modeled by the continuity constraints) at each time, the system has not only to support the management of the actions in the agenda, but also of each action belonging to the Responsibility Continuity Group ("RCG" in the following algorithm) of such actions. For each action A of such actions, a new data structure (called ***agent stack*** of A) has to be introduced, to store two different types of information: (i) the time window in which the action has to be executed, and (ii) a stack of the form $Stack_A$: $<(X_1, role_1), \ldots, (X_k, role_j)>$ where X_i is a specific agent, and $role_h$ her role in the management of the action A (i.e., responsible (R), delegate (D), or executor (E))[2] storing the different agents involved in the management of such an action, and the window of time.

---

[2] At the time of the execution of an action A, its agent stack $Stack_A$ should contain the responsible (bottom of the stack), a certain number of delegates (zero delegates in case no delegation has been performed; more than one delegate is possible, to support delegation of delegations), and one executor (which might also be the last delegate, or the responsible).

An important issue regards the evaluation of the time windows associated with (i) the actions in the agenda, and with (ii) the actions in the RCG of the agenda actions. Both windows (i) and (ii) are evaluated by the temporal reasoner, as discussed in Sect. 4. However, there is a subtle but important difference. The formers are evaluated whenever an action is entered in the agenda, i.e., whenever it has actually to be executed. Therefore, the time window exactly indicates to the executor the range of time when the action has to be performed. On the other hand, the actions in the RCG groups are actions which do not necessarily have to be executed soon: for instance, the RCG of a neurologist visit may include all the following neurologist's visits included in the CIG. From one side, it is important that the window of time in which such visits will have to be executed is evaluated soon. In such a way, when asking a neurologist to accept the responsibility\execution of such actions, we can also indicate her\him the (approximate) window of execution. This is an important information, since the agent may accept or reject also on the basis of her\him time availabilities. However, such a window is generally a quite approximate one. Notably, in principle, whenever a new CIG action is executed, the temporal window of each RCG action can be restricted (by adding the time of execution of the action executed last to the previous set of constraints, and propagating the resulting set of constraints through the temporal reasoner).

Thus, an important choice we have to take in our approach is whether and when we have to update the time windows associated with actions. Since temporal reasoning is quite computational expensive, we have chosen to evaluate such windows only twice:

(i)   First, they are evaluated whenever an action becomes part of an RCG group (so that we can show the windows to agents while asking them to accept to manage them);

(ii) Second, they are evaluated whenever actions enter into the agenda (i.e., when actions have actually to be executed next). At such a time, it is fundamental to give to the executor the precise window of execution (considering the constraints in the CIGs and its current execution status).

The execution of a CIG starts with an initialization phase (see Algorithm 2 in the following). All the initial actions are inserted into the agenda, together with the window of time in which they must be executed. For each one of such actions, and for each action belonging to the Responsibility Continuity Group ("RCG" in the following algorithm) of such actions, the approximate time window is evaluated, and the agent stack is initialized.

Notably the responsibles of the first actions are predetermined and provided as input to the execution engine.

The CIG execution engine operates as described by Algorithm 3. For each action A in the agenda, the CIG execution engine starts its execution by sending the *execute* message (line 2) to the agent on the top of the agent stack Stack$_A$, asking her to manage (according to her role) the action A in the time window T_A. Notably, as discussed above, the time window T_A is re-evaluated by META-GLARE at the time when A is inserted in the agenda (i.e., when the execution engine determines the CIG actions to be executed next). In case action A is executed (line 3), A is removed from the Agenda (line 4). Thus, the execution engine evaluates the set S of the next actions in the CIG to be executed, using the *get_next* function (line 5). Notably, identifying the next actions which have to be executed during the execution of a CIG is a standard operation (see [23], and consider [24] as regards the META-GLARE approach).

Each action B belonging to S is pushed onto the Agenda. Then, in the case that B has not yet a responsible (i.e., $Stack_B$ has not been created yet), the responsible of A has to find the responsible for B, and for all the actions in RCG(B). To find such a responsible, we first call the temporal reasoner to evaluate, for each action $C \in$ RCG(B), its temporal window. A message "next_responsible?" containing the resulting set of pairs (action, time-window) (denoted by RCG^T(B) in the algorithm -see line 12) is sent by the execution engine to the responsible of A (i.e. the agent stored at the bottom of $Stack_A$) to advise her\him to search for a responsible for B and the other actions in RCG^T(B) (line 12). Notably, since we manage continuity groups, the responsible of an action X in the CIG can be already determined before the time when X is inserted in

```
1.  let S={(A1,M_A1), …, (Ak,M_Ak)} be the set of the start-
       ing actions of CIG, and of their responsibles.
2.  for each action Ai∈S
        evaluate its temporal window Ti;
        push (Ai,Ti) onto the Agenda
3.  for each (A, T_A) in Agenda do
        for each B ∈ RCG(A) do
            evaluate the temporal window T_B
            initialize(Stack_B, M_A, "R", T_B)
```

Algorithm 2. Pseudocode of the initialization of the **CIG executor engine**.

```
1.    for each (A, T_A) in Agenda do
2.        OUT←send(top(Stack_A),execute(A,T_A))
3.        if (OUT == OK) then
4.            Remove A from Agenda
5.            S ← get_next(A)
6.            for each B in S do
7.                Evaluate the time window T_B
8.                push (B, T_B) onto the Agenda
9.                if B has no responsible then
10.                   for each C∈RCG(B)
11.                       evaluate its time window
12.                       send(next_responsible?
                              (bottom(Stack_A), RCG^T(B))
13.           Delete Stack_A
14.       else
15.           pop(stack of A)
16.           goto 2
```

Algorithm 3. Pseudocode of **CIG executor engine**.

the agenda (due to the fact that X belongs to the responsibility continuity group of another action already inserted in the agenda). Finally, the stack of A is deleted (line 13).

Otherwise, in case A is not executed (i.e. the agent on the top of StackA rejects its role), a pop on Stack$_A$ is performed (line 15). Thus, A remains in Agenda and the engine executor has to handle it again sending an execute message to the new top of the stack of A.

Notably, we support the fact that an agent accepts the responsibility, the delegation or the execution of a set of actions (all the actions in a continuity group) but, later on, stops to operate on some of the accepted actions. In such a case, the CIG execution engine "goes up" in the agent stack of the "rejected" actions to find new delegates or responsibles. Notably, though the current responsible may decide not to operate any more on the actions she previously accepted, before "retiring" she has to find a new responsible for them.

5.4   Support to Agents

As discussed above, in META-GLARE we distinguish among three different "roles" that agents can play in the management of a CIG action: *responsibles*, *delegates*, and *executors*. Each role has different rights and duties, so that META-GLARE provides a different support for each role.

A first set of facilities has the goal of supporting agents to find proper responsibles, delegates and executors of one or more CIG actions.

The *find_responsible* function allows an agent to find a "proper" responsible for an action or a set of actions (in a continuity group). First of all, it calls the *instance browsing* facility which returns the set of "candidate" agents that satisfy the requirements expressed by the CIG annotations (plus possible additional requirements introduced by the agent). The agent has to find in such a set a candidate willing to accept the new responsibility. Therefore, the agent selects one of the candidates and sends her\him an *accept_responsibility?({(A$_1$, T$_{A1}$)..., (A$_k$, T$_{AK}$)})* message, indicating all the actions and their time windows. If the candidate accepts them, the *agent stacks* of A$_1$, ..., A$_K$ are created, specifying the new responsible, otherwise the search for a responsible goes on, considering (in the order chosen by the agent) the following candidate.

The *find_delegate?* and *find_executor*? functions operate similarly, supporting the identification of appropriate delegates (if desired) and executors (compulsory) to actions (through the use of *accept_delegation?* and *accept_execution?* messages) and taking into account continuity groups.

In our approach, each agent has the possibility to receive and send different types of messages, depending on her current role (responsible, delegate, executor).

Responsible

Receipt of an execute(A, T$_A$) message. In our approach, the CIG execution engine only sends *execute(A, T$_A$)* messages to agents indicated in the agent stack of the action A, i.e., to agents that have already explicitly accepted to execute such an action. However, the acceptance time could be long before the time when the execute message is received. As a matter of facts, an agent may have accepted to execute all the actions in a continuity group, along a quite long range of time. Therefore, despite the fact that the agent has already accepted, we also support the case that, for any reason, at the time when A must be executed, the responsible wants\needs to decline (e.g., the responsible of a patient with a chronic disease may retire or move away). We allow her to do so, but with a restriction: before "retiring", the current responsible must find a new responsible for the action A and the other actions (not executed yet) in the responsibility continuity group of A (using the *find_responsible* function).

On the other hand, if the responsible still retains her responsibility, she still has several options: she can

(i)   **delegate** DCG(A) (i.e., A and all the other actions in the Delegate Continuity Group of A), through the *find_delegate* function,

(ii) **find an executor** for ECG(A) (i.e., A and all the other actions in the Executor Continuity Group of A), through the *find_executor* function,

(iii) directly **execute** A herself.

Receipt of a next_responsible?({(A1, T_{A1}),..., (Ak, T_{Ak})}) message
The current responsible is in charge of identifying an appropriate responsible for the actions $A_1 \ldots A_k$. To support her in this task, we provide the *find_responsible* function, described above.

Receipt of an accept_responsibility?({(A1, T_{A1}),..., (Ak, T_{Ak})}) message
The agent may accept or reject the new responsibility.

Notably, soon after the acceptance of the responsibility of a set of actions {(A1, T_{A1}),..., (Ak, T_{Ak})} (a Responsibility Continuity Group of actions), the new responsible can soon search for delegates or executors for such actions (considering their Delegate and Executor Continuity Groups respectively), using the *find_delegate* and *find_executor* facilities. In such a way, the mechanism of determining delegates and executors can proceed in a (partially) asynchronous way with respect to the actual execution of actions in the CIG.

Delegate
When a delegate receives an **execute(A, T_A)** *message,* she may decline. Such a situation is directly managed by the execution engine (see Algorithm 2), which pops the delegate from Stack$_A$ and sends the *execute(A, T_A)* message to the new top of the stack. On the other hand, if the delegate retains her role, she can **delegate** DCG(A), **find an executor** for ECG(A) or directly **execute** A herself. Additionally, she may accept or reject an *accept_delegation?({(A1, T_{A1}),..., (Ak, T_{Ak})}) request.*

Notably, as in the case of responsibles, soon after the acceptance of the delegation of a set of actions {(A1, T_{A1}),..., (Ak, T_{Ak})} the new delegate can look for delegates or executors for such actions.

Executor
When an executor receives an **execute(A, T_A)** *message,* she may decline. Such a situation is directly managed by the execution engine, as described above (concerning delegates). Otherwise, she must execute action A within the time interval T_A. Additionally, she may accept or reject an *accept_execution?({(A1, T_{A1}),..., (Ak, T_{Ak})}) request.*

6 A Case Study

In this section, we present an application of our approach to a GL for alcohol-related problems [10], adapted to the Italian context (see Figs. 4 and 5). First, we describe the first part of CIG that has been acquired in META-GLARE. Then, we show META-GLARE in action.

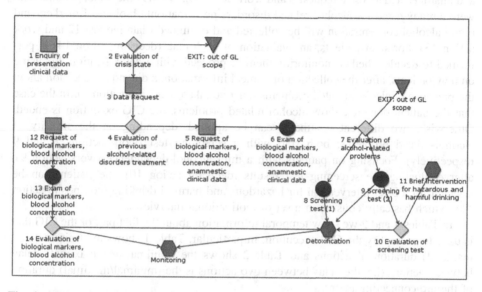

Fig. 4. META-GLARE graphical representation of part of the CIG on the treatment of alcohol-related disorders (original figure in [12]).

Responsibility Continuity Group : Responsible Qualification	Delegation Continuity Group : Delegate Qualification	Execution Continuity Group : Executor Qualification	Context	Action number
RG1 : R1, R4	DG1 : R1, R4	EG1 : R1, R2, R4	C1, C2, C3, C4, C5	1
			C1, C2, C3, C4, C5	2
	DG2 : R1, R4	EG2 : R1, R2, R4	C1, C2, C3, C4, C5	3
			C1, C2, C3, C4, C5	4
RG2 : R1	DG3 : R1	EG3 : R1	C1, C2, C3, C4	5
			C1, C2, C3, C4	7
RG3 : R1	DG4 : R1	EG4 : R5	C4	6
RG4 : R1	DG5 : R1	EG5 : R1	C1, C2, C3, C4	12
			C1, C2, C3, C4	14
RG5 : R1	DG6 : R1	EG6 : R5	C4	13
RG6 : R1	DG7 : R1	EG7 : R1, R2	C1, C2, C3, C4	8
	DG8 : R1	EG8 : R1, R2	C1, C2, C3, C4	9
			C1, C2, C3, C4	10
	DG9 : R1	EG9 : R1, R2	C1, C2, C3, C4	11

Fig. 5. The annotations of actions in Fig. 4 (original figure in [12]).

The CIG starts with the collection of the patient clinical data (query action 1). The data are used to diagnose whether the patient is currently experiencing a crisis state (decision action 2). Since the management of an alcohol-related crisis is outside the GL scope, the CIG ends. If, on the other hand, the patient is not experiencing a crisis, her clinical history is collected (query action 3), to distinguish whether it is the first time that the patient is in treatment for alcohol-related problems, or not (decision action 4). New patients require the collection of biological markers, blood alcohol concentration and anamnestic data (data request 5 and work action 6). On the other side, patients who were already cared for alcohol-related disorders need that only biological markers and blood alcohol concentration will be collected and examined (data request 12 and work action 13). For such patients, an evaluation of such data (decision action 14) is performed to decide whether monitoring them or proceed with a detoxification. Focusing on new patients, after the collection of clinical information, a diagnostic decision about the presence of alcohol-related problems must be taken (decision action 7). In the case that the patient does not show alcohol-related problems, the CIG execution is ended. Otherwise, two different treatments can be applied, depending on the severity of alcohol-related problems; both start with a screening test (work actions 8 and 9 respectively). Focusing on patients with a mild alcohol-dependence (work action 9), after evaluating the screening test results (decision action 10), the patient can be selected for a brief intervention for hazardous and harmful drinking (composite action 11), which basically consists in a set of motivational interviews.

In Tables 1 and 2 we show temporal information about the first part of the CIG that is used to exemplify the CIG execution. In particular, Table 1 shows the (minimal and maximal) duration of actions and Table 2 shows the (minimal and maximal) delay between actions (i.e. the delay between two actions is the (minimal/maximal) duration of the arc connecting them).

Table 1. Duration of the actions in the CIG.

Action number	Duration (min-max)
1	10–20 min
2	10–20 min
3	20–30 min
4	10–20 min
5	30–60 min
6	1–3 days
7	10–30 min
8	20–40 min
9	20–40 min
10	10–30 min
11	1–3 h
12	30–60 min
13	1–3 days
14	10–30 min

Table 2. Delay between actions in the CIG.

Delay between actions (from - to)	Duration (min-max)
1–2	0–20 min
2–3	0–30 min
3–4	20–60 min
4–5	1–2 days
4–12	1–2 days
5–6	1–2 days
6–7	1–2 days
7–8	1–6 h
8–9	1–6 h
9–10	1–2 h
10–11	1–3 days
12–13	1–2 days
13–14	1–3 days

Exploiting the annotation support (see Sect. 4.2), we have *annotated* all the actions defining the possible qualification(s) of its responsible, delegate (if any) and executor. Moreover, we have identified and specified the continuity groups in the CIG. In this specific application, possible values for the attributes in the annotations are the following:

- context: Community medicine (C1), SERT medicine (C2), in-patient care (C3), hospital ambulatory care (C4), social services (C5);
- qualification: physician (R1), nurse (R2), healthcare assistant (R3), social assistant (R4), laboratory technician (R5).

The treatment continuity criteria demand that all the actions corresponding to the initial evaluation of the patient status (actions 1–4) must have a unique responsible (responsibility continuity group RG1; see Fig. 5), which must be a physician (R1) or a social assistant (R4). The continuity group RG1 is further divided into two "subparts", corresponding to the two delegation continuity groups DG1 and DG2. In particular, DG1 corresponds to the identification of a crisis currently in progress (actions 1 and 2) and DG2 corresponds to the identification of previous alcohol-related disorder treatments (actions 3 and 4). Moreover, due to the execution continuity constraints, action 1 and action 2 belong to a single execution continuity group (EG1) and the actions 3 and 4 belong to a single execution continuity group (EG2). The executor of the actions in EG1 must be a physician (R1), or a social assistant (R4), or a nurse (R4). The actions in EG2 have the same constraints and the same annotations. After action 4, there are two alternative treatment paths. One path manages patients who are treated for alcohol correlated problems for the first time. Such a path is annotated with a responsibility continuity group RG2 on the actions to evaluate the patient's problem (action 5 and 7) and with a responsibility group RG3 on the exams needed for such an evaluation (action 6). RG2 and RG3 require a physician (R1) as responsible. Notably, a continuity group can contain non-contiguous actions (e.g., RG2 is composed by actions 5 and 7 which are not contiguous in the CIG).

In the following, we exemplify how META-GLARE extended execution engine can work on the above part of the CIG.

STEP 0: We suppose that the execution of the CIG starts at day 1 h 10 min 0. At the beginning, the META-GLARE executor engine identifies the first action (i.e. action 1) and puts it in the agenda. We suppose that agent A, a social assistant in the social services SS1, is the responsible of action 1. Since action 1 is in RG1, the responsibility of A regards all the actions belonging to such a continuity group (i.e., actions 1, 2, 3 and 4). Thus, the agent stacks of the four actions are created and initialized with X as responsible and with their time windows. In the initial step, the executor engine creates the agent stacks for actions 1-4 as follows (line 3 of Algorithm 1):

agent stack$_1$: (<(1, 10, 0), (1, 10, 0), (1, 10, 10), (1, 10, 15)>, <(A, R)>);
agent stack$_2$: (<(1, 10, 10), (1, 10, 25), (1, 10, 20), (1, 10, 45)>, <(A, R)>);
agent stack$_3$: (<(1, 10, 20), (1, 11, 15), (1, 10, 50), (1, 11, 55)>, <(A, R)>);
agent stack$_4$: (<(1, 11, 10), (1, 12, 55), (1, 11, 20), (1, 13, 15)>, <(A, R)>).

The agenda of the execution engine contains only action 1 and its temporal window, represented by the quadruple <(1, 10, 0), (1, 10, 0), (1, 10, 10), (1, 10, 15)>, that means that the action has to start between day 1 h 10 min 0 (i.e. the first triple) and day 1 h 0 min 0 (i.e. the second triple) and has to end between day 1 h 10 min 10 (i.e. the third triple) and day 1 h 10 min 15 (i.e. the last triple).

Agenda: <1, <(1, 10, 0), (1, 10, 0), (1, 10, 10), (1, 10, 15)>.

STEP 1: the executor engine sends an *execute* message for each action in the agenda (line 2 on Algorithm 2). In the agent there is only action 1, therefore the executor engine sends a message to the agent in the top element of the stack$_1$ (i.e., to A) to perform the execution of action 1. A receives the *execute* message and she decides to execute action 1 (i.e. she takes also the role of executor). Thus, A is put in the agent stack of action 1 as executor, and since actions 1 and 2 belong to the execution continuity group EG1, she has also the role of executor of action 2 (i.e. A is pushed as executor also onto the agent stack of action 2). At this point, the status of agent stacks and the agenda is the following:

agent stack$_1$: (<(1, 10, 0), (1, 10, 0), (1, 10, 10), (1, 10, 15)>, <(A, R), (A, E)>);
agent stack$_2$: (<(1, 10, 10), (1, 10, 25), (1, 10, 20), (1, 10, 45)>, <(A, R), (A, E)>);
agent stack$_3$: (<(1, 10, 20), (1, 11, 15), (1, 10, 50), (1, 11, 55)>, <(A, R)>);
agent stack$_4$: (<(1, 11, 10), (1, 12, 55), (1, 11, 20), (1, 13, 15)>, <(A, R)>).

A executes action 1 returning "OK" (line 2). The execution of action 1 lasts 10 min. Since action 1 has been executed, the executor engine removes it from the agenda (line 4). Then (line 5), the next action of the CIG is found (i.e. action 2) and it is put in the agenda with its time window and the agent stack of action 2 is updated with such a new time window (line 8). Action 2 has already a responsible, thus the agent stack of action 1 is simply deleted.

agent stack$_2$: (<(1, 10, 10), (1, 10, 20), (1, 10, 20), (1, 10, 40)>, <(A, R), (A, E)>);
agent stack$_3$: (<(1, 10, 20), (1, 11, 15), (1, 10, 50), (1, 11, 55)>, <(A, R)>);
agent stack$_4$: (<(1, 11, 10), (1, 12, 55), (1, 11, 20), (1, 13, 15)>, <(A, R)>).
Agenda: <2, <(1, 10, 10), (1, 10, 20), (1, 10, 20), (1, 10, 40)>>.

STEP 2: The above procedure is similarly repeated for action 2 in the Agenda. We suppose that, after receiving the message, A, who is registered as executor of action 2, executes it. A decides that the patient is not experiencing a crisis. Action 2 starts at day 1 h 10 min 10 and ends at day 1 h 10 min 30 (i.e. action 2 lasts 20 min). Thus, the next action is action 3 and then action 3 is put in the agenda with its time window and as consequence the time window in agent $stack_3$ is updated. Also in this case, action 3 has its responsible already defined (i.e. A).

agent $stack_3$: (<(1, 10, 30), (1, 11, 0), (1, 11, 0), (1, 11, 50)>, <(A, R)>);
agent $stack_4$: (<(1, 11, 10), (1, 12, 55), (1, 11, 20), (1, 13, 15)>, <(A, R)>).
Agenda: <3, <(1, 10, 30), (1, 11, 0), (1, 11, 0), (1, 11, 50)>>.

STEP 3: Action 3 is the only action in the Agenda and is managed by sending an *execute* message to its responsible A (i.e. A is on the top of stack in agent $stack_3$). In this case we suppose that A decides to ***delegate*** such an action. Exploiting the instance browsing facility of our navigation tool (see Sect. 4.1), A searches for an agent satisfying the requirements for action 3 (i.e. a social assistant or a physician in her context). Through the navigation tool, A obtains a list of possible agents. She selects a preferred one from the list and asks for acceptance, until she receives a positive reply. We suppose that (possibly after some negative replies of social assistants due to the time window associated to the action) the social assistant B accepts. Since actions 3 and 4 belong to the same delegation continuity group (i.e. DG2), B is also delegated for action 4.

agent $stack_3$: (<(1, 10, 30), (1, 11, 0), (1, 11, 0), (1, 11, 50)>, <(A, R), (B, D)>);
agent $stack_4$: (<(1, 11, 10), (1, 12, 55), (1, 11, 20), (1, 13, 15)>, <(A, R), (B, D)>).
Agenda: <3, <(1, 10, 30), (1, 11, 0), (1, 11, 0), (1, 11, 50)>>.

B decides to be the executor of action 3. Since actions 3 and 4 belong to the same execution continuity group EG2, B is nominated also as the executor of action 4 and she is put in the two stacks as executor.

agent $stack_3$: (<(1, 10, 30), (1, 11, 0), (1, 11, 0), (1, 11, 50)>, <(A, R), (B, D), (B, E)>);
agent $stack_4$: (<(1, 11, 10), (1, 12, 55), (1, 11, 20), (1, 13, 15)>, <(A, R), (B, D), (B, E)>).
Agenda: <3, <(1, 10, 30), (1, 11, 0), (1, 11, 0), (1, 11, 50)>>.

Y executes action 3. Action 3 starts at day 1 h 10 min 40 and lasts 40 min. Then action 4 is put in the agenda as next action with it is time window and as consequence the time windows in agent $stack_4$ are updated.

agent $stack_4$: (<(1, 11, 40), (1, 12, 20), (1, 11, 50), (1, 12, 40)>, <(X, R), (B, D), (B, E)>).
Agenda: <4, <(1, 11, 40), (1, 12, 20), (1, 11, 50), (1, 12, 40)>>.

STEP 4: The engine takes action 4 from the agenda, then it notifies to B (i.e. B is on the top of stack in agent $stack_4$) to execute action 4. Exploiting the instance browsing facility B identifies the agent C as executor of action 4. C satisfies the action annotations (i.e. she is a nurse and operates in SS1). When she accepts the assignments, she is put on agent $stack_4$ as executor.

agent $stack_4$: (<(1, 11, 40), (1, 12, 20), (1, 11, 50), (1, 12, 40)>, <(A, R), (B, D), (C, E)>).
Agenda: <4, <(1, 11, 40), (1, 12, 20), (1, 11, 50), (1, 12, 40)>>.

C executes action 4 at day 1 h 12 min 0 and its execution lasts 20 min. C identifies that the patient is treated for alcohol-related problems for the first time (i.e. the next action is action 5). Thus, action 5 is put in the agenda with its time window. Action 5 has not yet a responsible (line 9), thus the system asks A, the responsible of action 4 (i.e., the element at the bottom of the stack in agent $stack_4$) to find a responsible for such a new action. A must find a responsible who satisfies the action annotation (i.e. an agent who is a physician (R1) and works either in a Community medicine (C1) or in a SERT medicine (C2) or in-patient care (C3) or in a hospital ambulatory care (C4)). Using the instance browsing facilities, A finds a physician D, who works in the community medicine CM1, and asks her for the responsibility of action 5. D accepts the responsibility and, since action 7 belongs to the same responsibility continuity group (RG2), D is also nominated as responsible of both the actions in RG2.

agent $stack_5$: (<(2, 12, 00), (3, 12, 00), (2, 12, 30), (3, 13, 00), <(D, R)>>);

agent $stack_7$: (<(5, 12, 30), (10, 13, 00), (5, 12, 40), (10, 13, 30), <(D, R)>>).

Agenda: <5,<<(2, 12, 00), (3, 12, 00), (2, 12, 30), (3, 13, 00)>>.

Then, the CIG execution goes on in a similar way.

7   Comparisons and Conclusions

Clinical guidelines encode the "best" evidence-based procedures to treat specific diseases, and are important in order to ensure the quality of healthcare treatments. However, they usually involve the activity of multiple healthcare agents, operating in different contexts, having different qualifications and competences, and playing different roles (e.g., responsible vs. executor of an action). In our research, we have extended META-GLARE, our system to manage CIGs, to provide users with a comprehensive and homogeneous set of facilities to manage the above phenomena. In particular, META-GLARE allows to distinguish among different "roles" that an agent can play in the management of a CIG action: *responsible*, *delegate* and *executor*. For each action, META-GLARE supports the specification of the *qualification* and of the specific *competences* that each responsible, delegate and executor must have to manage it, as well as the *context* in which the action has to be managed. We also support a set of *facilities for agent coordination* to grant that, at each time during the execution of a CIG on a specific patient, each action to be executed "next" has a "proper" responsible and an executor (and, possibly, some delegate), and is executed in a "proper" context. Additionally, we also support "continuity constraints", to grant that, whenever possible, actions requiring the same qualification and competences are managed by the same agent. Last, but not least, our approach deeply takes into account the temporal dimension. Temporal reasoning is exploited in order to indicate the time window when actions have to be executed. Such an information is provided to executors, but is also used to find responsibles and delegates (accepting to manage the actions in the indicated time window).

Notably, we have described our approach on the basis of META-GLARE, but it is worth stressing that our methodology is completely general and system\ application-independent (i.e. other CIG systems can be extended applying our approach).

The approach described in this paper is the result of a stream of research in the area of CIG agent coordination, that we started already in [25]. In such an approach, we only considered the *responsibles* of actions. We have proposed to annotate (*colour*, in the terminology in [25]) CIG actions with *context, qualification* and *competences* for the responsible, and we have proposed several facilities to acquire and query annotations, and to execute coloured CIGs. In [26] we have extended such an initial approach along two main directions:

(1) we have considered the distinction between responsibles, delegates, and executor, and proposed facilities to support the coordination of such different "roles";
(2) we have taken into account continuity constraints, representing them and considering them in the agent coordination process.

In this paper we propose a further step forward of our approach: to make our support fully applicable in the real practice, we also considered the ***temporal dimension***. Considering time is essential for the practical applicability of CIG systems, but deeply affects the complexity of the phenomena to be coped with. First of all, we had to enrich our approach with temporal reasoning capabilities, to evaluate the window of time in which the CIG actions have to be managed, according with the temporal constraints in the CIG, and with the time of execution of the previously executed CIG actions. Second, we had to properly integrate such temporal reasoning capabilities within the agent coordination process. Indeed, we suggest the agent coordination process is deeply affected by the temporal analysis, since the temporal windows of execution have to be evaluated not only when actions enter in the agenda (i.e., when actions have to be actually executed), but also at coordination time, when agents are requested to accept the responsibility, delegation, or execution of CIG actions, so that they can accept or reject also considering the estimated time when such actions will have to be carried on. To consider such fundamental issues, in this paper we have proposed the temporal reasoning facility (Sect. 4), and we have deeply extended the coordination facilities (Sect. 5), and the CIG executor engine (Sect. 5) presented in our previous work in [26].

While in the literature there is no other approach to CIGs that has provided a support considering all the aspects above, several approaches have faced at least few of them.

First of all, the treatment of the temporal dimension of CIG has attracted quite a lot of attention within the medical informatics community. For instance, GLIF [27, 28] deals both with temporal constraints on patient data elements and with duration constraints on actions and decisions. In PROforma [29], guidelines are modelled as plans, and each plan may define constraints on the accomplishment of tasks, as well as task duration and delays between tasks. Moreover, temporal constructs can also be used in order to specify the preconditions of actions. DILEMMA and PRESTIGE [30] model temporal constraints within conditions. EON [31] uses temporal expressions to allow the scheduling of guideline steps, and deals with duration constraints about activities. Moreover, by incorporating the RESUME system, it provides a powerful approach to cope with temporal abstraction. In EON, the Arden Syntax allows the representation of delays between the triggering event and the activation of a Medical Logic Module (MDL), and between MDLs [32].

Within the AI community, it is widely recognized that temporal constraints are almost useless if they are not paired with adequate temporal reasoning mechanism to draw proper inferences from them [19], and many temporal reasoning approaches have been devised (see, e.g. the survey in [19]; Indeed, also the authors of this paper have been very active in the area [33–42]). However, the CIG community has paid only a (very) limited attention to temporal reasoning. This is quite surprising to us since, as discussed in [11] and in this paper, temporal reasoning is *necessary* to determine the time when next actions have to be executed (given the temporal constraints in the CIGs). Notable exceptions are represented by the approaches by Shahar [43] and by Duftschmid et al. [44].

In Shahar's approach, the goal of temporal reasoning is not to deal with temporal constraints (e.g., to check their consistency), but to find out proper temporal abstractions to data and properties. Therefore, temporal reasoning is not based on constraint propagation techniques, in fact, e.g., interpolation-based techniques and knowledge-based reasoning are used.

Miksch et al. have proposed a comprehensive approach based on the notion of temporal constraint propagation [43, 44]. In particular, in Miksch et al.'s approach, different types of temporal constraints – deriving from the scheduling constraints in the guideline, from the hierarchical decomposition of actions into their components and from the control-flow of actions in the guideline – are mapped onto an STP framework [20]. Temporal constraint propagation is used in order to (1) detect inconsistencies, and to (2) provide the minimal constraints between actions. In [44], there is also the claim that (3) such a method can be used by the guideline interpreter in order to assemble feasible time intervals for the execution of each guideline activity. Moreover, advanced visualization techniques are used in order to show users the results of temporal reasoning [45].

Notably, however, none of the above approaches have considered temporal reasoning in conjunction with the agent coordination phenomena discussed in this paper. Moreover, while several approaches to agent coordination have been proposed in the CIG literature (as widely discussed below), none of them takes into account the temporal reasoning facilities we propose in this paper.

In the formalism in [46], Fox's group has proposed an extension of the PROforma formalism to specify who will execute an action. However, the authors do not focus on agent coordination and action execution in different contexts. The goal of such a work is that of exploiting the pieces of information concerning agents for the sake of CIG contextualization (considering local human resources), and for flexibly adjusting them through delegation.

[47] have proposed a workflow-based solution to manage chronic patients over long time periods. Such an approach aims at allowing patients to obtain the necessary healthcare services by accessing different locations/organizations, which have to exchange/communicate health data whenever needed. The final goal of such an approach is to support cooperative work between different healthcare organizations; moreover, the authors model organizational knowledge (i.e. qualifications, resources etc.) by means of ontologies – as we do. However, their approach is not as flexible as ours, because interactions between agents, and allocations of the next action to a specific responsible, are strictly predetermined by a contract and cannot be determined dynamically during the CIG execution. On the other hand, we allow the responsible of the current action to navigate the ontology, and to dynamically and freely identify the responsible and\or the executor of the next action on the basis of the available

knowledge and constraints. Moreover, they do not support delegation, and do not take into account temporal reasoning issues.

[48] propose an ontology-driven execution of CIGs. Their approach relies on a *multi-agent* system, where agents in a medical center include not only persons, but also structures. In such an approach, the description of each CIG action includes a *hasResponsible* relation relating the action to one agent or to a set of agents. The main contribution of such an approach regards the delegation issue in a supervised fashion and the automation of the coordination of internal activities using a medical-organisational ontology. Since their approach is meant to be applied within a specific medical centre, it is focused on supporting interaction in a distributed environment, where the coordination between actors cannot be managed automatically.

Grando et al. [49] formalize cooperative work in CIG execution (but not distributed executions across different contexts). Their approach mainly focuses on the delegation of tasks to specific members of the working team, on the basis of their competences. Specific attention is devoted to cope with the assignment of the responsibility to enact services, and to exception handling. Specifically, they extend the design pattern framework introducing the types *role* (qualification in our approach) and *actor,* and a set of relations between key concepts. Since actors have roles and competences, they recall our notion of *agent.* Therefore, the authors take into account notions that are quite similar to our annotations. However, they do not consider the use of an ontology to formalize and standardize them. On the other hand, Grando et al. do not consider contexts: in this sense, their approach is more limited than ours, and not straightforwardly extendable to deal also with *distributed* (and not just *cooperative*) CIG executions. Moreover, temporal reasoning issues are not taken into account by Grando et al.

[50] have proposed a framework to support coordinated CIG execution by interdisciplinary healthcare teams. They distinguish among team managers, practitioner assistants, patient representatives (notably, such classes do not correspond either to our *qualification* classes, or to our roles). They have the concept of *capability,* which strictly resembles the notion of *competence* in our approach. They annotate actions, but their annotations are only related to the capability requirements. A main difference with respect of our approach is that Wilk et al. only consider CIG action *executors,* while they do not take into account *responsibles* and *delegates.* Moreover, they have the concept of team, i.e. a set of agents (defined using a hybrid approach) who manage the execution and are coordinated by a team manager, i.e. the responsible of execution for the whole CIG. The identification of executor of an action is not as general as the one in our approach: only the team manager can identify the executors and she has to take into account the agents in her team first. Only in the case that there are not any suitable and available agents in the team, she can search an external agent to execute the action and can add it to the team. Additionally, they do not cope with the notion of context of execution, as well as with temporal reasoning.

In summary, despite a huge interest of the Medical Informatics community in the CIG agent coordination phenomena, no approach in the literature has been devised until now coping with all the different issue covered by the approach we have proposed in this paper. In particular, to the best of our knowledge, our approach is the first CIG approach to agent coordination facing the temporal dimension through temporal reasoning, to determine the execution time of CIG actions.

Acknowledgments. The authors are very grateful to Prof. Gianpaolo Molino and Dr. Mauro Torchio of Azienda Ospedaliera San Giovanni Battista in Turin (one of the largest hospitals in Italy) for their constant support, and for their help in the definition of the case study.

References

1. Committee to Advise the Public Health Service on Clinical Practice Guidelines, Institute of Medicine: Clinical practice guidelines directions for a new program. National Academy Press, Washington, D.C. (1990)
2. Fridsma, D.B.: Special issue on workflow management and clinical guidelines. J. Am. Med. Inform. Assoc. **22**, 1–80 (2001)
3. Gordon, C., Christensen, J.P. (eds.): Health Telematics for Clinical Guidelines and Protocols. IOS Press, Amsterdam (1995)
4. Peleg, M.: Computer-interpretable clinical guidelines: a methodological review. J. Biomed. Inform. **46**, 744–763 (2013)
5. Terenziani, P., Montani, S., Bottrighi, A., Torchio, M., Molino, G.: Supporting physicians in taking decisions in clinical guidelines: the GLARE "what if" facility. In: Proceedings of AMIA Symposium, p. 772 (2002)
6. Montani, S., Terenziani, P.: Exploiting decision theory concepts within clinical guideline systems: Toward a general approach. Int. J. Intell. Syst. **21**, 585–599 (2006)
7. Isern, D., Moreno, A.: A systematic literature review of agents applied in healthcare. J. Med. Syst. **40**, 43 (2016)
8. Bottrighi, A., Terenziani, P.: META-GLARE: a meta-system for defining your own computer interpretable guideline system - architecture and acquisition. Artif. Intell. Med. **72**, 22–41 (2016)
9. Terenziani, P., Montani, S., Bottrighi, A., Molino, G., Torchio, M.: Applying artificial intelligence to clinical guidelines: the GLARE approach. Stud. Health Technol. Inform. **139**, 273–282 (2008)
10. Scottish Intercollegiate Guidelines Network: Management of harmful drinking and alcohol dependence in primary care. https://lx.iriss.org.uk/sites/default/files/resources/sign74.pdf
11. Anselma, L., Terenziani, P., Montani, S., Bottrighi, A.: Towards a comprehensive treatment of repetitions, periodicity and temporal constraints in clinical guidelines. Artif. Intell. Med. **38**, 171–195 (2006)
12. Bottrighi, A., Piovesan, L., Terenziani, P.: Supporting multiple agents in the execution of clinical guidelines. In: Zwiggelaar, R., Gamboa, H., Fred, A.L.N., and i Badia, S.B. (eds.) Proceedings of the 11th International Joint Conference on Biomedical Engineering Systems and Technologies (BIOSTEC 2018) - Volume 5: HEALTHINF. pp. 208–219. SciTePress (2018)
13. Terenziani, P., Montani, S., Bottrighi, A., Torchio, M., Molino, G., Correndo, G.: A context-adaptable approach to clinical guidelines. Stud. Health Technol. Inform. **107**, 169–173 (2004)
14. Montani, S., Terenziani, P., Bottrighi, A.: Exploiting decision theory for supporting therapy selection in computerized clinical guidelines. In: Miksch, S., Hunter, J., Keravnou, Elpida T. (eds.) AIME 2005. LNCS (LNAI), vol. 3581, pp. 136–140. Springer, Heidelberg (2005). https://doi.org/10.1007/11527770_19

15. Bottrighi, A., Giordano, L., Molino, G., Montani, S., Terenziani, P., Torchio, M.: Adopting model checking techniques for clinical guidelines verification. Artif. Intell. Med. **48**, 1–19 (2010)

16. Holzmann, G.: SPIN Model Checker: The Primer and Reference Manual. Addison-Wesley Professional, Boston (2003)

17. Piovesan, L., Molino, G., Terenziani, P.: Supporting physicians in the detection of the interactions between treatments of co-morbid patients. In: Healthcare Informatics and Analytics: Emerging Issues and Trends. pp. 165–193. IGI Global (2014)

18. Piovesan, L., Terenziani, P., Molino, G.: GLARE-SSCPM: an intelligent system to support the treatment of comorbid patients. IEEE Intell. Syst. **33**, 37–46 (2018)

19. Vila, L.: A survey on temporal reasoning in artificial intelligence. AI Commun. **7**, 4–28 (1994)

20. Dechter, R., Meiri, I., Pearl, J.: Temporal constraint networks. Artif. Intell. **49**, 61–95 (1991)

21. Brusoni, V., Console, L., Terenziani, P., Pernid, B.: Later: managing temporal information efficiently. IEEE Expert. **12**, 56–64 (1997)

22. Meiri, I.: Combining qualitative and quantitative constraints in temporal reasoning. In: Proceedings of the ninth National conference on Artificial intelligence-Volume 1, pp. 260–267. AAAI Press (1991)

23. Isern, D., Moreno, A.: Computer-based execution of clinical guidelines: a review. Int. J. Med. Inf. **77**, 787–808 (2008)

24. Terenziani, P., Bottrighi, A., Rubrichi, S.: META-GLARE: a meta-system for defining your own CIG system: architecture and acquisition. In: 6th International Workshop on Knowledge Representation for Health Care, pp. 92–107 (2014)

25. Bottrighi, A., Molino, G., Montani, S., Terenziani, P., Torchio, M.: Supporting a distributed execution of clinical guidelines. Comput. Methods Programs Biomed. **112**, 200–210 (2013)

26. Bottrighi, A., Piovesan, L., Terenziani, P.: Supporting multiple agents in the execution of clinical guidelines. In: Proceedings of the 11th International Joint Conference on Biomedical Engineering Systems and Technologies (BIOSTEC 2018) - Volume 5: HEALTHINF, pp. 208–219. SciTePress (2018)

27. Ohno-Machado, L., et al.: The guideline interchange format: a model for representing guidelines. J. Am. Med. Inform. Assoc. **5**, 357–372 (1998)

28. Peleg, M., et al.: GLIF3: the evolution of a guideline representation format. In: Proceedings of the AMIA Symposium, p. 645. American Medical Informatics Association (2000)

29. Fox, J., Johns, N., Rahmanzadeh, A.: Disseminating medical knowledge: the PROforma approach. Artif. Intell. Med. **14**, 157–182 (1998)

30. Gordon, C., Herbert, I., Johnson, P.: Knowledge representation and clinical practice guidelines: the DILEMMA and PRESTIGE projects. Stud. Health Technol. Inform. 511–515 (1996)

31. Musen, M.A., Tu, S.W., Das, A.K., Shahar, Y.: EON: a component-based approach to automation of protocol-directed therapy. J. Am. Med. Inform. Assoc. **3**, 367–388 (1996)

32. Sherman, E.H., Hripcsak, G., Starren, J., Jenders, R.A., Clayton, P.: Using intermediate states to improve the ability of the Arden syntax to implement care plans and reuse knowledge. In: Proceedings of the Annual Symposium on Computer Application in Medical Care, p. 238. American Medical Informatics Association (1995)

33. Terenziani, P., Carlini, C., Montani, S.: Towards a comprehensive treatment of temporal constraints in clinical guidelines. In: Proceedings Ninth International Symposium on Temporal Representation and Reasoning, pp. 20–27 (2002)

34. Anselma, L., Bottrighi, A., Montani, S., Terenziani, P.: Extending BCDM to cope with proposals and evaluations of updates. IEEE Trans. Knowl. Data Eng. **25**, 556–570 (2013)

35. Anselma, L., Piovesan, L., Terenziani, P.: A 1NF temporal relational model and algebra coping with valid-time temporal indeterminacy. J. Intell. Inf. Syst. **47**, 345–374 (2016)
36. Anselma, L., Terenziani, P., Snodgrass, R.T.: Valid-time indeterminacy in temporal relational databases: semantics and representations. IEEE Trans. Knowl. Data Eng. **25**, 2880–2894 (2013)
37. Anselma, L., Bottrighi, A., Montani, S., Terenziani, P.: Managing proposals and evaluations of updates to medical knowledge: theory and applications. J. Biomed. Inform. **46**, 363–376 (2013)
38. Anselma, L., Stantic, B., Terenziani, P., Sattar, A.: Querying now-relative data. J. Intell. Inf. Syst. **41**, 285–311 (2013)
39. Piovesan, L., Anselma, L., Terenziani, P.: Temporal detection of guideline interactions. In: HEALTHINF 2015 - 8th International Conference on Health Informatics, Proceedings; Part of 8th International Joint Conference on Biomedical Engineering Systems and Technologies, BIOSTEC 2015, pp. 40–50 (2015)
40. Anselma, L., Piovesan, L., Terenziani, P.: Temporal detection and analysis of guideline interactions. Artif. Intell. Med. **76**, 40–62 (2017)
41. Anselma, L., Mazzei, A., De Michieli, F.: An artificial intelligence framework for compensating transgressions and its application to diet management. J. Biomed. Inform. **68**, 58–70 (2017)
42. Anselma, L., Piovesan, L., Sattar, A., Stantic, B., Terenziani, P.: A general approach to represent and query now-relative medical data in relational databases. In: Proceedings of the Artificial Intelligence in Medicine - 15th Conference on Artificial Intelligence in Medicine, AIME 2015, Pavia, Italy, 17–20 June 2015, pp. 327–331 (2015)
43. Shahar, Y., Miksch, S., Johnson, P.: The Asgaard project: a task-specific framework for the application and critiquing of time-oriented clinical guidelines. Artif. Intell. Med. **14**, 29–51 (1998)
44. Duftschmid, G., Miksch, S., Gall, W.: Verification of temporal scheduling constraints in clinical practice guidelines. Artif. Intell. Med. **25**, 93–121 (2002)
45. Kosara, R., Miksch, S.: Metaphors of movement: a visualization and user interface for time-oriented, skeletal plans. Artif. Intell. Med. **22**, 111–131 (2001)
46. Sutton, D.R., Fox, J.: The syntax and semantics of the PRO forma guideline modeling language. J. Am. Med. Inform. Assoc. **10**, 433–443 (2003)
47. Leonardi, G., Panzarasa, S., Quaglini, S., Stefanelli, M., Van der Aalst, W.M.: Interacting agents through a web-based health serviceflow management system. J. Biomed. Inform. **40**, 486–499 (2007)
48. Sánchez, D., Isern, D., Rodríguez-Rozas, Á., Moreno, A.: Agent-based platform to support the execution of parallel tasks. Expert Syst. Appl. **38**, 6644–6656 (2011)
49. Grando, A., Peleg, M., Glasspool, D.: Goal-based design pattern for delegation of work in health care teams. In: MedInfo, pp. 299–303 (2010)
50. Wilk, S., et al.: MET4: supporting workflow execution for interdisciplinary healthcare teams. In: Fournier, F., Mendling, J. (eds.) BPM 2014. LNBIP, vol. 202, pp. 40–52. Springer, Cham (2015). https://doi.org/10.1007/978-3-319-15895-2_4

Realistic Synthetic Data Generation: The ATEN Framework

Scott McLachlan[1]([⊠]) [iD], Kudakwashe Dube[2] [iD],
Thomas Gallagher[3] [iD], Jennifer A. Simmonds[4],
and Norman Fenton[1] [iD]

[1] Queen Mary, University of London, London, UK
s.mclachlan@qmul.ac.uk
[2] Massey University, Palmerston North, New Zealand
[3] Missoula College, University of Montana, Missoula, MT, USA
[4] NSW Health, Sydney, NSW, Australia

Abstract. Getting access to real medical data for research is notoriously difficult. Even when data exist they are usually incomplete and subject to restrictions due to confidentiality and privacy. *Synthetic data* (SD) are best replacements for real data but must be *verifiably realistic*. There is little or no investigation into systematically achieving *realism* in SD. This work investigates this problem, and contributes the *ATEN framework,* which incorporates three component approaches: (1) THOTH for synthetic data generation (SDG); (2) RA for characterising realism is SD, and (3) HORUS for validating realism in SD. The framework is found promising after its use in generating the *realistic synthetic EHR* (RS-EHR) for labour and birth. This framework is significant in guaranteeing realism in SDG projects. Future efforts focus on further validation of ATEN in a controlled multi-stream SDG process.

Keywords: Synthetic data generation · Knowledge discovery

1 Introduction

The McGaw-Hill dictionary of Scientific and Technical Terms describes Synthetic Data as *any production data applicable to a given situation that are not obtained by direct measurement* [1]. Prior to [2] the domain of statistics, especially population statistics, primarily viewed synthetic data to be larger datasets that result from merging two or more smaller datasets [3, 4]. The earliest direct reference to synthetic data is a 1971 article describing creation of tables of synthetic data for use in testing, modifying, and solving problems with marketing data [5]. Other works present methods for creating fully synthetic data based on observed statistics [6, 7]; predicting and testing observational outcomes [8]; and generation driven by probability models for use in simulations [9]; and forecasting [10]. The *reasons for generating synthetic data* include software testing [11–14], population synthesis [15], hypotheses testing or generation of seed data for simulations [16, 17]. Recently, the major reason for generating synthetic data is limiting the release of confidential or personally identifiable information inherent to the use of real data sources [13, 18–20]. Some *synthetic data generation*

© Springer Nature Switzerland AG 2019
A. Cliquet jr. et al. (Eds.): BIOSTEC 2018, CCIS 1024, pp. 497–523, 2019.
https://doi.org/10.1007/978-3-030-29196-9_25

(SDG) approaches use *real data* either directly, or as seed data in their SDG methods [11, 21, 22]. Caution should be used prior to release of such synthetic datasets as a poorly designed or inappropriate model can still carry the risk of exposing confidential or personally identifiable information. Most contemporary research works have focused heavily on data *anonymization*, that is, isolating and replacing personally identifiable data with the concomitant goal of maintaining integrity of the data that an organisation may wish, or be required, to publish [23]. Anonymization has been dogged by modern methods for *re-identification of anonymised data* using a person's linkages to publicly available personal information sources, such as the electoral roll and newspaper articles [24–26]. As a result, some SDG methods also risk suffering inverse methods and re-identification attacks that ultimately breach personal privacy.

It is not enough to generate random data and hope it will be suitable to the purpose for which it will be used [27]. The data values may be required to fall within a defined set of constraints. For example, the *heart rate* should be a numerical value that falls within healthy resting (60–100), exercising (100–160) or disease state (40–60 or 160+) ranges. Some projects require increasingly more complicated datasets where not only the values of single attributes must be valid, but all values and interrelationships must be indistinguishable from observed data [28, 29]. *This is where the problem of realism becomes imperative,* yet it remains unexplored in current SDG literature [30]. The common sense implication of the term *realistic* is as [31] succinctly puts it: synthetic data that becomes *"sufficient to replace real data"*. The property of realism brings a greater degree of accuracy, reliability, effectiveness, credibility and validity [22]. Most researchers recognise the need for realism [18, 22, 31], however many leave realism unexplored in their works with only two authors giving some attention to it [18, 19]. In both cases this was vague and limited only to hinting that the aim of realism was that the synthetic data should be a representative replacement for real data [19], and comparably correct in size and distribution [18]. Neither handled validation of realism in the synthetic data they created. The lack of research attention makes it difficult to imbue realism into SDG methods, and to verify success in doing so. *Realism should only be asserted if it has been verified* [32, 33]. Scientific endeavours should always be concerned with testing and verification, yet few published approaches present systematic ways for validation [34, 35]. We find many SDG methods that claim success in the absence of a systematic ways of scientific validation [12, 36–38]. Some form of validation is necessary to support claims for realism in resulting synthetic data [32, 38, 39]. Otherwise, reliability of the approach must be questioned [40]. This work addressed these challenges and hereby presents the ATEN framework that allows realism to be inherent in SDG methods while also incorporating validation of realism in the resulting synthetic data.

The rest of this chapter is organised as follows: First, a review of related works focusing on SDG methods and realism is presented. Second, the ATEN framework and its component approaches, namely, THOTH, RA and HORUS, are covered in detail. Third, the ATEN framework is evaluated by applying it to the case of generating the synthetic electronic healthcare record (EHR) for labour and births. Fourth and finally, the chapter is concluded and summarised.

2 Related Works

A literature search was conducted to identify works describing methods or approaches for synthetic data generation (n = 7,746). This collection was reduced to works that also used the terms realistic (n = 290) or realism (n = 6) in describing either the need or purpose for synthetic data, their method, or the resulting synthetic dataset. The resulting collection included works that identified realism as a primary concern in the generation of synthetic data generally [12, 22, 41], or that discussed developing synthetic data that would be sufficient to replace, or be representative of, real data [13, 19, 31, 42]. Due to the low number of works that identified realism as a factor in synthetic data, a random selection of excluded works was included. This review found that one third of SDG articles focused on common goals, namely, *authenticity* [11], *accuracy* with respect to real structures [21], and the *replacement of real data* [43]. A key observation is the conspicuous absence, in the literature, of an investigation of **realism** for synthetic data, along with the lack of rigorous explanation of the approaches used to produce what authors claim to have been realistic datasets. *In the absence of a clear definition and framework for realism in the context of SDG, any process seeking to verify and validate realism in synthetic data is severely challenged.*

Works in the literature present common narrative for describing their SDG problem justification, operational method, and claimed results. This narrative consists of a common sequence of themes, each presented with two components. The themes are presented in Table 1. For the justification theme, research challenges include limited available data [44, 45] and privacy protection [37, 43]. Uses include testing of learning algorithms [45], enabling release of data [43], and prediction [37]. The operation theme includes SDG inputs such as network structures [45], observational statistics [44], and configuration files [37]. Methods ranged from random selection [45] and change behaviour modelling [37], to stochastic simulation using Markov models [44]. The result theme covers actions such as the use of benchmark and performance test simulation [45], comparative graphs [44], and performance analysis [46] used to assess published SDG methods. Resemblance to real networks [45], model advantages and capabilities [44] and likeness of the synthetic data to the synthetic scenario [37] were all reasons claimed by authors for claiming their SDG method was promising or successful.

Table 1. The common SDG narrative.

Narrative themes	Narrative components
Justification	It is difficult because of [*some difficulty*] to get real data for [*some use*], so we developed a new method to generate synthetic data for this purpose
Operation	Our method uses [*some input*] to generate the synthetic data using [*some method*]
Result	We performed [*some action*] and believe that the synthetic data created by our method is promising for [*some reason*]

SDG approaches set the goal of simply producing synthetic data that is a suitable replacement for real data. The focus is heavily weighted toward the outcome, the synthetic data. **Validation** of realistic aspects of synthetic data tended to be absent or singular or simplistic, ranging from direct comparisons between either the entire dataset or fields within the synthetic data to observations drawn from the real data [22], or graphical and statistical comparisons between the two [21, 44, 47]. The majority did not discuss validation at all [36, 48, 49]. Disclosure of the validation approach in research work completes and improves understandability of their work. It would also allow researchers to adequately assess whether or not a project met its goal; and the success claimed is truly justified [50]. This characteristic ensures that SDG experiments can be independently verified to the same standard as other scientific endeavours.

3   ATEN: The Framework for Realistic Synthetic Data Generation

It is common to see methodologies with multiple separate, combined, or sequential components presented as a framework [51]. This section presents the ATEN framework shown in Fig. 1. The ATEN framework is a synthesis of three interdependent component approaches, THOTH, RA, and HORUS which, when used together infuse realism into synthetic data. Each component of the ATEN framework seeks to answer the related questions in Table 2. The sections that follow describe in detail each of the components of ATEN.

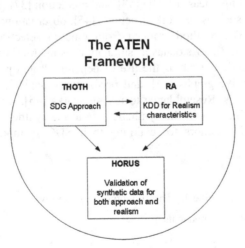

Fig. 1. The ATEN framework [52].

Table 2. ATEN component aims.

THOTH	How should we generate this synthetic data?
RA	What knowledge is necessary to achieve realism in the synthetic data?
HORUS	When THOTH operates using RA's knowledge, was realism achieved in the resulting synthetic data?

3.1 THOTH: The Enhanced Generic Approach to SDG

A review of the way authors described data generation approaches yielded a generic four-step SDG approach, which incorporates the minimum common structural elements shared by all SDG methods. The approach is presented as a waterfall model, primarily due to its cumulative and sequential nature. Thus, the next phase is undertaken solely through completion of the previous [53]. Verification, a required step of any scientific endeavour but one rarely seen in the context of SDG, can only occur during limited opportunities at the end of each step of the approach [53] and after the SDG operation is complete. The following paragraphs present the four-step SDG approach.

1. *Identify the need for synthetic data:* This step involves recognising both the need and justification, or reason, for creating synthetic data. The most commonly expressed justification across the contemporary literature was that the synthetic data being created was necessary to replace real data containing personally identifiable, sensitive or confidential information.
2. *Knowledge gathering:* This step can involve a number of sub-steps assessing the requirements for the synthetic dataset being created. It usually begins with analysis of the data to be generated, identifying such things as necessary fields to be generated, the scope, and any constraints or rules to be imposed.
3. *Develop the method or algorithm:* It is not unusual for researchers to identify common solutions that have become preferred for a given research method or field; a method or algorithm that has drawn significant focused attention or is considered more reliable to producing a particular outcome. Many of these algorithms have operational steps or processes requiring focused attention, or for which data must be properly prepared. Developing the generation solution is as important as the need, and the level of attention paid during this step has a direct relationship to the quality of the output.
4. *Generate the synthetic data:* The process of generation involves presenting any seed data, conditional requirements, rules, and constraints to the generation algorithm that will perform the processes that output synthetic data.

This four-step approach represents a simple method, which are favoured due to its usefulness, reduced complexity, and experiment time; all of which reduces cost [54–57]. However, the approach suffers the waterfall model weakness; flowing unidirectionally, lacking flexibility, meaning any change in requirements or issues identified necessitate expensive and time consuming redevelopment and retesting [58]. For this reason, a more adaptable and agile approach to SDG development should be encouraged. Pre-planning and preparation may mitigate the weaknesses of the generic SDG waterfall model. This is where THOTH will assist. THOTH encourages the synthetic data creator to perform decisive steps prior to engaging in the generation process. THOTH begins with characterisation, that is, identifying the level of synthetic-ness desired in the data to be generated. The synthetic-ness required of generated data can range from anonymisation of personally identifiable components in real data, through to truly synthetic data relying on no personally identifiable information during the creation process. The five primary characterisation types are shown in Table 3.

The characterisation level provides an element that aids in the second step, selection of the classification, or generation model, from the following five categories of synthetic generation methods: (i) data masking models that replace personally identifiable data fields with generated, constrained synthetic data [13, 43, 59], (ii) those that embed synthetic target data into recorded user data in a method known as Signal and Noise [11, 18, 60], (iii) Network Generation approaches that deliver relational or structured data [21, 41, 45], (iv) truly random data generation approaches like the Music Box Model [61], and (v) probability weighted random generation models like the Monte Carlo [12], Markov chain [61], and Walkers Alias methods [62].

Table 3. Characteristics of synthetic data.

Truly synthetic data	Data generated where no confidential or sensitive data has been directly used. Approaches may rely on algorithms that populate a dataset with generic seed data based on statistical probability, or acute randomness. An example of Truly Synthetic Data can be seen in CoMSER [62]
Fully synthetic data	Data generated using real data in the knowledge discovery (pre-generation) phase, but where no real data carries across into the synthetic dataset. Examples include capturing and breaking up real-world data into elemental components, rebuilding these into entirely new rows of data. Another uses the real data to construct a database architecture, populating that database with synthetic data based on observation [12]
Partially synthetic data	Datasets containing some form of synthetic data intermixed or aggregated with unaltered real data. An example is the Outbreak-Detection system using simulated 'signals' superimposed on real background 'noise' [63]
Anonymised-only data	Projects that identify and replace, remove, or scramble sensitive fields within a dataset, leaving the remaining fields unchanged
Real data	Real or observed data in which no attempt has been made to anonymise, conceal or synthesise any values

When combined with the generic SDG approach discussed earlier, the resulting THOTH-enhanced generic approach is shown in Fig. 2. With these steps complete, the synthetic data creator engages the remaining steps from the generic SDG approach described previously. However, they are beginning with an additional level of wisdom that comes from knowing where they are going (the level of synthetic-ness required of their efforts) and the framework for how they are going to get there (the informed selection of a generation model).

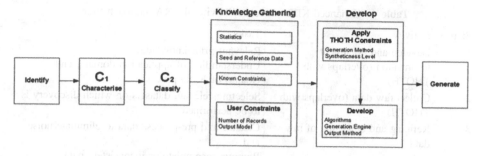

Fig. 2. THOTH integrated into the generic approach to SDG [52].

Summary of THOTH: We found a generic four-step waterfall approach is common to most SDG methods. This approach moves through identifying a need for synthetic data, gathering knowledge necessary to its generation, developing or customising an algorithm or generation method common to their domain or solution needs, before generating the synthetic data. Incorporation of THOTH benefits the researcher, providing greater awareness of their requirements and guiding the direction of the overall synthetic data generation approach.

3.2   RA: Characterising Realism for SDG

RA provides a structured approach to identifying and characterising realism elements, or knowledge, for use in SDG. The RA process, including the steps of enhanced knowledge discovery, are shown in Fig. 3 and described in Table 4. RA identifies extrinsic and intrinsic knowledge following a logical progression of steps, with increased focus on elements drawn from [64–67]. The following subsections present the processes used within the KDD data mining in Step 5 of Table 4.

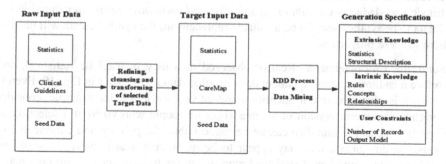

Fig. 3. Overview of the RA approach to realism in SDG [52].

Table 4. Enhanced KDD process following the RA approach [52].

Step	Activity	Tasks
1	Develop and document information (overlaps with THOTH)	Relevant prior knowledge Understanding of application domain, and Goal(s) of KDD process
2	Collect raw data (overlaps with THOTH)	Selecting relevant datasets on which discovery is to be performed
3	Refining and cleansing of raw data	Cleanse and pre-process data to eliminate noise, and Remove incomplete or inconsistent data
4	Create target data	Integrate data from multiple sources Transform raw data Project data by identifying useful features for representing the data, and Reduce variables to those that are necessary for KDD process
5	KDD and data mining	Identify data mining method to search for patterns within the target data (summarisation, classification, regression, clustering, web mining and others as described in Fayyad et al. [64]) Perform concept hierarchy analysis, formal concept analysis, rule identification methods used in HORUS
6	Interpret and evaluate mined patterns	Identify truly interesting and useful patterns
7	Presentation	Make knowledge available for use in synthetic data generation

RA: Extrinsic Knowledge

Extrinsic knowledge is the *sum of quantitative and qualitative properties* found in the real data to be synthesised. To be a suitable replacement, the synthetic data will need to adhere to these properties.

Quantitative Characteristics: Real or observed data may in itself be statistical, and therefore quantitative, such as patient demographic data shown later in Fig. 10. Even if it is not, it is often possible to identify quantitative knowledge, for example; consider generating a synthetic version of a spreadsheet of people who voted at a selection of polling booths, as the real data cannot be made public for privacy and confidentiality reasons. On the surface this may appear to be qualitative data however it would be possible to draw a number of statistical representations from it, such as: (a) how many people of each genealogical nationality voted in (b) each hour, (c) the percentage that were male, (d) the percentage of the overall population as found in census data voted in each polling booth, and so on.

Qualitative Characteristics: The qualitative characteristics of real or observational data should be identified and documented for any SDG project, but especially for those projects seeking realistic synthetic data. One example of qualitative characteristics may be to identify and describe the database schema. The database schema explains how the data is structured [68]. In the relational database example this includes expression of the tables, the fields within those tables, constraints such as those identifying the primary key or limiting field values along with any referential integrity constraints, or foreign keys [68].

Summary: Extrinsic Knowledge: These quantitative and qualitative observations of real data, once identified and documented, represent the characteristics that should be created and validated in synthetic data. This is especially true if authors present that there is a requirement for, or claim of, realism.

RA: Intrinsic Knowledge

Knowledge Discovery in Databases: While traditional methods of data mining often involved a manual process of scouring through databases in search of previously unknown and potentially useful information, these processes can be slow and an inefficient use of time [64, 66, 67]. Modern approaches, where the human is accentuated by machine learning or neural network algorithms are considered more expedient for realising insights from today's extremely large datasets [64, 66, 67].

Concept Hierarchies: Concept Hierarchies (CH) are a deduction of attribute-oriented quantitative rules drawn from large to very large datasets [69]. CH allow the researcher to infer general rules from a taxonomy, structured as general-to-specific hierarchical trees of relevant terms and phrases. For example: "bed in ward in hospital in health provider in health district" [67, 69, 70]. Developing a concept hierarchy involves organizing levels of concepts identified within the data into a structured taxonomy, reducing candidate rules to formulas with a particular vocabulary [69]. CH are used by RA to identify an entity type, the instances of that entity and how they relate to each other; they help to ensure identification of important relationships in the data that can be used to synthesise meaningful results [71].

Once the concept hierarchy tree is identified, a second pass across the source data is performed to provide an occurrence count for each concept. This second pass allows the researcher to enhance the concept hierarchy with statistical knowledge to improve accuracy of the generation model.

Formal Concept Analysis: Formal Concept Analysis (FCA) is a method of representing information that allows the researcher to easily realise concepts observed recognised from instances of relationships between objects and attributes. For example: occurrences of different nosocomial infections across the wards of a hospital. FCA starts with a formal context represented as a triple, where an object {G} and attribute {M} are shown with their incidence or relationship {I} [72]. A table is created displaying instances where a relationship exists between the object and its corresponding attribute(s).

Concept creation, represented as rules, occurs from the context table. For example, one might seek to identify the smallest or largest concept structures containing one particular object.

The second step to FCA involves creating the concept lattice. A concept lattice is a mapping of the formal context, or intersections of objects and attributes. The concept lattice allows easy identification of sets of objects with common attributes as well as the order of specialisation of objects with respect to their attributes [73].

Characteristic and Classification Rules: [69] provides a set of strategies that can be used to learn characteristic and classification rules from within a dataset. These rules can be applied as constraints during generation, and later as tools to compare against the resulting synthetic data to validate its accuracy and realism.

Characterisation Rules: The development of characteristic rules entails three steps. First, data relevant to the learning process is collected. All non-primitive data should be mapped to the primitive data using the concept hierarchy trees as shown in Fig. 5 (e.g. Forceps would be mapped to Assisted, Elective would map to Caesarean and so on). Second, generalization should be performed on components to minimize the number of concepts and attributes to only those necessary for the rule we are working to create. In this way, the *name* attribute on a patient record would be considered too general and not characteristic to a set of data from which we could make rules about the treatment outcomes for a particular ethnicity. The final step transforms the resulting generalization into a logical formula that identifies rules within the data. These rules are the sum of four elements, where if the values of any three of those elements are found to be consistent to the rule for a given instance in the dataset, the fourth element will always be true.

Classification Rules: Classification knowledge discovery discriminates the concepts of a target class from those of a contrasting class. This provides weightings for the occurrence of a set of attributes for the target class in the source dataset, and accounts for occurrences of attributes that apply to both the target and contrasting class. To develop a classification rule, first the classes to be contrasted, their attributes and relevant data must be identified. Attributes that overlap form part of the generalisation portion of the target class only. Attributes specific to a target class form the basis of classification rules.

RA: Summary
The RA enhanced and extended KDD method identifies realistic properties from real data, providing improved input data quality and constraints that improve the output of generation algorithms used to create synthetic data. An obvious benefit is that generation methods using this knowledge should deliver data that is an accurate replacement for real data. Another benefit is a set of knowledge and conditions that can be used in validation of realism in the data created. Its use for this last purpose is discussed in the next section.

3.3   HORUS: An Approach to Validating Realism

One of ancient Egypt's earliest precursor national gods, Horus, was revered as the god of the sky; that which contains both the sun and the moon. In the same way, the Horus approach to realism validation draws on both THOTH's enhanced generic SDG and RA's enhanced KDD approaches, effectively containing both the sun and moon as a means to validate for realism in synthetic data.

The validation approach incorporates five steps that analyse separate elements of the SDG method and resulting synthetic data. These steps are identified as the smaller square boxes in Fig. 4, with their descriptions below. Collectively, the five steps provide the information necessary for confirmation of whether synthetic data is consistent with and compares realistically to real data that the SDG model seeks to emulate.

Input Validation: Input validation concerns itself only with that knowledge coming from the generation specification in the form of data tables and statistics. The input validation process verifies each item, confirming that the right input data in the correct form is being presented to the generation engine, thus ensuring smooth operation of the data synthesis process [74]. Input validation is intended to prevent corruption of the SDG process [75].

Realism Validation 1: The first realism validation process verifies concepts and rules derived from the HCI-KDD process, along with any statistical knowledge that has been applied. Realism validation reviews and tests both the premise and accuracy of each rule to ensure consistency with the semantics of any data or guidelines used in their creation.

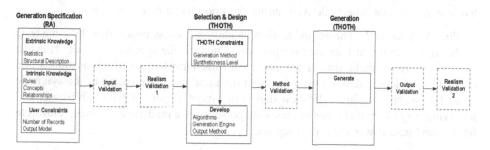

Fig. 4. HORUS approach to realism validation, showing touch points with THOTH and RA [52].

Method Validation: Method validation reviews the efforts of others inside and outside of the research domain. Attention is drawn to methodological approaches common for that domain, as well as methods other domains have employed for similar types of SDG. Evaluating the entire scope of method application ensures that which is chosen should be the most appropriate for the particular need and solution. Method validation also seeks to verify that the algorithm being used is correctly and completely constructed, and free of obvious defect [76].

Validation is not a search for absolute truth, more correctly, and in this instance, it is a search to establish legitimacy [76]. Table 5 provides the six key questions that should be asked of any SDG methodology the researcher may propose to use.

Table 5. Method validation questions [77].

Validation type	Validation focus
Conceptual	Does the theoretical model adequately represent the real world?
Internal	Is the algorithm and computer code that employs it free from error?
External	Does the algorithm and computer code adequately and accurately represent the real world?
Alignment	How does this model's output compare to that of other models?
Data	How does the synthetic data compare to real observed data?
Security	Have there been any undocumented changes or manipulations to the model or code that may contribute to or alter the results?

Output Validation: Output validation evaluates the output data and verifies its basic statistical content. This step demonstrates the difference between the two terms: validation and verification. Validation ensures the model is free from known or detectable flaws and is internally consistent [76]. Verification establishes whether the output, or predictions, of the SDG model are consistent with observational data. The output validation step ensures that the synthetically generated data conforms to the quantitative and qualitative aspects derived during the knowledge discovery phase.

Realism Validation 2: The second realism validation process undertakes the same tests as the first, except that tests are now performed against the synthetic dataset. This test aims to ensure synthetic data is consistent with the knowledge (rules, constraints and concepts) previously derived from the input data and used in creation of the synthetic data. The second realism validation step is the most important for establishing, and justifying, any claim that this synthetic data presents as a realistic and proper substitute for the real data it was created to replace.

3.4 Summary: Benefits of the ATEN Framework

There are a number of ways that ATEN benefits those engaging in SDG. First, it is a complete SDG lifecycle that considers every element before, during and after data generation. Second, it encourages more complete level of self-documentation than most presented in the SDG literature. The third benefit is cumulative from the first two, in that when applied during an SDG project, THOTH and RA provide the necessary knowledge to validate realism using HORUS. ATEN supports claims of success, realism, and enables repeatability. All of which are fundamental to the scientific method. Works found in the literature do not conform to the ATEN Framework, as significant gaps are evident in most SDG literature. The framework provides for additional knowledge discovery and documentation processes, which could be automated. However, this is dependent on the type of data being analysed, generation method, synthetic data sought, and the use to which that data will be applied. The knowledge discovery component leads to greater accuracy and help to support validation of realism.

4   Evaluating the ATEN Framework: The Labour and Birth EHR

This section evaluates ATEN by applying it to the **domain of midwifery**. While ATEN is intended to be generally applicable for use with any defined group of patients and chosen health problem or disease that has a Caremap, for the purposes of evaluating the ATEN framework, this work now focuses on the problem of generating the RS-EHR for only the delivery episodes for female patients who are giving birth in the Counties Manukau District Health Board (CMDHB) catchment area of Auckland in New Zealand. The practical advantages, to the authors, of focusing on delivery episodes for the purpose of this evaluation only are that: (1) deliveries take relatively short periods of time; (2) comprehensive statistics are readily available that cover a long period of time; (3) clinical guidelines as well as locally specified midwifery practice protocols derived from localisation of international clinical practice guidelines are widely available; (4) the delivery episode can range from being very simple to being very complex with a wide variety of complicating factors that include the health of the mother and that of the baby; and, (5) the authors had ready access to midwives on a regular basis throughout this research work. The rest of this section presents the prototype system, results of evaluation, and discussion of these results.

The labour and birth EHR contains a record of the labour and birth events starting at onset of labour and ending when delivery is complete and the new child is presented to her parents. To generate the labour and birth EHR in such a way that realism is achieved we apply the ATEN framework's components: THOTH, RA and HORUS. The next sections present this application, which leads to the synthetic labour and birth EHR that has the realistic properties that are guaranteed by the ATEN Framework.

THOTH is a combination of the generic method for SDG, combine with the pre-planning elements that characterise and classify the synthetic data being sought, in this case, the synthetic labour and birth EHR. Table 6 summarises the application of THOTH to the labour and birth scenario leading to the ingredients, method and context for the generation of the synthetic labour and birth EHR. In the context of the labour and birth EHR, the characterisation (truly synthetic data) was selected to meet with the ideal that we do not rely on access to the real EHR in the context of our generation approach. This ensures the highest degree of patient privacy as, unlike most other methods in this domain, no real patient records are necessary to this generation approach.

Analysis of SDG literature demonstrated that a probability weighted random generation approach was more likely to generate the synthetic records required. Also, other methods including the data masking and the signal and noise models required access to some amount of real (seed) EHR data, which discounted their use in this example.

RA is the knowledge discovery and characterisation approach seeking to identify realistic elements of the data gathered during THOTH. Application of RA specifically to the Labour and Birth problem required identification of the care process (Caremap) for labour and birth, as well as its concepts and contexts.

Table 6. Application of THOTH in the context of midwifery EHR generation.

Aspect of THOTH	Application to Labour & Birth context
Identify	Midwifery EHR in the context of the Labour and Birth event
Characterisation	Truly Synthetic Data
Classification *(method/algorithm)*	Probability Weighted Random Generation
Knowledge Gathering *(used in data/knowledge-driven generation algorithm)*	Clinical Practice Guidelines & organisational caremaps Ministry of Health (MoH) Labour and Birth statistics Expert Clinical Knowledge from Midwives and Obstetricians Population (census) demographic data Clinical Vocabulary Clinical Notes Library (authored by midwives)

Extrinsic Knowledge *Quantitative Properties:* The quantitative properties in the domain of midwifery included a range of demographic statistics regarding the mother and baby. Essentially they were not as simple as looking at the examples in blue contained in Fig. 10, presented later in this section, and saying that 22% of mothers were European, or that 24% of mothers were aged between 20–24 years. There were inter-relationships between these values that also needed to be modelled, including that of the 24% of mothers between 20 and 24 years of age, only 8% were identified as European. Other statistics included how many mothers delivered naturally versus by caesarean section, and the spread of clinical interventions across ethnicity, age, and gestation.

Qualitative Properties: A range of qualitative properties were assessed within the knowledge gathered for generating midwifery EHRs. These included the structure of the source data being used, as well as the structure and appearance of how the synthetic data should be presented on generation. A truncated example of how demographic data was structured in one midwifery EHR system is shown in Table 7. Other qualitative aspects might include: (a) logical internal consistence between the dates reported in different fields (last menstrual period, estimated due date, and so on), (b) whether fields have been misappropriated as placeholders for other data types, and (c) the completeness of fields within the dataset.

Table 7. Application of THOTH in the context of midwifery EHR generation [52].

Patient		
PK	patientID	INT
	title	TEXT(10)
	lastName	TEXT(30)
	firstName	TEXT(30)
	dateOfBirth	DATETIME
	gender	CHAR(10)
	ethnicity	CHAR(20)
	primaryLanguage	VARCHAR(100)

Intrinsic Knowledge Concept Hierarchy for Labour and Birth Domain: An extract focusing on child birth from the concept hierarchy (CH) developed for the labour and birth domain is presented in Fig. 5. The general term Childbirth breaks down into the two modes by which birth occurs, Caesarean and Vaginal. As an example; Caesarean births break down even further into the two specific types that occur, the elective or requested/planned caesarean and the emergency caesarean. In this way we are moving from the most general concept at the top to the most specific at the bottom. This is extended with the addition of quantitative statistics (in brackets) identified from the Ministry of Health (New Zealand) source data.

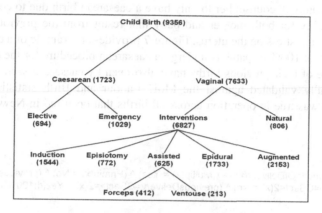

Fig. 5. Concept hierarchy enhanced with statistics [52].

The CH provides structural understanding of primary or significant concepts, from most general to most specific, within the domain being modelled. In RA, is also used to provide statistical understanding of the incidence of each concept. The CH provides constraints, or weights, that are applied during the generation phase, as well as forming one component used to verify statistical accuracy, and in turn realism, within the resulting synthetic data.

Constraining Rules: Characteristic Rule: Fetal heart monitoring is used in midwifery to assess the health, and stress being suffered, by the baby. In the domain of midwifery, we found that only those pregnancies clinically described as low risk receive intermittent fetal heart monitoring. However, clinical practice guidelines (CPGs) necessitate continuous monitoring for a higher risk pregnancy. Properties of this rule would be expressed as the sum of the four elements. The characteristic rule expressed in the conditional formula is shown in Fig. 6 containing the values: *Sex: Female, Pregnant: Yes; Pregnancy Status: Low Risk; Fetal Heart Monitoring: Intermittent in Labour.* This rule was validated against, and found to be consistent with, the CPGs for several hospital birthing facilities in New Zealand.

$$\forall \chi \ (\text{midwiferyPatient}(x) \rightarrow ((\text{Sex}(x) = \text{female}) \wedge (\text{Pregnant}(x) = \text{Yes}) \wedge (\text{pregnancyStatus}(x) = \text{Low Risk}) \wedge (\text{fetalHeartMonitoring}(x) = \text{Intermittent})))$$

Fig. 6. Example of a characteristic rule [52].

Classification Rule: The CPGs for Labour and Birth provide that where an expectant mother has had a previous caesarean birth, she may elect in this subsequent birth to still (safely) attempt a vaginal birth (known in medical terms as a VBAC - vaginal birth after caesarean). However, where she has had two or more previous caesarean births the obstetric team will counsel her to only have a caesarean birth due to considerations of risk and safety for both mother and baby that result from the previous caesarean scars and potential stress on the uterus. Figure 7 provides an example of a classification rule showing that 100% of patients undergo a caesarean procedure for the current birth if two or more of their previous births have also been by caesarean section. This rule was successfully validated against the MoH Labour and Birth statistics, with the finding that it was true in operation across all births that occurred in New Zealand for that year.

$$\forall \chi \ (\text{modeOfDelivery}(x) \rightarrow ((\text{Multip}(x) = \text{Yes}) \wedge (\text{Primip}(x) = \text{No}) \wedge (\text{previousDelivery=CSect<2}(x) = \text{No}) \wedge (\text{previousDelivery=CSect>=2}(x) = \text{Yes}[d{:}100\%])))$$

Fig. 7. Example of a classification rule [52]

Characterisation rules describe reduced collections of generalised attributes for a class occurring together in the dataset; where for any query of the dataset specifying n-1 attributes from the rule, the remaining attribute is the only one that can be true.

Classification rules describe specific collections of attributes that differentiate one class from one or more remaining classes; where the target class is the only response for a query against the dataset specifying all of the attributes defined in the rule. These rules are used to constrain generation, ensuring consistency between real-world and the synthetic. They are used during validation to identify instances where synthetic records may be inconsistent, for example, if the midwifery patient being generated was male.

Formalisation of Labour and Birth CPG into Labour and Birth Caremaps

The core set of constraints in the CoMSER Method [62] are CPGs, Health Incidence Statistics (HIS), patient demographic statistics and the Caremap, all formalised in an integrated way into the state transition machine (STM) following the process shown in Fig. 8 [51]. The STM is the constraint enforcement formalism for generating the RS-EHR entries satisfying the constraints.

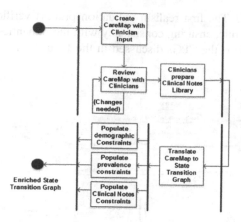

Fig. 8. UML activity diagram: process of creating and integrating constraints into State Transition Machine for the midwifery Caremap [62].

Figure 9 presents the UML State Diagram (USD) for the State Transition Machine (STM) that integrates the core constraints for generating the RS-EHR for delivery episodes within the Counties Manukau District Health Board (CMDHB) of Auckland, New Zealand (NZ).

The transition from one state to the next is determined by the pseudo-random selection of one state in the STM in which is stored the health incident prevalence constraint that is formally specified as the 2-tuple, $<P, O>$, such that P is the total number of patients who are known to enter the state according to statistics within the CMDHB catchment area, and O is the number of patients expressed as a percentage of the immediately preceding parent state. The caremap formalised by the STM in Fig. 9, covers the midwifery delivery event, which is also referred to, in this work, as the delivery episode. The caremap begins temporally at the point where the pregnant patient is established as 'in labour'. It follows the sequence of possible states, that is, clinical events or decisions or both, consistent with the locations, interventions and outcomes that are currently available to the patient or her treating clinicians until the birth process concludes in one of the possible outcomes. Thus, the Caremap and hence its STM form the basis of the integrated constraint framework and also the basis for the algorithm for the RS-EHR generation.

In validating the midwifery RS-EHR, **HORUS** was applied, adhering to the steps as presented in Fig. 4. The following subsections describe the results observed.

Input Validation: In creating the midwifery EHRs for the Labour and Birth event we used CPGs along with treatment and outcome statistics. Input validation necessitated ensuring statistics could be located or extracted that correctly applied to each part of the processes described in the CPGs. Also, cross-validation of those statistics was performed through comparison against more than one source. Where any difference in terminology existed between input datasets, clinicians were involved to ensure these data were correctly linked together [62].

Realism Validation 1: The first realism validation process verified both the premise and accuracy of each rule, ensuring consistency with the semantics of knowledge used in their creation, such as the CPGs discussed in the Input Validation example above.

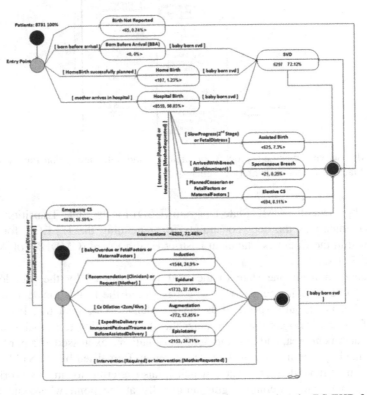

Fig. 9. UML State Diagram that integrates constraints for generating the RS-EHR for delivery episodes within the CMDHB catchment area of NZ [62].

They were tested in real circumstances to ensure they were not rendered irrelevant through interaction with the original source or observed data. Where any knowledge is at issue, the researcher should return to the knowledge discovery phase.

Method Validation: Method validation for these midwifery EHRs concluded that the use of caremaps extended with descriptive rules and statistics, presented as State Transition Machines, and a probability weighted generation model were appropriate given the available input knowledge, purpose and output data required of the CoMSER model.

Output Validation: As one example of output validation, statistical values from within the synthetic data were validated and verified against those identified in the knowledge gathered prior to generation. This comparison is shown as the orange line in Fig. 10, demonstrating that the values contained in the CoMSER synthetic midwifery records were consistent with the MoH statistics used in their production.

Realism Validation 2: In the example of RS-EHR, if a synthetic patient were to be treated in a manner contradictory to the principles or application of a CPG, this could invalidate the entire dataset. In the same instance, if seeking validation by clinicians, it may be necessary to present the synthetic EHR in a clinician-familiar manner.

Using the caremap STM in Fig. 9, the prototype system was used to generate midwifery RS-EHR for 1000 synthetic patients. Figure 11 presents a sample RS-EHR that has been generated by the CoMSER Method prototype. It should be noted that the

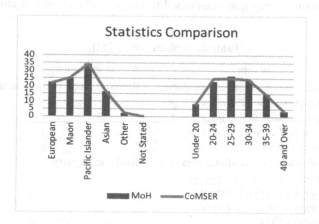

Fig. 10. A comparative quantitative example using patient demographics from the Ministry of Health (NZ) statistics with output validation from our prototype RS-EHR. (Color figure online)

Brianna Allen

Gender:	Female
Ethnicity:	European
DOB:	15 May 1978
NHI:	XX1234

Clinical Records View

Date	Time	Node	Clinical Note	Clinician
18 November 2014	9:05 AM	Start	G4P3	A.Midwife
18 November 2014	9:50 AM	>	Pt presenting to Labour and Birthing. Reports SRM 2 days ago, now reports brownish coloured fluid draining. CTG commenced. FH 188bpm. IV luer sited, bloods sent. IV plasmalyte commenced 500mL/hr. Mec liquor seen on pad, SRM confirmed. T 37.9, P 110 bpm, BP 102/66. Contracting 3:10, strong to palpate. VE: Cx 8 cm, St +1. Plan: commence IV fluids, for IV Abs for PROM, awaiting Obstetric review.	A.Midwife
18 November 2014	9:50 AM	Hospital Birth	Pt presenting to Labour and Birthing.	A.Midwife
18 November 2014	10:50 AM	>	BP 160/98. Call to obstetric consultant. Will attend shortly, meanwhile requesting that epidural be sited. CTG commenced, call to anaesthetist, who will attend shortly.	A.Midwife
18 November 2014	11.20 AM	Epidural	Epidural sited. BP following test dose 106/66. Epidural appears effective, pt now comfortable with contractions. BP stable.	A.Midwife
18 November 2014	2:20 PM	>	VE: Fully dilated, St +1, OA Clear liquor, normal CTG. Epidural remains effective. Plan: allow 1 hour for passive descent, then begin pushing.	A.Midwife
18 November 2014	3:50 PM	SVD	Spont delivery, live baby in poor condition. Cord clamped and cut, emergency bell rung for assisstance. Baby to Resuscitaire. 1mL Syntometrine to left thigh. Placenta and membranes delivered CCT, appear complete. Labial lacerations sutured, 4.0 vicryl. Fundus firm and central, EBL 300mL.	A.Midwife

Fig. 11. Sample realistic synthetic EHR generated by CoMSER.

column in the screenshot entitled "Node" indicates either the state or the transition in the STM from which the synthetic entry has been generated. The column has been inserted only for debugging purposes and may or may not be meaningful to the clinician.

A convenience survey of clinicians from New Zealand's midwifery discipline was conducted to assess the realistic characteristic of synthetic records generated using the CoMSER prototype application. The survey instrument used a forced choice Likert scale in which the clinician examined clinical and temporal notes independently and jointly. The realism survey questions posed to midwife clinicians is found in Table 8.

Table 8. Realism survey [62].

Ref	Survey response prompt	Aspect evaluated
Q1	After reviewing the record of a randomly selected patient, *I find the clinical notes for the record identical to the notes a clinician would expect to find in an actual patient EHR*	Realistic property for clinical notes
Q2	After reviewing the record of a randomly selected patient, *I find the temporal (day/time) information identical to what the clinician would expect to find in the actual patient EHR*	Realistic property for the temporal model
Q3	After reviewing the record of a randomly selected patient, *I find the clinical notes and temporal (day/time) information, when read together, has neither conflicts nor inconsistencies as would be expected in the actual patient EHR*	Realistic property for the entire RS-EHR and hence for clinical logic flow (*all constraints taken together*)

A total of n = 45 randomly selected records were examined (15 records each by 3 clinician experts) in answering whether the synthetic EHR possessed the same qualities as the clinician would expect to find in actual EHR. The results of this survey demonstrate that clinical and temporal notes, when examined independently, were identical in 93% (Q1) and 93% (Q2) of the records respectively, while 87% (Q3) of the records were identical when examined jointly. In assessing inter-rater reliability among the experts, inconsistencies between the RS-EHR and the actual EHR were identified in 0% (Expert 1), 7% (Expert 2), and 33% (Expert 3) of the records. This survey, involving practicing midwife clinicians, indicates that realism is found in the majority of clinical notes and temporal information, when examined independently and jointly, in synthetic EHRs produced by the CoMSER prototype application. This analysis substantiates our claim that the characteristic of realism does exist in the majority of RS-EHRs developed through the CoMSER method, thus demonstrating the promising usefulness for secondary use.

Summary of Application of ATEN Framework

This section has presented application of the ATEN framework to the generation of the synthetic EHR for the labour and birth domain. The most significant challenge in RS-EHR generation is ensuring that the generated RS-EHR is realistic. The prototype system for generating RS-EHR for midwifery uses an integrated constraints framework, which is formalised using the State Transition Machine (STM). The guideline-based Caremap for the labour and birth domain for which the RS-EHR is to be generated is embodied within the STM. Computations that makeup the RS-EHR are driven by STM execution using pseudo-random transition selection within defined frequency distributions based on local HIS. The quality of the generated RS-EHR is guaranteed by recognition and use of direct interaction with experienced and practising midwives. The development of methods and techniques for measuring the extent of realistic properties of the generated RS-EHR was necessary. Generating RS-EHRs using publicly available health statistics and CPGs ensures patient privacy and confidentiality while also benefiting many uses including: research, software development and training. The ATEN framework provided a structured approach that ensured procedural steps and documentation were not overlooked, and that validation was a consideration from inception through prototype production to evaluation of the resulting synthetic EHR.

While all random number generation methods apply statistics and therefore can be considered as applying the statistics in generation that the researcher intends to find in the result, most still have some variation from true. Many set only one or two parameters (for example, heads or tails), which simplifies their models and limits potential variation in the expected result. Ours set a large number of constraints that all had to be within statistical limits, such as: age, ethnicity, age at pregnancy, age at pregnancy by ethnicity, the type of birth, incidence of each node in the caremap, and the overall patient outcomes. There were more than 15 variables, some interrelated, being handled by the SDG algorithm. Each to be statistically similar at the end of the generation cycle. Validation using HORUS has shown that the prototype system designed with THOTH and RA has achieved the realism that the overall ATEN framework sets out to produce.

5 Discussion and Future Work

ATEN provides a comprehensive way to achieve realistic synthetic data through three inter-dependent approaches, THOTH, RA, and HORUS, that respectively cover (1) a generic approach to SDG with enhancement (THOTH); (2) knowledge discovery (RA); and (3) validation of realism in the resulting synthetic data (HORUS). To the best of our knowledge, no other work in this domain has produced a generic model for SDG, a framework for realism, or a unified approach to validation of synthetic data.

The main *benefit* of **THOTH** is the guarantee of a best plan for the generation method, as well as ensuring best preparation of the knowledge elements and techniques to be used in creation of synthetic data. The THOTH approach is easily implemented and comes with little resource overhead. A *limitation* of THOTH is the unidirectional linear nature of its waterfall-type model, however classification and characterisation may greatly mitigate the effects of this limitation.

With adherence to THOTH, **RA** *benefits* through assurance as to the quality of synthetic data being created. This is achieved through establishment of elements and characteristics that define realism for the generation project; the extrinsic quantitative and qualitative properties, and intrinsic knowledge aspects that inhabit the input data. Another benefit of RA is that as additional items of input or seed data are introduced, the statistics, knowledge, constraints, and rules become further refined, increasing the potential accuracy and realism of resulting synthetic data. A *limitation* that arises is that it is presently conducted manual, requiring the researcher to possess an eye for detail along with sound logic, analytical, and problem solving skills.

HORUS *benefits* through being an inherently straight-forward model for validation and verification of synthetic data. HORUS identifies rules, constraints, or data that may be causing issues; reducing the accuracy, realism, and utility of synthetic data being delivered. It is possible that fewer SDG iterations may be required, significantly reducing the time taken to produce accurate and realistic synthetic data. No directly comparable works were located during this research. However, the closest relatable work encountered was that of [35], whose work presented four separate approaches to validation of synthetic data produced in the domain of computational modelling. Each of these approaches appears, even in that authors' own summation, not to be representative of a single validation solution. The strength of HORUS is that it represents a single operational validation solution. HORUS has a significant *limitation* in that it is wholly dependent on having already engaged RA to identify the statistics, knowledge, and rules that will be significant in assuring that the synthetic data is suitably representative. Another limiting issue is that the case study conducted in this work identified that where the extrinsic quantitative aspects of the synthetic data are found wanting, continued engagement in the HORUS validation approach looking at the intrinsic knowledge, rules and constraints may be of little additional benefit until those extrinsic issues are resolved.

There are a number of avenues open for **future work**, including use of ATEN during the entire lifecycle of a significant real-life SDG project. This would necessitate the considered operation of a new SDG project where every element was documented rigorously, and where two streams are conducted concurrently. This new project due to the incompleteness of every SDG project reviewed during this research. In the first, or normal stream, the SDG project would operate in the manner that the majority do now, following the SDG generic approach described in Fig. 2. No input or other validation steps would be taken and realism would be given no more consideration than it is in the majority of SDG cases reviewed. In the second stream, another researcher would collect the same input materials and documentation from the first and use them to follow the complete and validated SDG approach described in this work. The second researcher would ameliorate his input materials and generation method through operation of ATEN. Both synthetic datasets could then be validated using HORUS. Another avenue for future work would be development of machine learning models to automate some or all of the KDD and validation.

6 Summary and Conclusion

This chapter has presented and demonstrated the ATEN framework, a triangle of three interdepended approaches: THOTH, RA and HORUS. The triangle is one of the strongest structures seen in engineering and nature. The components communicate with their adjacent neighbours; each enhanced through interaction with and engagement of its counterparts. THOTH provides framework and approach knowledge that improves RA, RA provides the extrinsic and intrinsic knowledge to seed HORUS, and the results of engaging HORUS either identify where an issue may exist in the first two and therefore target where additional work is required, or confirms their successful operation and therefore justify the claim of realism in the synthetic data.

The approach proposed in this work, first, draws on, expands and enhances established methods to result in a complete end-to-end validation solution. This ensures a complete analysis of the source data leading to useful knowledge, which greatly improves the generation method leading to better realism in synthetic data. Second, the knowledge gathered prior to synthetic data generation provides a solid base with which to validate the synthetic data, ensuring its ability to actually replace real data. Third, the approach presented here is simple, intuitive and not overly burdensome, with many of the component steps being activities that data synthesisers may already be undertaking in an albeit unstructured or unconsidered way.

References

1. McGraw-Hill: McGraw-Hill Dictionary of Scientific and Technical Terms, 6th edn. McGraw-Hill, London (2003)
2. Rubin, D.: Discussion: statistical disclosure limitation. J. Off. Stat. 9, 461–468 (1993)
3. Alter, H.: Creation of a synthetic data set by linking records of the Canadian survey of consumer finances with the family expenditure survey. Ann. Econ. Soc. Meas. 3(2), 373–397 (1994)
4. Wolff, E.: Estimates of the 1969 size distribution of household wealth in the US from a synthetic data base Trans.). In: Smith, J. (ed.) Modelling the Distribution and Intergenerational Transmission of Wealth. University of Chicago Press, Chicago (1980)
5. Green, P.E., Rao, V.R.: Conjoint measurement for quantifying judgmental data. J. Mark. Res. 8(3), 355–363 (1971)
6. Birkin, M., Clarke, M.: SYNTHESIS – a synthetic spatial information system for urban and regional analysis: methods and examples. Environ. Plan. 20(1), 1645–1671 (1998)
7. Stedinger, J., Taylor, M.: Synthetic streamflow generation: model verification and validation. Water Resour. Res. 18(4), 909–918 (1982)
8. Geweke, J., Porter-Hudak, S.: The estimation and application of long memory series models. J. Time Ser. Anal. 4(4), 221–238 (1983)
9. Graham, V.A., Hollands, K., Unny, T.E.: A time series model for Kt with application to global synthetic weather generation. Sol. Energy 40(2), 83–92 (1988)
10. Delleur, J., Kavvas, M.: Stochastic models for monthly rainfall forecasting and synthetic generation. J. Appl. Meteorol. 17, 1528–1536 (1978)
11. Barse, E., Kvarnstrom, H., Jonsson, E.: Synthesizing test data for fraud detection systems. Paper presented at the 19th Annual Computer Security Applications Conference (2003)

12. Houkjaer, K., Torp, K., Wind, R.: Simple and realistic data generation. Paper presented at the VLDB 2006 (2006)
13. Mouza, C., et al.: Towards an automatic detection of sensitive information in a database. Paper presented at the 2nd International Conference on Advances in Database Knowledge and Database Applications (2010)
14. Whiting, M., Haack, J., Varley, C.: Creating realistic, scenario-based synthetic data for test and evaluation of information analytics software. Paper presented at the 2008 Workshop on Beyond Time and Errors: Novel Evaluation Methods for Information Visualisation (BELIV 2008) (2008)
15. Gargiulo, F., Ternes, S., Huet, S., Deffuant, G.: An iterative approach for generating statistically realistic populations of households. PLOS ONE 5(1), e8828 (2010)
16. Srikanthan, R.M.T.: Stochastic generation of annual, monthly and daily climate data: a review. Hydrol. Earth Syst. Sci. Discuss. 5(4), 653–670 (2001)
17. Wan, L., Zhu, J., Bertino, L., Wang, H.: Initial ensemble generation and validation for ocean data assimilation using HYCOM in the Pacific. Ocean Dyn. 58, 81 (2008)
18. Killourhy, K., Maxion, R.: Toward realistic and artefact-free insider-threat data. Paper presented at the 23rd Annual Computer Security Applications Conference (CSAC) (2007)
19. Sperotto, A., Sadre, R., Van Vliet, F., Pras, A.: A labelled data set for flow-based intrusion detection. Paper presented at the 9th IEEE International Workshop on IP Operations and Management (IPOM 2009) (2009)
20. Zanero, S.: Flaws and frauds in the evaluation of IDS/IPS technologies. Paper presented at the Forum of Incident Response and Security Teams (FIRST 2007) (2007)
21. Ascoli, G., Krichmar, J., Nasuto, S., Senft, S.: Generation, description and storage of dendritic morphology data. Philos. Trans. R. Soc. Lond. 365, 1131–1145 (2001)
22. Bozkurt, M., Harman, M.: Automatically generating realistic test input from web services. Paper presented at the 6th International Symposium on Service Oriented System Engineering (2011)
23. Drechsler, J., Reiter, J.: An empirical evaluation of easily implemented, non-parametric methods for generating synthetic datasets. Comput. Stat. Data Anal. 55(12), 3232–3243 (2011)
24. Gymrek, M., McGuire, A., Golan, D., Halperin, E., Erlich, Y.: Identifying personal genomes by surname. Science 339(6117), 321–324 (2013). https://doi.org/10.1126/science.1229566
25. Ohm, P.: Broken promises of privacy: responding to the surprising failure of anonymisation. UCLA Law Rev. 57, 1701 (2010)
26. Sweeney, L., Abu, A., Winn, J.: Identifying Participants in the Personal Genome Project by Name. Data Privacy Lab, Harvard University (2013)
27. Lundin, E., Kvarnström, H., Jonsson, E.: A synthetic fraud data generation methodology. In: Deng, R., Bao, F., Zhou, J., Qing, S. (eds.) ICICS 2002. LNCS, vol. 2513, pp. 265–277. Springer, Heidelberg (2002). https://doi.org/10.1007/3-540-36159-6_23
28. Stratigopoulos, H., Mir, S., Makris, Y.: Enrichment of limited training sets in machine-learning-based analog/RF test. Paper presented at the DATE 2009 (2009)
29. Wu, X., Wang, Y., Zheng, Y.: Privacy preserving database application testing. Paper presented at the WPES 2003 (2003)
30. McLachlan, S., et al.: Learning health systems: the research community awareness challenge. BCS J. Innov. Health Inform. 25(1), 038–040 (2018)
31. Jaderberg, M., K. Simonyan, A. Vedaldi and A. Zisserman. (2014). Synthetic data and artificial neural networks for natural scene text recognition. arXiv:1406.2227
32. Penduff, T., Barnier, B., Molines, J., Madec, G.: On the use of current meter data to assess the realism of ocean model simulations. Ocean Model. 11(3), 399–416 (2006)

33. Putnam, H.: Realism and reason. In: Proceedings and Addresses of the American Philosophical Association, vol. 50, no. 6, pp. 483–498 (1977)

34. Barlas, Y.: Formal aspects of model validity and validation in system dynamics. Syst. Dyn. Rev. **12**(3), 183–210 (1996)

35. Carley, K.: Validating Computational Models. Carnegie Mellon University, Cambridge (1996)

36. Brinkhoff, T.: Generating traffic data. IEEE Data Eng. Bull. **26**(2), 19–25 (2003)

37. Giannotti, F., Mazzoni, A., Puntoni, S., Renso, C.: Synthetic generation of cellular network positioning data. Paper presented at the 13th Annual ACM International Workshop on Geographic Information Systems (2005)

38. Stodden, V.: The scientific method in practice: reproducibility in the computational sciences. SSRN Paper 1550193. MIT Sloan School of Management (2010)

39. Collins, H.: Changing Order: Replication and Induction in Scientific Practice. University of Chicago Press, Chicago (1992)

40. Moss, P.: Can there be validity without reliability? Educ. Res. **23**(2), 5–12 (1994)

41. Tsvetovat, M., Carley, K.: Generation of realistic social network datasets for testing of analysis and simulation tools. Technical report 9. DTIC (2005)

42. Richardson, I., Thomson, M., Infield, D.: A high-resolution domestic building occupancy model for energy demand simulations. Energy Build. **40**(8), 1560–1566 (2008)

43. Domingo-Ferrer, J.: Marginality: a numerical mapping for enhanced exploitation of taxonomic attributes. In: Torra, V., Narukawa, Y., López, B., Villaret, M. (eds.) MDAI 2012. LNCS (LNAI), vol. 7647, pp. 367–381. Springer, Heidelberg (2012). https://doi.org/10.1007/978-3-642-34620-0_33

44. Efstratiadis, A., Dialynas, Y., Kozanis, S., Koutsoyiannis, D.: A multivariate stochastic model for the generation of synthetic time series at multiple time scales reproducing long-term persistence. Environ. Model. Softw. **62**, 139–152 (2014)

45. Van den Bulcke, T., et al.: SynTReN: a generator of synthetic gene expression data for design and analysis of structure learning algorithms. BMC Bioinform. **7**(1), 43 (2006)

46. Mateo-Sanz, J.M., Martínez-Ballesté, A., Domingo-Ferrer, J.: Fast generation of accurate synthetic microdata. In: Domingo-Ferrer, J., Torra, V. (eds.) PSD 2004. LNCS, vol. 3050, pp. 298–306. Springer, Heidelberg (2004). https://doi.org/10.1007/978-3-540-25955-8_24

47. Gafurov, T., Usaola, J., Prodanovic, M.: Incorporating spatial correlation into stochastic generation of solar radiation data. Sol. Energy **115**, 74–84 (2015)

48. Brissette, F.P., Khalili, M., Leconte, R.: Efficient stochastic generation of multi-site synthetic precipitation data. J. Hydrol. **345**(3), 121–133 (2007)

49. Gainotti, S., et al.: Improving the informed consent process in international collaborative rare disease research: effective consent for effective research. Eur. J. Hum. Genet. **24**, 1248 (2016)

50. Arifin, S.M.N., Madey, G.R.: Verification, validation, and replication methods for agent-based modeling and simulation: lessons learned the hard way! In: Yilmaz, L. (ed.) Concepts and Methodologies for Modeling and Simulation. SFMA, pp. 217–242. Springer, Cham (2015). https://doi.org/10.1007/978-3-319-15096-3_10

51. Greene, J.C., Caracelli, V., Graham, W.F.: Toward a conceptual framework for mixed-method evaluation designs. Educ. Eval. Policy Anal. **11**(3), 255–274 (1989)

52. McLachlan, S., Dube, K., Gallagher, T., Daley, B., Walonoski, J.: The ATEN framework for creating the realistic synthetic electronic health record. Paper presented at the 11th International Joint Conference on Biomedical Engineering Systems and Technologies (BIOSTEC 2018), Madiera, Portugal (2018)

53. Lydiard, T.: Overview of the current practice and research initiatives for the verification and validation of KBS. Knowl. Eng. Rev. **7**(2), 101–113 (1992)

54. Ishigami, M., Cumings, J., Zetti, A., Chen, S.: A simple method for the continuous production of carbon nanotubes. Chem. Phys. Lett. **319**(5), 457–459 (2000)

55. Mahmoud, E.: Accuracy in forecasting: a survey. J. Forecast. **3**(2), 139–159 (1984)

56. Nicoletti, I., Migliorati, G., Pagliacci, M., Grignani, F., Riccardi, C.: A rapid and simple method for measuring thymocyte apoptosis by propidium iodide staining and flow cytometry. J. Immunol. Methods **139**(2), 271–279 (1991)

57. Rosevear, A.: Immobilised biocatalysts – a critical review. J. Chem. Technol. Biotechnol. **34** (3), 127–150 (1984)

58. Parnas, D., Clements, P.: A rational design process: how and why to fake it. IEEE Trans. Softw. Eng. **2**, 251–257 (1986)

59. Winkler, W.E.: Masking and re-identification methods for public-use microdata: overview and research problems. In: Domingo-Ferrer, J., Torra, V. (eds.) PSD 2004. LNCS, vol. 3050, pp. 231–246. Springer, Heidelberg (2004). https://doi.org/10.1007/978-3-540-25955-8_18

60. Andoulsi, I., Wilson, P.: Understanding liability in eHealth: towards greater clarity at European Union level. In: George, C., Whitehouse, D., Duquenoy, P. (eds.) eHealth: Legal, ethical and governance challenges, pp. 165–180. Springer, Heidelberg (2013). https://doi.org/10.1007/978-3-642-22474-4_7

61. Mwogi, T., Biondich, P., Grannis, S.: An evaluation of two methods for generating synthetic HL7 segments reflecting real-world health information exchange transactions. Paper presented at the AMIA Annual Symposium Proceedings (2014)

62. McLachlan, S., Dube, K., Gallagher, T.: Using CareMaps and health statistics for generating the realistic synthetic electronic healthcare record. Paper presented at the International Conference on Healthcare Informatics (ICHI 2016), Chicago, USA (2016)

63. Cassa, C., Olson, K., Mandl, K.: System to generate semisynthetic data sets of outbreak clusters for evaluation of outbreak-detection performance. Morb. Mortal. Wkly Rep. (MMWR) **53**, 231 (2004)

64. Fayyad, U.M., Piatetsky-Shapiro, G., Smyth, P.: Knowledge discovery and data mining: towards a unifying framework. KDD **96**, 82–88 (1996)

65. Fernandez-Arteaga, V., et al.: Association between completed suicide and environmental temperature in a Mexican population, using the KDD approach. Comput. Methods Programs Biomed. **135**, 219–224 (2016)

66. Holzinger, A., Dehmer, M., Jurisica, I.: Knowledge discovery and interactive data mining in Bopinformatics: state-of-the-art, future challenges and research directions. BMC Bioinform. **15**(6), I1 (2014)

67. Mitra, S., Pal, S., Mitra, P.: Data mining in soft computing framework: a survey. IEEE Trans. Neural Netw. **13**(1), 3–14 (2002)

68. Nijssen, G.M., Halpin, T.A.: Conceptual Schema and Relational Database Design: A Fact Oriented Approach. Prentice Hall Inc., Upper Saddle River (1989)

69. Han, J., Cai, Y., Cercone, N.: Data-driven discovery of quantitative rules in relational databases. IEEE Trans. Knowl. Data Eng. **5**(1), 29–40 (1993)

70. Sanderson, M., Croft, B.: Deriving concept hierarchies from text. Paper presented at the 22nd Annual International ACM SIGIR Conference on Research and Development in Information Retrieval (1999)

71. Barnes, C.A.: Concepts Hierarchies for Extensible Databases. Naval Postgraduate School, Monterey (1990)

72. Ganter, B., Willie, R.: Applied lattice theory: formal concept analysis. In: General Latice Theory. Birkhauser, Basel (1997)

73. Rodriguez-Jiminez, J., Cordero, P., Enciso, M., Rudolph, S.: Concept lattices with negative information: a characterisation theorem. Inf. Sci. **369**(51), 51–62 (2016)

74. Bex, G., Neven, F., Schwentick, T., Tuyls, K.: Inference of concise DTDs from XML data. Paper presented at the 32nd International Conference on Very Large Databases (2006)
75. Laranjeiro, N., Vieira, M., Madeira, H.: Improving web services robustness. Paper presented at the IEEE International Conference on Web Services ICWS 2009 (2009)
76. Oreskes, N., Shrader-Frechette, K., Belitz, K.: Verification, validation and confirmation of numerical models in the earth sciences. Science **263**(5147), 641–646 (1994)
77. McLachlan, S.: Realism in synthetic data generation. Master of Philosophy in Science MPhil, Massey University, Palmerston North, New Zealand (2017). Available from database

Author Index